COMPLICATIONS IN ORTHOPAEDIC SURGERY

Volume Two

COMPLICATIONS IN ORTHOPAEDIC SURGERY

Second Edition

Edited by

CHARLES H. EPPS, JR., M.D.

Professor and Chief
Division of Orthopaedic Surgery
Howard University College of Medicine and Howard University Medical Center;
Consultant, Handicapped and Crippled Children's Unit
District of Columbia General Hospital
Washington, D.C.

With 72 contributors

J. B. Lippincott Company
Philadelphia
London   Mexico City   New York
St. Louis   São Paulo   Sydney

Sponsoring Editor: Richard Winters
Manuscript Editor: Lee Henderson
Indexer: Ann Cassar
Design Director: Tracy Baldwin
Design Coordinator: Earl Gerhart
Designer: Katharine Nichols
Production Supervisor: J. Corey Gray
Production Assistant: Kathleen R. Diamond
Compositor: TAPSCO, Inc.
Printer/Binder: Halliday Lithograph

Second Edition

6   5   4   3   2   1

Library of Congress Cataloging in Publication Data
Main entry under title:

Complications in orthopaedic surgery.

   Includes bibliographies and index.
   1. Orthopedic surgery—Complications and sequelae.
I. Epps, Charles H. (Charles Harry), DATE.
[DNLM: 1. Orthopedics.   2. Postoperative Complications—
prevention & control.   3. Postoperative Complications—
therapy.   4. Wounds and Injuries—complications.
WE 168 C739]
RD732.C65   1986   617'.3   84-28861
ISBN 0-397-50638-4 (set)

The authors and publisher have exerted every
effort to ensure that drug selection and dosage
set forth in this text are in accord with current
recommendations and practice at the time of
publication. However, in view of ongoing research, changes in government regulations, and
the constant flow of information relating to drug
therapy and drug reactions, the reader is urged
to check the package insert for each drug for any
change in indications and dosage and for added
warnings and precautions. This is particularly
important when the recommended agent is a new
or infrequently employed drug.

Contributors

John P. Adams, M.D., M.P.H.
Professor and Chairman
Department of Orthopaedic Surgery
George Washington University School of
    Medicine and Health Sciences
Washington, D.C.

Russell L. Anderson, Jr., M.D.
Chairman of Orthopaedic Section
Tallahassee Regional Medical Center
Tallahassee, Florida

George I. Baker, M.D.
Major General, U.S. Army (Ret.);
Clinical Professor of Surgery
Uniformed Services University of the Health
    Sciences
Bethesda, Maryland;
and Attending Orthopaedic Surgeon
Community General Hospital
Syracuse, New York

Henry H. Bohlman, M.D.
Associate Professor of Orthopaedic Surgery
Case Western Reserve University;
Chief, Acute Spinal Cord Injury Service
Veterans Administration Medical Center
Cleveland, Ohio

Bruce Butler, Jr., M.D.
Consultant, Hand Surgery
Walter Reed General Hospital,
    Howard University School of Medicine, and
    Virginia State Crippled Children's Bureau;
Chief, Orthopaedic Department
Northern Virginia Doctor's Hospital
Arlington, Virginia

Peter G. Carnesale, M.D.
Assistant Professor
Department of Orthopaedic Surgery
College of Medicine
University of Tennessee Center for Health
    Sciences;
Staff Member, The Campbell Clinic
Memphis, Tennessee

Jerome M. Cotler, M.D.
Professor, Orthopaedic Surgery
Jefferson Medical College of Thomas Jefferson
    University
Philadelphia, Pennsylvania

John J. Csongradi, M.D.
Assistant Professor
Orthopaedic Surgery
Stanford University School of Medicine
Stanford, California;
Chief, Orthopaedic Section
Palo Alto Veterans Administration Hospital
Palo Alto, California

Thomas B. Dameron, Jr., M.D.
Associate, Raleigh Orthopaedic Clinic
Raleigh, North Carolina;
Clinical Professor
Orthopaedic Surgery
University of North Carolina School of
    Medicine
Chapel Hill, North Carolina

Roger Dee, M.D., Ph.D.
Professor and Chairman
School of Medicine
State University of New York at Stony Brook
Stony Brook, New York

James H. Dobyns, M.D.
Professor of Orthopedic Surgery
Mayo Medical School;
Consultant in Orthopedics and Surgery of the
    Hand
Mayo Clinic
Rochester, Minnesota

Charles C. Edwards, M.D.
Professor of Orthopedic Surgery
University of Maryland
Baltimore, Maryland

Charles H. Epps, Jr., M.D.
Professor and Chief
Division of Orthopaedic Surgery
Howard University College of Medicine and
  Howard University Medical Center;
Consultant, Handicapped and Crippled
  Children's Unit
District of Columbia General Hospital
Washington, D.C.

E. Burke Evans, M.D.
Professor and Chief
Orthopaedic Surgery
The University of Texas Medical Branch at
  Galveston
Galveston, Texas

C. McCollister Evarts, M.D.
Dorris H. Carlson Professor and Chairman
Department of Orthopaedics
University of Rochester Medical Center
Rochester, New York

William Patrick Fortune, M.D.
Professor of Orthopaedic Surgery
Department of Orthopaedic Surgery
George Washington University Medical Center
Washington, D.C.

Victor H. Frankel, M.D.
Director, Department of Orthopaedic Surgery
Hospital for Joint Diseases Orthopaedic
  Institute
New York, New York

Vincent F. Garagusi, M.D.
Professor of Medicine and Microbiology and
Director, Infectious Diseases Division
  and Clinical Microbiology and Serology
  Laboratories
Georgetown University
Washington, D.C.

Stuart A. Green, M.D.
Chief, Osteomyelitis Service
Rancho Los Amigos Hospital
Downey, California

John E. Hall, M.D.
Professor of Orthopaedic Surgery
Harvard Medical School;
Senior Associate in Orthopaedic Surgery
Boston Children's Hospital; and
Associate in Orthopaedic Surgery
New England Baptist Hospital
Boston, Massachusetts

Sigvard T. Hansen, Jr., M.D.
Professor and Chairman
Department of Orthopaedics
University of Washington
Seattle, Washington

James H. Herndon, M.D.
Professor and Chairman
Department of Orthopaedics
Brown University;
Surgeon-in-Chief
Department of Orthopaedic Surgery
Rhode Island Hospital
Providence, Rhode Island

Mason Hohl, M.D.
Clinical Professor of Orthopaedic Surgery
University of California at Los Angeles School
  of Medicine;
Consultant in Orthopaedics
Wadsworth Veterans Administration Facility
West Los Angeles, California

Robert W. Jackson, M.D., M.S., F.R.C.S.(C)
Professor, Department of Surgery
University of Toronto;
Chief, Division of Orthopaedics
Toronto Western Hospital
Toronto, Ontario, Canada

Alfred Kahn III, M.D.
Assistant Clinical Professor
Department of Orthopaedic Surgery
University of Cincinnati School of Medicine
Cincinnati, Ohio

Tamas Kallos, M.D.
Anesthesiologist
South Miami Hospital;
Clinical Associate Professor of Anesthesiology
University of Miami School of Medicine; and
Consultant, Veterans Administration Hospital
Miami, Florida

William J. Kane, M.D., Ph.D.
Professor of Orthopaedic Surgery
Northwestern University Medical School;
Attending Orthopaedic Surgeon
Northwestern Memorial Hospital and
  Children's Memorial Hospital
Chicago, Illinois

Peter I. Kenmore, M.D.
Professor and Chief
Orthopaedic Surgery
Georgetown University
Washington, D.C.

Robert L. Larson, M.D.
Orthopedic Surgeon
Orthopedic and Fracture Clinic of Eugene;
Orthopedic Consultant
University of Oregon Athletic Department
Eugene, Oregon; and
Clinical Assistant Professor of Surgery
Division of Orthopedics and Rehabilitation
School of Medicine
Oregon Health Sciences University
Portland, Oregon

Roger N. Levy, M.D.
Clinical Professor of Orthopaedic Surgery
Mount Sinai School of Medicine
New York, New York

Ronald L. Linscheid, M.D.
Professor of Orthopaedic Surgery
Mayo Medical School;
Consultant in Orthopaedic Surgery and
    Surgery of the Hand
Mayo Foundation and Mayo Clinic
Rochester, Minnesota

J. Drennan Lowell, M.D.
Associate Professor of Orthopaedic Surgery
Harvard Medical School;
Assistant Director
Department of Orthopaedic Surgery
Brigham and Women's Hospital
Boston, Massachusetts

Henry J. Mankin, M.D.
Orthopaedist-in-Chief
Massachusetts General Hospital;
Edith M. Ashley Professor of Orthopaedic
    Surgery
Harvard Medical School
Boston, Massachusetts

Roger A. Mann, M.D.
Associate Clinical Professor
Department of Orthopaedic Surgery
University of California Medical School
San Francisco, California

Philip J. Mayer, M.D.
Head, Section of Spine Surgery
Department of Orthopaedics
Marshfield Clinic
Marshfield, Wisconsin

Newton C. McCollough III, M.D.
Professor and Chairman
Department of Orthopaedics and Rehabilitation
University of Miami School of Medicine;
Chief, Orthopaedics and Rehabilitation
Jackson Memorial Hospital
Miami, Florida

Paul R. Meyer, Jr., M.D.
Professor of Orthopaedic Surgery
Northwestern University Medical School;
Director, Acute Spinal Cord Injury Center
Northwestern Memorial Hospital
McGraw Medical Center of Northwestern
    University
Chicago, Illinois

Lyle J. Micheli, M.D.
Associate Professor, Orthopedic Surgery
Harvard Medical School;
Director, Division of Sports Medicine
Children's Hospital Medical Center
Boston, Massachusetts

Edward H. Miller, M.D.
Clinical Professor
Department of Orthopaedic Surgery
University of Cincinnati
Cincinnati, Ohio

David G. Murray, M.D.
Department of Orthopedic Surgery
Upstate Medical Center
State University of New York
Syracuse, New York

John A. Murray, M.D.
Professor, Surgeon, and Chief
Orthopaedic Service
M. D. Anderson Hospital and Tumor Institute
Houston, Texas

Donald A. Nagel, M.D.
Professor
Division of Orthopaedic Surgery
Stanford University School of Medicine
Stanford, California

Robert J. Neviaser, M.D.
Professor of Orthopaedic Surgery;
Director of the Hand and Upper Extremity
    Service
George Washington University Medical Center
George Washington University School of
    Medicine and Health Sciences
Washington, D.C.

St. Elmo Newton III, M.D.
Clinical Professor of Orthopedics
University of Washington
Seattle, Washington

George E. Omer, Jr., M.D., M.Sc.
Professor and Chairman
Department of Orthopaedics and Rehabilitation
Professor of Surgery
Chief, Division of Hand Surgery
Professor of Anatomy
Medical Director of Physical Therapy Program
School of Medicine
University of New Mexico
Albuquerque, New Mexico

Raymond O. Pierce, Jr., M.D.
Professor of Orthopaedic Surgery
Indiana University Medical Center;
Chief of Orthopaedic Surgery
Wishard Memorial Hospital
Indianapolis, Indiana

Melvin Post, M.D.
Chairman, Department of Orthopaedic Surgery
Michael Reese Medical Center;
Professor, Rush Medical College
Department of Orthopaedic Surgery
Chicago, Illinois

Mark E. Pruzansky, M.D.
Assistant Professor of Orthopaedics
Mount Sinai School of Medicine
New York, New York

Edward A. Rankin, M.D.
Associate Professor of Orthopaedic Surgery
Howard University Medical Center;
Chief, Orthopaedic Surgery
Providence Hospital;
Consultant, Handicapped and Crippled
    Children's Service
District of Columbia General Hospital
Washington, D.C.

Norman M. Rich, M.D.
Professor and Chairman
Department of Surgery
F. Edward Hebert School of Medicine
Uniformed Services University of the Health
    Sciences
Bethesda, Maryland

Robin R. Richards, M.D., F.R.C.S.(C)
Lecturer, Department of Surgery
University of Toronto;
Attending Orthopaedic Staff
St. Michael's Hospital
Toronto, Ontario, Canada

Brian A. Roper, M.A., B.M., F.R.C.S.
Consultant Orthopaedic Surgeon
The London Hospital, Whitechapel;
Consultant Orthopaedic Surgeon
King Edward VII Hospital for Officers; and
Honorary Consultant Orthopaedic Surgeon
The Hospital for Sick Children
London, England

Aaron G. Rosenberg, M.D.
Clinical Instructor
Rush Medical College;
Adjunct Attending Surgeon
Department of Orthopaedic Surgery
Rush Presbyterian-St. Luke's Medical Center
Chicago, Illinois

Steven D. K. Ross, M.D.
Assistant Professor of Orthopaedics
University of Southern California
Los Angeles, California

Augusto Sarmiento, M.D.
Professor and Chairman
Department of Orthopaedics
University of Southern California School of
    Medicine
Los Angeles, California

Arnold D. Scheller, M.D.
Assistant in Orthopedics
Department of Orthopedic Surgery
Tufts New England Medical Center;
Clinical Assistant Professor
Department of Orthopedic Surgery
Tufts University School of Medicine; and
Director, Implant Service
Boston Veterans Administration Hospital
Boston, Massachusetts

Marvin L. Shelton, M.D.
Associate Professor of Clinical Orthopaedic
    Surgery
Columbia University College of Physicians and
    Surgeons;
Director, Department of Orthopaedics
Harlem Hospital
New York, New York

Herbert S. Sherry, M.D.
Associate Professor of Orthopaedics
The Mount Sinai School of Medicine
New York, New York

Edward H. Simmons, M.D.
Head of Orthopedics
Buffalo General Hospital;
Professor of Orthopedics
State University of New York at Buffalo
Buffalo, New York

Marcus J. Stewart, M.D.
Chief of Orthopaedics
Veterans Administration Hospital;
Clinical Professor of Orthopaedics
University of Tennessee Center for the Health
    Sciences
Memphis, Tennessee

Alfred B. Swanson, M.D.
Director of Orthopaedic and Hand Surgery
    Training Program
Grand Rapids Hospitals;
Director of Orthopaedic Research
Blodgett Memorial Medical Center
Grand Rapids, Michigan; and
Professor of Surgery
Michigan State University
Lansing, Michigan

Genevieve deGroot Swanson, M.D.
Coordinator
Orthopaedic Research Department
Blodgett Memorial Medical Center
Grand Rapids, Michigan;
Assistant Clinical Professor of Surgery
Michigan State University
Lansing, Michigan

Rodney L. Teichner, M.D.
Anesthesiologist
Department of Anesthesiology
South Miami Hospital
Miami, Florida

Robert E. Tooms, M.D.
Professor, Department of Orthopaedic Surgery
University of Tennessee Center for Health
  Sciences;
Active Staff Member
Campbell Clinic
Memphis, Tennessee

Joseph S. Torg, M.D.
Professor of Orthopaedic Surgery
Director, Sports Medicine Center
University of Pennsylvania School of Medicine
Philadelphia, Pennsylvania

Roderick H. Turner, M.D.
Clinical Professor of Orthopaedic Surgery
Tufts University School of Medicine;
Secretary, Medical Staff
New England Baptist Hospital
Boston, Massachusetts

James R. Urbaniak, M.D.
Professor and Chief
Division of Orthopaedic Surgery
Duke University Medical Center
Durham, North Carolina

Michael C. Welch, M.D.
Assistant Clinical Professor
Department of Orthopaedic Surgery
University of Cincinnati College of Medicine
Cincinnati, Ohio

R. Geoffrey Wilber, M.D.
Instructor, Department of Orthopaedics
Case Western Reserve University
Cleveland, Ohio

Ross M. Wilkins, M.D., M.S.
Assistant Clinical Professor
Department of Orthopaedics
University of Colorado Health Sciences Center;
Medical Director
Mile High Transplant Bank; and
Attending Physician
Veterans Administration Hospital
Denver, Colorado

Robert A. Winquist, M.D.
Associate Clinical Professor in Orthopaedics
University of Washington School of Medicine
Seattle, Washington

William G. Winter, M.D.
Chief, Orthopedic Surgery
Denver Veterans Administration Medical
  Center;
Associate Professor
Department of Orthopedic Surgery
University of Colorado Health Sciences Center
Denver, Colorado

George Wortzman, M.D.
Professor of Radiology
University of Toronto Faculty of Medicine;
Radiologist-in-Chief
Mount Sinai Hospital
Toronto, Ontario, Canada

Contents

Part Two: Complications of Trauma

VOLUME TWO

COMPLICATIONS IN
ORTHOPAEDIC SURGERY

24 Complications of Treatment of Fractures and Dislocations of the Dorsolumbar Spine

Paul R. Meyer, Jr.

Trauma to the dorsolumbar (or thoracolumbar) spinal column, direct or indirect, can produce injury to the spinal cord, the conus medullaris, the cauda equina, or a combination of the three. The result may produce an extensive list of systemic complaints. These include loss of bone substance (by means of traumatic, infectious, or neoplastic involvement of the vertebral column), loss of structural stability, injury to an intervertebral disc, or again, a combination of the above with associated concomitant neurologic injury.

Neurologic injury, when it does occur, may be either *complete and irreversible* (with complete loss of function distal to, and in some instances, above the site of the injury), resulting in side-effects that in one way or another may affect almost every organ system, or *partial or incomplete*, with partial preservation of neurologic function below the level of injury and functional neurologic recovery a possibility.

Vertebral column injuries that result in neurologic disability often result in physical disabilities requiring one period or more of extended hospitalization or surgery. The most common complications are loss of skin sensitivity, resulting in skin breakdown through the development of pressure decubiti; joint contractures; limb fractures; acute or chronic urinary tract infections; rectal and urogenital disorders with loss of voluntary bowel and bladder function; impotence in men; psychosocial instability; and total and permanent physical impairment, resulting in unemployment and terminating in total societal dependency.

Fractures and dislocations of the dorsolumbar spine, even in the absence of neurologic injury, may also produce complications in adjacent organ systems. Examples include spinal deformity with disfigurement (scoliosis), leading to embarrassed cardiac or pulmonary compliance, or the development of secondary neurologic involvement where none existed before.

This chapter has been organized in such a manner as to present to the reader those complications that may result from injury to the dorsolumbar spine and the sequelae that may follow. Although there may be complications or residual disabilities not mentioned in the chapter, this should not be interpreted as implying a level of lesser importance, rather a lesser frequency.

HISTORY OF MANAGEMENT

The earliest known documentation of spinal cord trauma and its manifestations is in the Surgical Papyrus.[50] This early medical report, estimated to have been written between 2500 and 3000 B.C., began with the comment that spinal cord injury is ". . . an ailment not to be treated." Even today, similar opinions are occasionally expressed.

Hippocrates (approximately 400 B.C.) made mention of his method of managing vertebral column injuries. His technique described the use of an "extension-bench," made known by Celsius as a *scamnum* in the 1st century of the common era. Galen also reported on the effects of trauma to the vertebral column and the spinal cord. He noted that longitudinal incision of the spinal cord produced little apparent neurologic injury, whereas transverse incision across the substance of the spinal cord produced definite paralysis below the level of injury. The importance of this work went unnoticed until the 7th century, when Paulus Aegenita first recommended surgery for fractures of the spine. Even then, his advice was ignored.[32,46] Other early authors who recommended surgical management of spinal injuries included Fabricius Hildanus and Lewis.[95] This latter surgeon is reported to have been the first to perform surgery for the care of spinal injury.

Since ancient and medieval times, forceful and brisk manipulative procedures of the spine for spinal deformity (usually secondary to tuberculosis) were described. The most famous of these writings is Vidus Vidius' translation of Orabasius' *De Laqueiset* (1544). With the victim lying prone on a bench, the spine was pulled from a position of kyphosis into extension by means of upward traction on the shoulders while simultaneous traction was applied distally from the hips or lower extremities. To correct the spinal deformity, an attendant applied direct pressure over the area of spinal deformity by standing or sitting on the area of the spinal gibbus or by means of direct pressure with a crossbar. Guttmann and Silver reported on the 19th-century work of Jean François Calot, whose modifications of this technique included the use of the hands as the preferred method of manipulation of spine fractures or dislocations, particularly when associated with paraplegia.[69]

During the 1920s and 1930s, postural reduction of fractures and dislocations of the dorsolumbar spine with hyperextension used as the method of gaining spinal correction was begun. The patient was placed in the prone position and hyperextended over slings, frames, or hammocks.[40,136] Another method of obtaining correction was to hang the patient in an inverted position, allowing the weight of the body to serve as a means of countertraction. This method was used by Bohler,[15] and prone placement between two tables was used by Watson-Jones.[167,168] Following manipulation, most patients required the application of a plaster jacket that extended from the pubic symphysis to the clavicle to maintain hyperextension of the vertebral column. Another method was the use of postural reduction

in a "plaster bed." Particularly in the presence of the loss of skin sensation, it soon became obvious that this method of bringing about spine stability was unsatisfactory. The consequence was the frequent appearance of pressure sores, with disastrous consequences.

Until after World War I, little hope was offered to those rendered paraplegic through trauma. The attitude of the time was recorded by Courville as "a matter of preserving life by constant and meticulous care when the life was of little value to the patient and costly to his relatives."[35] Cushing, in his report as Senior Consultant of Neurological Surgery to the American Army during World War I, discussed patients with spinal cord injuries only to lament their invariably pitiful fate and early death.[78] Kuhn, giving American figures for World War I, noted that only 20% of patients who sustained spinal cord injury survived to be evacuated to America, and only 10% lived another year.[95] It was estimated that only 1% survived more than 20 years. Today, this figure has markedly changed. The annual mortality rate for the first year following trauma is now only *4.93%*, and the annual mortality rate for each year thereafter is *1% per year.*[110]

The care provided for patients with spinal cord injuries has undergone drastic philosophical and objective changes since World War II. During the early days of the war, British authorities designated specific hospitals to be spinal cord injury centers to which all patients with such diagnoses were referred. Munro, in 1943, wrote of paraplegics: "Nothing less than an active self-supporting wheel-chair life is to be considered for a moment as an end result."[118] His philosophy was principally responsible for the establishment of special paraplegic centers by the United States Army during World War II. The credit, however, for the development of specialized centers for the care of spinal cord injuries lies with Sir Ludwig Guttmann, director of the famous Spinal Injury Center at Stoke Mandeville, England.[63-69] It was through Sir Ludwig's efforts that the frequently fatal and disastrous complications resulting from spinal cord neurologic injury were recognized and efforts directed toward their solution.

MORTALITY AND COST

The mortality rate resulting from spinal cord injury varies from study to study. Meyer found 4.93%,[110] Barber and Cross 5.2%,[11] and Hoffman and Bunts 25.2%.[80] Acute causes of death differ from those producing late loss of life. Death following acute injury is usually the result of multiple trauma, acute respiratory distress syndrome, acute renal disease resulting directly from trauma or from the by-products of trauma, the effects of head trauma, hemorrhage, and pulmonary embolism.[154,173,174] On the other hand, the two most common causes of late death are pulmonary and urinary sepsis. In the past, less common causes of late death were renal amyloidosis secondary to long-standing urinary tract sepsis or skin pressure (decubiti) problems and late pulmonary embolism.[37,56,159]

Historically, spinal injury has been known as a very costly illness.[32] Young, in 1970, reported initial hospital costs for the care of spinal cord injury to be $30,000 to $40,000 per patient.[174] By 1983, these figures ranged from $56,000 to $64,000, according to Northwestern University statistics.[115] Lifetime costs during the same period were between $700,000 and $1.4 million. Naturally, the age of onset of the disease is a great factor, as is the level of injury. Talbot, as early as 1971, reported statistics gathered by Liberty Mutual Insurance Company, describing the initial medical costs for traumatic paraplegia at $65,000, and three times that figure for quadriplegics.[153] Somewhere in this area lie the real figures.

The life expectancy of a patient rendered paraplegic is estimated to be approximately *7% less than that of a healthy person.* A number of variables affect this figure, most importantly, the level of injury and the age of onset.[97]

Many spine-injured patients return to gainful employment. Approximately 18% rejoin the ranks of the tax-paying employed, and 56% return to some type of gainful societal endeavor.[115]

INCIDENCE

If one considers only those who survived 1 year after the initial trauma, the incidence of spinal cord injury in the U.S. population is estimated to be between 25 and 35 per million.[110] If, however, one considers both those who failed to survive the initial injury and those who survived 1 year after trauma, one will find the incidence of spinal cord injury to be close to 50 per million. This latter figure becomes increasingly more important as initial trauma care at the roadside continues to improve. This means that one can anticipate an increasing number of survivors. Thus, the annual incidence of spinal cord injury in the U.S. is probably between 8,750 and 12,000. Approximately 60% are quadriplegics, and 40% paraplegics. Accompanying the annual increase in the number of spinal cord injury patients is the estimated 150,000 to 250,000 existing spine-injured patients presently surviving.

ETIOLOGY

Fractures and dislocations of the dorsolumbar spine are generally the result of direct violence. In the thoracolumbar spine the primary causes include falls, injuries from falling objects, direct injuries to the vertebral column, and gunshot wounds. Because of the violent force associated with such injuries and because of the anatomy of the spinal canal, neurologic injury most often accompanies such injuries.

The etiology and incidence of injuries to the thoracolumbar spine vary with geography (rural vs. urban population) and the nature of the industry present in a given area (farming, construction, or heavy industry). Statistics derived from the combined activities of the Illinois State Trauma System[112] and the Midwest Regional Spinal Cord Injury Care System,[110] which includes the 200-mile catchment area encircling Chicago (to include all of the state of Illinois), reveal that for the years 1972 through 1975, industrial accidents represented a significant share of the 109 dorsolumbar injuries treated between November 1973 and October 1975. Twenty-six were secondary to falls from a height (23.9%), and 12 patients had been struck by a falling object (11%); these two represented 35% of the dorsolumbar injuries in this series. Motorcycle and pedestrian accidents accounted for 33 (30.2%), and there was an unusually high incidence of gunshot wounds (37 or 34%). This latter figure increased between 1974 and 1975. This is most likely due to improved reporting and data retrieval;[120] however, other spinal injury centers in the U.S., particularly those representing large metropolitan areas, noted a similar rise. Other miscellaneous causes for injury to the dorsolumbar spine include water accidents 0.9% (see Table 24-1).

Statistics on injury to the dorsolumbar spine between 1972 and October 1984 have recently been updated. They reveal the following number of thoracolumbar injuries managed between 1972 and 1984, and their etiologies. Of the 109 dorsolumbar spine injuries managed between 1972 and 1975, 23 (21.1%) required operative intervention. Of the 23, 10 (43%) were of such severity that closed reduction was performed shortly following admission. This latter group represented industrial-type accidents; 60% were caused by falling objects. Comparative data for the period between 1972 and October 1984 are found in Table 24-1.

Freed and associates reported on 243 paraplegic and quadriplegic patients and noted a ratio of thoracic to lumbar spine injuries of 9 to 3; 37.8% of his patients were construction workers who had sustained their injuries in falls or from direct blows to the spinal column.[55] Meinecke, reviewing 340 paraplegics in a multiple-injury population composed principally of coal miners and steel workers, noted that 81% of the injuries resulted from work-related accidents, 14% from traffic accidents, and 5% from miscellaneous causes.[109] Of the work-related injuries, approximately 55.5% resulted from falling objects, 18.2% from falls, and another 7.6% from automobile accidents. Miscellaneous causes accounted for 18.4%.

Silver reported 50 spinal injury cases, 21 (42%) of which were dorsolumbar spine injuries.[146] The causes were as follows: automobile—50%, falls—38%, falling objects—8%, miscellaneous—4%. Munro reported 52.5% of injuries to result from falls, 25% from automobile accidents, 10% from gunshot wounds, and 12.5% from miscellaneous causes.[118] The significance of reporting these two somewhat outdated series

Table 24-1. Breakdown by Etiology of 728 Dorsolumbar Spinal Injuries, Midwest Regional Spinal Cord Injury Care System— 1972–October 31, 1984

ETIOLOGY	NO. OF CASES	PERCENTAGE
Fall	194	26.76
Automobile injury	185	25.52
Gunshot wound	143	19.72
Motorcycling	58	8.00
Falling/flying object	32	4.41
Pedestrian injury	19	2.62
Medical, NEC	16	2.21
Other	16	2.21
Other vehicular injury	11	1.52
Penetrating wound	8	1.10
Person-to-person injury	6	0.83
Fixed-wing aircraft	5	0.69
Winter sports	4	0.55
Snowmobiling	4	0.55
Air sports	4	0.55
Unknown etiology	3	0.41
Diving	3	0.41
Football	3	0.41
Horseback riding	3	0.41
Hang gliding	2	0.28
Bicycling	2	0.28
Spinal tumor/cancer	2	0.28
Skiing	1	0.14
Rotating-wing aircraft	1	0.14
Other sport	1	0.14
Explosion	1	0.14
Low back pain	1	0.14
Totals	728	100.00

is the variation in their ratios, most likely due to the differences in geography and occupation.

The orthopaedic literature of the 1950s and 1960s[27,59,84,96,157] seemed to reveal, with increasing frequency, injuries to the lumbar and lumbosacral spine due to either the non-use or improper use of manual automobile seat restraints. This trend did not seem to have changed as of October 1984, though new national seatbelt legislation was passed in July 1984, along with widespread adoption (by 49 states) of mandatory child seat restraint laws. A close follow-up of automobile-related injuries should reveal a change in these statistics.[158]

Atraumatic Injuries to the Spine

Atraumatic processes are known to affect and inflict injury to the dorsolumbar vertebral column. Those more commonly recognized as doing so are hereditary or idiopathic scoliosis;[95] congenital scoliosis secondary to developmental errors such as hemivertebra, spinal hypoplasia, or achondroplasia;[4] and the normal aging or "wear and tear" process of degenerative osteoarthritis with bony overgrowth (spondylosis). Each is capable of producing neurologic encroachment that could lead to neurologic injury. Another disease entity that could—but not within the more advanced nations of the world—produce spinal column and neurologic involvement is tuberculous osteomyelitis.[71,78,79] Bacterial vertebral osteomyelitis is even more rare, though it must always be thought of in the patient expressing severe symptoms of pain in the area of the spine unrelieved by anything but total immobilization. It is often associated with disc space infections secondary to urologic or pulmonary sepsis, rheumatoid ankylosing spondylitis with progressive vertebral deformity,[126] or chest or spinal column surgery in which extensive laminectomy produces an unbalanced spinal deformity from which a secondary neurologic encroachment can arise. Neurologic involvement (paraplegia) has also been reported secondary to such procedures as sympathectomy[117,143] and resection of abdominal aortic aneurysms.[34,52,148] This unusual cause of spinal cord involvement apparently results from retrograde occlusion of the anterior spinal artery.

Fractures of the dorsolumbar spine may be described in terms of the force that produces the injury: flexion, extension, rotation, axial loading, translation, or a combination of the above. Depending on the extent of injury to the anterior and posterior longitudinal ligaments and the integrity of the anterior (vertebral) column, the middle (pedicle and facets) column, and the posterior (lamina and spinous process) column, such fractures may be either *stable* or *unstable*.

Stable Fractures

When the mechanism of injury and the forces exerted on the dorsal or dorsolumbar spine are of such magnitude and direction as to leave the posterior bony elements (the lamina and spinous process) and the posterior and, in particular, the anterior longitudinal ligaments intact, the forces will most likely be directed through the disc space or to the vertebral body directly. The type of fracture most likely to result under such a circumstance is the vertebral body compression fracture. The result is an "impacted" or "compression" vertebral fracture, a stable fracture. Angulation of the vertebral column on lateral projection (kyphosis) may be the result, depending on the extent and location of the vertebral fracture. Translation of one vertebral process on another is not likely to be present when the integrity of the anterior longitudinal ligament has been maintained, or if so, only a minute degree of displacement will occur. The spinal canal will be minimally compromised, and neurologic injury (paraplegia) is rare, though, due to the vascular anatomy of the thoracic spinal cord, it is possible. Should the symptoms come on slowly or incompletely, the changes should remain incomplete or transient.[81] With the inherent stability of the dorsal spinal column provided by the thoracic cage (the ribs and intercostal muscles), along with the spinal ligaments and muscular attachments, angular deformity to the spine will remain limited and scoliosis minor if the injury to the vertebral body is bilateral. If the injury is only to one side of the vertebral body and to the pedicle and facet on that side, the resulting scoliosis may be greater.

Lumbar roots usually escape injury following minor degrees of dorsolumbar compression fracture. On occasion, fragments of the posterior border of a vertebral body may extrude into the spinal canal posteriorly (bursting injury), resulting in direct upper motor spinal cord injury in the dorsal spine between D1 and D10, a mixed upper and lower motor neuron injury between D11 and L1, and a root (lower motor neuron) injury when the injury to the vertebral body or posterior elements occurs below the level of L2. Surgery is indicated if there is obvious evidence that an incomplete neurologic injury complicated by bone or disc extruded into the canal (as identified by myelography, CT, or magnetic resonance imaging) is producing the neurologic injury. If the neurologic change is the result of a vascular injury, surgery will not be of any help whatsoever.

It is not uncommon, following the fracture of a dorsal or lumbar vertebra, to note the presence of an abdominal ileus during the early days after injury. This can often be treated by allowing only intravenous fluids and nothing by mouth during the period of ileus, or it may be managed by the application of transcutaneous electrodes on the abdominal wall.[133] Recumbency in the absence of neurologic injury is required only during the period of maximum discomfort and is seldom required for more than a week. Management depends on the extent of the injury. Such fractures may require little or no orthotic support. If an orthosis is needed, the devices most often prescribed are the three-point (Jewett) hyperextension orthosis (supporting the sternum, pubis, and dorsolumbar pad), the Knight-Taylor orthosis, or the hyperextension body cast for injuries between D5 and L3. The orthosis or cast is worn for 3 months. When the vertebral injury lies above D5 (the upper limit of the usefulness of a three-point hyperextension orthosis), a cervical extension must be applied to the orthosis to maintain proximal spine support and stability.

Flexion injuries to the dorsal and lumbar spine, resulting in disruption of the posterior ligamentous structures with separation of the posterior bony elements and anterior vertebral body fracture, frequently result in uncomplicated facet dislocations. When reduced, they are stable provided that they are maintained in hyperextension. I feel that this fracture should be surgically stabilized. Although this injury is produced by an anterior compression–posterior distraction force to the vertebral elements and can result in embarrassment to the blood supply of the spinal cord, this does not often occur in the absence of fractures.[81,83]

Maxwell and Kahn,[102] Nicoll,[120] and O'Connell[122] have reported on the "filum terminali syndrome" and its traction effects on the vascular supply to the spinal cord.[59] Schneider,[142] in 1960, noted that between maximum flexion and extension of the cervical spine, the spinal canal increased 5 cm in length (from the foramen magnum to the first dorsal vertebra). When this motion into flexion and extension involved the neck and torso, it produced a change in length of the spinal cord of 7.5 cm (*18–24% in the cervical cord*), as measured between the brain stem and the conus medullaris. Thus, as with the filum terminale syndrome, in the presence of spinal cord traction, the maximum neurologic deficit will be closest to the point of terminal fixation. The major deficit would therefore be found in the lower extremities.

When disruption of the anterior and posterior longitudinal ligaments is associated with fractures of the anterior, middle, or posterior vertebral column, neurologic injury is seen more frequently. Management includes the early use of chemotherapeutic agents such as corticosteroids, mannitol, or dextran.[110,112,114] Clinical evidence does not yet substantiate the use of naloxone.[53] The rationales behind the use of these drugs are that corticosteroids assist in the reduction of intracellular neural tissue edema and provide some protection to the cell membrane, as well as providing protection to the cellular lysosomes; that mannitol reduces extracellular edema; that dextran increases intravascular capillary blood flow by reducing sludging; and that naloxone is believed to increase capillary blood pressure, thus enhancing the blood flow to the smaller vessels and to the tissue directly within the spinal cord.

Unstable Fractures

Maximum motion (flexion and extension) of the dorsal and lumbar spine occurs at the D12–L1 junction. The reason why it is here rather than at some other location is that in this location the lower facet of D12 and the superior facet of L1 face more medially and laterally than elsewhere, allowing for more unrestrained flexion-extension. A second major reason is the loss of the inherent stability provided by the tho-

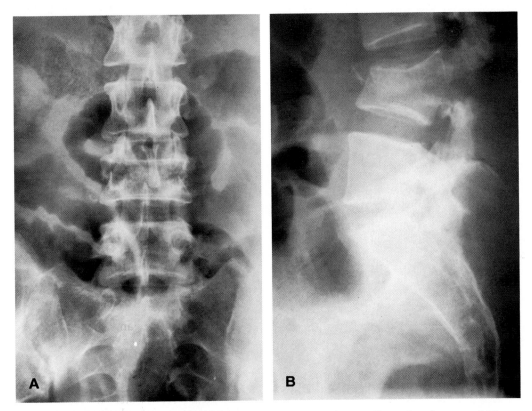

FIG. 24-1. Anteroposterior (*A*) and lateral (*B*) views of a flexion-distraction fracture of L4 without neurologic injury, resulting from a lap (abdominal-only) seatbelt upon sudden deceleration following a motor-vehicle accident.

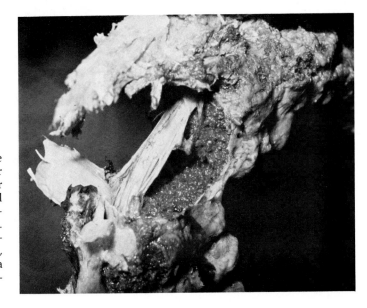

FIG. 24-2. Note the fracture through this fresh cadaver spine at the dorsolumbar junction, with rupture of all posterior ligamentous structures and rupture of the dura. This demonstrates the susceptibility of the spinal cord, conus medullaris, and cauda equina to direct injury or injury to their vascular supply.

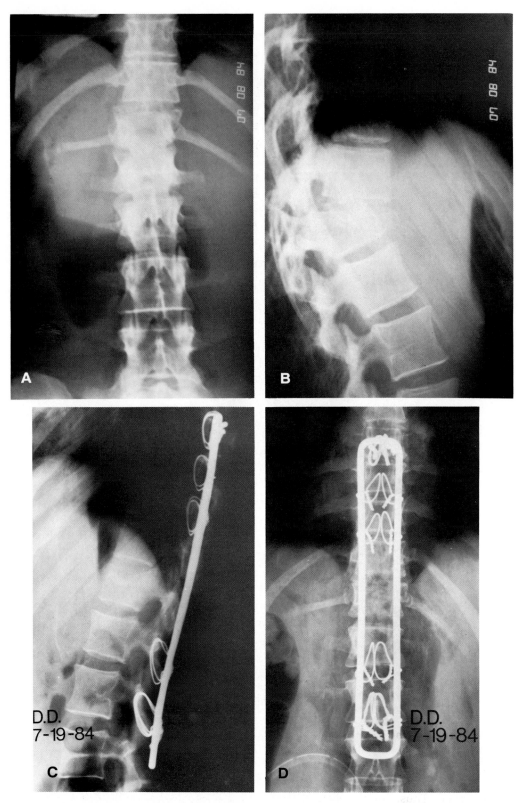

FIG. 24-3. Anteroposterior (*A*) and lateral (*B*) views of a fracture-dislocation at T11–12. Note on the lateral view the complete anticipated disruption of the posterior longitudinal ligament and the fractures of the posterior and anterior elements. (*C*) Lateral roentgenogram following open reduction with Luque-rod internal fixation. (*D*) Anteroposterior view.

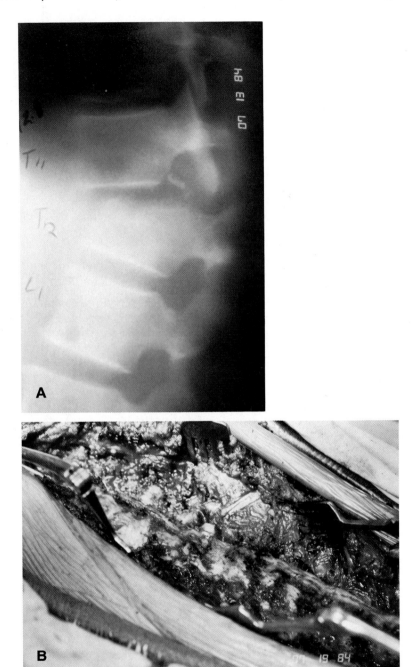

FIG. 24-4. (*A*) Fracture-dislocation at T11–12 with dislocation of the T11 inferior facets and fracture of the superior facet of T12. (*B*) Surgical view of the exposed superiorly dislocated facet of T12 in the middle of the picture. Note the depression in the interspinous ligament just superior to the facet. There is evidence of dislocation of the upper segment.

racic rib cage. Thus, hyperflexion injuries occur most commonly in the D12–L1 area of the dorsolumbar spine (Fig. 24-1). So-called dorsolumbar spine injuries often extend from the junction of the thoracic-lumbar spine to the level of L2. The level of injury often reported by many authors is D12–L1.[82] In my own series, the levels of injury at or near the dorsolumbar junction were D12, 13.3%; L1, 7.6%; and T11, 4.7%

(Fig. 24-2). Owing to the hypermobility at the D12–L1 junction, torsional injuries to the vertebral column also frequently occur here. These injuries have been well described by Holdsworth,[81,82,83] Hardy and Dixon,[71] and McSweeney.[106]

The type of vertebral process injuries commonly associated with flexion and torsion injuries to the lower dorsal and upper lumbar spine are fractures of one or both articular processes with forward displacement and rotation of the upper vertebra on the lower member. Another, seemingly more common, injury to the vertebral column, particularly in those driving while wearing lap seatbelts but not shoulder harnesses at the time of injury, is the "slice"-type fracture through the upper surface of the vertebral body, extending through the posterior element (through the facets and transverse processes), then through the upper third of the lower vertebra, extending from posterior to anterior. Frequently occurring along with this is a posterior rupture of the interlaminar (ligamentum flavum) and interspinous ligaments, with a palpable defect produced by the widening of the space between the posterior spinous processes, due to angular displacement of the vertebra above on the one below (Figs. 24-3 and 24-4). If the facet joints are not dislocated, this fracture is best maintained in proper alignment by maintaining the spine in a position of hyperextension. Guttmann was the greatest proponent of conservative management, which avoids the potential neurologic injuries (paraplegia) often associated with hypermobile spine injuries.[69] When the injury can be easily reduced, or when the reduced position, once obtained, is lost, this is a significant indication of gross spine instability! Fractures that can be easily reduced by "postural positioning" following injury often fall into this class. Some authors recommend similar conservative management in conjunction with a protracted period of immobilization (see Indications for Myelography). It is for this reason that Holdsworth and Hardy,[83] Kaufer and Hayes,[92] Leidholt and co-workers,[98] and others[110,112,113] recommend internal fixation for certain types of injuries, although they often prefer conservative management.

Unstable fracture-dislocations of the spine at the junction of D12–L1 are capable of producing injury to the conus medullaris and cauda equina (a mixed upper motor and lower [root] motor neuron injury). Philosophical differences exist as to the most appropriate means of managing these injuries. Some advocate postural reduction and recumbency until the fracture is stable (8–14 weeks).[69] This is, admittedly, an older approach to the management of such fractures and expresses the European influence. Other authors are more inclined to perform open procedures with internal fixation.[81,110,113]

MYELOGRAMS: INDICATIONS AND INTERPRETATION

Over the 13 years that the Spinal Cord Injury Program has been in place, greater than 2130 patients with spine injuries have been admitted. From this group of patients has come the development of a protocol relevant to the indications for obtaining myelograms. Every new admission is considered for such evaluation. Thus, the question is answered depending on whether the patient falls into one of the five categories (see Indications for Myelography).

Indications for Myelography

Changing neurologic pattern
  Deteriorating
  Improving
Preoperative evaluation of incomplete
  neurologic injury
Inconsistency between bone injury and
  neurologic injury
Unanticipated early neurologic recovery
  plateau
Inconsistency between somatosensory-evoked
  responses and neurologic examination

When the myelogram reveals an obstruction the question then arises, How is the treatment plan altered? Holdsworth and Hardy[83] and Bedbrook[13] are of the opinion that the presence of an obstruction on a myelogram, whether in the patient with a complete neurologic injury or in one with an incomplete neurologic injury, is of little or no significance. I am in complete disagreement with this belief. There are only two or three indications for an early or immediate surgical response:

A patient with radiologic evidence of the cause of a finding of progressive neurologic deterioration

A patient with evidence of progressive loss of neurologic function and an unreducible dislocation

A patient with an incomplete neurologic injury who, on myelography, reveals a complete obstruction to the flow of the contrast column in the presence of a reduced fracture-dislocation

Spinal fluid manometrics? Are they useful? Certainly, many readers are familiar of cases in which the patient with a complete neurologic injury was found on myelography to have normal manometrics! Therefore, it is my belief that manometrics give little indication of the presence or absence of spinal cord compression, whether extrinsic and intrinsic, nor does it indicate the cause of the spinal block (*i.e.*, blood clot, bone, or edema). The presence of such a finding in trauma without other substantiating findings in the neural canal may only give cause and concern for the need for surgical exploration (*i.e.*, laminectomy).[28,29,69]

The neurologic injury produced by the violence of the trauma (fracture-dislocation) is different from the mechanism of injury of a slow-growing tumor.[91] With trauma, the vascular supply to the spinal cord, the conus medullaris, and the cauda equina is disrupted by direct injury resulting from concussion, contusion, laceration, or obstruction. Such vascular injury may result in complete or incomplete neurologic injury, just as does complete or incomplete cord transection at the time of injury. The neurologic injury is thus often commensurate with the initial trauma. Early surgery in the presence of a complete neurologic injury is never successful in returning neurologic function. With incomplete neurologic injuries, indiscriminate surgery may result in further loss of neurologic function.[11,33,63,73,82,122] It is for this reason that I (representing both neurosurgery and orthopaedics) have found it appropriate not to perform surgery within the first 1½ to 2 weeks because of the inherent danger of

altering the existing blood supply to the spinal cord. Most surgeons agree that in the presence of an advancing neurologic injury, anterior or posterior decompression may be indicated.[54,59] Bricher and associates describe what they believe are irrefutable indications for immediate laminectomy: (1) debridement of open, highly contaminated wounds (*e.g.*, shrapnel injuries); (2) the presence of open wounds with evidence of dural laceration and obvious dural leakage that are uncontrolled by the usual methods of skin approximation, pressure, and so forth; and (3) spinal cord compression by bony fragments in the presence of an incomplete neurologic injury.[18] The problem with the latter is that seldom, except in the presence of tumor, does posterior decompression restore adequate blood flow to the spinal cord (the source of such blood supply, the anterior spinal artery, lies anteriorly). Thus, relief of such embarrassment must come from the direction of compression.

THE ROLE OF THE NUCLEUS PULPOSUS

The role of the nucleus pulposus in the pathogenesis of so-called recoil injuries of the spine refers primarily to the cervical spine, and to a lesser degree to the dorsolumbar spine. Cramer and McGowan report rupture of the anterior longitudinal ligament at tensile loads near 37 pounds.[36] They note that vertebral bodies are less strong than the ligaments and that fractures occur before the ligaments rupture. It has been found that the posterior longitudinal ligaments are more elastic than the anterior ligaments and have a different shape by virtue of the increased anterior width of the intervertebral disc. Therefore, with excessive hyperflexion, the posterior ligaments rupture, along with the posterior arch of the disc, resulting in extrusion of the nucleus pulposus. Although such an explanation is anatomically plausible, I have found this to be the case in only two injuries in the area of the cervical spine (in 1250 cervical injuries). Likewise, I have found posterior extrusion to be present in only the most severe fracture-dislocations of the lumbosacral spine.

LUMBAR FRACTURE-DISLOCATION

Injury to the lumbar spine is most often the result of violent trauma resulting from automobile accidents, falls, or falling objects.[92,110] In my experience between 1972 and October 1984, the primary causes of injury were falls (26.8%), automobile accidents (25.5%), and gunshot wounds (19.8%). An injury recently reported to be on the increase is the "fulcrum fracture,"[84] which is induced by improper placement of automobile seatbelts.[59,96,157] The incidence of associated injury is noted to be low,[92] although some authors[18,106,123] report associated serious intra-abdominal injuries (pelvic fractures, intermittent partial obstruction of the ileum due to adhesions secondary to mesenteric tear,[84] splenic rupture,[27] small-bowel perforation,[156] and in one case, pancreatic and duodenal rupture[60]). I agree with the potential findings. In the early part of 1984, two patients with fulcrum fractures were admitted to the Acute Spine Injury Service, one with an injury to the small bowel, requiring an iliostomy, the other sustaining a large-bowel injury, requiring a colostomy. Garrett and Braunstein, in a review of 2778 accidents, reported 944 injuries in victims who wore seatbelts.[60] Eight compression fractures of the lumbar spine occurred in this group as a result of the pelvis being held firmly in the seat, allowing sharp flexion of the spine to occur with sudden deceleration. This resulted in lumbar compression fractures. In that series, no "split" fractures of the vertebral bodies were noted.[60] Howland and colleagues[84] and Watson-Jones[168] report vertical fractures through L3 as viewed laterally. The fractures were treated closed in hyperextension casts. In both of their two reported cases the vertebral bodies were "split" in the form of "chance" fractures.

Lumbar dislocations are estimated to account for 10% to 20% of dorsolumbar fractures[92,110,120] and 4% to 9% of all spine injuries.[92,110] Kaufer and Hayes report that 53% of their cases had neurological involvement, with 13 of the 21 patients (63%) having D12–L1 dislocations.[92] The second highest level of injury in their series was L12. In my own series of 728 dorsolumbar spine injuries admitted to the acute unit

Table 24-2. Incidence of Fracture-Dislocations of the Dorsolumbar Spine by Level of Injury

HIGHEST LEVEL OF INJURY	NO. OF PATIENTS	PERCENTAGE
T1	12	1.83
T2	16	2.44
T3	30	4.57
T4	29	4.41
T5	34	5.18
T6	27	4.11
T7	15	2.28
T8	26	3.96
T9	33	5.02
T10	68	10.35
T11	100	15.22
T12	131	19.94
L1	30	4.57
L2	24	3.65
L3	19	2.89
L4	36	5.48
L5	22	3.35
S1	0	0.00
S2	5	0.76
Total valid cases	657*	

* Of 728 patients with dorsolumbar spine injuries, 71 had neurologic deficit with no fracture.

between 1972 and October 1984, the primary level of injury was T12, and the secondary area was T11 (Table 24-2). Of all injuries to the dorsolumbar spine, 40.4% were in the dorsal spine, 39.1% were dorsolumbar, 19.2% were lumbar, and 0.7% were sacral. In this series of dorsolumbar spine injuries, D12 was most often involved (13.1%), L1 next (7.7%), followed by L2 (4.7%) and D11 (3.5%). In another series by the author in 1974, the three most common sites were D12 (15.6%), L1 (13.8%), and D10 (10.1%) (see Fig. 24-1).[110]

Although it has been stated that closed manipulation and reduction of dislocations of the dorsal and dorsolumbar spine may cause extension of the neurologic loss,[92] this has not been my experience (Figs. 24-5 and 24-6).[11] Of 2032 total spine injuries, 728 were dorsolumbar (39.1%), and 68 (9.3%) were complete fracture-dislocations treated by closed reduction. No complications resulted (Fig. 24-7). In each case, internal fixation was performed in 2 to 3

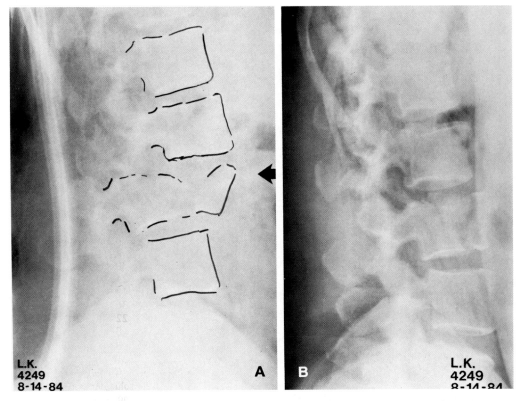

FIG. 24-5. (*A*) Lateral view of a comminuted fracture at L3 with dislocation of L2 on L3. Facet fractures are present. (*B*) Lateral view following closed reduction reveals accurate realignment of both the vertebral column and the comminuted fracture fragment at L3.

weeks with one of several methods. In our present series, 346 patients (47.5%) required surgery: Weiss springs (42.6%), Harrington rods (40.0%), and Luque rods (10.2%) were used, each in association with a spine fusion. Comparative figures for Weiss springs[110] and Harrington rods[72] were noted in 1976. At that time, the Luque-rod system did not yet exist. Bohler,[15] Rogers,[136] and Stanger[150] also advocated open reduction for the management of such fractures. Kaufer reports six closed reductions in ten patients without ill effects.[92] He also reports five of 11 patients (gathered from other than his own personal series) who required a late secondary spine fusion to obtain spine stabilization. Kaufer's conclusions were in opposition to conservative, nonoperative treatment, closed reduction, laminectomy, or surgical reduction without the use of internal fixation of fracture-dislocations of the dorsolumbar spine.

Injuries to the lumbar vertebral column differ from those of the dorsal and dorsolumbar junction in that most severe lumbar fracture-dislocations are unstable.[90,92] Because of their instability, these fractures have the potential of producing cauda equina (peripheral) nerve root injuries rather than upper motor neuron injuries, as might be seen occurring to the cord or conus medullaris with a dorsal or dorsolumbar spine injury. This occurs because the cauda equina is below the termination of the spinal cord, which is located at the level of D12–L1. Injuries to the cauda equina are therefore unpredictable. This explains why it is so often impossible to predict accurately whether an injury to the cauda equina is a complete or an incomplete injury. It is for this reason that I call injuries to the cauda equina *incomplete*. Often within minutes or hours of trauma there will be a complete absence of motor and sensory function be-

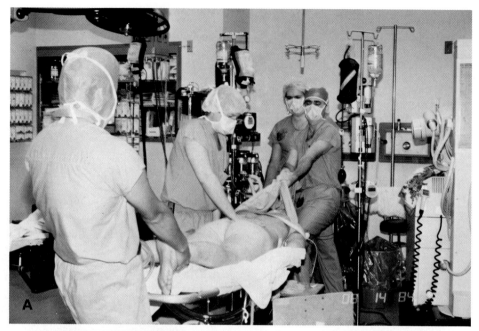

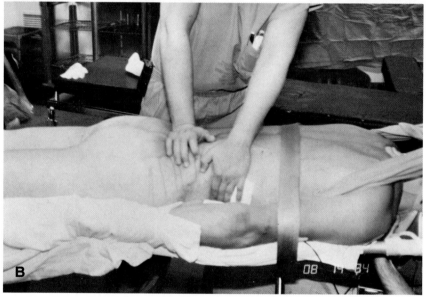

FIG. 24-6. (*A*) Operating room view of the closed reduction technique. The patient is placed prone on Stryker frame. Traction is applied to the upper thoracic spine (through the axilla) and both lower extremities. Direct pressure is applied over the lumbar gibbus. Neurologic status at admission: complete injury. (*B*) When spine instability is great, lateral pressure can be used to correct lateral spine malalignment.

low the level of injury, only to be followed within days or weeks by some return of motor or sensory function. This kind of neurologic return is indicative of a tempo-

rary incomplete nerve injury known as *neurapraxia.* Unlike the spinal cord, nerve roots are very resistant to trauma. This is probably due to their mobility and their

FIG. 24-7. Fracture-dislocation with a comminuted vertebral body fracture of L3. (*A*) Note the complete posterior dislocation of L3 beneath the fragment of L3 remaining with the proximal spine. Note the extent of posterior structure disruption. (*B*) Lateral view immediately after reduction.

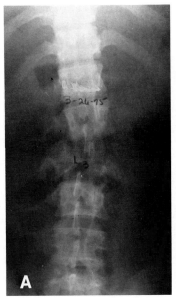
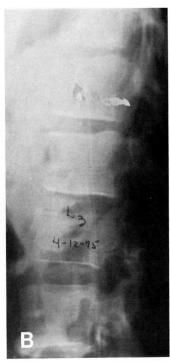

anatomical composition (axonal fibers enclosed in an axonal sheath). Thus, it requires a more violent injury to produce nerve "tearing."[14] As a rule, axons whose epineuria remain intact will recover if they are motor nerves. This is not necessarily true of the sensory components of the cauda equina. Here, the nerve arises from a sensory ganglion outside the spinal cord. When the injury lies between the spinal cord and the ganglion cell, regeneration does not occur in the unipolar, single-process central (dichotomous) branch. The peripheral branch, which forms the sensory fiber of a peripheral nerve, will regenerate.

LUMBOSACRAL FRACTURE-DISLOCATION

Traumatic dislocations at the L5–S1 interval are relatively rare. Such cases have been described by Dewey and Brown,[44] Evans,[51] Meyer and Dobozi,[111] and Watson-Jones.[168] Dewey and Brown report two cases of L5–S1 dislocation in which motor-sensory function was initially decreased below the level of S1.[44] One was the result of an automobile accident, the other the result of

a falling object. Closed manipulation was attempted in both cases and failed. Surgical decompression revealed bilateral dislocation of the particular facet, requiring excision for reduction. I have reported success with closed reduction but have found similar pathologic facet disruption at the time of internal fixation (see Figs. 24-5 and 24-6).[111] Watson-Jones describes the mechanism of injury of this fracture as one of hyperextension, resulting either from a blow over the knees with the hips and knees flexed or from a direct blow over the lumbosacral joint, producing hyperextension (a position that might be expected in a coal miner on his hands and knees during a cave-in).[168] All authors agree that open reduction and/or stabilization is required. Dewey and I have described the presence of an associated incomplete neurologic injury with progressive improvement. Dewey suggests traction as a means of treatment.[44] Neuman is of the opinion that traction and manipulation exacerbate neurologic involvement and recommends only open reduction.[119] I initially recommended closed manipulation and reduction if the L5–S1 dislocation was acute, followed by placement of the patient in a position of flexion on a wedge Stryker frame for a 2- to 3-week period prior to spine stabilization.[113] This gave time for the neurologic injury to stabilize before surgery. Having identified the pathology, that of an associated extrusion of the intervertebral disc against the anterior aspect of the dural sack at the level of L5–S1, I would now suggest an early approach to this surgical problem.

OPEN INJURIES AND INFECTIONS

Infections of the spinal column are more often the result of hematogenous and transmeningeal invasion than of direct trauma. The following case is illustrative. The patient, a 79-year-old man, had had a prostatectomy 3 months prior to his admission with an impending paraplegia, and a neurologic level at L2. There was roentgenographic evidence of possible tumorous involvement of both L1 and L2. Needle biopsy was thought to have revealed tumorous tissue. Because of an increasing root deficit, a wide laminectomy was performed at D12–L1 and L2. Spontaneous anterior subluxation of L3 under L2 followed immediately (Fig. 24-8). The patient was placed in halo-femoral traction for 4 weeks, followed by an anterior interbody fusion. Cultures obtained at the time of surgery revealed gram-negative *Escherichia coli.* The infection remained external to the dura. The patient was aggressively treated with appropriate antibiotics. Six weeks postoperatively, spontaneous rupture of a large flank abscess occurred, along with rupture of portions of unabsorbed vertebral end plate. This was followed by a spontaneous healing of the bone graft and closure of the sinus. The source of this patient's vertebral body and disc space infection was believed to have been his prostatectomy (see Fig. 24-7).

Infectious complications of fracture or dislocation of the dorsal or lumbar spine secondary to open wounds are rare. Only a few cases were observed during World War II and the Korean and Vietnam conflicts. Comarr, in a review of the records of 858 military patients rendered paraplegic secondary to war injuries between 1946 and 1955, reports that 579 (67%) had a posterior debridement (laminectomy) at some point following their injury, while 279 (32.5%) were followed without exploration.[28] Of the laminectomized patients, 16% showed neurologic improvement postoperatively. *Of those managed nonoperatively, 29% improved neurologically.* In neither case was there any discussion of complications (infections) secondary to gunshot wounds. A recent review of patients with gunshot wounds admitted to the Acute Spinal Cord Injury Service between 1972 and January 1984 revealed osteomyelitis secondary to the gunshot wounds in fewer than 1%. Such an occurrence generally followed the concomitant injury of a hollow viscus such as the esophagus or large bowel. Both are highly contaminated areas.[115]

Jacob and Berg describe combat injuries as largely the result of bullet wounds in the largest areas of the body (D1 through D12) and of shell fragments passing upward from the ground involving the lower lumbar spine.[85] Ninety-four percent of their patients underwent laminectomy, 90 of whom (78.9%) had sustained open injuries. Of the complications, only three of the surgical group had documented gram-negative sepsis; however, lower urinary tract infection was present in 85 patients (80.2%). Seventy-five percent of their infections were related to Proteus variants. No mention was made of spinal infections.

GUNSHOT WOUNDS

The orthopaedic and neurosurgical management of trauma that terminates in fracture, dislocation, and instability of the dorsolumbar spine is discussed by the following authors: Bedbrook,[13] Comarr and Kaufman,[30] Cramer and McGowan,[36] Dewey and Browne,[44] Hardy,[70] Holdsworth,[81-83] Howland and associates,[84] Jacobson and Bors,[86] Kaufer and Hayes,[92] McSweeney,[107] Meineke,[108] and Yashon and co-workers.[172] Spinal instability is in great part determined by and related to the mechanism of the injury and the structures involved. *The same does not apply to gunshot wounds, even when produced by high-velocity missiles.* Although such wounds may produce great destruction, they seldom disrupt all surrounding structures, so as to produce gross instability. On the other hand, it is not at all uncommon for even the low-velocity gunshot wound to produce neurologic injury. Such injuries

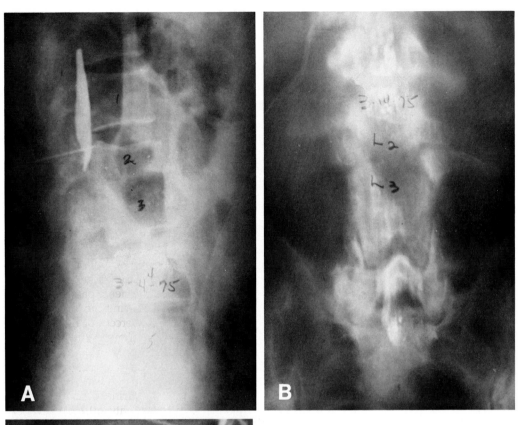

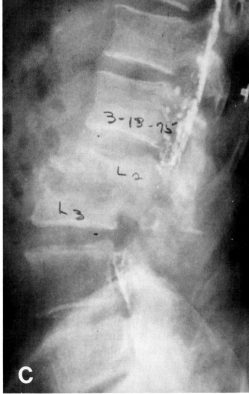

FIG. 24-8. Disc space and vertebral body in a 79-year-old man with paraparesis of both legs. (*A*) Lateral view of the lumbar spine reveals the suspected obstruction to contrast media and loss of disc space at L2–3. (*B*) Follow-up tomogram reveals the area from which the posterior process has been surgically excised. (*C*) Subluxation occurred after laminectomy of L3 anterior to L2. Note the disruption of the disc space and the involvement of the adjacent vertebra.

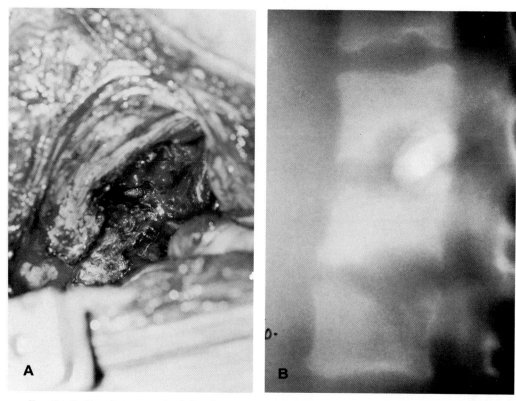

FIG. 24-9. Gunshot wound of the thoracic spine (T10) with osteomyelitis of the adjacent vertebra T9–11. *A,* clinical appearance; *B,* preoperative roentgenogram.

are frequently thought to be complete at first examination; however, careful evaluation frequently reveals the injury to be incomplete—only sensory or motor. A recent review of all gunshot wounds admitted to the Acute Spinal Cord Injury Service between 1972 and January 1984 reveals that 228 gunshot wounds were admitted. Of these, 145 (64%) were injuries to the thoracic, thoracolumbar, or lumbar spine. Of those gunshot wounds to the thoracic and lumbar spine, 105 (74%) were complete and 37 (26%) incomplete (Fig. 24-9).[115]

When significant neurologic involvement exists, the chances of its recovery are small. Gunshot wounds are capable of producing significant cord injury by either direct or indirect (blast) effects. The latter is more likely to occur with a high-velocity missile (*i.e.,* a missile traveling with a muzzle velocity of greater than 1350 feet per second). Yashon and colleagues report 54% of gun-shot victims in their series as having had complete absence of motor and sensory function on admission.[172] Those patients found to have complete neurologic injury on admission seldom experienced return of function. This observation was also made by Comarr,[28] Benassy and co-workers,[14] Carey,[22] Covall and associates,[32] Davidoff,[39] Harris,[73] Matson,[101] Mayfield and Cazan,[103] and Morgan and colleagues.[116] As stated earlier, I am no longer as confident in this finding, for I have, in several instances, observed patients who demonstrated significant neurologic recovery following admission for management of a gunshot wound. No specific reason can be identified for such recovery, other than early retrieval and appropriate supportive management, including the prevention of shock, the management of acute associated injuries, and the administration of corticosteroids, if their administration has any effect at all.

A major unresolved question in the management of gunshot wounds is, is laminectomy indicated? In my series, only 6 laminectomies were performed in 228 (3%) acute and chronic gunshot injuries.[115]

Comarr[28] and Yashon and colleagues,[172] discussing gunshot wounds, note that in their experience laminectomy was seldom indicated. When it was performed, no evidence of return of function followed. The presence or absence of a positive Queckenstedt's sign (failure of CSF pressure to rise or fall when, during lumbar puncture, the jugular vein is compressed) had little significance as an indicator for laminectomy, regardless of the cause of injury (fracture, gunshot wound, etc.).[44] Those who advocate or consider laminectomy more or less uniformly agree that it might be indicated when, shortly after injury to the spinal cord or nerve roots, an incomplete lesion and progressive loss of function are revealed during the period of early observation.[40,44,141,163] The findings of bony fragments or foreign bodies in the spinal canal, a positive Queckenstedt's sign, and a complete loss of motor and sensory function are not indicators of a need for laminectomy. Bedbrook, reviewing the pathologic process of traumatic spinal paralysis, notes that compression of the spinal cord was not the most common mechanism of irreversible injury.[12] Rather, he found crushing, stretching, and rotational shearing stresses more often to be the cause of permanent cord damage. I believe the latter correct.

Examination of the spinal cord at autopsy, according to Bedbrook, revealed that neural damage frequently extended over a distance of 1 cm to 5 cm opposite the site of spinal injury. This followed fracture of the posterior-superior border of the vertebral body below, with the intervertebral disc debris serving as a fulcrum over which the spinal cord was stretched, thus producing secondary cord compression. The pathologic changes that occurred subsequent to trauma were noted to be a continuous process. Initially, the cord appeared normal (between 1 and 24 hours). Thereafter, there was increasing evidence of gliosis and fibrosis associated with necrosis and liquifaction and death of the central gray matter. These changes may have been the result of direct trauma, followed by edema and ischemia. In some instances, infection was noted with these changes. These pathologic findings of spinal cord trauma are not amenable to improvement by surgical decompression, except in specific instances of well-localized spinal cord hematomyelia or spinal cord compromise secondary to cord compression, and even then, the correct surgical approach is from the direction of the compression, not categorically by means of laminectomy.

In dorsolumbar and lumbar spinal trauma, in which nerve root injury results in a completely flaccid (motor-sensory) loss of function, the nerve root has likely been torn in a "ragged" fashion, with disruption of both the axonal fibers and the nerve sheath (neurotmesis). Bedbrook has noted that only those rootlets having intact sheaths surrounding the axonal fasciae were capable of recovery.[12] Should the sheath be intact and the axon disrupted (axonotmesis), axonal regeneration will occur provided that the cell body is intact.

Trauma produces other findings. Cord edema may produce evidence of progressive or transitory extension of paralysis. This same edema may also be responsible for occlusion of the neural canal and obstruction of the flow of cerebrospinal fluid. The latter finding is also usually transitory. Following initial trauma, extension of neurologic injury over a wide area will seldom result unless major spinal cord or nerve root vascular insufficiency occurs. A contributing factor might be vertebral fracture instability, causing cord compression or compromise of the root blood supply. Occasionally, retrograde intercostal or radicular artery thrombosis will occur following dorsolumbar fracture, even when early fracture reduction has been attained. It may also follow laminectomy, particularly when the surgery is in the vicinity of the dorsal spinal vertebra D10–11, resulting in injury to the vessel of Adamkiewicz.[34,97]

It is known that spinal column malalignment may contribute to further embarrassment of the anterior spinal artery as it descends or ascends through the anterior sulcus of the dorsal and dorsolumbar segments of the spinal cord (Fig. 24-10). It is

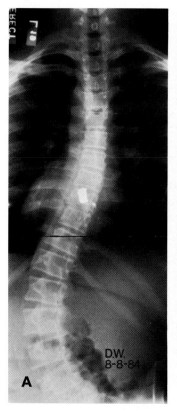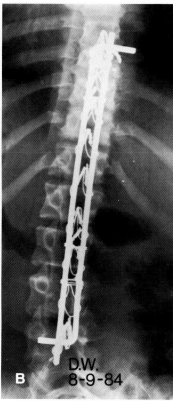

FIG. 24-10. (*A*) Preoperative posteroanterior view of the dorsolumbar spine 1 year after a gunshot wound at T9 in a 23-year-old man. (*B*) Postoperative radiograph of the same spine following Luque-rod instrumentation from T8 to L4.

also recognized that the vascularity to that portion of the spinal cord between T4 and L2 is, at best, precarious. Further discussion of the blood supply to the spinal cord follows.

HISTOPATHOLOGIC CHANGES IN SPINAL CORD ISCHEMIA

Allen, in 1908 and 1911, described the histopathologic changes that appeared in the spinal cord secondary to experimental impact.[5-7] The experiment consisted of dropping a known weight a known distance onto the exposed dorsal surface of an anesthetized animal's thoracic spinal cord. Allen followed and recorded the sequential changes that occurred in this traumatized spinal cord following animal sacrifice. His works are classics, quoted and reverified to this date.[47,124,125]

Immediately (in the first hour) following impact on the dorsal spinal cord of a force of 540 g-cm (30 g × 18 cm), Allen found

edema and hemorrhage to the superficial area overlying the dorsal column. There was associated hemorrhage in the pia mater and bluish purple discoloration overlying the dorsal columns. At *2 hours,* hemorrhage was noted within the central gray matter. There seemed to be little of the gray matter not invaded by red blood cells. Portions of the white matter were likewise involved. The most central portion of the cord had taken on the appearance of hyaline degeneration. Edema of the white matter was found to be extreme. At *4 hours,* additional changes were noted. Numerous swollen axis cylinders were seen within the white matter, particularly in the lateral and posterior columns. Whether this was the result of injury from impact or biochemical changes from outpouring of serum or blood could not be ascertained. At *5 to 6 hours* there was only an exaggeration of the findings described above. At *6 hours,* obvious evidence of spinal cord destruction was noted.

Again it was Allen, in 1914, who first reported the experimental midlongitudinal sectioning of the spinal cord (myelotomy) in animals to allow a "great outpouring of blood from the injured area posteriorly through this incision."[8] He found improvement (in both gross examples and microscopic sections) in the state of preservation of the substance of the cord—"a decompressed cord." The implications of these findings led him to perform this procedure on three human patients who had traumatic fracture-dislocations of the dorsal and dorsolumbar spine. Although two of the patients died postoperatively of causes apparently secondary to the spinal injury, Allen's conclusion was that surgery must be performed in the early hours after trauma for any chance of success.[8] This conclusion arose because it was also Allen's opinion that "the lot of the spinal-cord injured was death and those that did not die, the last state was far worse than the first."

Unfortunately, others have not found laminectomy or myelotomy as successful as Allen anticipated.[22,29,73,116,171]

ASCENDING NEUROLOGIC LOSS FOLLOWING SPINAL CORD INJURY

Of 109 dorsolumbar injuries resulting in paraplegia, three patients (2.8%) were found on admission to have the injury level at D12–L1, while their neurologic level was at the D6–8 interval.[113] Two of the three cases demonstrated ascending neurologic deficits (decreased sensation) within the first few hours following admission. The injuries remained complete, having reached their level of maximum deterioration by the third day after trauma. Each was diagnosed as a complete injury (by the absence of sacral sparing on initial neurologic evaluation) within 4 hours of trauma. It was interpreted that these ascending lesions were the result of progressive vascular ischemia to the conus medullaris and the lower third of the dorsal spinal cord. The most plausible cause was interruption of the anterior spinal artery by way of the radicularis magnus artery (the vessel of Adamkiewicz).

It is not possible to ascertain accurately the cause of an ascending lesion. In the absence of a more proximal vertebral body injury with obvious evidence of fracture-dislocation at the D12–L1 or D11–12 level, the most logical cause of neurologic extension is progressive spinal cord vascular ischemia. The above findings appeared in patients who on admission were found either to have no evidence of bony injury or to have had an injury that apparently reduced spontaneously. None demonstrated any indication for laminectomy, although one demonstrated (on myelogram) a medullary obstruction to contrast media seven vertebral levels above the site of injury. This obstruction resolved spontaneously on a repeat myelogram at 3 weeks (Fig. 24-11).

Frankel, discussing the problems of ascending cord lesions in the early stages following acute spinal cord injury, notes that the onset of neurologic changes in his series was within the first days to weeks following injury.[54] He reports seven patients who had sustained injuries to the dorsal and dorsolumbar junction that resulted in ascending lesions between 2 and 18 days after injury. Five bony injuries were at the level of D12, one at D11, and one at D4. Although the incidence was only seven in 808 reported cases (0.8%), Frankel is of the opinion that closer review of lesions involving the lower dorsal spine would in all likelihood reveal an incidence between 1.5% and 2%. (The incidence was 2.8% in my 1976 series.[113]) The most common improvements were a "complete" lesion becoming "incomplete" and an incomplete lesion decreasing in neurologic level by one or two segments. This usually occurred within the first 4 days. I have noted that in the presence of a slow but progressive deterioration in neurologic function, *the deterioration is almost always temporary.* In Frankel's experience, the most unusual change was an incomplete lesion that became complete.

In all likelihood, the most common cause of an ascending level of neurologic impairment is some form of vascular embarrassment, ascending hematomyelia, or the presence of an inflammatory or necrotizing lesion. Six of Frankel's cases were accompanied by hyperpyrexia above 102°F (38.9°C).

Frankel and others describe varied approaches to the management of these as-

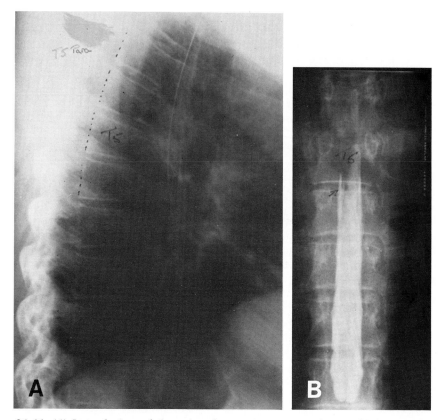

FIG. 24-11. (*A*) Lateral view of the spine demonstrates no evidence of bone injury. The patient had sustained a known injury at D11–12, with initial paraplegia at D12. With advance of the paraplegia, a myelogram (*B*) was obtained on the third day, which revealed obstruction of contrast material at T5. The shape of the obstruction was interpreted as cord edema. The contrast material was left in place; at 3 weeks the obstruction had resolved spontaneously.

cending lesions. Guttmann discusses the possibility of surgery, particularly when an ascending lesion is due to an epidural hematoma, or in the more rare presence of a subdural or medullary hematoma with associated cord edema.[63] Each of these may result in a vascular catastrophe as a consequence of either intrinsic (hematomyelia) or extrinsic pressure on the anterior spinal artery, resulting in anterior spinal artery thrombosis. Hardy[70] is of the opinion that when an ascending lesion occurred, it was the result of one rather than two radicular vessels supplying the cord. In seven similar cases he reports that heparin therapy was not successful. Harris reports the use of 20% mannitol and dexamethasone.[73] This regimen is also advocated by the author.[110,112,114] Hardy and his neurophysiol-

ogist co-worker note obliteration of the spinal artery system under such circumstances. These changes were also noted in a paper by Buss and Greenfield in 1919.

NEUROLOGIC AND RADIOLOGIC ASSESSMENT

From an anatomical viewpoint, it is good to recall that the spinal cord ends with the conus medullaris, posterior to the vertebral bodies of D12 and L1. This portion of the spinal cord contains the lower two segments of the lumbar spinal cord (L4–5) and the five sacral segments. Since the lumbar roots have already begun to exit from the spinal cord at a level adjacent to the T10 vertebral body, this allows for the passage of lumbar nerve roots lateral to the conus medullaris

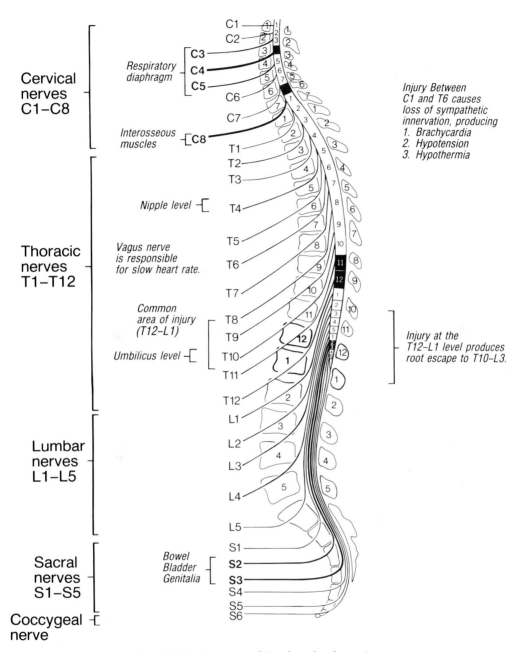

Fig. 24-12. Anatomy of the dorsolumbar spine.

and thus accounts for the mixed upper motor neuron–lower motor neuron injuries associated with fracture-dislocation at D12–L1 (Fig. 24-12).

Injuries distal to the L1 vertebral body produce pure nerve root (lower motor neuron) injuries. When upper motor neuron injuries occur, spasticity results. When combined upper and lower motor neuron injury occurs, spastic changes occur in the bowel and bladder from involvement of the sacral segments, while flaccid involvement of the lower extremities results from injury to the cauda equina (which at this level consists of peripheral nerves).

Immediately following injury to the dorsal

Table 24-3. Perianal Signs in Neurologic Assessment of Acute Spinal Cord Injury*

NEUROLOGIC LOSS	RECTAL TONE	RECTAL SENSATION
Complete	Absent	Absent
Complete	Present	Absent
(In the presence of bulbocavernous reflex)†		
Incomplete‡	Absent	Present
Incomplete§	Present	Present

* The finding of "sacral sparing" indicates incomplete spinal cord injury; neurologic improvement is possible.
† Involuntary spinal reflex
‡ Neurologic improvement possible
§ Significant improvement anticipated

spinal cord, neurologic examination may reveal a complete absence of motor, sensory, and reflex function below the level of the injury (spinal shock). Such injury may be the result of either functional or anatomical transsection of the spinal cord and will reveal absence of voluntary perianal motor and sensory function (also the result of spinal shock). The first reflex to return (often within minutes to hours) following trauma to the spinal cord portion of the nervous system will be the bulbocavernous reflex. Generally, the absence of perianal sensation, in the presence of a bulbocavernous reflex without voluntary muscle function in the perianal area or within the lower extremities, is evidence of a complete and, most likely, permanent spinal cord injury (Table 24-3). *Without question, the most important neurologic finding is the presence or absence of perianal sensation or voluntary perianal motor control.* If all other muscle or sensory function is absent yet perianal sensation persists ("sacral sparing"), this is substantial evidence of an *incomplete* injury. With this finding, there does exist a chance for the return of either sensory or motor function, though it may not seem likely. Also recognized as important signs of neurologic incompleteness in the immediate period following injury are the following: (1) testing for and identifying the presence of *intra-anal proprioception.* In the absence of perianal pinprick sensation, voluntary perianal muscle contractions, or the

bulbocavernosus reflex, as poor as it may seem, the finding of intra-anal proprioception is an indication of incompleteness. (2) The presence of *patellar or ankle reflexes* in the immediate postinjury period (*i.e.,* within the first 10–18 hours after injury) is also a very important and positive finding. When all else seems nonfunctioning, this single finding may be the cardinal finding of partial intactness and will require appropriate early evaluation. Some authors state that this latter finding indicates only a cessation of "spinal shock." I personally do not know the importance of "spinal shock" and therefore place no prognostic value on its presence or absence. Similarly, the involuntary "bulbocavernosus reflex" is almost always present, is the first reflex to be found following trauma, and when not present tends to indicate a vascular injury to the sacral segment of the area of the conus medullaris of the spinal cord.

It is not uncommon with cauda equina injuries below the level of L2 to find flaccid loss of motor function along with loss of sensation below the level of injury. These traumatized roots frequently reveal themselves to be only temporarily or partially traumatized, and thus will reveal partial return of function over a period of weeks to months. This is a classic example of *neurapraxia:* nerve sheath and axon trauma without anatomical disruption.

An extensive review of the literature in the 1960s revealed only two verifiable cases in which return of neurologic function below the level of injury occurred more than 24 hours after the diagnosis of complete neurologic injury.[12] It is therefore appropriate to state emphatically that in the face of failure of return of any neurologic function within the first 24-hours after injury, complete and permanent neurologic injury is likely.

Interpretation of the Findings

Having observed and assessed the patient with acute neurologic trauma, one must interpret the findings.

Should repeated neurologic examination during the first 24 hours after trauma fail to reveal evidence of motor or sensory function, the spinal cord injury has most likely sustained a complete and permanent injury.

Reflex return below the level of injury, without voluntary motor or sensory function, can, as stated above, be an indication that the spinal cord has not been *totally* traumatized or is no longer in a so-called state of spinal shock and that the spinal reflex arc remains intact. It does not indicate any kind of return of voluntary motor control.

The presence of motor or sensory function below the level of injury is evidence of an incomplete or partial neurologic injury, and the patient has the potential for neurologic improvement.

Emergency surgery is rarely indicated when a complete neurologic injury exists, even in the face of spinal malalignment, bony fragmentation of the canal, or obstruction to contrast media. Surgery will not alter the finding of a complete neurologic injury. If, on the other hand, upon neurologic reassessment it is noted that an "incomplete" injury reveals an extension of neurologic loss, careful interpretation is required, and appropriate surgical relief may be considered.

Roentgenographic assessment follows initial cardiopulmonary and neurologic evaluation. Initially, only routine anteroposterior and lateral views are required. When one is using the Stryker wedge frame with the patient in the prone position, lateral films of the thoracic and lumbar spine can be readily obtained without obstruction from frame supporting structures. This position also provides access to the traumatized spine and allows for proper positioning of the patient (into hyperextension when indicated) and assists in maintaining the reduction of an unstable fracture-dislocation.

Care must be taken to observe for pulmonary injuries and multiple rib fractures when placing the patient into the prone position. These findings do not contraindicate placing the patient into the prone position, but one should be aware of the findings and treat accordingly. Thus, the routine schedule of prone-supine positioning (every 2 hours) as prescribed on my unit might be altered. When pulmonary compromise is a major consideration, the patient may require maintenance in the supine position on an oscillating Rotorest bed or on a standard bed with three-quarter rolls, so as to unweight all skin areas.[68]

Prognosticators of Intact Neurologic Status

It is extremely difficult to differentiate between the neurologically complete (irreversible) injury and the "temporary" complete injury, which, in reality, is an undiagnosed incomplete injury. Until such time as evoked cortical responses become the standard by which complete and incomplete neurologic injury can be differentiated, the routine neurologic assessment will have to suffice. This examination, therefore, will ultimately supply the answers. Tarlov points out that the thick motor fiber is most sensitive to compression; proprioceptors, less sensitive; and the thin pain fibers, least sensitive.[154] Thus, the presence of pain, position "sense," or motor function, no matter how slight, is a favorable clinical prognosticator.

Wannamaker, in a review of spinal cord injuries from the Korean conflict, notes that a patient who had lost both motor and sensory function occasionally had return of some function following decompressive surgery.[165] Most likely, the injury was incomplete prior to surgery. Wannamaker does report one case of such neurologic return of function after 24 hours of complete absence of motor and sensory function. This case stands as one of two spinal cord cases in the world literature to have such a return. Wannamaker interprets the above as a suggestion that a more prolonged "safety" period exists in the human spinal cord than research in laboratory animals has indicated.[97,165]

In view of this, the following postulations can be made. In the presence of a complete motor-sensory paralysis resulting from vertebral fracture and/or dislocation, precious time must not be lost in attaining reduction so as to relieve spinal cord compression and ischemia. Nonsurgical manipulation and reduction should be attempted. Laminectomy should be performed only in the presence of a degenerating neurologic state in which there is roentgenographic or myelographic evidence of cord compression in the presence of a reduced fracture. Disruption of nerve tissue results in irreparable injury, and surgical or conservative care will not alter the result. Incomplete injuries, on the other hand, should be treated by conservative means such as fracture reduction, corticosteroid therapy, administration of osmotic diuretics, and spine fusion following neurologic stabilization. Occasionally, significant return of function will occur to the patient whose injury is neurologically incomplete—without surgery.

THE VASCULAR SUPPLY OF THE SPINAL CORD

The classic description of spinal cord vertical arterial pathways as composed of one anterior and two posterior longitudinal arteries reinforced at each level by *"rami radiculares"* was corrected by the observations of Adamkiewicz (1882), Kadyi (1889), and Pamon (1908). In brief, the anterior artery has been noted not to be continuous. Moreover, the radicular branches are of unequal length, and certain of them supply more than one segment (Fig. 24-13).

Lazorthes and associates have described the 31 pairs of radicular branches that penetrate the vertebral canal through the intervertebral foramen to be of three types:[97]

Proper radicular branches, which end within the roots or on the dura mater before reaching the spinal cord
Piamatral radicular branches, which do not penetrate beyond the arterial system surrounding the spinal cord
Spinal branches, which are the only ones that truly vascularize the spinal cord

Of the 62 left and right radicular branches, seven or eight, at most, truly participate in the vascularization of the spinal cord. Lazorthes and associates observe that their situation and distribution are more or less fixed, making it possible to distinguish three large arterial areas: the superior or cervical thoracic area, the intermediate or mid-thoracic area, and the thoracolumbar area.[97]

Intermediate or Mid-thoracic Area

The mid-thoracic area corresponds approximately to the 4th through the 8th thoracic segments. Its vascularization generally arises from a single artery situated at T7. This accounts for the interesting finding of an injury at the T7–8 bony level producing a motor-sensory lesion at the T4 level.

Lower or Thoracolumbar Area

The lower, or thoracolumbar, area includes the last three or four thoracic segments and the lumbar sacral segment of the spinal cord. It is an area of rich vascularity and depends on a single artery coming from one of the last dorsal or first lumbar arterial branches of the aorta. Adamkiewicz (1882) named this vessel *magnus ramus radicularis anterior*. Its importance, however, went unrecognized. In 1957 Lazorthes and co-workers proposed calling the vessel of Adamkiewicz *arteria intumescentia lumbalis*.[97] This vessel is characterized by its importance and fixity at the lumbar enlargement. The intumescentia lumbalis artery has variable importance, depending on its origin—superior, middle, or lower. More generally, it is found in the vertebral canal in company with one of six nerves: the 9th, 10th, 11th, or 12th thoracic nerves (75%) or the 1st or 2nd lumbar nerves (10%). Occasionally it is as high as the 5th, 6th, 7th, or 8th dorsal nerve (15%). In such cases there is a supplementary artery below it known as the *arteria conus medullaris*.

At the level of the conus medullaris there is a constant anastomosis between the princeps "trident": the anterior spinal and two posterior spinal arteries. This loop, known as the anastomotic loop of the conus medullaris, is constant.

Intermedullary Arterial Distribution

There is a constant nature to the intermedullary arterial distribution, which contrasts with the variability of the afferent arterial tracts. Peripheral arteries, which descend from the radicular branches, supply the pia mater and the spinal cord to vascularize the white matter. Central arteries from the anterior median sulcus, provided by the spinal branches alone, vascularize a

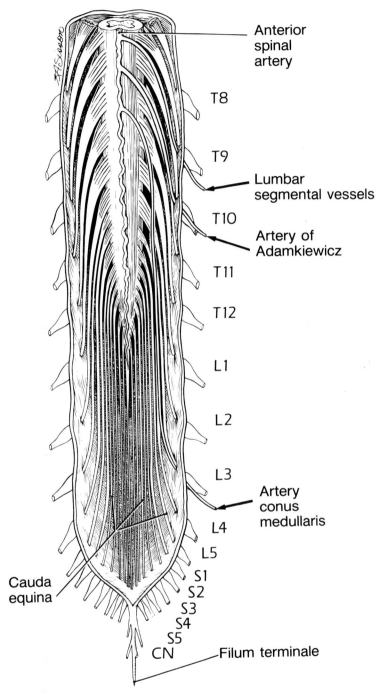

FIG. 24-13. Vascular supply of the spinal cord.

central area of the spinal cord made up of gray matter and the most central portion of the white matter. No separation of the spinal system into anterior and posterior parts with different organizations and circulations is possible.

Mid-thoracic Area.   The superficial anastomotic network in the mid-thoracic area is poor. The central arteries are small, few, and widely spaced (approximately 16 in 20 cm).

The superficial anastomotic network in the thoracolumbar area is rich. The central arteries are large and numerous (about 100 in 10–20 cm).

Thoracolumbar Area.   The clinical relevance of the didactic discussion of vascularity is the recognized fact that surgical approaches to the chest and flank may cause and are recorded as having caused interruption in the arterial blood supply to the spinal cord. The result is incomplete or complete paraplegia. This is particularly so with the lateral chest approach at the level of the 11th or 12th rib. When the approach is from the left (Hodgson and associates[77,78,79]), one is immediately brought down on the thoracic or lumbar radicular arteries exiting the aorta. Lazorthes and colleagues have demonstrated that the closer to the aorta that these arteries (carrying the arterial supply to the lumbar enlargement) are ligated, the greater the chance of successful anastomotic substitution.[97] This is not the case with radicular branches destined for the spinal cord. Also, the slower the obstruction, the greater the "surprise," and the less the chance for alternate pathways.

Further clinical information in the area of spinal cord vascularity has been gathered by pathological evaluation of posttraumatic and autopsy animal and human spinal cords. Histologically, and by electron microscopy, the posttraumatic cord reveals isolated hemorrhage in the central gray matter very early.[8,10] Central necrosis occurs as described by Bedbrook,[12] Ducker and Hamit,[47] and Osterholm and Matthews.[124,125] This hemorrhage migrates into the white matter and long tracts within hours. It is worth mentioning that in both humans and animals the progressive course of paraplegia has on some occasions been modified by preserving the diminished spinal cord circulation and maintaining neuron oxygenation during the early hours after trauma. Techniques such as general cardiovascular support, occasionally with controlled hypertension,[93] local hypother-

mia,[171] myelotomy,[5–8] laminectomy,[29,116] and administration of urea[88] and corticosteroids,[47,114,123,124] have been used in specific instances with occasional success.

It should be noted that injury to the anterior spinal artery, resulting in significant neurologic deficit and paraplegia, may follow situations other than trauma: scoliosis,[142] Pott's disease,[72–74] resection of abdominal aortic aneurysms (thought to be secondary to disruption of the vessel of Adamkiewicz),[34,52,148] and sympathectomy for hypertension.[117,144] This latter case apparently resulted from the innocent interruption of a peripheral intercostal vessel while the surgeon was approaching the anterior lateral chest via the 11th rib. This resulted in an apparent retrograde thrombosis of the intercostal vessel, followed by secondary radicular artery thrombosis, which was in turn followed by accidental sudden loss of blood supply to the anterior spinal artery.

Ferguson and colleagues, in 1975, reported five additional cases of spinal cord ischemia secondary to resection of abdominal aortic aneurysms, bringing the number of these complications in the world literature to 23.[52] Although this consequence does not relate to fracture or dislocation of the dorsolumbar spine, it does relate to the vascular consequences that may affect the spinal cord secondary to trauma. Ferguson and co-workers demonstrated in their cases that hypotension, or the "steal phenomenon"—not emboli—produced the syndrome under discussion.[52] Their patient population was older and did demonstrate some changes in the anterior spinal artery, along with evidence of anterior spinal artery syndrome, resulting in motor-sensory paraplegia with associated rectal and urinary incontinence and loss of pain and temperature sensation. Vibratory and proprioceptive senses were spared. These latter tracts lie in the posterior spinal cord, which receives its blood supply from the posterior spinal arteries. In contrast to the lumbar segment of the cord, in the thoracic region the vascular supply to the posterior arteries is in large part derived from the anterior spinal artery. When the anterior spinal artery undergoes occlusion, so may the blood supply to the posterior vessels. Should this occur, loss of vibratory and proprioceptive senses will also result.

Normally, the anterior and posterior spinal arteries are anastomotic channels that arise from the intercommunicating branches of the segmental arteries from the aorta.[97] In the thoracic region there is a reduced number of anterior radicular arteries arising from the intercostal and lumbar arteries that supply the thoracic spinal cord. The main blood supply to the lowermost portion of the spinal cord is through the "arteria radicularis magna," or vessel of Adamkiewicz.[2] It commonly enters from the left between the levels of T8 and L4 and is not normally subject to trauma during abdominal aortic surgery, though such injury may occur. When the vessel of Adamkiewicz has a lumbar origin (and this cannot be known beforehand without an arteriogram), it may become involved and result in neurologic injury to the conus medullaris and cauda equina.

The posterior spinal arteries described above depend in large part on the anterior spinal arteries in the lower thoracic and upper lumbar region. These vessels form an anastomotic loop about the conus medullaris. The vessel of Adamkiewicz contributes significantly to this loop to provide filling to the anterior spinal artery, the radicular branches of the cauda equina, and the posterior spinal arteries.

Several contributing factors, relating to the sensitivity of the spinal cord to vascular embarrassment, particularly when occasioned by alterations in anterior spinal arterial blood flow, are proposed. These include

Direct compression of artery with resulting ischemia

Interruption of arterial collateral flow

Occlusion of an intercostal vessel with retrograde thrombosis of a radicular artery, reducing flow to the anterior spinal artery

Occlusion of the abdominal aorta for varying periods to excise an abdominal aortic aneurysm, resulting in a decrease in blood flow through the vessel of Adamkiewicz when this vessel happens to reveal itself as an anatomic variant and appears as a lumbar rather than a lower thoracic segmental artery. It is possible, then, that

this aberrant vessel may be the principle blood supply to the anterior spinal artery. The result of normal anatomic variations occurring in the vessels providing major contributions to the anterior spinal artery, secondary to unequal growth between the spinal column and the spinal cord. Such unequal growth may result in an abrupt right-angle branching of the vessels from the aorta. This sharp change in vascular direction may produce partial vascular stenosis and with it a reduction in the orifice size of the vessels. The result will be a decreased intravascular blood pressure in the radicularis magna. Although this may reduce the flow in the anterior spinal artery, it may not become clinically pathologic unless there is further embarrassment to this vascular system.[52]

CLOSED MANAGEMENT

Rationale for Chemotherapy in the Early Treatment of Spinal Cord Injury

The synthetic corticosteroid dexamethasone (Decadron) is used principally to protect and maintain cellular membrane integrity. It is also a very effective anti-inflammatory agent. The use of mannitol (a very effective osmotic diuretic) has been recommended for some time in the presence of cerebral edema.[38,42,114,124] Though it has never been shown to be equally effective in reducing edema in the spinal cord, it is used for this purpose.

Dexamethasone continues to be administered to all patients with acute spinal injuries as soon as possible following injury and neurologic trauma. Although mannitol is still thought to be effective, there is such a high incidence of associated head injury with spinal cord injury (36% in my series) that it is no longer administered routinely.

Every effort should be made to maintain a normotensive to mildly hypertensive cardiovascular state in the patient with acute spinal cord injury.[92] This may be accomplished by the administration of crystalloids such as Ringer's lactate, normal saline, or dextrose and water, or colloids such as fresh frozen plasma, whole blood, or packed cells.

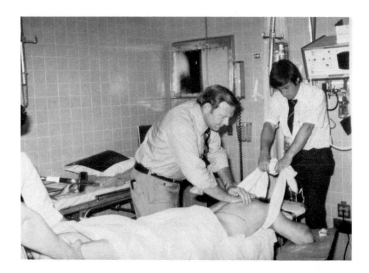

FIG. 24-14. Closed manipulation and reduction of a fracture-dislocation of the dorsal spine. Following neurologic assessment, with the patient prone on a Stryker frame and diazepam and morphine administered for relaxation, traction is applied proximally by means of a sheet around the chest and under the arms and distally on each extremity. The physician applies pressure over the area of maximum deformity. After manipulation, roentgenograms are best obtained with the patient prone. Hyperextension of the spine is maintained by pillows beneath the chest and pelvis when the patient is prone, and under the area of injury when the patient is supine.

Reduction by Manipulation

Closed, forceful manipulative reductions of spinal deformities were first advocated as early as 2000 to 3000 B.C. and were discussed in the literature as early as A.D. 1544.[69] Some authors in more recent times have questioned the advisability of this procedures in the presence of fracture-dislocations, particularly when the neurologic injury is incomplete.[69,81,118] To date, in my series of more than a dozen such cases (Figs. 24-14, and 24-15), none has revealed any evidence of neurologic deterioration secondary or attributable to fracture manipulation. One author recommended open reduction and internal fixation (Fig. 24-16).[76] Others have categorically denied any increase in neurologic deficit following closed manipulation and reduction.[102,110,113]

Minor angulations of the dorsolumbar spine are not considered bothersome, though they are often associated with comminuted fractures of the vertebral body or their posterior elements. I believe that an angular deformity up to 25° to 35° observed and given sufficient time will heal spontaneously. Greater than this, however, the deformity will most likely require internal fixation. Some fractures may be frankly unstable and likely to displace. These will also require internal fixation. Some physicians accept this displacement and allow such fractures to heal by postural reduction and prolonged recumbency.

OPEN MANAGEMENT

Side-Effects of Anesthesia in the Spinal Cord–Injured Patient

During the past decade, surgeons providing care for spine-injured patients have become acutely aware of the major complications that may accompany general anesthesia in these patients without careful and coordinated preoperative planning. In addition to the common complications of drug sensitivity and blood volume changes is the now-recognized hazard of administering such a drug as succinylcholine (suxamethonium) for pre-induction paralysis prior to intubation if administered to the spinal cord–injured patient within 3 to 6 weeks of injury. Desmeules,[42] Roth and Wuthrich,[138] and others have demonstrated that in the normal patient the administration of succinylcholine produces no problems. However, in patients with significant burns, tetanus, massive trauma, or other neurologic disorders, cardiac arrhythmias and cardiac arrest may result from administration of

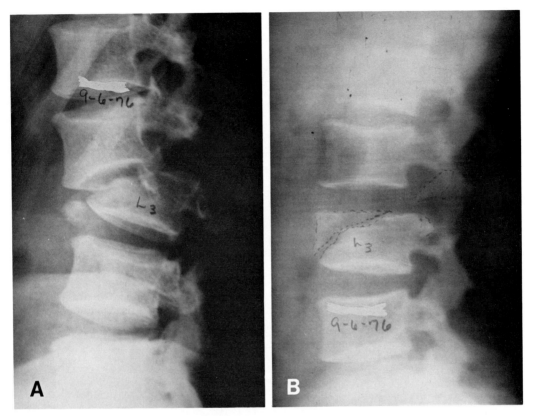

FIG. 24-15. (*A*) Lateral roentgenogram reveals a posttraumatic fracture and subluxation of L2 on L3. Note the significant disruption of the posterior elements and a comminuted fracture of the anterior superior plate of the body of L3. (*B*) This view shows spinal alignment following closed manipulation and reduction. On admission the patient was paraplegic (L2) without perianal sensation. Following reduction, in 12 hours the patient had complete return of sensation and eventual bilateral return of lower-extremity motor function.

this drug.[161] The cause is apparently a central denervation hypersensitivity below the level of the spinal cord lesion, resulting in excessive end-plate depolarization in hypotrophic muscle and excessive potassium release so severe as to cause cardiac arrest. Roth and Wuthrich reported the case of a 3-year-old and an adult who had circulatory arrest following the administration of succinylcholine.[138] Both were attributed to hyperkalemia (from the sudden release of potassium into the vascular system) secondary to the administration of the drug.

Two patients with uremia responded similarly to the administration of suxamethonium, as did a patient with tetanus and one who had received the drug 3 weeks after multiple trauma. One patient had a serum potassium level of 3.8 mEq/liter, which rose to 7.4 mEq/liter within 2 minutes after suxamethonium was given.

The question still exists whether this syndrome is the result of ion exchange that takes place during depolarization in the region of the motor end plate or is a direct result of damaged muscle. The latter is more likely. It is known that during normal voluntary muscle action, at least 1000 muscle fibers are stimulated per motor end-plate depolarization. It has been postulated that asynchronous muscle depolarization inflicts injury on muscle cells, liberating potassium by mechanical injury to the muscle cell itself. Others have reported on

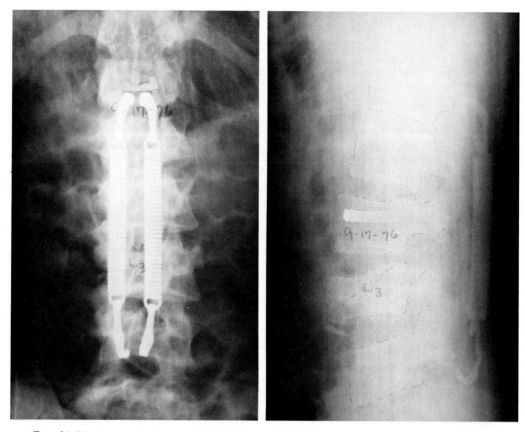

Fig. 24-16. Anteroposterior and lateral postoperative views of a dorsal spine fracture treated with a Weiss-spring procedure on D12 to L4, with bone grafting from the tibia. Note the maintenance of reduction of the fracture and the subluxation noted in Figure 24-15.

elevation in serum phosphokinase and myoglobinuria following the administration of suxamethonium in pathologic states, as noted herein. Because of problems related to hyperkalemia or excessive release of potassium into the circulation following administration of suxamethonium, tubocurarine, a nondepolarizing relaxant, is recommended if required during the induction phase of anesthesia. The best recommendation, in light of this complication, is not to administer any neurodepolarizing agent to any patient with multiple trauma, spinal injury, or other nervous system injury. The appearance of this complication is prevalent in spinal cord–injured patients between 3 and 6 weeks after injury, owing to the rapid loss of muscle mass secondary to denervation and loss of central control.[138]

Surgical Decompression

Schneider reviewed indications for and contraindications to laminectomy in spine-injured patients and found that the single most important and generally agreed to reason for immediate surgery, by neurosurgeons and orthopaedic surgeons alike, was "if the patient was becoming progressively worse, as demonstrated by a deterioration in neurologic function."[143] This statement is generally correct, but it must be weighed against the findings of the neurologic examination at admission. This is particularly true of the incomplete neurologic injury revealing progressive deterioration. Progressive ascending neurologic changes may, and frequently do, occur secondary to cord edema and are generally associated with a concomitant change in the vascular supply to the spinal cord. Although this is a worrisome finding, I have found that when neurologic symptoms deteriorate insidiously, they will generally improve just as quickly. On the other hand, when the neurologic picture changes rapidly and neurologic deterioration results, such function is less likely to return. Thus, unless there is more conclusive evidence as obtained from somatosensory-evoked potentials, myelograms, CT scans, magnetic resonance imaging, polytomograms, and so forth, surgical intervention should be withheld and the progress of the neurologic symptoms carefully followed. At the same time, it is important to observe for the probable cause of vascular embarrassment to the cord (bone encroachment or intervertebral disc protrusion). Then, if surgical decompression becomes necessary, the correct direction of the surgical approach can be made, based on positive findings, not suppositions. Thus, the real problem comes in recognition of these surgical indicators. Likewise, it is important to recognize that many injuries admitted as incomplete will, with time, undergo significant neurologic recovery without surgery.

Indicators for Laminectomy Schneider[143] and others[14,22,114,116,155,172] have been of the opinion that (besides neurologic deterioration) the most plausible indication for surgery is complete obstruction of the subarachnoid space in the patient whose neurologic injury is incomplete. If, on admission, the patient has a complete neurologic injury, regardless of what the radiographic or neurologic examinations demonstrate, there is little indication for exploratory surgery. Again, the opinion of Schneider, the author, and others is that an obstruction on myelogram within the subarachnoid space is most likely due to hematoma or medullary swelling, will be self-limiting, and will not require surgical intervention.

Munro is of the opinion that fractures of the dorsolumbar spine resulting in obstruction of the neurocanal should be treated in hyperextension for 4 to 7 days rather than surgically managed.[118] It is his opinion that fractures resulting from compression were better relieved by this means. Those not

relieved were the result of lateral dislocation and might indicate a need for surgery, though he does not qualify the neurologic state as a consideration.

The question arises as to the indications for surgery in the presence of open fractures or penetrating wounds of the spine. Most authors[143,165] are of the opinion that surgical debridement of gunshot wounds produced by the "civilian," low-velocity handgun are probably not in need of debridement surgery, owing to the less-tissue-destructive nature of such wounds. Their management would thus require only local debridement of the site of bullet entrance (and exit, if present) and appropriate antibiotic coverage. However, patients who sustain highly destructive high-velocity gunshot wounds of the spine do require consideration of surgical debridement, owing to the extensive soft tissue damage. They will require definitive intravenous antibiotic therapy. Evidence of the best rates of improvement in neurologic function following gunshot wound debridement is reported by Comarr and Kaufman:[30] 16% improvement following surgery and 28.9% improvement without surgery. Wannamaker reported 29% improvement following laminectomy; however, he studied patients with war injuries secondary to gunshot wounds sustained in the Korean conflict.[165] His statistics also revealed numerous complications that resulted from surgery, such as wound infection, dural cutaneous fistula, staphylococcal meningitis, and grand mal seizures.

Indications for myelography and emergency decompressive surgery, particularly in the patient with injury of the cervical spine, have been described by the author.[114] These same indicators apply to any area where there is significant possibility that a vascular or otherwise vital structure has occurred.

The most appropriate means of management of the fresh dorsal or lumbar fracture-dislocation is early postural reduction if there are no other indications for immediate surgery. Surgery, on the other hand, may be required in the presence of a neurologically incomplete injury in which there is demonstrable evidence of bone in the neural canal and obstruction of the subarachnoid space on myelogram, and in which reduc-

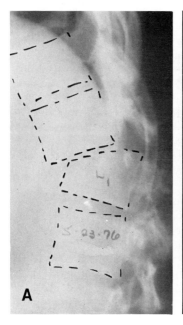 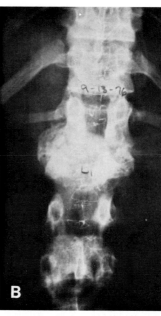

FIG. 24-17. Fracture and sub-luxation of D12 on L1 was treated by laminectomy. (*A*) Lateral view of the dorsolumbar junction. Note the posterior subluxation of L1. The patient was completely paraplegic (L1) on admission. (*B*) Because of spinal displacement and paraplegia, laminectomy was performed (D12–L1–L2).

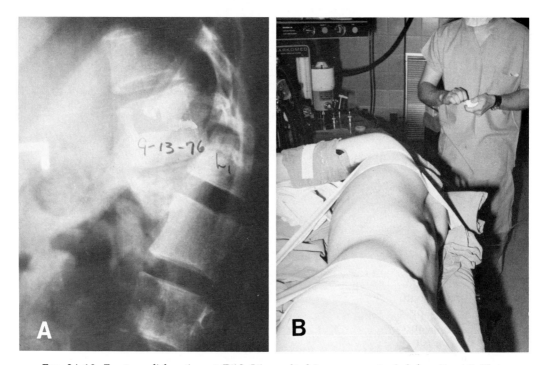

FIG. 24-18. Fracture-dislocation at D12–L1 resulted in severe spinal deformity. (*A*) Note the displacement. Previous films revealed only subluxation, now dislocated owing to posterior instability secondary to injury and laminectomy. (*B*) Because of the severe spinal deformity, the patient developed gibbi, which prevented supine positioning.

FIG. 24-19. Three types of internal devices: (*A*) Harrington distraction rods, (*B*) Weiss springs, and (*C*) Maurig-Williams spine plates. Note the laminar-hook fixation of the Harrington and Weiss apparatuses and the spinous-process fixation of the plates. Of the three devices, the Maurig-Williams plates (*C*) are no longer used as a means of internal fixation, and the Weiss springs (*B*) are used only for facet joint dislocation in the thoracic and lumbar areas of the spine.

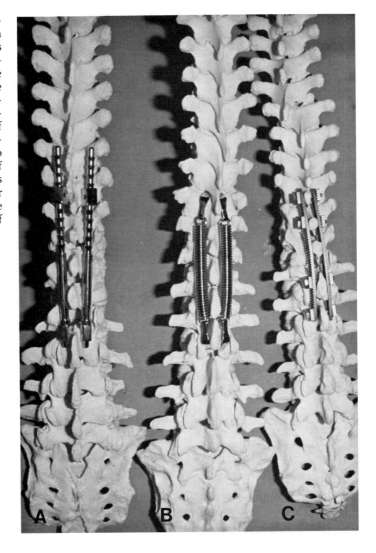

tion by conservative means fails, leading to the conclusion that a surgical decompression (from the appropriate direction) will enhance neurologic recovery. Attempts at relief of anterior pressure by a posterior laminectomy, with or without dentate ligament sectioning, are inappropriate when the primary pathology is anterior.[89] In the presence of complete motor-sensory loss, with or without anatomic reduction of a fracture-dislocation, surgical stabilization is probably best delayed for 10 to 14 days, giving the effects of trauma time to subside. When posterior internal fixation surgery is performed, posterior decompression should not be combined, for fear that it may aggravate preexisting spinal instability (Figs. 24-17 and 24-18).

Contraindications to Surgery

Surgery on the dorsal or lumbar spine need rarely be performed for stabilization within the first week or week and a half. This is particularly so in the face of multisystem trauma.

Other contraindications to the performance of major spinal surgery might be the nonavailability of a spine trauma surgeon or surgeons and other personnel (anesthesiologist, thoracic surgeon, neuro-

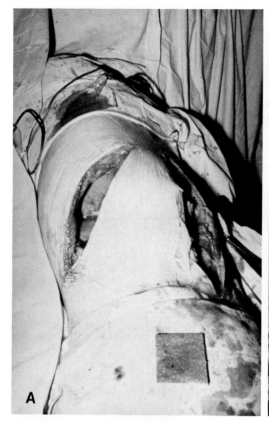

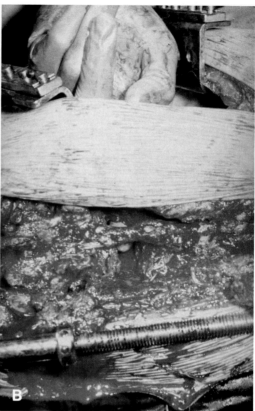

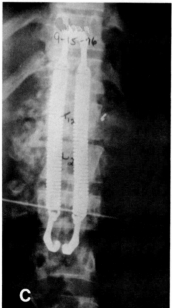

FIG. 24-20. Combined transpleural and posterior approach to a long-standing fracture-dislocation at D12–L1. (*A*) Simultaneous left transpleural and posterior approaches to the spine were employed to allow dissection and protection of the aorta anteriorly and the dura (*B*) and its contents posteriorly. (*C*) The body of L1 was excised, and Weiss springs were placed (with a bone graft), bringing D12 into bony opposition to L2.

surgeon, orthopaedic surgeon) who are accustomed to working together as a team, managing similar problems on numerous previous occasions. Included within this team are spinal cord–neurologically trained nurses, therapists, social workers, and other

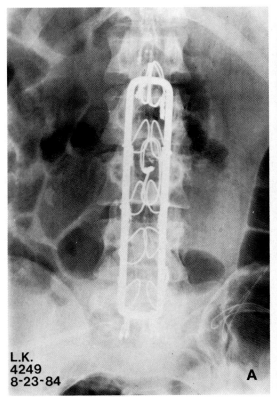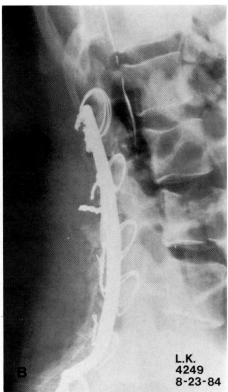

FIG. 24-21. Internal fixation of L1–S1 with a Luque rectangular rod. (*A*) Anteroposterior view. (*B*) Lateral view of the Luque-rod L1–S1 fusion extended to the sacrum owing to a pars interarticular defect at L5.

paraprofessionals, each of whom is comfortable working within an evironment with which he or she is familiar because of the frequency of the admission of such cases (greater than 50 to 100 spinal cord admissions per year).[62] The surgical team should be familiar with various methods and techniques of spine stabilization and fusion (Fig. 24-19).

Historical Considerations

As early as 1940, Alby advocated internal fixation of spine fractures by bone grafting.[3] Wilson, of the U.S., introduced fixation of fractures of the spine using Maurig-Williams-type plates and screws. His procedure, because of unsound mechanical reasons (though theoretically logical), did not receive wide general acclaim in either the orthopaedic or neurosurgical communities. In 1953 Holdsworth and Hardy, who had

condemned manipulative reduction as unsafe, became advocates of open reduction and internal fixation, using plates and bolts (similar to Wilson).[83] These were placed across one or more spinous processes above and below the level of dislocation. This procedure was particularly advocated for unstable fracture-dislocations at the dorsolumbar junction. It was Holdsworth's contention that this procedure was effective in promoting cord and root recovery by preventing further damage.

Dick agreed that internal fixation stabilized the spine, prevented further nerve root injury, and simultaneously facilitated nursing care.[45] In 1954 Holdsworth withdrew the statement that "the method [spine stabilization with plates] is simple." This repudiation followed a review by Guttmann of 100 cases treated by open reduction and internal fixation. He reports that Maurig-

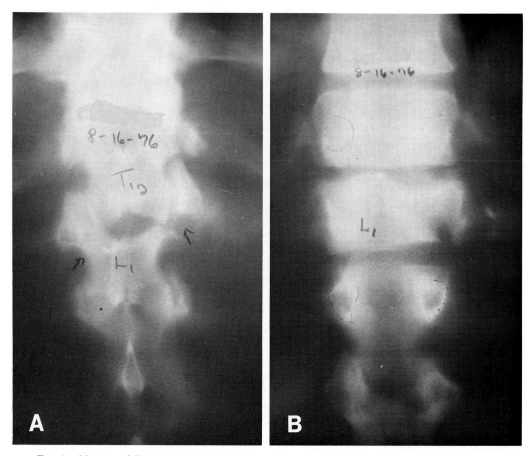

FIG. 24-22. (*A* and *B*) Tomograms reveal that this unilateral fracture of a posterior superior facet and pedicle includes a portion of the adjacent vertebral body. (*C*) Scoliosis developed secondary to insertion of a Weiss-spring compression device across the unilateral facet–pedicle fracture. (*D*) The most appropriate means of internal fixation in the presence of a unilateral facet–pedicle–vertebral body fracture is Harrington distraction rods.

Williams plates did not prevent redislocation or angulation and contributed to increased rigidity of the spine, pain, and further collapse of initially extended vertebral fractures. Thus, it was noted that plates did not effectively prevent progressive angulation of the vertebral column and that gibbi developed in spite of internal fixation. Once mobilized, the internal fixation loosened by breaking or tearing loose the bolts from the spinous processes, resulting in the need for removal. Several patients developed hematoma and infection, and there was little neurologic evidence that surgery promoted root escape or improved recovery any better than conservative treatment.[70] Holdsworth, noting instances in which clinical symptoms deteriorated following internal fixation, be-

came more conservative. He eventually advocated operative procedures for only the most unstable fractures. Guttmann regarded open reduction and internal fixation with plates and bone grafts in traumatic paraplegia as indicated only in the "most excessive fracture-dislocation."[64] Bedbrook, noting avascular necrosis of the vertebral body following severe compression fracture, advanced the opinion that this was probably the cause of progressive spinal angulation following internal fixation.[12] Holdsworth's continued opinon was that unstable fractures could not be stabilized in early stages by conservative means alone.[82] On the other hand, Guttmann advocated postural reduction only, and if redislocation occurred, later surgery might be considered. Holds-

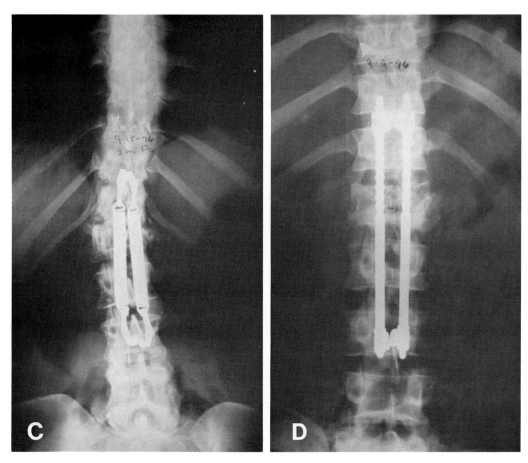

FIG. 24-22. (*Continued*)

worth found that many of his internal fixation patients required continued bed care for periods of 8 to 12 weeks, during which time adequate bone healing occurred.[81] This immobilization period was comparable to the conservative care suggested by Guttmann. All authors—while appreciating that surgical reduction may fail and is fraught with hazards of both instability and neurologic deterioration—agreed that dislocations with neurologic involvement required great care and that long-standing fracture-dislocations cannot be reduced by closed manipulation alone.

Procedures and Selection Criteria for Internal Fixation Devices

Selecting the appropriate internal fixation device for stabilization of the spine is sometimes difficult because absolute guidelines for their use do not exist. Ultimately, the decision hinges on a consideration of a number of important variables, not the least of which is the surgeon's preference.

Rightly or wrongly, the orthopaedic surgeon more familiar with the Harrington-rod procedure in the management of scoliosis will more often use rods for internal fixation than some other equally appropriate, or better, method. The difference in the approach to the problem is not so much the type of internal fixation that the surgeon selects as its appropriate application for biomechanical reasons. Other factors also require consideration: (1) the presence or absence and severity of associated neurologic injury, (2) the presence of vertebral body bone fragments within the neural canal, (3) the severity of the vertebral body fracture, (4) whether the fracture is a wedge compression, burst (see Figs. 24-5 and 24-15), unilateral, or bilateral body–pedicle–

facet–posterior element fracture (see Fig. 24-18), and (5) the integrity of the anterior and posterior ligamentous structures (see Figs. 24-4 and 24-5).

Harrington-Rod Internal Fixation.   The literature offers information on the use of, indications for, and results of Harrington-rod instrumentation in the stabilization of dorsolumbar vertebral fractures.[45] Criteria for its use are better established today than in the past, although as alternate methods of fixation (*e.g.,* Weiss springs, Luque rods) have become available, their hard and fast indications are less well defined (Figs. 24-20 and 24-21).

From 1972 through October 1984, 728 patients with thoracolumbar fractures were admitted to the Acute Spinal Cord Injury Service. Of these, 83.6% were neurologically involved. Of the patients with neurologically incomplete injuries, 51.2% were treated surgically and the remainder conservatively. Of the surgical group, 43.0% were managed with Harrington rods. Of the patients admitted with neurologically complete injuries, 38.4% were managed surgically. Of those, 21.1% were managed with Harrington rods, the remainder by some alternative manner. Likewise, of the patients who were neurologically normal on admission, 60.1% were managed surgically, 30.4% of whom were managed with Harrington rods, the remainder by some alternate method.

Indications.   Probably the sure indication for the use of Harrington rods is the presence of an unbalanced fracture of the vertebral body. Usually associated with hemifracture of the vertebra is a unilateral fracture of one pedicle and facet (on the same side). Harrington rods provide a stable, balanced means of internal fixation (Fig. 24-22).

Another prominent indication for the use of Harrington rods is the presence of a "burst" fracture of the vertebral body. In spite of the severity of the fracture, when there has not been significant translatory displacement of one vertebra on another, the anterior and posterior longitudinal ligaments will have remained intact. By means of the Harrington rods, the biomechanical force of distraction very often produces a significant reduction (Fig. 24-23). The only problem with this reduction is that it often occurs, or appears to occur, because of distraction of fragments of the vertebral body. This leads to late deformity, owing to failure of the fragments to heal together. In this instance, Harrington rods may be the culprit.

Harrington rods are indicated in the presence of significant spinal malalignment resulting from fracture or dislocation. Such injuries may be stable or unstable. They may also be several weeks old and not possible to reduce. Nonetheless, Harrington rods are the appropriate method of stabilization (Fig. 24-24).

Falling within the category of instability and benefiting from the use of Harrington rods is the spine having had previous wide laminectomy (see Fig. 24-23, *E*) resulting in further spinal instability. Both Dickson and Bradford have expressed the belief that at least two intact lamina must be present above and below the injury site in order that the tendency for kyphosis to occur will be counteracted. In such cases, Weiss springs have been used as a means of both preventing and correcting the presence of kyphosis (Figs. 24-25 and 24-26).

Contraindications.   Probably one of the easiest contraindications to identify is the spine that demonstrates gross ligamentous instability. This can usually be suspected if there has been significant lateral translation of one vertebral body on another.

A second easy contraindication (though one might get away with using the rods in certain instances, as described later), is when it can be readily identified that a bilateral facet dislocation exists, with or without a vertebral body fracture.

Because of the problem of fragment distraction, in spite of the radiographic evidence of successful reduction, Harrington rods should probably not be used in the presence of a burst fracture with an associated complete neurologic injury. The problem is distraction of the vertebral body fracture fragments, which prevents good fracture healing. Some other type of internal fixation (Luque rods) could better provide both improved spinal alignment and stabilization.

When fractures involve the dorsal spine, particularly in the presence of a moderate

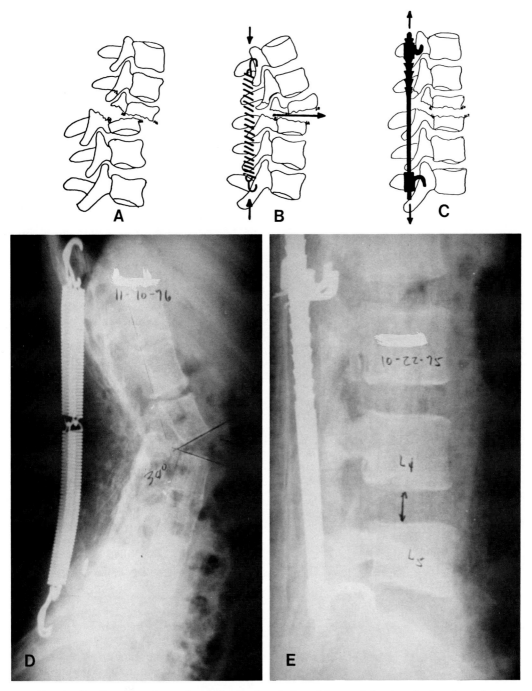

FIG. 24-23. Considerations of stability in the choice of internal fixation devices for spinal injuries. (*A*) The gross displacement in some spine injuries often results in disruption of both the anterior and posterior longitudinal ligaments and the posterior elements. *B* demonstrates the potential for displacement when a compression device (Weiss spring) is used for a fracture such as that in *D* (see Figs. 24-29 and 24-30, the same patient). (*C*) Overdistraction at the fracture site may occur when distraction rods are used (see roentgenogram, *E*). The surgeon must consider the state of ligamentous stability when choosing the appropriate method of internal fixation.

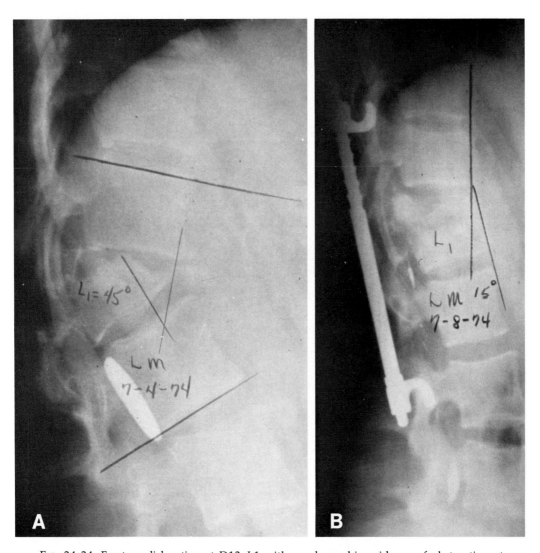

FIG. 24-24. Fracture-dislocation at D12–L1 with myelographic evidence of obstruction at L1. (*A*) Posterior displacement of L1 caused obstruction of the neural canal and marked angulation of the spine. (*B*) Postoperative (Harrington distraction rod) internal fixation position of the dorsolumbar spine. A wide laminectomy was immediately performed because of an "incomplete" neurologic injury. Owing to the patient's condition, spine fusion was not performed immediately.

dorsal kyphosis, Harrington rods cannot be used unless they are bent to match the dorsal spine anatomy. In such situations, either Weiss springs or the Luque rods should be used (see Figs. 24-20 and 24-21).

A Modification of the Harrington-Rod Procedure–Luque-Rod System. A technique now used with great regularity is to combine Harrington distraction rods with Luque sublaminar wires. This combination has

come about with the realization that in certain instances the use of Harrington rods alone produces spine instability by distraction. Also, their use in the area of the highly mobile lower lumbar spine frequently leads to the dislodgment of the lower hooks of the device, either at the rod–hook interface or at the hook–lamina interface. This situation generally results when the patient is allowed out of his restraining orthosis

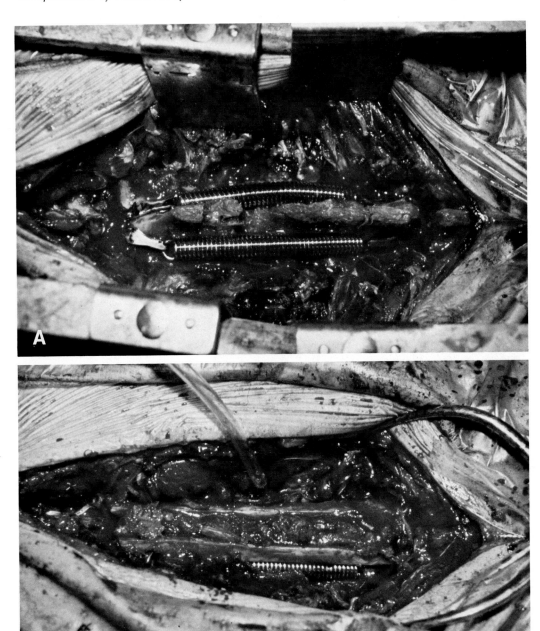

FIG. 24-25. Surgical views of the dorsolumbar spine at operation for Weiss-spring internal fixation. (A) Weiss-spring hooks have been inserted two levels above and two levels below the injury site, following reduction of a fracture-dislocation and maintenance under compression. (B) Either tibial or iliac bone grafts are placed about the vertebral spinous processes and lamina for spine fusion along with the Weiss-spring procedure (see Fig. 24-27, B).

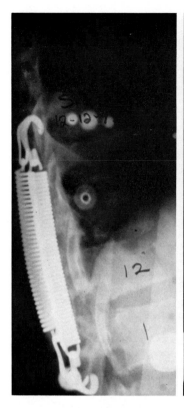 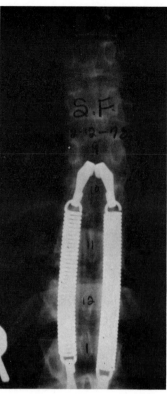

FIG. 24-26. On these postoperative roentgenograms of Weiss-spring internal fixation of a fracture-dislocation of the dorsolumbar spine, note the spinal alignment and the distance fused (D10–L1).

and flexion of the lumbar spine is resumed. To circumvent this complication, many surgeons now combine the use of Luque sublaminar wires at the most superior intact lamina beneath the upper hook, and likewise, at the lower end. It is the surgeon's choice whether this technique is carried out on both of the laminae above and below the injury site. Although the inherent concern is the placement of sublaminar wires into the neurocanal in the patient who is neurologically intact or who has an incomplete neurologic injury, this technique has definitely reduced the problem of dislodgment of the rod-hooks from the laminae.

One final note. As noted by Edelstein, Meyer, and associates,[48] when bone fragments lie within the neural canal in the patient with an incomplete neurologic injury, an anterior decompression may be indicated if there is obstruction of the canal. In such instances, when the fracture of the spine lies at the dorsolumbar junction, an 11th-rib anterolateral transthoracic ap-

proach will provide adequate access for vertebral body fragment decompression of the dura at the T12–L1 level. I frequently perform a combined anterior-posterior procedure. This allows for the simultaneous insertion of posterior stabilizing Harrington rods while the anterior vertebral body is excised, followed by an anterior inlay rib of fibular bone graft between the remaining adjacent vertebrae.

Weiss-Spring Internal Fixation. The use of Weiss dynamic compression springs as an adjunctive internal fixation procedure in the management of traumatic spinal injuries began in the U.S. in 1972 in cooperation with and at the request of the now-deceased Professor Marian Weiss of Konstancin, Poland. Professor Weiss developed the procedure after the first use of the device by Dr. Weiss's mentor, Professor Grusa, who had utilized the springs in the management of juvenile scoliosis arising either from poliomyelitis or congenitally. Although the springs were not effective in the prevention of or the progression of scoliosis, they were found to be an effective means of stabilizing certain spine fractures. During the early years when the Weiss springs were used, their success was varied and their specific indications ill-defined. Today, Weiss springs are still used, but their indications are now better identified. The operative procedure that competes most with the use of the springs is the Luque-rod procedure.

Indications. The primary indication for the use of Weiss springs is the traumatic spine injury in which a flexion-distraction injury to the dorsal-lumbar or lumbar spine has resulted in a bilateral dislocation of the facets *without fracture* and a forward subluxation of the superior vertebra on the inferior vertebra, *with or without neurologic injury.* Obviously, in this instance, the injury will have resulted in a traumatic spinal kyphosis and gibbus formation.

The second indication for use of the springs is the patient who has sustained a wedge compression fracture of the vertebra of 25% to 50% of the anterior body, without fracture of the posterior vertebral body wall. Again, in this case a traumatic kyphosis will be present. The important aspect of this indication is that the posterior wall of the affected vertebral body not be fractured and, if placed under compression, would not cause bone to be extruded into the neural canal. This is of paramount importance if the patient's neurologic examination reveals that the injury remains neurologically incomplete. The same holds true for the lumbar spine, as well as the dorsal or dorsolumbar spine. It is *not* a factor if the patient has sustained an injury to the dorsal spinal cord and has suffered a neurologically complete injury.

I have found this procedure very effective in the management of fracture-dislocations of the lumbosacral joint, with or without neurologic injury, when the facets may have been fractured and forward subluxation of the superior vertebra on the lower one has resulted. In this case, the lower hooks of the device are inserted into the second sacral foramen below and over the lamina at the elected level above.

Contraindications. There are, in my opinion, contraindications to the use of the springs:

The neurologic examination reveals that the patient has an incomplete injury, and the injury to the vertebral body has resulted in a fracture to the posterior vertebral body wall.

The patient has, on anterior-posterior roentgenograms, an unbalanced fracture, resulting in a unilateral fracture of one side of the facet–pedicle–vertebral body. In this case, the application of a compression load across the fracture site would result in an iatrogenic scoliosis on the side of the fractures.

The springs would be inserted in the area of the lumbar spine lordotic curve, resulting in an exaggerated hyperextension of the lumbar spine.

The anterior longitudinal ligament is obviously disrupted or highly suspected of being disrupted. The use of Weiss springs in this situation would again produce an exaggerated hyperextension deformity.

Insertion Technique. The routine insertion of Weiss springs includes the creation of a small, bilateral laminotomy site on the superior border of the superior lamina onto which the surgeon believes the upper hooks should be applied. The same technique is performed on the lower border of the lower lamina selected for insertion of the lower hooks. Normally, two intact laminae above the level of injury and two laminae below the fracture site are selected for insertion of the hooks. An attempt is made, as when using Harrington rods, to have two intact laminae above and below the fracture site against which the springs, like the rods, can lie. Upon these an anteriorly directed fulcrum is applied. Occasionally, if the superior lever arm is thought to be long, the upper hook might be applied three laminae above, rather than two. The same may hold true if one of the intervening laminae above is fractured.

Care is taken to notch the laminae centrally on the surfaces to which the hooks are applied to allow easy and accurate insertion when the system is under maximum tension and to ensure stable hook fixation (see Figs. 24-25 and 24-26).

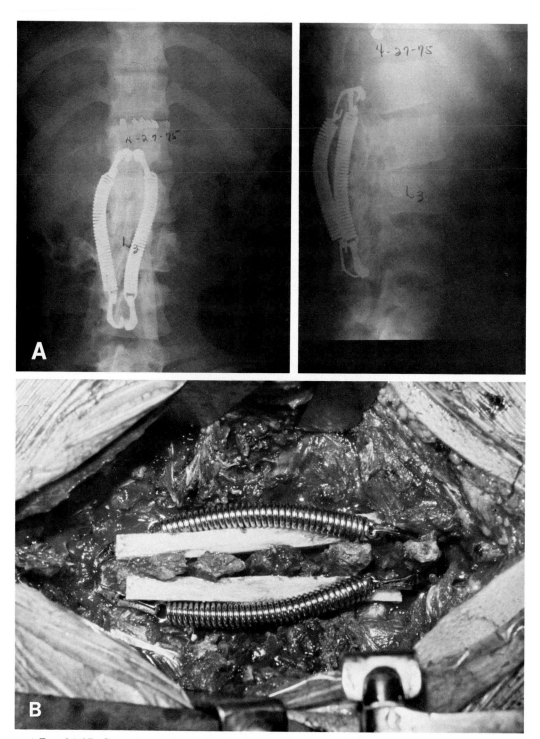

Fig. 24-27. Operative and postoperative views of Weiss-spring internal fixation and an alternate method of spine fusion. (*A*) Note the position of the spine following insertion of Weiss springs and the apparently intact posterior wall of the body of L3. (*B*) A tibial bone graft was inserted beneath the Weiss springs. This technique allows for compression of the bone graft against the posterior elements and assists in mechanical maintenance of spinal correction.

When to Use Weiss Springs Instead of Harrington Rods. Weiss-spring fixation is indicated instead of Harrington-rod fixation in the following situations:

When a gibbus or traumatic kyphosis has resulted from a vertebral body wedge compression fracture (with maintenance of the posterior vertebral body border)

When there is disruption of the posterior structures (the posterior longitudinal ligament, ligamentum flavum, or interspinous ligament) (Fig. 24-27). Although in some cases vertebral element displacement may not exist even in the presence or suspected presence of ligamentous disruption (without fracture), such injuries are potentially unstable. Although surgery is not absolutely indicated, when there is neurologic injury, surgical stabilization allows an earlier entrance of the patient into an active rehabilitation program, with less concern for extension of the neurologic injury. In this type of spinal deformity, the use of springs not only applies a corrective hyperextension moment on the spine, but also places a compression moment across the posterior elements and a distractive (corrective) force anteriorly.

When other methods of internal fixation (rods or plates) have been used and failed.

When fracture-dislocation of one dorsal vertebra on another requires reduction and stabilization. Although internal fixation of the upper dorsal spine is less often indicated than is internal fixation of the lower dorsal spine because of the inherent internal stability provided by the rib cage, there are fracture-dislocations of one dorsal vertebra on another that require reduction and stabilization to prevent significant gibbus formation at the injury site and possible cardiovascular compromise. The Weiss spring has been very effective in maintaining the reduction. The advantage here is that the device conforms to the normal upper dorsal kyphosis while applying a corrective moment. Harrington distraction rods require bending before insertion, and this may accentuate the deformity and set up stress or fatigue risers in the rod. Also, Harrington compression rods are more difficult to insert and less likely to produce the correction sought.

In the presence of a comminuted fracture of a vertebral body and a complete neurologic injury, the Weiss-spring procedure may be used; however, the better procedures to use would be the Harrington-rod or Luque-rod procedures.

In the spine that has been operated on and on which a one- or two-level laminectomy has been performed, there is potential spinal instability. In the presence of exposed dura, consideration and care must be taken when one is using Weiss springs, Harrington rods, or Luque rods not to apply internal fixation components or bone grafts directly against the exposed dura. Before either bone graft or internal fixation is inserted, a free graft of subcutaneous fat or Gelfoam should be applied across the surface of the dura. Similarly, the bone graft, if obtained as strips from the posterior ilium or the tibia, can be applied beneath the springs (see Fig. 24-27).

Maurig-Williams (Spinal) Plates. A brief note concerning the use of Maurig-Williams plates as a method of internal fixation. *This method of spine stabilization is no longer recommended.* The presence of a flexion moment (from whatever cause) across the fracture site frequently causes a loss of fixation of the plate's bolts from the spinous processes owing to the cutting out of the metal bolt from the bone. This results in the loss of internal fixation, prominence of the metal plate under the skin, the possible occurrence of an area of skin breakdown over this area of subcutaneous prominence, and ultimately, with the loss of internal fixation, the occurrence of an increased kyphotic deformity at the level of the fracture site (Fig. 24-28). Although this can occur in both the thoracic and lumbar areas, Weiss springs can be used as a countermeasure only in the thoracic area for biomechanical reasons.

Loss of Internal Fixation

The only real complication that has arisen from the use of Weiss springs or Harrington rods has been loss of fixation of the hooks at the hook–bone interface. The most likely reason for this failure is the lack of stable placement of the hook to the lamina at the

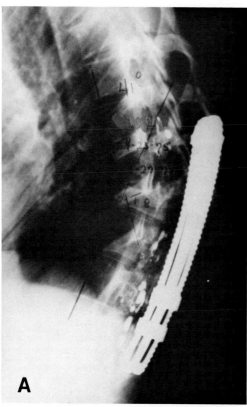

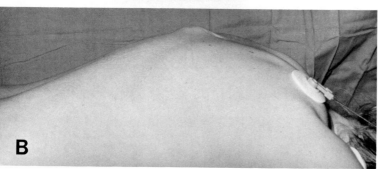

FIG. 24-28. Loss of internal fixation with Maurig-Williams plates. (*A*) Note the loss of fixation at D6–7, resulting from bone failure (spinous processes). (*B*) A gibbus was caused by the metal prominence beneath the skin. This type of internal fixation device is no longer used.

time of hook placement. Another reason for failure may be the application of excessive distraction forces on the hook, particularly when using the Harrington distraction apparatus. Only one significant spine malalignment has resulted from the use of Weiss springs (Fig. 24-29). This occurred in a tumorous spine and resulted in removal of the springs and replacement by Harrington distraction rods (Fig. 24-30). In the 153 operations performed, none of the devices have required removal for infection. Several Maurig-Williams plates have been removed

because of the prominence of the plate beneath the skin. This is associated with failure of internal fixation (see Fig. 24-28).

ORTHOTIC CONSIDERATIONS

Spinal Orthoses

Dorsolumbar fractures, managed both conservatively and surgically, regardless of the presence or absence of neurologic changes or the extent of the spinal instability, all require some type of external

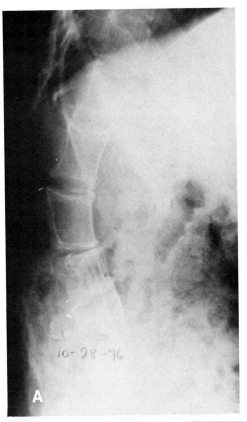

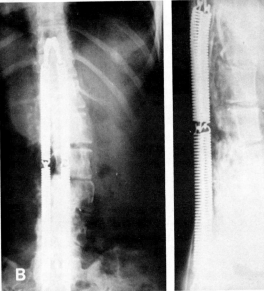

FIG. 24-29. Tumor (neurofibroma) of the lumbar spine with deformity and internal (Weiss-spring) instrumentation. (A) Lateral view shows kyphosis developing owing to intraspinal erosion of the posterior elements. (B) Postoperative anteroposterior and lateral views of the dorsolumbar spine after insertion of internal fixation (Weiss spring); scoliosis had been present for 12 years. Note the correction of the kyphosis in the lateral view (see Figs. 24-23, D and 24-30, the same patient).

orthosis for a prescribed period, usually 3 months. The following considerations dictate the requirements for the specific orthosis to be used.

D1–6. High dorsal spine fractures, at or above D6, cannot be managed by a "hyperextension" orthosis alone (Fig. 24-31) for anatomical reasons. The rationale is

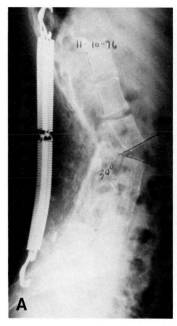
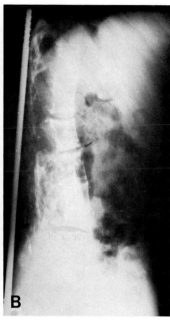

FIG. 24-30. Failure of the anterior longitudinal ligament resulted in spine malposition. (*A*) Posterior compression produced a hyperextension moment on the spine, resulting in spontaneous rupture of the anterior longitudinal ligament at L2–3. This produced a significant lordosis and neurologic embarrassment. (*B*) The Weiss springs were removed and replaced with Harrington distraction rods from T10 to the foramen of S2. Postoperatively, the patient was immobilized in a body cast that included the pelvis, after which he was allowed to ambulate (see Fig. 24-33).

that to be effective the sternal and pubic rami pads (at the upper and lower ends of the orthosis, respectively) must have a broad area for pressure. This implies that the pad must be at the level of D5–6 superiorly. For an orthosis to be effective above D6, a cervical extension must be applied to the Knight-Taylor or Jewett hyperextension orthosis. In patients who sustain axial load–rotatory fractures at D6 and above (Fig. 24-32), it is customary to apply this kind of extension to the Knight-Taylor orthosis (see Fig. 24-31, *C*) to maintain head–cervical spine–upper dorsal spine alignment during the period required for healing and stability.

D6–L5. Injuries to the dorsal or lumbar spine between D6 and L5, whether managed conservatively or operatively, require orthotic support with either a three-point hyperextension Jewett orthosis or a Knight-Taylor orthosis (see Fig. 24-31, *A* and *B*). For fractures of the upper dorsal spine, particularily in the area of D6–8, the orthotic device that has provided the best stability is the Knight-Taylor orthosis, with the addition of anterior pectoral horns. These additions assist in maintaining the spine in an upright, or hyperextended, position (Fig. 24-31, *E*).

When spinal fractures are unstable for whatever reason (increased mobility at the fracture site, patient unreliability, etc.), a plaster body cast (see Fig. 24-31, *D*) is suggested in place of either of the two previously mentioned orthoses. The only concern with the use of a plaster or plastic orthosis is that both cover the skin, and in the spinal cord–injured/insensitive-skin patient, one must be concerned with a greater possibility of skin breakdown, particularily in the area of the iliac crests.

The major complications with plaster casts are related to its weight and the hazards of using it over insensitive skin. If adequate precautions are not taken, pressure areas may result in skin pressure problems over the sacrum and iliac crests.

It is recommended before flexion-extension radiographs are taken to determine the state of bony healing that the patient wear the orthosis a minimum of 3 months. It has been my observation in managing 2032 spine injuries (728 [40%] dorsolumbar and 1304 [60%] cervical) from 1972 to October 1984 that 3 months is the average period required for healing of spine fractures.

L5–S1. Management of injuries at the lumbosacral junction is difficult because of the anatomy of the area and the compound motion across these joints. Not only do flexion and extension occur across the lumbosacral joints, but there is motion in both

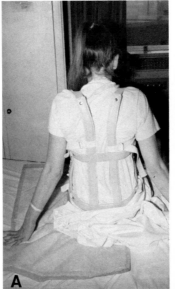

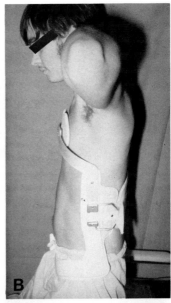

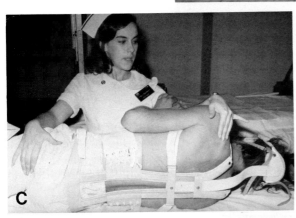

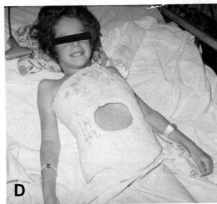

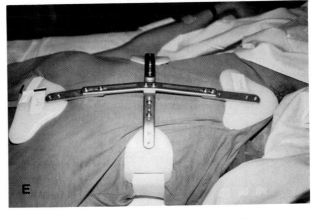

Fig. 24-31. (A) The Knight-Taylor thoracic lumbosacral orthosis (TLSO), modified by the addition of pectoral horns. This orthosis is used primarily for conservative and postoperative stabilization of spine fractures between T6 and L5. The primary attribute of this orthosis over others are the posterior upper thoracic extension, the anterior pectoral horns, and the abdominal apron. (B) The Jewett three-point (TLSO) hyperextension orthosis. This orthosis is best used for less severe (and more stable) compression fractures of the thoracic-lumbar vertebra with intact posterior elements. The basic stabilizing principle of this orthosis is hyperextension. (C) For fractures of the upper dorsal spine (D1–6) the Taylor orthosis with a cervical extension is used. It assists in preventing forward displacement of the head, neck, and upper thorax at the fracture site, during the period of healing from 4 weeks to 3 months, and allows for early mobilization of the "high" paraplegic. (D) The body cast with three-point hyperextension, or flexion, is used in place of the standard orthosis in patients for whom removal is contraindicated or in whom stability is more precarious. (E) The Jewett-type (cruciate) hyperextension (TLSO) orthosis.

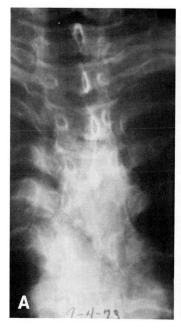
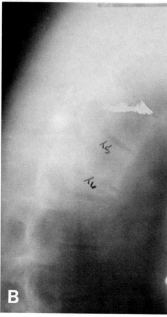

FIG. 24-32. An axial load flexion injury to the proximal thoracic spine (D5–6). (*A*) Note that the fracture is oblique and extends through both vertebra. (*B*) Kyphotic deformity of proximal dorsal spine resulted in compromise of the spinal canal and anterior small artery thrombosis and paraplegia.

of the sacroiliac joints. Also, pelvic motion in relation to the lumbosacral joint is influenced by hip flexion and extension. Therefore, surgical fusion in this area of the vertebral column requires more rigid immobilization than a thoracolumbosacral orthosis can provide.

On numerous occasions, a plaster-of-paris "pantaloon" one-legged body spica, from the sternal notch to the pubic symphysis and down to the supracondylar region of one femur, has been successfully utilized when fusing the lumbosacral joint. Two such cases were for traumatic dislocation (Fig. 24-33).

Lower-Extremity Orthoses

A question often asked is, Which dorsolumbar spine–injured patient, having sustained a complete neurologic injury, will ambulate? The answer lies in the level of injury.[99]

Above D10. Certainly there will be exceptions to a rule, but it can generally be said that the spinal cord–injured patient having sustained a neurologic injury above the level of D10 will probably not find it energy-economical or efficient to attempt ambulation. For one to be a successful ambulator, it is necessary to have pelvic control. The patient that has sustained an injury to the spinal cord above the neurologic level of D10 will have neither paraspinal muscle control nor upper and lower abdominal muscle control. Both of these muscle groups provide pelvic girdle control, which is required for pelvic stability sufficient for ambulation. Because attempted ambulation in the presence of such muscle weakness is so tiring (the body's weight being born on the patient's upper extremities and hand, specifically), the patient turns to the full-time use of a wheelchair. Lower-extremity orthoses are indicated for extremity control, prevention of joint contractures, and protection of and control of flail extremities.

D10–L1. Injuries to the spine between D10 and L1 produce neurologic injuries that have components of both an upper motor (spinal cord) injury and a lower motor (cauda equina) neuron injury. The anatomy of the spinal cord in this area is important. Because the L1 nerve exits from the spinal cord at or opposite the bony level of D10, the L1 nerve root often escapes injury, although injury to the spinal cord occurs. This is called *root escape*. Thus, it is not uncommon that a patient with an injury in this area may retain sufficient motor control to ambulate with a "swing-to" or "swing-through" gait assisted by crutches

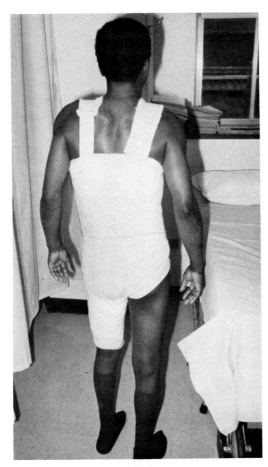

FIG. 24-33. This unilateral hip spica with body cast is recommended for injuries to the lumbar and lumbosacral area in which reduction of pelvic motion is indicated to block lumbosacral flexion. This type of immobilization is recommended for injuries to the lumbar and lumbosacral spine whenever pelvic motion is likely to result in failure of healing, or when internal fixation crossing the lumbosacral joint may be disrupted at the L5–S1 level owing to spine–pelvis motion (see Figs. 24-23, *D* and *E;* 24-29, *B;* and 24-30).

and bilateral above-knee orthoses (see Fig. 24-34, *right*) to provide knee and ankle stability in the presence of flaccid paralysis. The ankle unit on the orthosis should be placed in approximately 5° to 10° of dorsiflexion to allow for a smooth swing-to gait.

Below D12. Patients whose spinal and neurologic injuries fall below the level of D12 have a significantly better chance of

ambulation than the two above groups. The reason for this is that there is preservation of the three muscle groups required for ambulation: the paraspinal muscles, the upper and lower abdominals, and the iliopsoas, which is important in swing-to movement of the advancing extremity during ambulation. To provide knee stability and at the same time allow ambulation with only the use of a cane, a below-knee (ankle–foot) orthosis (Fig. 24-34, *left*) is suggested. Again, the foot and ankle should be placed in approximately 5° of plantar flexion. This will produce a mild knee recurvatum, which will aid knee stability and obviate the need for an above-knee orthosis.

There are many types of ankle–foot orthoses. The type prescribed depends greatly on the neurologic status of the distal extremity.[99]

SYSTEMIC INJURIES ASSOCIATED WITH TRAUMA TO THE DORSOLUMBAR SPINE

Incidence

A review of my statistics on the incidence of associated multiple trauma in more than 728 acute dorsolumbar spine–injured patients admitted between 1972 and October 1984 reveals the following. There is a 58.2% incidence of multiple trauma in patients sustaining a spine or spinal cord injury— injury to the head and face, 24.6%; injury to the chest (with hemothorax and pneumothorax injuries), 28.3%; extremity and pelvic girdle injuries, 26.5%; and injuries to the abdomen and other vital organs, 15.5% (Table 24-4).

It is of particular interest that in my series, almost on a one-on-one basis, where there was significant fracture and/or dislocation involving the dorsal spine, particularly when the injury was above D7, multiple rib fractures, pneumothorax, hemothorax, and fractures of the scapula, clavicle, or shoulder girdle occurred. The frequency with which such injuries are associated with dorsal spine fractures indicates that they must be looked for.

Silver reports 50 cases of chest injuries and other complications seen in the acute phase following spinal injury.[146] He notes a high incidence of chest injuries associated

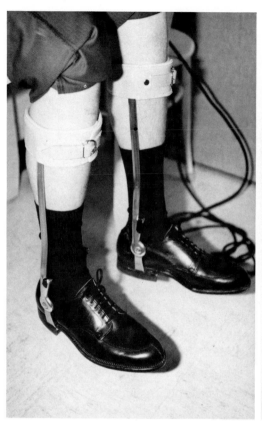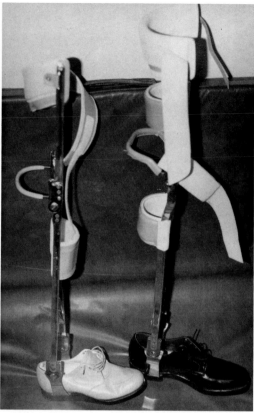

FIG. 24-34. Lower-extremity orthoses. (*Left*) There are a number of ankle–foot orthoses available to control loss of lower-extremity motor activity below the knee: double-upright, Klenzak ankle, Becker ankle, and blocked-ankle. The choice of the device depends on the residual motor function. (*Right*) Above-the-knee orthoses (knee–ankle orthoses) are necessary when both knee and ankle stability are required in the absence of thigh and calf muscle function. For patients using orthoses with a swing-to type of gait, placing the foot in 5° dorsiflexion assists in toe clearance and at mid-stance, enhances hip extension and stability (through the ligament of Bigelow).

Table 24-4. Incidence of Systemic Injuries Associated With Trauma to the Dorsolumbar Spine

LOCATION	NO. OF CASES*	PERCENTAGE
Head	179	24.6
Chest	206	28.3
Abdomen	113	15.5
Extremities	193	26.5
Incidence of multiple trauma	324	58.2

* From a total of 728

with dorsal spine injuries, of which 20% resulted in hemothorax and pneumothorax. Of 16 head injuries in his series, 12 were associated with cervical spine injuries, two with thoracic and two with lumbar spine injuries. (Fifty percent of the patients reported in this series were victims of automobile accidents; 38% had falls from heights. My own statistics on dorsolumbar spine injuries associated with head trauma are similar: 54.1% from motor-vehicle accidents, 28.6% from falls or falling objects, and 6.4% from gunshot wounds.)

Meinecke reported a large series of injuries that occurred in a highly industrial area in Germany, principally the steel and coal industry. Most of the accidents that produced spinal injuries also produced a high incidence of head and chest injuries.[109] Of 340 patients, 57% had injuries other than the spinal. When a significant portion of the victim's body was buried at the time of the accident, it was not unusual to find the chest and vertebral spine injured. Forty-five percent of the workers in Meinecke's series sustained injuries from falling objects, and 11% of these were buried by them. Eighteen percent suffered falls from heights, 11% sustained crushing injuries, and 26% were injured in automobile or other accidents.

Tricot and Hallot reported 462 patients with associated spinal injury and paraplegia. Of these, 14.5% had associated fractures.[160] Tricot expressed the opinion that because of the problems of management of long-bone fractures in spine-injured patients, particularly when there has been a loss of skin sensation, the fractures should be managed surgically. Although this opinion is not universally accepted, I agree, particularly when both the spine fracture and the extremity fracture are acute.

Chest Trauma

Chest trauma is the most common (28.3% vs. 24.6% for head trauma) trauma seen in the dorsolumbar spine–injured patient. Therefore, it is incumbent on the initial examiner to be aware of the extremely high frequency of injuries that should be anticipated. Interestingly, many of these injuries are *silent.* Injury to the dorsal spine above D7 very often reveals, on close inspection, multiple rib fractures over rather wide areas, and more often bilaterally than is appreciated (observe for paradoxical chest motion associated with unstable segmental rib fractures). Also frequently present are fractures of the 1st rib and clavicle, almost always associated with hemothorax or pneumothorax. Decreased respiratory sounds and an imbalance in chest excursion may signal such a complication. Not infrequently, a second fracture of the spine in some other location (cervical, dorsal, or lumbar[20]) will also be present.

Chest motion may be severely compromised owing to intercostal nerve paralysis, particularly if the spinal cord injury involves the lower cervical or upper dorsal spine. Such an injury results in a loss of intercostal function, leaving effective respiration only by means of the diaphragm and the accessory respiratory muscles that originate in the neck and have their insertion over the uppermost ribs. During the initial hospital evaluation of the patient, roentgenographic evaluation of the chest should accompany the examination of the spine. The finding of increased density in a lung field may be indicative of either atelectasis due to retained secretions, a foreign body, or overlying hemothorax. The absence of vascular markings along the upper lateral lung field (particularly over the apex of the upper lobe) is indicative of a pneumothorax and requires an immediate consultation with a chest surgeon and the insertion of a chest tube connected to a water-trap (Pleurovac) system at 20 mm H_2O suction.

The examining physician should also observe the position of the tracheal shadow on a well-positioned anteroposterior chest film. Deviation of the mediastinal and tracheal structures may indicate the presence of some of the complications mentioned above. Tricot and Hallot report a high incidence of rib fractures in association with spinal fractures involving the upper dorsal spine, particularly in the patient revealing neurologic injury.[160]

Gunshot injuries to the chest, with associated or anticipated complications, take precedence over associated injuries to the dorsal spinal. Again, it is recommended that thoracic surgery consultation be obtained and that a chest tube be inserted when there is evidence of pneumothorax or hemothorax.

Following injury to the dorsolumbar spine, it is customary to find a significant decrease in pulmonary function.[18] For this reason, early consultation with the respiratory therapy service is suggested.

Cheshire and Coats, in a review of 237 injuries to the vertebral column, describe only five deaths among 109 patients with dorsal and lumbar spine injuries (4.6%) (Table 24-5).[24]

Of the deaths reported, only one was the result of an acute respiratory problem. The others were secondary to head injury, ce-

Table 24-5. Death Rates From Fracture-Dislocation of the Dorsolumbar Spine

Total no. of dorsolumbar fractures	109	(100.0%)
No. of deaths	5	(4.6%)
Acute	2	(1.8%)
Subacute	3	(2.8%)
Death rate—total system	26	(7.0%)

* Total deaths, all levels, all patients, 4 years (1972–1976) (Data from Midwest Regional Spinal Cord Injury Care System)

rebral abscess, congestive heart failure, myocardial infarction, pulmonary embolism, hepatic failure, and aortic thrombosis. The death rate was quite similar (4.9%) in my series, in which and the primary etiologic factors causing death were pneumonia, pulmonary embolism, and respiratory failure.

Venerando and associates have noted that there is a marked deficiency in the respiratory dynamics of the ribs and diaphragm in the paraplegic whose spinal cord injury lies above D10.[162] Paraplegics with lesions below this level, however, demonstrate a larger than normal chest excursion in both axillary and xiphoid circumferences. Spirographic investigations reveal that paraplegics with high lesions maintain a satisfactory respiratory efficiency in spite of the deficit imposed by the loss of the abdominal muscles and rib activity. Guttmann and Silver demonstrated by means of serial electromyographic studies of quadriplegics that the intercostal and abdominal muscles seem to participate in an act of respiration on a reflex basis.[69] This has relevance for those with injuries close to the upper dorsal spine, which closely mimic injuries to the cervical spine.

Silver also found that in quadriplegic patients with paralysis of respiratory muscles who had complete lesions, there was a higher mortality rate from pulmonary embolism.[146,147] Although the incidence of pulmonary embolism in complete and incomplete injuries is similar, Walsh[164] and Tribe and Watson[167] found the incidence of venous thrombosis in the legs no higher among those with cervical injuries than among other groups of paraplegic patients.

In my series, 18 patients (2.5%) had deep venous thrombosis, and the number of patients undergoing pulmonary embolism was 59 (8.1%). Both series revealed that the highest incidence of deep venous thrombosis was in the patients with injury to the dorsal spine. When pulmonary embolism occurs in the patient with a cervical injury, it is almost always fatal. Bertrand notes that in the presence of "severe shock or serious injury" associated with spinal cord injury, particularly with injury to the chest or abdomen, early elective spinal surgery should not be considered, owing to alterations in pulmonary and metabolic functions.[118] Silver notes that 67% of his patients with dorsal spine injuries had pulmonary complications.[146]

Jacobson and Bors reviewed 114 spinal injuries in Vietnamese combat soldiers, 57 (50%) by gunshot wound.[86] Of the 43 patients who sustained gunshot wounds of the chest (all resulting in hemopneumothorax), 35 (81%) had injuries between D1 and D12. Of 18 gastrointestinal tract wounds, 13 resulted in associated lesions involving the lumbar and sacral regions.

Abdominal Injuries

The assessment of the abdomen in the patient with an injury of the dorsal or lumbar spine can be difficult. If there is paralysis of both the intercostal and abdominal muscles and an associated loss of sensation, the physical findings commonly associated with catastrophic blunt trauma to the abdomen will be absent. There will be an absence of muscle rigidity, an absence of the "rebound" tenderness test (even in the conscious victim) and an absence of bowel sounds (frequently a condition seen following acute spinal and spinal cord injury)—all of which make examination of the abdomen difficult and confusing. The etiology of posttraumatic bowel atony is poorly understood; the difficulty of distinguishing between autonomic and pathologic disturbances in intestinal mobility secondary to the interruption of sympathetics or parasympathetics during the early period of so-called spinal shock was described by O'Hare.[123] In the presence of hypotension and bradycardia (both vital signs also commonly associated with traumatic sympathectomy and injury to the upper thoracic spinal cord), it is difficult to be sure that there isn't an intra-abdominal disorder rather than just an autonomic reflex producing the findings.

Shoulder pain without other evidence of injury can be indicative of diaphragmatic irritation. Peritoneal lavage in the emergency room after standard prepping of the abdomen and via a "mini-lap" incision, using 1000 ml 0.1% normal saline, is a safe and effective method of determining the presence or absence of intra-abdominal bleeding. The return of nonclotting sanguineous fluid is evidence of significant intra-abdominal injury and requires early exploration. If blood does not return immediately, the lavage solution should be allowed to run in completely, followed by withdrawal of the fulid by reverse gravity flow (*i.e.*, placing the same IV bottle and the still-attached tubing onto the floor). This allows the fluid from the abdomen to flow via the tube into the bottle on the floor by means of both gravity and the increased intra-abdominal pressure produced by the fluid. If the fluid that returns is so tinted that newsprint cannot be read through it, sufficient blood is present within the abdomen to warrant an exploration. Of course there are always traps that one can and will fall into. In the presence of an acute and extensive burst fracture of a vertebra involving the lumbar spine, an extensive retroperitoneal hemorrhage will often occur and seep into the intra-abdominal space. Although retroperitoneal hemorrhages may be anticipated, they are not an indication for surgery. As a matter of fact, the finding is a contraindication for surgery. Nonetheless, the finding of significant blood in the abdominal cavity indicates the need for surgical exploration.

Another similar technique used in the emergency room or on the unit, should the patient's findings begin to change and concern over the occurrence of intra-abdominal bleeding be present, is the use of the so-called four-quadrant tap, in which the needle is inserted into each of the four abdominal quadrants in a search for evidence of free blood within the peritoneal cavity.

It is not unusual to find some evidence, in a patient admitted with an acute spinal injury, of either gastric bleeding or some small quantity of blood within the upper gastrointestinal tract. Because it is routine to request that a nasogastric tube be inserted before the patient is transferred to the spinal injury center to prevent gastric dilation (which results from apprehension, swallowing air, or from secondary reflex ileus, this tube is normally left in place on low suction until reflex bowel activity begins. Generally around the third to fifth day the fluid will test positive for blood. Because this phenomenon has frequently been observed over the years, numerous investigations with a fiberoptic gastroscope have been undertaken. These have revealed irritation at the tip of the nasogastric tube, where it has come into contact with the side wall of the stomach. In this area there will be some small amount of bleeding. Rarely is bleeding so severe as to require blood replacement. The question of whether corticosteroids produce an increased incidence of gastric bleeding always arises. My opinion is that they do not. Corticosteroids are used in 100% of the patients admitted to the Acute Spinal Cord Injury Center with neurologic injury. The incidence of gastric bleeding in patients with dorsolumbar spine injuries is 2.1% (15 patients). Whether this is due to excessive vagus outflow, producing increased gastric acidity, in the presence of traumatic sympathectomy, is still an unanswered question. Whatever the cause, it is my belief that the incidence has been either reduced or maintained low by three means: early removal of the nasogastric tube, routine prophylactic administration of 30 ml of aluminum hydroxide (Amphojel) per 1 to 2 hours via the nasogastric tube, and routine administration of cimetidine 300 mg four times a day. If there is no obvious or known cause for the absence of peristalsis and the condition persists, bowel activity can often be reactivated by the application of a TENS (transcutaneous electrical nerve stimulation) unit. This unit, which functions by means of electrodes applied to the abdominal wall, has been noted to produce early gastric motility and has allowed discontinuation of the nasogastric tube because of the presence of persistent gastric or small-bowel dilatation.

In deciding whether to explore the abdomen of a patient with a spine or spinal cord injury, the general surgeon must take into consideration the hazards and potential injury that can occur to the nervous system should the patient have an unstable spine injury and require transfer to an operating table. It is for this reason, along with numerous others, that it is recommended that a spinal cord– or spine-injured patient be placed on a wedge Stryker frame when first seen in the emergency room.

Bricher and associates reported on 18 patients with spinal cord injuries and associated abdominal or chest injuries, 13 of which were secondary to gunshot wounds.[18] One of four deaths occurred in the operating room secondary to hemorrhage. Should abdominal surgery be required, a neurosurgeon or orthopaedic surgeon should be available to take advantage of the exposure and the availability of the general surgeon to evaluate the anterior spine, should it be necessary. Rarely is it. Of course, in the face of an incomplete neurologic injury and a projectile having produced anterior compression on the canal, particularly with a deteriorating neurologic status, an anterior approach to the dura and spinal cord would be indicated. (This applies, likewise, to thoracotomies for exposures of the base of the neck, the chest, and the upper lumbar spine, where the chest surgeon may be performing the exploratory surgery.)

Cardiovascular Response to Spinal Cord Trauma

As noted previously, the patient with acute spinal cord injury resulting from trauma to the upper dorsal spine will almost always demonstrate the expected peripheral cardiovascular changes seen with injuries to the cervical spine. Cardiovascular shock reveals itself with hypotension, tachycardia, and diaphoresis; head injury will result in hypotension (or normotension), a normal pulse rate, and no diaphoresis. The cardiovascular responses to be anticipated with acute spinal cord injury include the following:

Bradycardia secondary to traumatic loss of sympathetic autonomic influences to the myocardium and overriding parasympathetic (vagal) nerve influences (spinal injury between C6 and D6)
Hypotension produced by loss of sympathetic influences, resulting in peripheral vasodilatation. This results in a lower cardiac output and a concomitant drop in blood pressure.
Hypothermia secondary to peripheral vasodilatation as a result of the blood's being closer to the surface of the skin.

These findings have been confirmed by Troll and Dohrman in acute quadriplegia and in patients with injuries to the dorsal spine between D1 and D6. Bradycardia and hypotension, along with an increase in venous compliance, occurred.[161] With hypotension as the symptom, treatment is often the administration of excessive fluids. Caution is advised. What has been noted with excessive fluid administration is a lag in the central venous pressure behind the pulmonary artery wedge pressure, resulting in congestive heart failure or pulmonary edema.

Pulmonary Embolism. One of the more common—and potentially the most dangerous—complications that occurs in a patient having had either multiple injuries or spine injuries, both producing and requiring prolonged recumbency, is pulmonary embolization. All emboli are worrisome, but those originating in the common femoral and the iliac vessels of the pelvis are potentially the most lethal. With embolization, the emboli may progress through the vena cava to the lung to obstruct the main pulmonary artery ("saddle emboli") or one of its major branches. This produces a rapid cardiopulmonary decompensation and death secondary to obstruction of blood flow through the lungs.[146] Lesser emboli may produce partial pulmonary vascular occlusion, resulting in small areas of parenchymal infarction, but these are not accompanied by collapse of the cardiovascular system.

The mystery to this pathologic process is that the patient may be totally symptom free yet will indicate a sensation of "impending doom." There are a number of characteristic findings on the physical examination: swelling of one affected extremity, a history of and the finding of pink-tinged sputum (hemoptysis), pain on the affected side of the chest with inspiration, elevation in temperature with no apparent cause, and a friction rub on auscultation of the chest. A chest x-ray may initially be negative or may reveal reduced vascular markings as the first changes. The most accurate method of making the diagnosis is by means of the technetium (VQ) scanning procedure.[93] Areas of increased density on the scan indicate pulmonary embolization. It must again be emphasized that patients with high spinal cord injuries, particularly in the upper dorsal area, may not experience respiratory discomfort. Again, depending on the severity of the symptoms and the extent of the treatment required, the clinical symptoms usually dissipate within 3 to 4 days, although pulmonary consolidation may persist and roentgenographic changes may continue for several weeks.

Fatal pulmonary emboli are most commonly associated with older patients. In my series the incidence of pulmonary embolism was 2.5% (18 patients). An increased incidence of pulmonary emboli in older patients is postulated to be the result of reduced endogenous heparin as the number of mast cells are reduced by aging. It may also be attributed to the presence of incipient circulatory failure, again the result of aging. Such problems as venous stasis, recumbency, surgery, and blood loss all contribute to Selye's theory of a decreased clotting time associated with increased platelet concentration during episodes of increased stress. Some believe the pulmonary embolism to be secondary to dehydration (possibly induced by surgery), a lack of nutrition, or the presence of a postoperative alteration in plasma with an increased number of platelets.[164,166,167,168] This latter occurrence is believed to increase the propensity for intravascular clotting and is particularly associated with long-bone fractures, which themselves frequently provide ample "excuse" for the occurrence of pulmonary embolization. Wesseler and colleagues note a temporary thrombotic state in relation to idiopathic intravascular coagulation and describes contributing causes in older patients as the presence of preexisting atrial fibrillation, malignant disease, and cardiac decompensation.[170] Each may contribute to the intravascular clotting phenomenon.

Patients with vertebral and spinal cord injury cannot be accurately evaluated for the presence of a positive Homan's sign because of the absence of pain sensibility in the lower extremities. It is therefore important to inspect the thighs and calves frequently, observing for swelling, increased heat, or redness. Unfortunately, pulmonary embolism results from thrombosis within the deep venous system; therefore, it will only occasionally reveal outward, visible physical findings. On the other hand, superficial venous thrombosis is a complication more easily managed because it is detectable early and responds rapidly to therapy.

The question of prophylactic anticoagulation is frequently raised. Obviously, the very fact that the question continues to arise is indication enough of the differences in opinion. One thing on which all agree is that aggressive therapy is not required for patients with superficial venous thrombosis.[145] Measures effective for this process are use of compression stockings (thigh-length), elevation of the legs or the foot of the bed, and aspirin, phenylbutazone (Butazolidin), or dextran therapy. Heparin may be required when there is evidence of potential of obvious pulmonary embolization. If repeated embolization occurs during the course of the therapy (including heparin therapy), it may become necessary either to ligate the vena cava (which has lymphedema of the lower extremities as it major complication) or to insert an "umbrella." Of 56 spinal cord–injured patients in Shull and Rose's series (23 dorsal, six lumbar), 16 were thought to have "pneumonia"; only *one* was diagnosed as having pulmonary embolism and treated with anticoagulants.[145] Of the 56 spinal cord injuries, 31 were incomplete, and most patients were mobilized within 7 to 10 days.

Of 188 deaths in which the diagnosis of pulmonary embolism was made at autopsy, 35.6% were secondary to malignancy, 27% secondary to acquired heart disease, and 3.2% secondary to fracture.[145] The site of origin of pulmonary emboli was unknown in the highest percentage of cases (43.6%); 18% were found arising in the femoral vessels, 13% from the heart, and 12.7% from the periprostatic plexus and iliac veins.

Walsh and Tribe reported on 500 paraplegics, among whom they found 66 cases of phlebothrombosis and pulmonary embolism (13.2%), with a fatal outcome in 15 (3%).[164] At autopsy, 15 of 31 traumatic paraplegics who died of causes related to the paraplegia demonstrated massive pulmonary embolism as the primary cause of death. Fatal embolism in this series was found to occur between the fourth and eighty-fifth days after trauma. I frequently question whether there isn't a relationship between the onset of deep venous thrombosis (with or without pulmonary embolism) and the presence of urinary sepsis (due to emboli arising from pelvic veins in patients with urinary sepsis). Shull and Rose[145] and Walsh and Tribe[164] note a high incidence of pulmonary embolism (16.5%) in complete spinal injuries, compared to that in incomplete spinal injuries (9%), as well as a very high incidence of embolism in dorsal lesions (19.1%). This information brings to the forefront the question of whether there is value in daily passive exercising of the lower limbs during the first 6 weeks following injury. The patients in these series had exercised, but the exercise failed to prevent the complication. The authors raise the question as to the use of prophylactic anticoagulants. Without much question, more clinicians than before are beginning to recommend low-dose heparin (5000 units subcutaneously three times a day). Tribe reports finding stress ulcers involving the gastrointestinal tract at autopsy, raising concern over the use of prophylactic heparin.[159]

Rossier reported in 1965 on 32 cases of acute spinal injury. Seven patients died, five as the result of pulmonary embolism (16%). Again, my recent statistics reveal that embolism occurred in 17 (2.5%) dorsolumbar spine injuries.

In a 10-year study of 431 patients with acute spinal cord injury, Watson found a 5% incidence of pulmonary embolism in those with complete neurologic injuries involving the dorsal spine and a 7% incidence in those with complete lumbar spine injuries.[167] Of patients with incomplete neurologic injury, 11% of those with dorsal lesions had pulmonary embolism, as did 3% of those with lumbar injury. The left leg (68%) was found to be involved twice as often as the right (32%). Phillips reported a similar finding, left greater than right.[127]

Watson also reported that of the 99 patients having pulmonary embolism, 14% occurred in the first week and 18% in the second week.[167] Among patients who had pulmonary emboli, thrombophlebitis had been diagnosed in approximately half (45%). The average age of patients at the time of pulmonary embolism was 41 years;

at death, 45 years. *The age of maximum risk was 40 years.* Eighty-six percent were male, 14% female. The incidence of complications and deaths was no higher in the presence of an associated chest injury. Of 16 associated injuries, 13 were to the chest (81%), and one was fatal (0.6%). Of particular interest and importance was the finding that the incidence of fatal thrombophlebitis and pulmonary embolism was higher in the unoperated patients (18%) than in the operated (7%). This gives credence to the belief that pulmonary embolism develops in those patients managed without surgery, who require a longer period of enforced recumbency. This probably gave rise to venous thrombosis in Watson's series. Prophylactic anticoagulation was not recommended.

Long-Bone Fractures

Eichenholz reported on a series of 700 chronic paraplegics cared for at the Bronx Veterans Hospital between 1946 and 1962.[49] Fewer than 4% sustained long-bone fractures. Of 32 treated, 30 were managed conservatively with soft, padded (pillow) splints that were frequently removed while the patient was on the Stryker frame.

Although the first consideration in management is a patient's general condition, and although early fracture stabilization is a consideration, maintenance and preservation of the patient's normal physiological functions and prevention of decubiti are also important. Anatomic reduction of a fracture is not a primary consideration.

In the chronic paraplegic, time and experience have demonstrated an inability of denervated tissue to withstand the insult of pressure and repeated trauma. As testimony to this, wound and fracture healing in the chronic or long-standing paraplegic is often delayed. Because tissues and muscles are either flaccid or intermittently spastic, vascular tone in the muscles themselves, as well as in the muscle–tendon attachments to bone, is likewise disturbed. This results in excessive hemorrhage at the fracture or operative site, the occurrence of large hematomas, and a chance for secondary infection (often from a distant source of contamination such as the bladder, decubiti, etc.).

Eichenholtz noted that the use of skin

traction in the long-standing paraplegic was hazardous and should be not used.[49] The prolonged use of skeletal traction also posed problems of osteoporosis and decubiti and rapidly fell into disuse. Open reduction and internal fixation of fractures in the presence of atrophic, osteoporotic, avascular bone and functionless muscle frequently sets the stage for loss of internal (plate-and-screw) fixation, particularly in the presence of unprotected mechanical forces across an insensitive fracture site.

Freehafer and Mast reported a similar study in which they reviewed 46 fractures, of which 37 (80%) were managed by minimum immobilization with pillow splints, simple positioning, casts, or braces.[57] The latter mechanism was used least. Five (10%) of the fractures were treated open, two patients were treated in skeletal traction, and two were treated with skin traction on a Foster frame. Pillow splints were used for fractures below the middle third of the femoral shaft, plaster casts were used for the fractures of the tibia, and orthoses were used for fractures in the supracondylar area of the femur or proximal tibia. Of nine hip fractures in paraplegics, two were treated surgically. One required removal of the femoral prosthesis following sepsis.

Freehafer and Mast were of the opinion that the long-standing, nonambulatory paraplegic who sustains a hip fracture and radiographically demonstrates significant bone atrophy should not be a candidate for prosthetic replacement. I agree with this concept completely in the chronic or long-standing paraplegic. On the other hand, I believe that the acute dorsal or lumbar spine–injured patient, suffering paraplegia along with multiple trauma (to include long bones), does require early fracture surgery. This is a must if the patient is to be mobilized rapidly to prevent the many complications discussed in this chapter.

Freehafer states that one of the few indications for internal fixation of a fracture in a paraplegic with a long-standing high dorsal spine injury is the presence of severe spasticity. Shortening of an extremity does occur when a fracture is managed conservatively but has not been found to be a problem. Although abundant callus develops across fracture sites in chronic paraplegics, periarticular bone (not to be confused with heterotopic bone ossification) does not occur. When nonunion of a fracture occurs in the chronic paraplegic, particularly when it involves the middle to distal thirds of the femur, amputation may be a consideration, particularily when there is circulatory insufficiency in the presence of infection, severe pressure areas, or repeated fractures. It should be stressed that for patients who were ambulatory prior to fracture (whether their injury is complete or incomplete neurologically), surgery should be designed to provide anatomic reduction to allow return to full capacity. When the patient has not been ambulatory, treatment should be conservative. If the extent of return of neurologic function is unpredictable, management of long-bone fractures should be aimed at providing the patient with maximum function, should he be able to return to a near-normal neurologic status.

McMaster and Stauffer advocate routine operative management of acute fractures in the acute spine-injured patient.[105] This circumvents the use of plaster over insensitive skin. I am in complete agreement, as stated above.

Secondary Scoliosis

Interestingly enough, scoliosis secondary to trauma was not a problem that I initially thought required consideration, particularly in the adult following spinal cord injury. However, it is! My first experience with such secondary scoliosis came in a 46-year-old man with a bone injury at D11 and neurologic impairment at D12. Within a year following his initial trauma, the patient required management for a posttraumatic scoliosis due to the presence of an unbalanced fracture with a resulting lateral angulation (scoliosis) or to a combination problem of mechanical scoliosis secondary to fracture, to an associated unbalanced paralysis of the paraspinal muscles, or to both.

The appearance of scoliosis in adolescents following spinal cord injury is a known problem. The complication usually occurs in those young people who have sustained their spinal cord injury prior to age 16.[21,94,104] The actual incidence of this complication is low when one takes into account the entire population with spinal column and spinal cord injuries.

Familial Scoliosis. The radiographic shape of a scoliosis curve is usually helpful in identifying the curve's origin, though not always. Certainly it is possible that the scoliosis may have been present at the time of the spine trauma, but again, most likely not. When the anteroposterior x-ray reveals an S-shaped curve composed of a primary and a secondary component, the origin is not trauma; rather, it is a form of juvenile (idiopathic or "familial") scoliosis.

Traumatic Scoliosis. A review of the literature reveals that Roaf, in 1970, reported on 12 traumatic paraplegics with secondary scoliosis in which the apex was within the dorsolumbar region.[134] All 12 cases occurred before the age of 15 (average age at onset—8; average age at evaluation—16). Roaf noted that adults who develop scoliosis and trunk deformity secondary to neurologic lesions rarely develop marked changes in bone shape or severe scoliosis. As noted above, this has not been my experience.

Paraplegic scoliosis is primarily the result of the unequal action of the postural muscles of the trunk, principally the rotator muscles of the erector spinae group. If the deformity remains untreated, alteration in the shape of the vertebral bodies and articular processes occurs as a result of impeded growth of the articular processes, the development of hypoplasia of the laminae on the concave side, and excessive growth of the vertebral body on the convex side. The presence of a unilateral or asymmetric fracture of the vertebral body also contributes to the appearance of the scoliosis. Either way, there is an asymmetric inclination of the articular processes above and below the apical vertebra.

A major contributor to the development of posttraumatic paraplegic scoliosis is asymmetric rib action. The area most often affected is the upper mid-dorsal spine, which deforms on its own secondary to asymmetric muscle paralysis. Alteration in sitting and standing balance also contributes to the development of scoliosis and severe lordosis in the spastic and flaccid paraplegic. It may progress in young patients to produce cardiopulmonary compromise, which may result in decreased pulmonary compliance and an inability to sit or function in a wheelchair without an orthotic device. Many of these patients will require a spine fusion to prevent significant deformity and to enable them to maintain a good cardiopulmonary status. Unbalanced sitting, secondary to scoliosis, also contributes to the development of unilateral decubitis ulcers over the ischium and/or greater trochanter. Severe dorsal or dorsolumbar scoliosis may affect the paraplegic's ability to ambulate. If the deformity causes the pelvis to shift, the patient may lose balance during the swing-to or stance phases of gait. A deformity that affects the paraplegic's balance may also affect his ability to drive a car.

Pain Below the Level of Spinal Cord Injury

Pollock and co-workers reported on a study of pain below the level of spinal cord injury in 246 patients with injuries to the spinal cord itself, the conus medullaris, and the cauda equina.[130] Their findings revealed that the spontaneous pain of which these patients complain is of three types: mentioned pain, visceral referred pain, or paresthesia.

"Mentioned" pain is pain in an area or segment adjacent to the lesion. It is probably best described as root pain. Certainly, in the postoperative patient, one might anticipate the complaint of pain in the area of surgery. A similar distribution of pain is also seen in other problems affecting the spine: tabes dorsalis, tumors, disc syndromes, and the like.

Visceral referred pain occurs in dysfunctions seen to occur secondary to disease or trauma of the viscera. It is not unlike the garden-variety pain often observed in normal people. It occurs in both the neurologically intact and the neurologically injured patient. One theory on the presence of such pain has been presented. With bowel distention or compromise, pain is evoked owing to recruitment and participation of the autonomic nervous system. This pain perception can and does occur even in the patient with a known complete neurologic injury.

Paresthesia is a difficult-to-describe pain found to occur distal to the level of the lesion and is imperfectly localized. The patient may describe the perceived sensations as burning, tingling, stinging, or "pins-and-needles." This sort of pain is difficult to differentiate from that of a cauda equina lesion with root symptoms, particularily if the injury is in the same area. Patients complaining of severe distal burning pain were closely observed, and when spinal anesthesia was induced below the level of the lesion, suppression of all spasm and reflex activity was noted. With this came the disappearance of the patient's symptoms. Interrupting sensory impulses entering the spinal cord below the level of the lesion, through any pathway, did not abolish pain. Therefore, there seems to be some indication that distal burning pain originates in the distal end of the segment, proximal to the injury of the spinal cord. This phenomenon is similar to that of pain referred from a neuroma at the end of the proximal segment of an injured peripheral nerve.

"Burning pain" was noted by Pollock[130] to be the most common spontaneous pain complaint in 82% of the pain cases he reviewed. It was noted that, as time passed, the pain diminished, the patient's pain threshold increased, or the pain receded from the patient's conscious awareness. It was not uncommon to find increased pain with intercurrent disease, surgical procedures, or an environment change, and these recurrent complaints were not interpreted as evidence of sensory pathway integrity.

Four of 50 special study patients reported by Pollock perceived pain when they had a disease (kidney stones, orchitis, cystitis) or underwent an invasive procedure (cystoscopy). Each patient had a spinal lesion between the D10 and L1 neural segments. In each of these patients it appeared that the sensory fibers responsible for the reported pain entered the spinal cord above the level of the lesion. It was concluded from this special study that for both skeletal and visceral systems, stimuli for pain—even severe pain from blood vessels, bone, subcutaneous tissues, and viscera—send impulses over the ordinary sensory pathways in the spinal cord. There is no substantial evidence that the sympathetic nervous system played a significant role in pain perception. The following conclusions may be drawn. Distal burning pain associated with severe injuries to the spinal cord seems to originate in the caudad end of the segment, cephalad to the lesion. In cases of severe injury with functional or anatomical transection of the spinal cord,

no pain is felt when a structure below the level of the injury is diseased or injured.

Autonomic Dysreflexia

Autonomic dysreflexia is a pathologic process found to occur only in patients with spinal cord lesions between D1 and D6. The principal defect is the traumatic interruption of the sympathetic and autonomic nervous system accompanied by an abnormal, pathologic rise in blood pressure (to levels as high as 300/180) in the absence of any compensatory reflexes. As noted, the injury must lie in an area between D1 and D6, in which the sympathetic ganglia lie, for this pathologic reflex to occur. Such elevations in blood pressure can cause intracranial hemorrhage, should a vascular defect be present.

Involuntary (spastic) muscle hyperactivity below the level of injury, as may result from overdistention of the bladder or bowel, is the known factor that causes an established chain of events to occur, resulting in the clinical entity known as autonomic dysreflexia or hyperreflexia. This situation arises below the level of the spinal cord lesion, where afferent sympathetic activity from bowel or bladder distention stimulates the sympathetic efferent system—below the level of the spinal cord lesion. This pathologic sympathetic response is recognized as producing a significant constriction of the splanchnic vascular bed, terminating in a state of hypertension. Normally, in the presence of hypertension, regardless of the cause, central reflexes are activated via the carotid artery pressure sensors within the thalamus, stimulating these two areas to produce inhibitory impulses. The result is a suppression of the heart rate (via the vagus) and dilatation of the splanchnic vascular bed (via the parasympathetics). When injury exists above the level of D6, the central efferent pathway from the cerebral cortex to the spinal cord autonomic system is interrupted. Thus, the splanchnic vessels maintain their state of vasoconstriction unabated during this period of stimulation, and at the same time, by way of the carotid artery pressure sensors, stimulation of the vagus via the parasympathetics produces a slowing of the heart (owing to an absence of any sympathetic input to the heart). *This results in a state of hypertension with asso-*

ciated bradycardia. Other physical findings noted on examination are severe, excruciating headaches and excessive diaphoresis, resulting from vasodilation above the level of the spinal cord lesion. The latter finding is an example of a compensatory reflex.

Autonomic dysreflexia is an emergency. It must be managed promptly. The most successful method of management is to find and eliminate the cause of bladder or bowel distention. This is usually a plugged urinary catheter or a bowel overly distended with feces. Relieving this condition by replacing the catheter or by digital extraction of the rectal contents will bring about immediate relief and sequential reduction in the afferent sympathetic stimulation, relieving the vascular constriction within the splanchnic vascular bed and eliminating the process that produces the hypertension or autonomic dysreflexia. Should these two procedures fail to relieve the situation, preparation should be made for the immediate administration of intravenous fluids and the possible use of a ganglionic blocking agent (trimethaphan camsylate [Arfonad] 1 g/liter) with constant monitoring of the blood pressure by fluid titration. This latter procedure must be under the control of a physician. Usually, identification of the noxious stimulant is sufficient to relieve the hypertensive state. Seldom is spinal anesthesia or the instillation of a local anesthetic into the bladder required for the relief of this extreme situation.

Ciliberti and co-workers describe similar hypertensive states resulting from the administration of anesthesia in patients with paraplegia.[25] They interpret this anatomic reflex mechanism as an alarm system of abnormal visceral activity in a paralyzed part of the body. In 54 patients with lesions above D5, 50 torr or more of elevation in blood pressure during anesthesia was noted in 43%.

Secondary Amyloidosis

A former major secondary complication and *chronic* sequela of fracture-dislocation of the dorsal or lumbar spine with associated spinal cord and cauda equina injury was amyloidosis. The primary cause of amyloidosis, particularily in the post–spinal-cord–injured patient is the presence of repeated sepsis in some area (*i.e.,* urinary tract infections, decubiti, etc.).

It is documented that the combination of long-standing paraplegia (12 years or more) and chronic urinary tract sepsis (pyelonephritis and urinary calculi), particularly if accompanied by a repeated history of suppurative pressure decubiti, will lead to amyloidosis and result in renal insufficiency and death. Dalton and colleagues report a series of 89 such patients, of whom 26 (29%) developed amyloidosis and died.[37] Dalton and co-workers also found that of the acutely injured patients who succumbed within a year of injury, as well as those who died within 5 years of trauma, the incidence of subtle amyloidosis was 40% (26 of 65). Renal failure secondary to amyloidosis, with proteinuria as a major finding, was noted in 67%.

The significance of the presence of suppurative decubiti was not greatly appreciated in the past. Dalton and associates call attention to the fact that 23 of 26 patients (88%) having pressure decubiti in one series were noted to have amyloidosis.[37] In another series of patients in whom decubiti were noted, 22 of 35 (63%) had amyloidosis.

It is important to appreciate that the pyelonephritis is not associated with amyloidosis and should be considered a separate entity.

For paraplegic spinal cord–injured patients who came to autopsy, it was noted that the average life span following trauma was approximately 11.3 years. For those coming to autopsy with a pathologic diagnosis of amyloidosis, the average life span after trauma was noted to be 7.9 years.

Heterotopic Ossification

Heterotopic ossification, also known as neurogenic ossifying fibromyopathy,[149] myositis ossificans circumscripta neurotia,[1] and ectopic ossification, is a pathologic process identifiable in the spine injured patient,[75] although the statistical incidence in the acutely injured is low (0.5% in our series). It is a process that is also seen in other neurologic disorders, such as multiple sclerosis, meningioma involving the spinal cord, arachnoiditis,[101] poliomyelitis,[33,74,76] epidural abscess,[149] tetanus,[129] burns,[16] and occasionally in hemiplegia.[135] To date, there is still a lack of hard evidence as to the true cause of this condition. The new (pathologic) bone seen in these patients is not bone within a joint capsule, rather within the surrounding soft tissue. It cannot be considered an arthropathy.

In spite of more than 100 papers by various authors and authoritative surveys by Ceiller, the cause remains obscure.[23] This same conclusion was drawn by Hardy and Dixon in 1963.[71] Abramson proposed that in the presence of spinal-injury osteoporosis, there is excessive mobilization of calcium, which may contribute to the production of heterotopic ossification.[1] Weinmann and Sicker are of the opinion that osteoporosis is principally due to the loss of fundamental muscle stimulus to bone.[169]

It is known that the most common site for the deposition of great masses of bone is the area anterior to the hip joints[1] involving the iliopsoas muscle and tendon and resulting in extracapsular bony ankylosis of the joint. Heterotopic bone may also be found in great masses within the abductor or quadriceps muscles of the thigh, just proximal to the patella or along the medial side of the medial femoral condyle near the intersection of the abductor magnus muscle. It is particularly interesting that heterotopic ossification is seldom noted in the areas of the ankles, wrists, fingers, toes, or hip joint extensor muscle masses.

As stated earlier, the cause of this disease process remains obscure; however, Hardy and Dixon note a trait for the development of this abnormal process in patients having an extensive history of decubitus ulceration over bony prominences such as the ischium and the greater trochanter.[71] More often than not, such findings are more often identified in the chronic or long-standing spinal cord–injured patient than in the acute victim.

Hardy and Dixon report a 16.5% incidence of heterotopic ossification in their series,[71] Liberson[99] 53.3%, Abramson[1] 41%, and Soule[149] 37%. In Hardy's series of 100 patients, each of whom was classified as a complete paraplegic (42 spastic, 58 flaccid), 16 revealed abnormal bone deposition. Each of the abnormal depositions was below the level of the injury and between the upper border of the pelvis and the knee joint. Of Hardy's patients, 52 were noted to have extensive decubitus ulceration overlying bony prominences; the remaining 48 patients revealed no sepsis.

Furman and associates, in 1970, reported the finding of elevated alkaline phosphatase levels in the absence of fracture healing or liver disease as the possible *sine qua non* of heterotopic bone deposition.[58] In their series of 15 patients, 13 of whom were spastic, 7 (47%) developed heterotopic ossification. (The joints involved were the hip—7, knee—3, shoulder—1, and elbow—1. No mention was made of the time after injury.) The normal alkaline phosphatase level in their laboratory was between 3 and 14 King-Armstrong Units. In their series the onset of a mean maximum serum alkaline phosphatase level occurred in conjunction with radiographic evidence of ectopic bone formation. They also noted that when the elevation in the alkaline phosphatase level was not accompanied by ectopic bone formation, the level did not remain elevated longer than 3 weeks. The authors stressed the important finding that when the alkaline phosphatase level returned to normal, no further heterotopic or ectopic ossification developed. Similarly, localized swelling decreased, and the mass of deposited bone remained. Their interpretation was that the alkaline phosphatase level remains elevated only during the period of active new bone formation and deposition.

The clinical findings commonly associated with heterotopic ossification in the extremities or joints are edema and swelling of the lower extremity, particularly in the area of new bone deposition, and associated edema that is difficult to differentiate from the edema often associated with superficial thrombophlebitis or deep venous thrombosis. When the problem of differential diagnosis exists, the three most helpful findings for diagnosing heterotopic ossification are roentgenograms positive for new bone deposition, positive bone scans, and elevations in the serum alkaline phosphatase levels in the presence of normal serum calcium.

Management. The management of this pathologic process is difficult to describe because of the obscure etiology. It has already been stated that there appears to be a relationship between the onset of heterotopic ossification and the presence of decubitus ulcerations around bony prominences. Therefore, the prevention of this complication may simply be the reduction of the incidence of decubitus ulcers. It has been suggested that the protection of bony prominences may be a way of preventing skin breakdown in patients with insensitive skin.[71] It is not uncommon in the paraplegic patient with a complete neurologic injury to note marked internal rotation of one of the extremities, to the extent that potential dislocation, or certainly subluxation, of the femoral head from the acetabulum might occur. This is usually the result of an internal rotation contracture, associated with spastic adductors and "scissoring." This often results in a flexion deformity at the hip, with an extremely prominent greater trochanter and ischial tuberosity, particularly when there is significant atrophy of the gluteus maximus and hamstring muscle mass.

It is recognized that heterotopic ossification is very resistant to treatment. Bone removed surgically frequently redevelops.[9] Surgery may be followed by infection. It is recognized that if motion of a major joint is restricted, particularly the hips or knees, surgical excision of such ectopic bone must be considered if the patient is to be able to sit. Other operative procedures occasionally performed but rarely recommended are joint arthroplasties and, in the rarest of occasions, amputations.[71] Selecting the correct time for the excision of heterotopic or ectopic bone is extremely important and difficult to do accurately. Removal of heterotopic bone too early in the disease process frequently results in more extensive ossification, particularly in the presence of postoperative hematoma. The two obvious serious complications that can result are infection and recurring ankylosis.

The best time for surgical excision is when the palpable mass has ceased to enlarge, the alkaline phosphatase level has returned to normal, and there is evidence of significant joint restriction requiring surgical excision. Surgery should be designed to allow 90° of flexion at the hip. Because postoperative wound infections are a real risk, it is highly recommended that following surgical excision of heterotopic bone, antibiotic coverage be used, particularly when bone is being excised near the perineum (especially in the presence of rectal and bladder incontinence), when urinary sepsis with bacteremia has been a problem, or when laxity of soft tissues with hematoma production is anticipated. Hardy had a series of 603 spine-injured patients, 100 of whom developed heterotopic ossification. Only eight required excision surgery.[71] That indication was ankylosis.

Furman and associates have recommended that cobalt radiation may be indicated for the prevention of heterotopic bone formation.[58] One patient received 500 R, the other 1000 R per day for 5 days. These two patients were treated successfully with this method of therapy, revealing a reduction in alkaline phosphatase activity and a cessation of heterotopic ossification.

The more recent means of managing heterotopic bone formation and deposition is the use of diphosphonates.[139] Historically, interest in the pyrophosphates and diphosphonates began when it was noted that when these substances appeared in the plasma and urine, they inhibited the precipitation of calcium phosphate. One of the inhibitors in the urine was found to be inorganic pyrophosphate. Further work led to the development of diphosphonates (synthetic compounds that are structurally related to pyrophosphates), which are stable to enzymatic hydrolysis. Russell and Fleisch, reporting on the pyrophosphate activity of alkaline phosphatase, note that when pyrophosphate was administered parenterally to animals, it prevented various types of soft tissue calcification; however, when pyrophosphates were injected or ingested, they were noted to be destroyed rapidly.[139] Thus these latter compounds are not promising for the treatment of certain disorders of calcium metabolism. An important finding, however, was the affinity of pyrophosphate to hydroxyapatite. Because of this affinity, pyrophosphate has been linked with gamma-emitting isotopes[102] (technetium pyrophosphate) used as a bone-scanning agent.

It has been noted that a closely related compound, diphosphonate (EHDP), does affect the behavior of calcium salts *in vitro* and also the precipitation of calcium phosphate from solution. It blocks the transformation of amorphous calcium phosphate to hydroxyapatite without inhibiting the formation of the initial phase of matrix production. The actions of EHDP, therefore, are interpreted as inhibiting heterogeneous nucleation and the subsequent growth and aggregation of crystal nuclei of hydroxyapatite. Diphosphonates have been shown to bind strongly on the surface of crystals of hydroxyapatite. Here they displace orthophosphonate, slowing down the formation of crystals. This step is significant in the reduction of both soft tissue and urinary calcium deposition.

Diphosphonates are effective both orally and parenterally. There is good correlation between the individual diphosphonates and the inhibition of growth *in vitro* and the blocking of soft tissue calcification *in vitro.* Thus it has been proposed that EHDP may prevent periarticular calcification and inhibit some articular changes.[151]

EHDP has been used in treating myositis ossificans progressiva (MOP). This rare congenital disease is characterized by skeletal deformity and the extensive formation of ectopic bone in muscle, leading to severe crippling and early death. A daily dosage of EHDP of 3 mg to 30 mg/kg body weight/day was noted to prevent the mineralization of ectopic bone. These findings revealed the benefits to be present in more than half of the cases so treated. As predicted, EHDP seemed better at preventing new sites of calcification than in reversing existing lesions. Areas of swelling and inflammation still occur in the presence of ectopic bone formation, but these usually do not calcify and may subside without leaving a permanent trace. In adult patients, preoperatively administered EHDP has allowed the surgical removal of ectopic bone without the recurrence of calcification at the operative site, although in others, particularly children, calcification has recurred. However, this may be related to nests of growth cells remaining in the area of exostosis or ectopic bone excision.

In a well-documented trial in patients having ectopic calcification, it was noted the EHDP inhibited ectopic calcification in the area of the hip following total hip replacement; however, there was evidence of recurrence when the treatment was stopped 3 months following surgery. This suggests that EHDP blocked not production of ectopic matrix, but only mineralization. Thus, from a clinical point of view, it is possible that if the matrix is prevented from mineralizing for a long enough period, reasonable function may be achieved. This work, as described by Russell and Fleisch, is taken from their extensive bibliography.[139] Their findings are still considered theoretical and not yet proven. Diphosphonates have now been in use in the U.S. for several years and have been found very successful in the prevention of heterotopic ossification in the spinal cord–injured patient.

Spinal Stenosis

Spinal stenosis is a problem that, not infrequently, arises in the lumbar spine, affecting the cauda equina by compression (spondylosis). It may also occur following trauma or may follow surgery. The most common atraumatic etiologic factors, according to Alexander, are achondroplasia, kyphosis, short pedicles, thick laminae, and osteoarthritic spurs.[4]

Although the topic may not be related directly to fracture or dislocation of the dorsolumbar spine, it does involve the area of the spine adjacent to the lower dorsal spinal cord, conus medullaris, and cauda equina, and thus it warrants mention. I have reported one patient with spinal stenosis that resulted in a serious complication following dorsolumbar laminectomy. A 49-year-old achondroplastic woman, short, obese, and stocky, with impending paraplegia at a neurologic level of D11, was referred to the Acute Spinal Cord Injury Center at Northwestern University. The pathologic findings as observed on roentgenograms were short pedicles, thick laminae, and osteoarthritic spurs at all levels. The widest sagittal neurocanal space was at L5. (Normally in the achondroplastic, L5 is the narrowest.) Because of the pathology (D10–S1), it is often necessary in performing a myelogram to perform a cisterna magna puncture to delineate the neural canal. When progressive lumbar stenosis exists, the method of management is a central laminectomy. According to Alexander,[4] Harrington rods, combined with a lateral-mass spine fusion, are often required for stability. It should be recognized that bony spurs and disc material may lie anteriorly in a narrow spinal canal. If approached from a strictly posterior angle, neurologic injury may result, with permanent paralysis. It is therefore inadvisable to attempt significant decompression from a strictly posterior approach. In the case herein reviewed, following wide laminectomy (D10–L4) without dural manipulation or internal fixation, the patient awakened as a D11 complete paraplegic. In spite of blood pressure maintenance and the administration of corticosteroids and mannitol during surgery, but without the benefit of somatosensory-evoked potentials (not yet available as a surgical-assist tool at the time that this surgery was performed), no functional recovery occurred. The cause was most likely inadvertent surgical trauma to an aberrant vascular contribution to the anterior spinal artery via the vessel of Adamkiewicz.

MANAGEMENT CONSIDERATIONS

Caloric Costs in the Paraplegic

Clarke,[26] in a review of normal and paraplegic college students, evaluated the caloric costs of activities in the paraplegic. His findings revealed that for the average active yound adult, the recommended U.S. daily caloric intake should be set at 2900 calories per day. Extensive studies during all activities of the paraplegic patient's waking day and activities at rest revealed that the active paraplegic man's daily intake was approximately 2280 calories per day, while his caloric output was approximately 2245 calories per day. The control group of normal students averaged a caloric intake of 2700 calories per day. The principal recommendation from this study is the finding of low calorie expenditure during normal and occasionally excessive wheelchair and class activities (2245 calories per day), indicating a need for conservative caloric intake in the paraplegic patient and a regular program of physical activity.

Antibiotic Considerations in Spinal Injury

As with any major orthopaedic surgical procedure, the complication most feared by the surgeon is wound infection. So it is in spinal surgery. Because of the poor blood supply and lack of perfusion of antibiotics into infected long bones, chronic osteomyelitis is a real concern. However, in surgery of the spine, where the vascular supply is usually abundant, the most sinister effect of surgery could be acute sepsis involving the meninges and potentially resulting in meningitis and death. Fortunately, the dura is extremely resilient and resistant to infection. Should infection reach the subarachnoid space, host defense mechanisms are reduced, compared to systemic defense mechanisms. This is because the levels of complement and antibody are far lower than in the systemic circulation. Phagocytosis of bacteria by granulocytes is thus diminished because of reduced or absent opsonization mediated by complement and specific antibodies. Early in the course of bacterial meningitis, there may even be a delayed migration of granulocytes into the spinal fluid.[131,140]

Because of the reduction in host defense within the subarachnoid space, antibiotic choice is critical, since the outcome of infection is largely a contest between the antibiotic and invading bacterium. To be successful, the antibiotic chosen must not only be able to cross the blood barrier, but it must reach concentrations in the spinal fluid that exceed by eightfold to tenfold the minimal concentration required to kill the invading bacterium. Thus, antibiotics that are bacteriostatic (*i.e.*, erythromycin and tetracycline) are unsuccessful in treating bacterial meningitis. Likewise, the failure of chloramphenicol to treat many cases of Klebsiella, Proteus, Enterobacter and Serratia meningitis lies not in its ability to penetrate the blood–brain barrier, which it does well, but in its failure to reach concentrations within the spinal fluid that exceed eight to ten times the minimal bactericidal concentration.

Staphylococcus aureus and *S. epidermidis* are still common causes of bacterial meningitis in the neurosurgical patient and meningitis following head and neck trauma. These infections are most successfully treated with oxacillin or nafcillin given in high dosage (12–18 g/day intravenously). Although the penicillins do not cross the intact blood–brain barrier to any appreciable extent, in the presence of inflammation, they will penetrate in sufficient amount to kill staphylococci at dilutions of spinal fluid eight to ten times above baseline.

Over the past several years, meningitis produced by enteric gram-negative bacilli and *Pseudomonas aeruginosa* has become more common. This reflects our ability to treat seriously ill patients who have been exposed to broad-spectrum antibiotics and are frequently cared for in intensive-care units, with multiple intravenous lines, endotracheal intubation, and exposure to a fairly resistant local bacterial flora. Fortunately, with the development of third-generation cephalosporins (*i.e.,* moxalactam and cefotaxime), many of these gram-negative bacillary infections can be treated successfully. This is because these newer cephalosporin antibiotics penetrate the blood–brain barrier in much higher concentration than do the first- or second-generation cephalosporins and because the third-generation cephalosporins kill the invading gram-negative bacilli at much lower concentrations than do the earlier-generation cephalosporins.

Some sensitive gram-negative infections of the meninges may also be successfully treated with the combination of sulfamethoxazole-trimethoprim (Bactrim, Septra). These agents should be used only after identification and sensitivity studies of the isolated bacteria have been completed and not as initial therapy of gram-negative bacillary meningitis.

Meningitis in adults produced by *Pseudomonas aeruginosa* and *Acinetobacter* species cannot be treated by intravenous antibiotics alone. Intravenous therapy (*i.e.,* piperacillin or mezlocillin along with gentamicin or tobramycin) must be supplemented with daily intrathecal or intraventricular (via an Ommaya reservoir) gentamicin or tobramycin. This is necessary because the aminoglycosides (gentamicin, tobramycin) do not cross the blood–brain barrier to any appreciable extent, even in the face of meningeal inflammation, and because the antipseudomonas penicillins (piperacillin, mezlocillin) do not reach sufficient concentration within the cerebrospinal fluid. In patients treated as outlined above, the concentrations of gentamicin or tobramycin within the cerebrospinal fluid should be monitored, as should the spinal fluid bactericidal titer.[132]

Management of the Neurogenic Bladder

With little question, the organ system most often involved by complications following spinal cord injury is the urinary system. Infection is the most common offender and is probably the result of bladder atony secondary to neurogenic injury, resulting in urine stagnation and, in the presence of an indwelling catheter, repeated contamination from the outside. In spite of the ease of identification of the most probable cause of infection, it must be appreciated that in the management of the acutely injured patient, monitoring of fluid output is required.

The diagnosis of a urinary infection is somewhat pragmatic. After considerable discussion by the infectious-disease and urologic community, an arbitrary boundary (100,000 per mm^3) above which the urinary bacteria count establishes the diagnosis of urinary tract infection, and serves as an indicator for management with antibiotics has been established. No attempt should be made to sterilize the urine prophylactically just because of the presence of a urinary catheter. Rather, good urinary catheter care should be enforced by the nursing staff. To establish this care requires specific in-service training, particularly when the staff is required to manage a paralytic patient with a paralytic bladder.

An important step in the direction of eliminating the "expected" urinary tract infection is the early institution of an intermittent catheterization program as soon as feasible following admission. Such a program promotes urinary asepsis and the development of an automatic neurogenic or "reflexogenic" bladder.

Indwelling Catheter Management. Careful technique with the urinary catheter will ensure relatively problem-free use for short periods (see Technical Precautions for Long-Term Urinary Catheterization).

Technical Precautions for Long-Term Urinary Catheterization

Sterile technique is used for insertion of the catheter. Gloves are worn, the area around the entrance of the catheter into the urethra is cleansed adequately, and secretions and excretions around the urethra–catheter interface are cleansed periodically.

In male patients the catheter is taped to the lower abdomen to prevent the development of a penile–scrotal fistula or penile ulceration from uncontrolled pulling of the catheter on the penis and bladder. In female patients the catheter is taped to the inner thigh, for similar reasons.

The patient's fluid intake is increased (3000 ml/day). To prevent formation of bladder calculi, the patient takes acidifying juices (cranberry juice, 600 ml/day) and avoids citrus fruits and juices, which are alkaline. The patient also takes oral ascorbic acid (500 mg–1 g/day) to maintain an acidic urine.

The intake of carbonated fluids, which are bladder irritants, is reduced.

The patient's intake of high-calcium foods (*e.g.,* milk products, certain vegetables) is controlled to prevent pebblelike renal calculi.

The catheter is irrigated daily with normal saline solution or 30 ml of a 0.25% acetic acid solution with each catheterization.

The urinary catheter is changed every 7 to 10 days, with sterile technique.

Intermittent Catheterization Technique. In male patients with neurogenic bladder dysfunction, the following routine is suggested for conversion to an external "Texas" catheter from an indwelling catheter. With sterile catheterization technique, the bladder is initially emptied by pressure on the abdomen. The patient is then catheterized every 4 hours until the urinary bladder residual reaches 200 ml or less. Following this stage, the patient catheterizes *himself* every 6 hours until the residual is 150 ml or less; then every 8 hours until the residual is 100 ml or less. At the point at which the patient's urinary residual remains at or below 100 ml, the patient catheterizes himself once every 8 hours. When the residual is down to less than 60 ml, he may remain on the Credé program, catheterizing himself only once a week.

External "Texas" Catheter Management. Once a male patient begins the intermittent ("decath") catheterization program, an external catheter is worn during the intervals between catheterization. It is attached at one end to a collection bag and at the other end to a condom, which is applied to the penis. It is held in place by surgical tape or an appropriate fastener. Automatic (reflex) or passive urination (accomplished by the Credé maneuver) is allowed. As with an internal catheter, certain precautions are necessary (see Technical Precautions for Intermittent Urinary Catheterization).

Note that nowhere in this discussion of catheter management is the use of prophylactic antibiotic therapy suggested. Antibiotics are used only for the management of specific acute urologic infections of known bacterial strain and sensitivity. On the other hand, administration of acidifying medications such as methenamine mandelate (Mandelamine—4 g/day) or drinking cranberry juice in rather large quantities to maintain the acidity of the urine and reduce the hazards of urinary sepsis and urinary (bladder or renal pelvis) stone formation is recommended.

Technical Precautions for Intermittent Urinary Catheterization

Particularly in the patient with absent sensation, care must be taken not to apply the catheter-condom too tightly, which could cause skin necrosis on the penis.

The attachment of the catheter to the condom must not be applied directly against the glans penis for fear of skin breakdown.

The catheter system should be changed daily.

Should there be any sudden change in the character of the urine or an increase in the residual, the patient should immediately seek the attention of his physician.

Sexual Function

Males. One of the more devastating complications resulting from neurologic trauma to the dorsolumbar area of the spinal cord is the loss of male sexual function. This is particularly true in lower motor neuron paraplegics with flaccid paralysis. Talbot notes that differences in sexual function in patients with complete versus incomplete neurologic loss are great.[152] In a study of 56 patients with complete neurologic loss, all patients exhibited complete loss of both motor and sensory function, including control of bowel, bladder, and sexual function.[87] Determinations of spasticity or flaccidity were taken into account, and the following findings emerged. The patient with dorsal spinal cord injury who sustained a spastic or upper motor neuron lesion had, in 74% of cases, the capability of having a reflex erection. On the other hand, 90% with flaccid paralysis or a lower motor neuron lesion lost their ability to have an erection. No patient with a dorsal spine injury—whether of the upper or the lower motor neurons—had the capability of ejaculation or orgasm or had any libido. When patients sustained segmental injuries of the lumbar spinal cord with upper motor neuron lesions, 76% maintained the ability to have an erection. Of those patients sustaining a lower motor neuron (peripheral nerve) injury to the lumbar segment with flaccid paralysis, 68% lost the ability to have an erection. It was reported that 7% of patients with lumbar upper motor neuron (spastic) lesions maintained the ability to ejaculate, while 11% of those with lower motor neuron lesions maintained the ability to have an ejaculation. Of those with upper motor neuron lesions of the lumbar spine, 3.6% maintained the ability to have an orgasm, while none with lower motor neuron injury had this ability. Only 26% of the patients with upper motor neuron lesions of the lumbar spine maintained libido, while 5.6% of those with lower motor neuron lumbar lesions maintained libido.

It is difficult to explain why or how erections occur in flaccid (lower motor neuron) paralysis. Possibly, they are the result of restoration of sacral connections (between S2 and S5), or they may be what are described as "psychological erections." It is believed that three sexual centers exist: the thalamus, the thoracic spinal cord, and the lumbosacral spinal cord. Jacobson and Bors, in a review of 114 Vietnam combat injuries of the dorsolumbar spinal cord, revealed the presence of pseudospontaneous erections, reflex in nature, occasionally interpreted by the patient as psychological erections.[86] Patients with incomplete injuries (at all levels) reported psychological erections. The authors also found that in the presence of lower motor neuron (dorsal) injuries, only a small number of patients reported the ability to have an erection. In a review of 38 patients with complete lower motor neuron lesions, 16 (42%) reported psychological erections, and four (10.5%) reported dribbling emissions. Other series report such emissions in as high as 19% of cases.

Females. Paraplegia in no way affects fertility. Although spinal cord injuries may cause amenorrhea for varying lengths of time, after several months, the menstrual hormonal cycle again becomes regular,[30] and conception is unimpaired.[86] Similar findings were noted by Guttmann[66] and Hardy.[70] The only common complication noted during pregnancy in paraplegic women is the frequent occurrence of urinary tract infections. Fetal development is considered to be normal. No real impairment in uterine contractions has been observed during delivery in any of the patients having sustained dorsal spine or spinal cord injuries.

Labor pain is influenced by the presence of dorsal spinal cord injury. Labor pains are definitely less severe for a paraplegic than for a normal woman. Quite commonly, a paroxysmal increase in blood pressure (autonomic dysreflexia) will be noted along with bradycardia during delivery and expulsion of the placenta.[137] Concomitant with autonomic dysreflexia, facial flushing with or without diaphoresis (above the level of the injury) may occur. When it does, the patient may report headaches of varying types and ascending sensations synchronous with uterine contractions. Goller and Paeslak report that these physiological changes produce no danger for the mother or baby during delivery.[61]

It should be remembered that autonomic dysreflexia occurs only in patients who sustain neurologic injuries between C5 and D6 in which there is loss of control of the sympathetic nervous system by the cerebral cortex. This means that patients with injuries to the spine and spinal cord between C5 and D6 are most susceptible to this pathologic phenomenon. Spinal anesthesia is a very effective method of relieving splanchnic arterial vasoconstriction as a result of sympathetic nervous system stimulation. Likewise, delivery of the fetus and release of uterine distention is also an efficient and noninvasive means of managing autonomic dysreflexia. Treatment depends on the level of the hypertension and the severity of the patient's complaints.

There has been a question as to whether a paraplegic woman is more likely to give birth to a damaged or deformed baby, particularly if the mother was injured during the first trimester. There has been some suggestion that this might be true, but solid evidence does not exist. The treating physician must watch the woman carefully with x-rays and must monitor blood factors, which may indicate anemia. Also, maintenance of normal nitrogen balance to prevent pressure decubiti and good urinary care to reduce urinary tract infections are most important.

VASCULAR EXTENSION OF SPINAL CORD DYSFUNCTION

The blood supply of the spinal cord is a complicated and intricate system of 31 paired radicular arterial branches taking exit from the aorta throughout the thoracic and upper lumbar spine.[97] Accompanying these vessels are two particularly important radicular vessels: the superior and inferior anterior great radicular arteries. The position and level of origin of these two vessels vary. Complications secondary to spinal and vascular (aortic, intercostal) surgery and sympathectomy occasionally result in embarrassment of the blood supply to the spinal cord and can contribute to extension of the spinal cord lesion.

Regardless of the cause, the pathologic changes secondary to direct spinal cord contusion, crushing, or laceration have been described by numerous authors.[5–8,10,12,47,90,118]

An extremely confusing area of study is the question of the relationship between direct spinal cord injury and the reality of the problem of spinal cord autodestruction (or extension of posttraumatic neurologic dysfunction). There is definitely a correlation between spinal cord histopathologic findings and the passage of time following graded animal spinal cord experimental trauma.[8,47,124,125] Large areas of central hemorrhage secondary to external trauma lead to extensive destruction of the central gray matter. These changes progress outward from the central gray matter toward the more peripheral spinal cord white matter. During the stage of central hemorrhage, the white matter becomes edematous and in time undergoes necrotic changes similar to those noted in the central gray matter. The pertinent question is: What is the link between external spinal cord trauma and the presence (or reality) of an expanding central cord hemorrhage that with time demonstrates a progressive destruction of both the central gray matter and the peripheral white matter? Does the original trauma produce the histopathologic changes? Or, is the process of progressive autodestruction established following trauma, and is it the result of tissue hemorrhage, tissue hypoxia, adverse tissue pH, or enzyme release and lysis? Osterholm,[124,125] Ducker and Hamit,[47] and others[93] have addressed their research to the histochemical activities of the injured spinal cord.

Tarlov, doing spinal cord compression and vascular response research, noted the following finding: *Mechanical compression of the spinal cord, not anoxia, is the major cause of loss of neurologic function.*[154] This has been substantiated by others.[47,124,175] Although spinal cord compression does in all likelihood have a component of ischemia, Tarlov revealed that ischemia to the dog's spinal cord produced irreversible, extensive neurologic injury.[154] On the other hand, dogs subjected to compression of the spinal cord sufficient to produce loss of motor and sensory function recovered fully after withstanding up to 2 hours of compression. Similar observations on the dissimilar effects of pressure and ischemia are quoted by Lazorthes and associates.[97]

Kelly and colleagues have noted, following the production of a single lesion by experimental direct trauma, a drop in oxygen content in injured spinal cord tissue.[93] Within 1 hour, oxygen levels diminish below local needs, exacerbating necrosis of the central gray matter. One could anticipate that in the presence of a protracted hypoxia, a progressive necrosis and further spinal cord destruction will occur.

Osterholm and Matthews report finding excessive norepinephrine in the area of hemorrhage of the central gray matter following laboratory-induced spinal cord injury in animals. It is his belief that the presence of this substance produced an autodestruction of cellular structures and a blockage of neurotransmission.[124,125] This theory has been questioned and criticized. Zivin and associates make other observations.[174] They produced spinal cord injury in rabbits by a closed method—sudden inflation and immediate deflation of a balloon catheter placed epidurally at the L2–3 interspace. They then sacrificed the animals at 5, 15, 30, and 120 minutes and determined the biochemical levels of serotonin, norepinephrine, and dopamine. No significant difference in dopamine concentration was identified, and in this study, consistently low levels of norepinephrine were noted at the site of the lesion, both in the central gray matter and white matter of the cord. Serotonin concentrations in the central gray matter of the lesion were decreased, while serotonin concentrations in the white matter rapidly increased to 2.5 times those of the controls at 15 minutes. At edge of the lesion, the concentrations of serotonin in the white matter rose by a factor of 2.5 to 3 within 5 minutes and maintained that level.

Histochemically, Zivin and colleagues found that at 5 and 15 minutes the gray matter at the site of the lesion was enlarged and 75% replaced by blood. Little change was noted in the white matter. At 30 minutes, destructive changes began in the white matter, and at 2 hours, unequivocal evidence of yellow fluorescence was noted in the white matter. After 1 day, there was yellow fluorescence of smooth axons in the white matter and evidence of necrotic degeneration. The gray matter was completely destroyed by yellow autofluorescence. At 4 days destruction at the injury site was essentially complete. Of the amines measured, serotonin was highest in the gray and white matter. It was found that white matter serotonin increased to similar levels just above and below the center of the lesion. The authors note that only when the lesion extended from gray to white matter did permanent neurologic deficits result. It was therefore assumed that serotonin may play a role in injury propagation. In the gray matter at the center of the lesion, a decrease in norepinephrine (and to some extent, serotonin) levels may indicate release of the transmitters, either as a result of cell injury or as a release in excess of synthesis. Therefore, both the histochemical and the biochemical changes noted by Zivin and associates suggest that serotonin may influence injury propagation, that it has vasoactive properties, and that it is probably a motor neuron depressant. This suggests that reserpine, a serotonin antagonist, might be of benefit in treatment.

In hypoxia at the site of the lesion, which does occur, there may be some influence of oxygen levels over monoamine metabolism, inhibiting re-uptake and degradation and enhancing release—all contributing to changes in tissue concentrations of serotonin.[175] Ducker and Hamit evaluated therapeutic hypothermia and corticosteroid administration in the traumatized dorsolumbar spinal cords of dogs.[47] Their findings, which were statistically significant, indicated that improvement and recovery of neurologic function resulted from the use of corticosteroids (intramuscular dexamethasone) or local cord hypothermia. Zivin and associates found that the response of the spinal cord to trauma is edema, hemorrhage, and necrosis.[175] Use of corticosteroids and hypothermia minimizes these clinical findings and the subsequent pathologic changes. Mannitol and urea are suspected to be beneficial in the relief or prevention of edema.[88]

CORTICOSTEROID MANAGEMENT

The effectiveness and the role of corticosteroids in the management of acute spinal cord injury are now, more than ever, questioned.[17] For years, corticosteroids have been recommended in the early management of neurologic tissue injury[41,47,114,175] in the belief that they

Improve neuronal excitability and impulse conduction

Decrease post-injury tissue response to trauma (reduced inflammatory response), thereby maintaining and increasing blood flow

Preserve the spinal cord ultrastructure by reducing the occurrence of injury-induced, free radical–catalyzed lipid peroxidation

Other, less specific beneficial effects of corticosteroids reported are edema reduction and cell membrane and lysosome stabilization.

It is a policy of the Acute Spinal Cord Injury Center at Northwestern University to administer corticosteroids only to patients sustaining acute neurologic injuries. The protocol suggests the administration of 50 mg dexamethasone (Decadron) by IV push as soon after injury as possible. This is followed by a daily tapered dosage of dexamethasone, 10 mg IV every 6 hours, and decreased in amount each day by 2 mg. The taper is usually complete within 5 to 7 days.

Two indications for the continuation of corticosteroid therapy are

A demonstrated neurologic improvement. In such an instance, one may be reluctant to discontinue the medication within the prescribed 5 to 7 days.

Evidence of neurologic deterioration. In such cases, it is suggested that corticosteroids be either continued or reinstituted.

Several new revelations were reported in the recent study by Brachken and associates.[17] High-dose corticosteroids (methylprednisolone, 1000 mg/day for 10 days) were found to produce

An increased incidence of wound infections

An unexplained higher death rate (2–3 times) than in the low-dose group

A higher incidence of death due to cardiac arrest (whereas a cause in the low-dose group was respiratory arrest)

A 78% increased incidence of pulmonary embolism

A higher incidence of decubitus ulcers

Of interest, there is no evidence of an increased tendency for gastrointestinal bleeding to occur in either the high- or the low-dose group. Of the patients studied, 29.6% received cimetidine, 43.1% received cimetidine and some antacid, 23.7% received only an antacid, and the remaining 3.6% received no additional drugs.

The corticosteroid dexamethasone (Decadron) is widely used by those managing acute spinal cord injuries. Most of the evidence supporting the use of the drug has been derived from animal studies, which identified some beneficial effects.[47] A major question that yet remains to be answered is whether there are any beneficial effects to high- versus low-dose corticosteroid management. There does not appear to be any.[17] The most plausible rationale behind the use of corticosteroids is their known anti-inflammatory effects. The customary dosage is 50 mg by IV push initially, followed by a daily tapered dose.

Mannitol is a drug frequently administered to patients with acute spinal cord injury. Its effect is that of an osmotic diuretic. It has long been recommended by the neurosurgical community for the reduction of cerebral edema following head trauma.[38,42,114,124] Its osmotic effects have never been shown to have any direct influence over the reduction of posttraumatic spinal cord edema. Therefore, its suggested administration is no longer a recommendation in the spinal cord protocol. If it *is* administered, the recommended dosage is 500 ml of 20% mannitol administered over a 1- to 2-hour period shortly following the initial trauma.

Cimetidine hydrochloride is a known and effective drug whose action as an H_2 histamine receptor antagonist decreases both nocturnal and daytime basal gastric acid secretions. The usual dosage is 300 mg four times each day.

MANNITOL MANAGEMENT

Mannitol is a very effective osmotic, non-metabolized, long-chain (and high-molecular-weight glucose molecule) diuretic. It has a very long history of use by neurosurgeons, both preoperatively and postoperatively, for the prevention or control of cerebral edema. The dose used is 500 ml of 20% mannitol or 1000 ml of 10% mannitol.

Mannitol is administered intravenously over a 2- to 4-hour period. If effective, it may be repeated once or twice during the first 24 hours, but the patient's urinary output and electrolytes must be carefully monitored.

There is no real evidence that the use of mannitol is effective in the management of swelling of the spinal cord brought on by trauma (although it has been used for the past 14 years without any side-effects). For this reason, we now advise that the drug not be administered at the initial institution providing patient care. After patient arrival at the Acute Spinal Cord Injury Center and following evaluation by the neurosurgery service, if there is evidence of severe head trauma requiring mannitol administration, it will be requested by the neurosurgery service (see Chap. 7).

BIOMECHANICAL LABORATORY DATA: INTERNAL FIXATION DEVICES

A study by Pinzur, Meyer, and colleagues[128] has revealed that the vertebral load that the spine is able to withstand before failure is approximately 600 pounds. Vertical load tests of internal fixation devices such as Harrington compression or distraction devices and Weiss springs revealed that not one of the three even closely approximated (by half) the stiffness of a fresh cadaver dorsolumbar spine when measured on a load displacement chart (Fig. 24-35). The findings are in terms of stiffness rather than strength and reveal (when comparison is limited to the three devices noted above) that the Harrington compression rod has the greatest stiffness and can thus withstand the greatest dis-

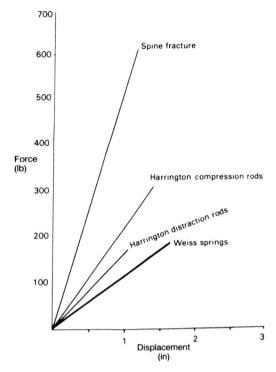

FIG. 24-35. Comparison of the stiffness of a fresh cadaver spine with that of three types of internal fixation devices. The initial internal stiffness of a fresh cadaver dorsolumbar spine is approximately twice that of any of the three internal fixation devices placed under similar loads.

placement before it fails. Second was the Harrington distraction rod. Of interest, there a consistent failure of the spine was noted at the level above the upper hook of the Harrington compression-rod apparatus (indicative of the stiffness of the apparatus) when the spine is under compression. Although the Harrington distraction-rod apparatus was second in this respect, it was least able to withstand angular deflection before failure. Again, of the three listed devices, the Weiss springs were the least stiff, yet were able to withstand the greatest angular deformity before failing. They were never found to fail at the bone–hook or spring–hook junction, which is where the Harrington distraction-rod apparatus usually failed. A component of this failure was a state of relative lengthening of the spine

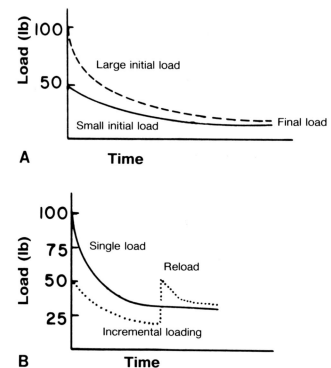

FIG. 24-36. Diagrammatic demonstration of load decay or stress relaxation. (*A*) This absorption of load occurs primarily in ligaments and soft tissue. In time, approximately half of the load is lost through decay. (*B*) Incremental application of an internal fixation load will result in a reduction of the amount of load decay and an overall increase in corrective forces.

during the application of a bending moment to the spine (as with bending forward of the trunk) combined with a distraction moment on the rods when in place.

These data may be interpreted as follows. Theoretically, one would expect greater angular correction (kyphosis to extension) with Harrington compression rods, yet this was not the case. Our findings substantiated the work of Elfstrom and Nachamson: the spine under load undergoes "load decay" or "stress relaxation" (regardless of the type of internal fixation device used). This holds true even when Luque rods are used, though here it has more to do with the type of fracture and the mechanical rationale for the occurrence of compression of the vertebral elements during vertical loading of the spinal column.

This mechanical reaction (load decay) to either distraction or compression is evidenced by a change in spinal alignment after application of a static load (Fig. 24-36, *A*). These changes also occur within the paraspinal soft tissues, allowing lengthening or shortening in excess to the original load.

Such a "decay" can be sufficient to allow loss of internal fixation and the recurrence of angular deformity. Thus, if adequate postoperative orthotic immobilization is not implemented, load-decay failure of the vertebral column, albeit minor, may lead to failure of internal fixation components (Harrington-rod compression or distraction) at the hook–bone interface. "Dynamic" devices such as Weiss springs (in which the implant has a tendency to return to its "resting length") will also demonstrate evidence of load decay. However, if the device has been appropriately used, under the correct conditions, the presence of load decay or stress relaxation may enhance the correction of the spinal deformity.[108] Again, the use of an external immobilizing orthosis is recommended until spine stability or fusion has been demonstrated (see Figs. 24-16 and 24-17). Figure 24-36, *B* demonstrates the application of a load at a lower initial limit, resulting in less load decay. By subsequent increases or "reloading," a greater force may be gradually induced to a level almost equal the amount initially applied.

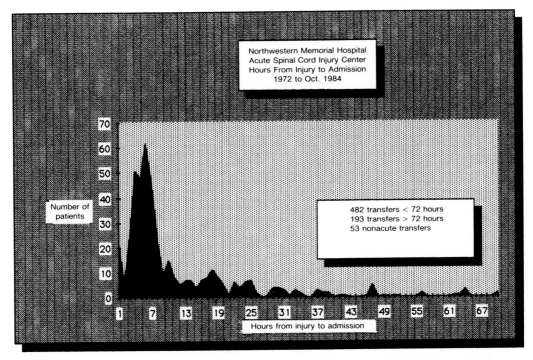

Northwestern Memorial Hospital
Acute Spinal Cord Injury Center
Hours From Injury to Admission
1972 to Oct. 1984

Number of patients

482 transfers < 72 hours
193 transfers > 72 hours
53 nonacute transfers

Hours from injury to admission

FIG. 24-37. Time from injury to admission, Midwest Regional Spinal Cord Injury Care System, 1972 to October 1984.

CAUSES OF DEATH AND SURVIVAL RATES IN PATIENTS WITH DORSAL AND LUMBAR SPINE INJURIES

The Edwin Smith surgical papyrus on spinal cord injury, written between 3000 and 2500 B.C., described the spinal cord–injured victim as one whose lot was "hopelessness and despair."[50] Comments on the care and survival of these patients in the early literature amounted to "bed care and little else can be done." As already noted, the 1-year survival rate of spine-injured patients following World War I was 10%. Following World War II, the average survival time was 10 years after injury. Matlack revealed in 1974 that patients who had sustained a spine injury at an average age of 27 had a mortality rate 3.9 times that of others of the same age, and that the life expectancy of these patients in the U.S. was estimated to be 59 years, or 32 years after the onset of their disability.[100]

The average 27-year-old in the U.S. has a life expectancy of 75 years; however, the life expectancy of a victim of spinal cord injury is lower by some 21%.[43] Matlack also quotes the 1974 annual mortality statistics for incomplete quadriplegics and paraplegics as 1% to 2% and for complete quadriplegics and paraplegics, 4% to 6%.[100] Thus, the annual mortality rate for patients with spinal cord injury in the six spinal injury centers he surveyed was estimated to be 10.7%. All of Matlack's statistics include both cervical and dorsolumbar injuries.

It is interesting to compare several large series of spinal injuries in which mortality rates are discussed. Barber and Cross's[11] rate was 5.2%; Bunts'[19] (in a composite of eight series) was between 9% and 23%; Nyquist's[121] was 10%; and that of Hoffman and Bunts[80] was 25%. The most significant mortality rate is that reported by Freed and associates[55] from a 23.6-year follow-up: 22.2%. Freed and colleagues also reports a Veterans Administration review covering 9.75 years with an estimated death rate of 13.9%.[31] In 1943 Munro reported a mortality rate of 57% in a series of 40 hospitalized patients; 23 died, two from pulmonary embolism in dorsolumbar injuries.[118] Of those with cervical injuries, 74% died between 3 and 6 weeks after injury (43% of these deaths were the direct result of sepsis).

Tribe, in reporting 16 patients with acute traumatic paraplegia, of whom 13 died within 1 month, noted the average age to be 49.5 years.[159] The average time between injury and death was 10 days; three patients lived to 7.5 weeks. Their deaths resulted from pulmonary infection. Tribe also reviewed 122 deaths in paraplegics, noting that 84 were directly related to the injury; 44 (52%) died of uremia secondary to renal failure with pyelonephritis and amyloidosis. This same author, reporting the deaths of 150 paraplegics between 1945 and 1962, noted that 28 patients (18.6%) died within the first 2 months. The principal cause of death in the patients with cervical injuries was respiratory complications, while in the other patients it was pulmonary embolism. The only reason for including these older statistics is to illustrate vividly the vast improvements that have resulted from the sophisticated care now available through and provided by today's specialized acute spinal cord injury centers, which include a trauma information retrieval system, allowing a median admission time for greater than 2000 patients over a 13-year period to be 10.6 hours (see Fig. 24-37). In my series of 728 patients with dorsolumbar spine injury, 23 patients (3.16%) died during acute care.

REFERENCES

1. Abramson, A.S.: Bone disturbances in injuries to the spinal cord and cauda equina. J. Bone Joint Surg., 30A:982, 1948.
2. Adamkiewicz, A.: Die Blutgefasse des menschlichen ruckeumarkes Tiel, die Gafesse der Ruckenmarkoberflache. S. B. Heidelberg, Akad Wiss., 85:101, 1882.
3. Alby, R.: Bone Graft Surgery. New York, Appleton-Century-Crofts, 1940.
4. Alexander, E., Jr.: Significance of the small lumbar spinal canal: Cauda equina compression syndromes due to spondylitis. 5. Achondroplasia. J. Neurosurg., 31:513, 1969.
5. Allen, A.R.: Injuries of the spinal cord. J.A.M.A., 50:941, 1908.
6. ———: The symptom complex of transverse lesion of the spinal cord and its relations to structural changes therein. Am. J. Med. Sci., 135:735, 1908.
7. ———: Surgery of experimental lesions of spinal cord equivalent to crush injury of fracture dislocation of spinal column. J.A.M.A., 57:878, 1911.
8. ———: Remarks on the histopathological changes in the spinal cord due to impact: An experimental study. J. Nerv. Ment. Dis., 41:141, 1914.
9. Armstrong, C.T., Ress, C.P., Weiss, A.A., and Ebel, A.: Results of surgical treatment of extra-ossification in paraplegia. N.Y. State J. Med., 59:2538, 1959.
10. Assenmacher, D.R., and Ducker, T.B.: Experimental traumatic paraplegia, the vascular and pathological changes seen in reversible and irreversible spinal cord lesions. J. Bone Joint Surg., 53A:671, 1971.
11. Barber, K.E., and Cross, R.R.: The urinary tract as a cause of death in paraplegia. J. Urol., 67:494, 1952.
12. Bedbrook, G.M.: Some pertinent observations on the pathology of traumatic spinal paralysis. Paraplegia, 1:215, 1963.
13. ———: Treatment of thoracolumbar dislocation and fractures with paraplegia. Clin. Orthop., 112:27, 1975.
14. Benassy, J., Blanchard, J., and LeCoq, R.: Neurological recovery rate in para-tetraplegia. Paraplegia, 4:259, 1967.
15. Bohler, L.: The Treatment of Fractures. Bristol, John Wright & Sons, 1935.
16. Boyd, B.M., Jr., Roberts, W.M., and Moore, G.R.: Periarticular ossification following burns. South. Med. J., 52:1048, 1959.
17. Brachken, M.B., Collins, W.F., Freeman, D.F. et al.: Efficacy of methylprednisolone in acute spinal cord injury. J.A.M.A., 251(1):45, 1984.
18. Bricher, D.L., Waltz, T.A., Jr., Telford, R.J., and Beall, A.C., Jr.: Major abdominal and thoracic trauma associated with spinal cord injury: Problems in management. J. Trauma, 2:63, 1971.
19. Bunts, R.C.: Presentation of renal function in the paraplegic. J. Urol., 81:720, 1959.
20. Calenoff, L., Chessare, J.W., Rogers, L.F. et al.: Multiple level spinal injuries: Importance of early recognition. A.J.R., 130:665, 1978.
21. Campbell, J., and Bonnett, C.: Spinal cord injury in children. Clin. Orthop., 112:113, 1975.
22. Carey, P.D.: Neurosurgery and paraplegia. Rehabilitation, 52(27):27, 1965.
23. Ceiller, P.: Para-Osteo Arthropathies des Paraplegiques par Lesion Belamoelle et de la Queve de Cheval. Paris, Imprimerie Generale Leheure, 1920.
24. Cheshire, D.J.E., and Coats, D.A.: Respiratory and metabolic management in acute tetraplegia. Paraplegia, 4:6, 1966.
25. Ciliberti, B.J., Goldfein, J., and Rovenstine, E.A.: Hypertension during anesthesia in patients with spinal cord injuries. Anesthesiology, 15:273, 1954.
26. Clarke, K.S.: Caloric costs of activity in paraplegic persons. Arch. Phys. Med. Rehabil., 47:427, 1966.
27. Cocke, W.M., and Meyer, K.R.: Splenic rupture due to improper placement of automobile safety belt. J.A.M.A., 183:693, 1963.

28. Comarr, A.E.: Laminectomy in patients with injuries to the spinal cord. J. Int. Coll. Surg., 31: 437, 1959.

29. ———: Interesting observations on females with spinal cord injury. Med. Serv. J. Can., 22:651, 1966.

30. Comarr, A.E., and Kaufman, A.A.: A survey of the neurological results of 858 cord injuries: A comparison of patients treated with or without laminectomy. J. Neurosurg., 13:95, 1956.

31. Controller, Department of Medicine and Surgery: Mortality Report on Spinal Cord Injury. Reports and Statistics Service, Veterans Administration, November 13, 1958.

32. Covall, D.A., Clipper, I.S., Hoem, T.I., and Rusk, H.A.: Early management of patients with spinal cord injury. J.A.M.A., 151:89, 1953.

33. Costello, R.B., and Brown, A.: Myositis ossificans complicating anterior poliomyelitis. J. Bone Joint Surg., 33B:594, 1951.

34. Coupland, G.A.E., and Reeve, T.S.: Paraplegia: A complication of excision of abdominal aortic aneurysm. Surgery, 64:878, 1968.

35. Courville, G.B.: In Tice, F. (ed.): Practice of Medicine, p. 139. Rogerston, Prior, 1932.

36. Cramer, F., and McGowan, F.J.: The role of the nucleus pulposus in the pathogenesis of so-called "recoil" injuries of the spinal cord. Surg. Gynecol. Obstet., 79:516, 1944.

37. Dalton, J.J., Jr., Hackler, R.H., and Bunts, R.C.: Amyloidosis in the paraplegic: Incidence and significance. J. Urol., 93:553, 1965.

38. d'Aubigne, M.R., Benassy, Y., and Ramadier, T.O.: Chirurgie Orthopedique des Paraplegia, pp. 235–242. Paris, Masson et Cie, 1956.

39. Davidoff, L.M.: Spinal cord injuries. Surg. Clin. North Am., 21:433, 1941.

40. Davis, A.G.: Fractures of the spine. J. Bone Joint Surg., 11:133, 1929.

41. de la Torre, J.C. et al.: Pharmacologic treatment and evaluation of permanent experimental spinal cord trauma. Neurology, 25:508, 1975.

42. Desmeules, H.: Hyperkalemia following succinylcholine. Can. Med. Assoc. J., 108:1527, 1973.

43. DeVivo, M.J., Fine, P.R., Maetz, H.M., and Stover, S.S.: Prevalence of spinal cord injury: A reestimation employing life table techniques. Arch. Neurol., 37:707, 1980.

44. Dewey, P., and Browne, P.S.H.: Fracture-dislocation of the lumbosacral spine with cauda equina lesion. J. Bone Joint Surg., 50B:635, 1968.

45. Dick, I.L.: The treatment of traumatic paraplegia in fractures of the lumbodorsal spine. Edinburgh Med. J., 60:249, 1953.

46. Dick, T.B.S.: Traumatic paraplegia pre-Guttmann. Paraplegia, 7:173, 1969.

47. Ducker, T.B., and Hamit, H.F.: Experimental Treatment of acute spinal cord injury. J. Neurosurg., 30:693, 1969.

48. Edelstein, D.L., Meyer, P.R., Schafer, M.F., and Wixson, R.L.: Combined simultaneous anterior posterior spinal column neural decompression and fusion for fracture-dislocation of the thoracic/lumbar spine. Orthop. Trans., 7:480, 1983.

49. Eichenholtz, S.N.: Management of long bone fractures in paraplegic patients. J. Bone Joint Surg., 45A:299, 1963.

50. Elsberg, C.A.: The Edwin Smith surgical papyrus and the diagnosis and the treatment of injuries to the skull and spine 5,000 years ago. Am. Med. Hist., 3:271, 1931.

51. Evans, E.M.: Some recent studies in spondylolisthesis. J. Bone Joint Surgery, 41B:430, 1959.

52. Ferguson, L.R., Bergan, J.J., and Yao, J.S.: Spinal ischemia following abdominal aortic surgery. Ann. Surg., 181:267, 1975.

53. Flamm, E.S., Young, W., Demopoulos, H.B. et al.: Experimental spinal cord injury: Treatment with naloxone. J. Neurosurg., 10:227, 1982.

54. Frankel, H.L.: Ascending cord lesion in the early stages following spinal injury. Paraplegia, 7:111, 1969.

55. Freed, M.D., Bakst, H.J., and Barrie, D.L.: Life expectancy, survival rates, and causes of death in civilian patients with spinal cord trauma. Arch. Phys. Med., 47:457, 1966.

56. Freehafer, A.A.: Sepsis of the hip in patients with advanced neurologic disease. Clin. Orthop., 29:180, 1963.

57. Freehafer, A.A., and Mast, W.A.: Lower extremity fractures in patients with spinal cord injury. J. Bone Joint Surg., 47A:683, 1965.

58. Furman, R., Nicholas, J.J., and Jivoff, L.: Elevation of the serum alkaline phosphatase coincident with ectopic bone formation in paraplegic patients. J. Bone Joint Surg., 52A:1131, 1970.

59. Garceau, G.J.: Filium terminale syndrome (the cord traction syndrome). J. Bone Joint Surg., 35A: 711, 1953.

60. Garrett, J.W., and Braunstein, P.W.: The seatbelt syndrome. J. Trauma, 2:220, 1962.

61. Goller, H., and Paeslak, V.: Our experiences about pregnancy and delivery of the paraplegic woman. Paraplegia, 8:161, 1970.

62. Guidelines for Facility Categorization and Standards of Care: Spinal Cord Injury. Chicago, American Spinal Injury Foundation, 1981.

63. Guttmann, L.J.: Surgical aspects of the treatment of traumatic paraplegia. J. Bone Joint Surgery, 31B:389, 1949.

64. ———: Statistical survey on one thousand paraplegics: Initial treatment of paraplegia trauma. Proc. R. Soc. Med., 47:1009, 1954.

65. ———: The management of the paraplegic patient. Practitioner, 176:157, 1956.

66. ———: New turning–tilting bed and head traction unit. Br. Med. J., 1:288, 1967.

67. ———: Spinal deformities in traumatic paraplegics and tetraplegics following surgical procedures. Paraplegia, 7:38, 1969.

68. Guttmann, L.J., and Robertson, S.: The paraplegic patient in pregnancy and labour. Proc. R. Soc. Med., 56:380, 1963.

69. Guttmann, L.J., and Silver, J.R.: Electromyographic studies on reflex activity of the intercostal and abdominal muscles in cervical cord lesions. Paraplegia, 3:1, 1965.

70. Hardy, A.G.: The treatment of paraplegia due to fracture-dislocations of the dorsolumbar spine. Paraplegia, 3:112, 1965.

71. Hardy, A.G., and Dixon, J.W.: Pathological ossification and traumatic paraplegia. J. Bone Joint Surg., 45B:76, 1963.
72. Harrington, P.R., and Dickson, J.H.: An eleven year clinical investigation of Harrington instrumentation. Clin. Orthop., 112:113, 1973.
73. Harris, P.: The initial treatment of traumatic paraplegia. Paraplegia, 3:71, 1965–1966.
74. Hausson, K.G., and Austlid, O.: Myositis ossificans in poliomyelitis: Two case reports. Arch. Phys. Med., 36:506, 1955.
75. Heilbrun, N., and Kuhn, W.G., Jr.: Erosive bone lesions and soft tissue ossification associated with spinal cord injury (paraplegia). Radiology, 48:579, 1947.
76. Hess, W.E.: Myositis ossificans occurring in poliomyelitis: Report of a case. Arch. R. Coll. Neurol. Psychiatr., 66:606, 1951.
77. Hodgson, A.R., and Stock, F.E.: Anterior spine fusion, a preliminary communication on the radical treatment of Pott's disease and Pott's paraplegia. Br. J. Surg., 44:266, 1956–1957.
78. Hodgson, A.R., Stock, F.E., Fang, H.S.Y., and Ong, G.B.: Anterior spine fusion, the operative approach and pathological findings in 412 patients with Pott's disease of the spine. Br. J. Surg., 48:172, 1960.
79. Hodgson, A.R., Yau, A., and Vim.: A clinical study of 100 consecutive cases of Pott's paraplegia. Clin. Orthop., 36:128, 1964.
80. Hoffman, C.A., and Bunts, R.C.: Present urological status of 5-year Korean war paraplegics. J. Urol., 88:60, 1961.
81. Holdsworth, F.W.: Symposium on Spinal Injury, p. 161. Edinburgh Royal College of Surgeons, 1963.
82. ———: Review article—fracture, dislocations and fracture-dislocations of the spine. J. Bone Joint Surg., 52A:534, 1970.
83. Holdsworth, F.W., and Hardy, A.G.: Early treatment of paraplegia from fracture of the thoracolumnar spine. J. Bone Joint Surg., 35B:540, 1953.
84. Howland, W.J., Curry, J.L., and Buffington, C.B.: Fulcrum fractures of the lumbar spine. J.A.M.A., 193:240, 1965.
85. Jacobs, G.B., and Berg, R.A.: The treatment of acute spinal cord injuries in a war zone. J. Neurosurg., 34:164, 1971.
86. Jacobson, S.A., and Bors, E.: Spinal cord injury in Vietnamese combat. Paraplegia, 8:263, 1970.
87. Jochheim, K.A., and Wahle, H.: A study of sexual function in 56 male patients with complete irreversible lesions of the spinal cord and cauda equina. Paraplegia, 8:166, 1970.
88. Joyner, J., and Freeman, L.W.: Urea and spinal cord trauma. Neurology, 13:59, 1963.
89. Kahn, E.A.: The role of dentate ligament in spinal cord compression and syndrome of lateral sclerosis. J. Neurosurg., 4:191, 1947.
90. Kakulas, B.A., and Bedbrook, G.M.: Pathology of Injuries of the Vertebral Column. In Vinken, P.J., and Bruyn, G.W. (eds.): Handbook of Clinical Neurology. New York, American Elsevier, 1976.
91. Kaplan, L., Towle, B.R., Grynbaum, B.B., and Rusk, H.: Comprehensive follow-up study of spinal dysfunction. Arch. Phys. Med., 47:393, 1966.
92. Kaufer, H., and Hayes, J.T.: Lumbar fracture-dislocaton: A study of twenty-one cases. J. Bone Joint Surg., 48A:712, 1966.
93. Kelley, D.L., Jr. et al.: Effects of local hypothermia and tissue oxygen studies in experimental paraplegia. J. Neurosurg., 33:554, 1970.
94. Kilfoyle, R.M., Foley, J.J., and Norton, P.L.: Spine and pelvic deformity in childhood and adolescent paraplegia: A study of 104 cases. J. Bone Joint Surg., 47A:659, 1965.
95. Kuhn, W.G.: The care and rehabilitation of patients with spinal cord and cauda equina injury. J. Neurosurg., 4:40, 1947.
96. Kulowski, J., and Post, W.B.: Intra-abdominal injuries from safety-belt and automobile accidents: Report of a case. Arch. Surg., 73:970, 1956.
97. Lazorthes, G. et al.: Arterial vascularization of the spinal cord. J. Neurosurg., 35:253, 1971.
98. Leidholt, J.D., Young, J.J., Hahn, R.H.E. et al.: Evaluation of late spinal deformities with fracture-dislocations of the dorsal and lumbar spine in paraplegics. Paraplegia, 7:16, 1969.
99. Liberson, M.: Soft tissue calcification in cord lesions. J.A.M.A., 152:1010, 1953.
100. Matlack, D.: Cost Effectiveness of Spinal Cord Injury Center Treatment, pp. 112–132. Thesis, Bernard Baruch College, Mount Sinai School of Medicine, City University of New York, October 1974.
101. Matson, D.D.: Craniocerebral trauma. In Bowers, F. (ed.): Surgery of Trauma. Philadelphia, J.B. Lippincott, 1953.
102. Maxwell, J.J., and Kahn, E.A.: Spinal cord traction producing an ascending, reversible, neurological deficit: Case report. J. Neurosurg., 26:331, 1966.
103. Mayfield, F.H., and Cazan, G.M.: Spinal cord injuries: Analysis of 6 cases showing subarachnoid block. Am. J. Surg., 55:317, 1942.
104. Mayfield, J.K., Erkkila, J.C., and Winter, R.B.: Spine deformity subsequent to acquired childhood cord injury. J. Bone Joint Surg., 63A:1401, 1981.
105. McMaster, W.C., and Stauffer, E.S.: Management of long bone fractures in the spinal cord injured patient. Clin. Orthop., 112:45, 1975.
106. McSweeney, T.: The early management of associated injuries in the presence of coincident damage to the spinal cord. Paraplegia, 5:189, 1968.
107. ———: The management of closed injuries of the spine. Phoenix, Combined International Medical Society–Paraplegia and Veterans Administration, October 1974.
108. Meinecke, F.W.: Early treatment of traumatic paraplegia. Paraplegia, 1:262, 1964.
109. ———: Frequency and distribution of associated injuries in traumatic paraplegia and tetraplegia. Paraplegia, 5:196, 1968.
110. Meyer, P.R.: Lower limb orthotics. Clin. Orthop., 102:58, 1974.
111. Meyer, P.R., and Dobozi, W.: Fracture-dislocation of the dorsolumbar spine. Hampartzoum Kelikian Symposium. Chicago, Northwestern University, December 1975.
112. Meyer, P.R., and Raffensperger, J.G.: Special centers for the care of the injured. Midwest

Regional Spinal Cord Injury Care System. J. Trauma, 13:308, 1973.

113. Meyer, P.R., Rosen, J.S., and Hamilton, B.B.: Midwest Regional Spinal Cord Injury Care System, RSA-OHD-HEW Grant 13P-55864/5-03, Progress Reports II, III, IV. Chicago, Northwestern University, 1973, 1974, 1975, 1976.

114. Meyer, P.R., Rosen, J.S., Hamilton, B.B., and Hall, W.: Fracture-dislocation of the cervical spine: Transportation, assessment, and immediate management. Instr. Course Lect., 25:171, 1976.

115. Midwest Regional Spinal Cord Injury Care System Grant Proposal, Grant #G008435139, U.S. Department of Education, Office of Special Education and Rehabilitative Services, Rehabilitation Services Administration. Chicago, Northwestern University, August 1984.

116. Morgan, T.H., Wharton, G.W., and Austin, G.N.: The results of laminectomy in patients with incomplete spinal cord injuries. Paraplegia, 9:14, 1971.

117. Mosberg, W.H., Jr., Voris, H.C., and Duffy, J.J.: Paraplegia as complication of sympathectomy for hypertension. Am. Surg., 139:330, 1954.

118. Munro, D.: Thoracic and lumbosacral cord injuries. J.A.M.A., 122:1055, 1943.

119. Newman, P.H.: A clinical syndrome associated with severe lumbosacral subluxation. J. Bone Joint Surg., 47B:473, 1960.

120. Nicoll, E.A.: Fractures of the dorsolumbar spine. J. Bone Joint Surg., 31B:376, 1949.

121. Nyquist, R.H.: Mortality in spinal cord injuries. Proceedings of the Ninth Annual Clinical Spinal Cord Injuries Conference, pp. 109–112, Washington, U.S. Government Printing Office, October 1960.

122. O'Connell, J.E.A.: Discussion on cervical spondylosis. Proc. R. Soc. Med., 49:202, 1956.

123. O'Hare, J.M.: The acute abdomen in spinal cord injury patients. Proceedings of the Fifteenth Annual Clinical Spinal Cord Injury Conference, Long Beach, California, Veterans Administration Hospital, pp. 113–117. Washington, U.S. Government Printing Office, 1966.

124. Osterholm, J., and Matthews, G.J.: Altered norepinephrine metabolism following experimental spinal cord injury. I. Relationship to hemorrhagic necrosis and post-wounding neurological deficits. J. Neurosurg., 36:384, 1972.

125. ———: Altered norepinephrine metabolism following experimental spinal cord injury. II. Protection against traumatic spinal cord hemorrhagic necrosis by norepinephrine synthesis blockade with alpha methyl tyrosine. J. Neurosurg., 36:395, 1972.

126. Paget, J.: On a form of chronic inflammation of bone (osteitis deformans). Med. Chir. Trans., 60:37, 1877.

127. Phillips, R.S.: The incidence of deep venous thrombosis in paraplegia. Paraplegia, 1:116, 1963.

128. Pinzur, M.S., Meyer, P.R., Lautenschlager, E.P. et al.: Measurement of internal fixation device support in experimentally produced fractures of the dorsolumbar spine. Orthop., 2:28, 1979.

129. Pitts, N.C.: Myositis ossificans as a complication of tetanus. J.A.M.A., 189:237, 1964.

130. Pollock, L.J. et al.: Pain below the level of injury of the spinal cord. Arch. Neurol. Psychiatr., 65:319, 1951.

131. Rahal, J.J., Simberkoff, M.S.: Host defense and antimicrobial therapy in adult gram-negative bacillary meningitis. Ann. Intern. Med., 96:468, 1982.

132. Resiberg, B.: Personal communication, December 1984.

133. Richardson, R.R., Meyer, P.R., and Cerullo, L.J.: Transcutaneous electrical neurostimulation in musculoskeletal pain of acute spinal cord injuries. Spine, 5:42, 1980.

134. Roaf, F.: Scoliosis secondary to paraplegia. Paraplegia, 8:42, 1970.

135. Roberts, P.H.: Heterotopic ossification complicating paralysis of cranial origin. J. Bone Joint Surg., 50B:70, 1968.

136. Rogers, W.A.: Cord injury during reduction of thoracic and lumbar vertebral body fracture and dislocation. J. Bone Joint Surg., 20:689, 1938.

137. Rossier, A.B., Ruffieux, M., and Ziegler, W.H.: Pregnancy and labour in high traumatic spinal cord lesions. Paraplegia, 7:210, 1969.

138. Roth, F., and Wuthrich, H.: Clinical importance of hyperkalemia following the suxamephonium administration. Br. J. Anaesth., 41:311, 1969.

139. Russell, R.G., and Fleisch, H.: Pyrophosphate and diphosphonates in skeletal metabolism. Clin. Orthop., 108:241, 1975.

140. Sande, M.A.: Antibiotic therapy of bacterial meningitis: Lessons we've learned. Am. J. Med., 71:507, 1981.

141. Schmorl, G.: Über die anden Wirbelbandscheiben vorkomnenden Ausdehnungs und Zessei Bungsvorgange und die dadurch an ihnen und des Wirbelspongiosa Hesvorgesufeneu Verzandesungen. Verh. Dtsch. Pathol. Ges., 22:250, 1927.

142. Schneider, R.C.: Transposition of compressed spinal cord in kyphoscoliosis patients with neurologic deficits. With special reference to vascular supply of the cord. J. Bone Joint Surg., 42A:1027, 1960.

143. ———: Surgical indications and contraindications in spinal cord trauma. Clin. Neurosurg., 8:157, 1962.

144. Shallat, R.F., and Klump, T.E.: Paraplegia following thoracolumbar sympathectomy. J. Neurosurg., 34:569, 1971.

145. Shull, J.R., and Rose, D.L.: Pulmonary embolism in patients with spinal cord injury. Arch. Phys. Med., 47:444, 1966.

146. Silver, J.R.: Chest injuries and complications in the early stages of spinal cord injury. Paraplegia, 5:226, 1968.

147. Silver, J.R., and Moulton, A.: Physiological and pathological sequelae of paralysis of the intercostal and abdominal muscles in tetraplegic patients. Paraplegia, 7:131, 1969.

148. Skillman, J.J., Zervas, N.T., Weintraub, R.M., and Mayman, C.I.: Paraplegia after resection of aneurysms of the abdominal aorta. N. Engl. J. Med., 281:422, 1969.

149. Soule, A.B., Jr.: Neurogenic ossification fibromyopathies: A preliminary report. J. Neurosurg., 2:485, 1945.

150. Stanger, J.K.: Fracture-dislocation of the thoracic lumbar spine. With special reference to reduction by open and closed operation. J. Bone Joint Surg., 29A:107, 1947.

151. Stover, S.L., Hahn, H.R., and Miller, J.M.: Disodium etidronate in the prevention of heterotopic ossification following spinal cord injury. (preliminary report). Paraplegia, 14:146, 1976.

152. Talbot, H.S.: A report on sexual function in paraplegics. J. Urol., 61:265, 1949.

153. ———: Spinal cord injury. Arch. Surg., 102:539, 1971.

154. Tarlov, I.: Acute spinal cord compression paralysis. J. Neurosurg., 36:10, 1972.

155. Taylor, R.G., and Cleave, J.R.N.: Injury to the cervical spine. Proc. R. Soc. Med., 55:1053, 1962.

156. Tinsley, M.: Compound injuries of the spinal cord. J. Neurosurg., 3:306, 1946.

157. Tolin, S.H.: Unusual injury due to seat-belt. J. Trauma, 4:397, 1964.

158. Traffic Safety Newsletter. U.S. Department of Transportation, National Highway Traffic Safety Administration, Washington, August 1984.

159. Tribe, C.R.: Causes of death in early and late stages of paraplegia. Paraplegia, 1:19, 1963.

160. Tricot, A., and Hallot, R.: Traumatic paraplegia and associated fracture. Paraplegia, 5:211, 1968.

161. Troll, G., and Dohrmann, G.J.: Anesthesia of the spinal cord injured patient: Cardiovascular problems and their management. Paraplegia, 13:162, 1975.

162. Venerando, A.M., Monte, A.D., and Lamberti-Bucconi, F.: Spirographic and thoraco-metric studies in paraplegic patients. Paraplegia, 4:116, 1966.

163. Verbiest, F.: Symposium on Spinal Injury, p. 119. Edinburgh Royal College of Surgeons, 1963.

164. Walsh, J.J., and Tribe, C.: Phlebo-thrombosis and pulmonary embolism in spinal cord injury. Paraplegia, 3:209, 1965.

165. Wannamaker, G.T.: Spinal injuries. A review of the early treatment of 300 consecutive cases during the Korean conflict. J. Neurosurg., 11:517, 1954.

166. Warren, R.: Medical progress: Post-operative thrombophilia. N. Engl. J. Med., 249:99, 1953.

167. Watson, N.: Venous thrombosis and pulmonary embolism in spinal cord injury. Paraplegia, 6:13, 1968.

168. Watson-Jones, R.: Fracture and Other Bone and Joint Injuries, 1st ed., p. 641. Edinburgh, E.&S. Livingston, 1940.

169. Weinmann, J.P., and Sicker, H.: Bone and Bones: Fundamentals of Bone Biology. St. Louis, C.V. Mosby, 1947.

170. Wesseler, S., Cohen, S., and Fleischner, F.G.: The temporary thrombotic state. N. Engl. J. Med., 254:413, 1956.

171. White, R.J. et al.: The technique of localized spinal cord hypothermia in the human, pp. 58–60. Proceedings of the 17th Veterans Administration Spinal Cord Injury Conference, Bronx, New York, 1969. Washington, U.S. Government Printing Office, 1971.

172. Yashon, D., Jane, J.A., and White, R.J.: Prognosis and management of spinal cord and cauda equina bullet injuries in sixty-five civilians. J. Neurosurg., 32:163, 1970.

173. Yaumans, G.P., Paterson, P.Y., and Sommers, H.M.: Antimicrobial Therapy: The Biologic and Clinical Basis of Infectious Disease. Philadelphia, W.B. Saunders, 1975.

174. Young, J.S.: Development of systems of spinal injury management with correlations to the development of other esoteric health care systems. Arizona Med., 27:1, 1970.

175. Zivin, J.A. et al: Biochemical and histochemical studies of biogenic amines in spinal cord trauma. Neurology, 26:99, 1976.

25 Complications of Pelvic Fractures and Their Treatment

William J. Kane

The recent increased attention of orthopaedic surgeons and the orthopaedic literature to fractures and dislocations of the pelvis can be demonstrated by a critical review of the indices of those journals dedicated to the management of trauma—both general soft tissue trauma and, more specifically, osteoarticular trauma. This increased interest is an indication of a much more aggressive posture toward pelvic fractures and their attendant injuries by all concerned with the care of such patients. This change of attitude from what might have been described as passive or reactive to one that can be characterized as active or anticipatory is the keystone to the improved care of the patient with a pelvic fracture. Management programs or algorithms now point the way for appropriate diagnostic workups and treatment plans. These workups have been facilitated by the evolution of computed tomography (CT) scans of the disrupted pelvis[79] and by the increased use of diagnostic angiography.[80,92] Therapy has been strengthened by the availability of angiographic embolization of arterial vessels and by the bolder use of open reduction of pelvic disruptions in conjunction with internal or external fixation devices. Although these changes in attitude and technique bespeak a growing confidence in the minds of surgeons treating pelvic disruptions and associated injuries, there are some aspects to this overall problem that do not seem to change.

Traffic injuries are still responsible for approximately two of every three pelvic fractures, and because of the kinetic energy involved, these injuries are frequently associated with severe bony disruptions and soft tissue damage. It is probably because of the association of severe vascular chest and head injuries that the mortality rate for pelvic fractures has not substantially moved from the 10% vicinity quoted a decade or more ago,[26,33,35,54,70,72,83,84,93,99] despite the improvements across the board in managing the multitrauma patient; the impact imparted by the mass and velocity of a moving motor vehicle simply disrupts too many critical systems for survival. Another continuing lesson that can be made from this statistic is that even with the improved diagnosis and therapy of the bony injuries (by means of the CT scan and various fixation devices), the major emphasis in severe pelvic fractures and dislocations should be on the associated soft tissues, not the hard tissues. This dictum cannot be repeated too often.[12,18,27,28,59,93,99,100]

Complications of a pelvic fracture or dislocation can be categorized anatomically as (1) osteoarticular, of the pelvis, (2) soft tissue, of the pelvic contents, and (3) associated hard and/or soft tissue, not directly associated with the pelvis and its contents but affecting and affected by the pelvic trauma. (This last category is discussed in other chapters of this text.)

Pelvic fracture complications may also be considered from a chronologic viewpoint: (1) acute—due to the initial force, (2) subacute—due to a later consequence of the initial force or to the therapy required for it, and (3) chronic—due to a persistent effect of acute or subacute complications or to a prolonged treatment program frequently necessitated by a pelvic disruption.

REGIONAL CONSIDERATIONS

The osseous pelvis is a semirigid basinlike structure made up of two innominate bones (formed on each side by an amalgamation of the ilium, ischium, and pubis, which each contribute to the formation of the acetabulum) and by the sacrum and the coccyx. The symphysis pubis, the two sa-

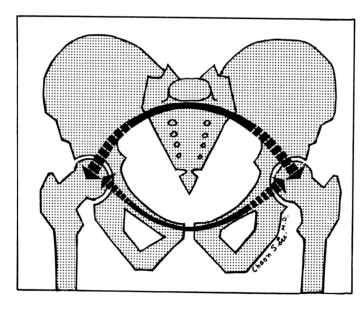

FIG. 25-1. In the erect position, weight-bearing forces are transmitted from the upper femora to the acetabula and then through the thick rings of the ilia, called the arcuate lines, which curve superiorly and posteriorly to the sacroiliac joints and then into the spinal column through the sacrum. This forms the femorosacral arch. This main arch is augmented by a subsidiary tie arch that joins the extremities of the femorosacral arch. The subsidiary arch is made up of the bodies of the pubic bones and their horizontal rami. (Kane, W.J.: Fractures of the pelvis. In Rockwood, C.A., Jr., and Green, D.P. [eds.]: Fractures, 2nd. ed., Vol. 2. Philadelphia, J.B. Lippincott, 1984)

croiliac joints, and the sacrococcygeal joint are virtually immobile but do allow for slight motion, particularly in the young and in pregnant women. The sacroiliac joint, variously described as a diarthrosis or an amphiarthrosis, derives its stability from the undulating concavoconvex surfaces of the sacrum and the ilium, and from the extremely strong and heavy posterior sacroiliac ligaments. Stability is not derived from a keystone shape. Quite the reverse is true: the posterior and superior dimensions of the sacrum are not greater than the anterior and inferior dimensions; therefore, the body weight pressing down on the sacrum does not increase stability as one would expect if the keystone-in-arch principle were at work. This fact is, in my opinion, one of the chief reasons why chronic subluxations of the sacroiliac joint following traumatic disruptions are so symptomatic: the lost stability through the weight-bearing femorosacral or ischiosacral arches allows for motion, and consequently for pain.

Anteriorly, the symphysis pubis, an amphiarthrosis, gains much of its stability from the anterior interpubic ligament, but it is a considerably weaker joint than the sacroiliac joints.[17] It forms a portion of the subsidiary tie arch, which joins the ends of the major weight-bearing, posterior arch; because it is not a weight-bearing arch, subluxations of the symphysis pubis after trauma are usually asymptomatic, and resections of the anterior pelvis may be performed without leading to instability or symptoms (Fig. 25-1).[70,93]

The named arteries of the pelvis are derived from the external and internal iliacs, which are branches of the paired common iliacs. The external iliac gives rise to the inferior epigastric and the deep circumflex iliac and traverses the iliacus and psoas muscles to exit the pelvis as the femoral artery. Since the muscles intervene between the external iliacs and the bony pelvis, these vessels are less often disrupted by sharp fracture edges than are the internal iliac vessels and their branches. The internal iliac artery, also called the hypogastric, supplies most of the pelvis and its contents after dividing into posterior and anterior divisions. The posterior division divides into iliolumbar, lateral sacral, and superior gluteal branches; the anterior division gives rise to the obturator, inferior gluteal, and internal pudendal, which are the parietal vessels, and the umbilical, superior vesical, and middle rectal, and either the male inferior vesical or female uterine–vaginal, which are the visceral branches.

The pelvis is served by nerve branches

of the lumbar and sacral plexuses, which give rise, respectively, to the femoral and sciatic nerves, which traverse the pelvis to the lower extremities. Muscular branches from the lumbar plexus to the quadratus lumborum and psoas and the iliohypogastric branch are usually not involved in fractures of the pelvis. The ilioinguinal, genitofemoral, lateral cutaneous nerve of the thigh, the obturator, and the femoral nerve are occasionally injured in association with pelvic fractures. Likewise, the sacral plexus and its branches, such as muscular branches to the quadratus femoris, gemelli, piriformis, obturator internus, coccygeus, and levator ani, or the pelvic splanchnics, pudendals, gluteals, posterior cutaneous nerve of the thigh, perforating cutaneous nerve, and perineal branch are damaged in conjunction with fractures of the pelvis.

The lower urinary tract is particularly susceptible to trauma in pelvic fractures. The bladder, lying directly behind the symphysis pubis and separated from it by the space of Retzius, is partially covered by peritoneum at its dome. Urinary extravasation from the bladder may therefore be intraperitoneal, extraperitoneal, or both, depending on the location of the laceration. In the male the first portion of the urethra is surrounded by the prostate; below the prostate, the urethra passes through the urogenital diaphragm, made up of the transverse perineal muscles, the bulbourethral glands, and the two investing fascial layers. The distal portion of the urethra passes into the corpus spongiosum of the penis. The female urethra is shorter and more mobile, since the urogenital diaphragm is not so well developed; both factors are responsible for the lower rate of urethral injury in females with pelvic fractures. Posterior to the female bladder are the uterus, cervix, and upper vagina.

The lower gastrointestinal tract within the pelvis consists of a small portion of colon, the rectum, and the anus. The colon has mobility owing to its well-developed mesentery, whereas the rectum, having no mesentery, is immobilized against the anterior sacrum and coccyx, at the distal tip of which it turns downward and backward becoming the anus, passing through the levatores ani.

PREVENTION

The recognition by the treating physician that complications of pelvic disruptions are common and can be lethal is the first step in their prevention and treatment. This awareness affects the priority and import that are given to their diagnosis and treatment in the welter of management of the multiple injuries of a typical multiple-system injury victim.

Basic resuscitative measures are directed toward obtaining a clear airway, adequate respiration, effective cardiac output and peripheral perfusion, and control of serious hemorrhage. A general history and overall physical examination, to the extent that such is possible and feasible, is taken for baseline purposes.

Many hospital emergency rooms insist that patients (1) who are unconscious owing to trauma or (2) who have sustained a fracture of a major bone of the lower extremity owing to trauma be assumed to have a fracture of the pelvis until proven otherwise. This precaution helps one to avoid missing such diagnoses as a fractured proximal femur or dislocated hip, especially in the presence of an ipsilateral fracture of the distal femur or tibia or a fracture-dislocation of the pelvis.

An important step in taking the history is to determine the approximate energy forces and vectors and the chronology of the accident and subsequent care leading up to the present complaints, if these data can be elicited. The state of the lower genitourinary tract can initially be estimated by determining pretrauma fluid intake, posttrauma voiding, if any, and the present state of bladder sensation. Blood within the vaginal vault must be assessed according to the woman's menstrual history and the possibility of pregnancy.

Examination for intra-abdominal and urinary tract injury by means of clinical, laboratory, and roentgenographic tests should be undertaken while similar studies are directed at osseous injuries. A very useful and too frequently omitted examination is the rectal examination, for not only may pelvic fragments be palpated, but a prostate that is mobile and high-riding is pathognomonic for a disruption of the posterior urethra (Fig. 25-2).

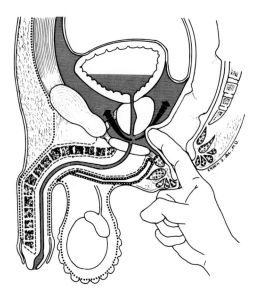

FIG. 25-2. Rectal examination reveals that the prostate is retracted upward and backward out of its normal position. This is pathognomonic of posterior disruption of the urethra. The mobility of the prostate is due to the fact that the puboprostatic ligaments have been disrupted. Extravasation of urine into the extraperitoneal perivesical space occurs. (Kane, W.J.: Fractures of the pelvis. In Rockwood, C.A., Jr., and Green, D.P. [eds.]: Fractures, 2nd. ed., Vol. 2. Philadelphia, J.B. Lippincott, 1984)

Radiographic studies of the pelvis should be simple and efficient at the outset and should consist of a plain AP view that will serve as a screening film. Later, special views such as tilt or oblique views can be obtained as warranted. Contrast studies of the urinary tract and vascular system may also be appropriate at this point.

It is perhaps worthwhile to remind oneself that during the diagnostic phase of the management, therapeutic steps may be taken: application of compression dressings for external hemorrhage, extremity splinting, and fluid replacement. Certainly, the patient should be protected from unneeded, uncomfortable, and unsafe movement of the pelvic fragments that could be brought about by frequent patient transfers and that, in turn, could lead to further damage to the bony fragments and the adjacent soft tissues.

CLASSIFICATION

This classification set forth below is useful, since it facilitates therapeutic and prognostic decisions. For example, the first two groups are stable, whereas the third group is unstable and requires a considerably longer period of protection from weight bearing. Also, patients in the third group, generally reflecting greater trauma, sustain much higher blood losses than those in the first two groups, and the identification of a Group III fracture alerts the physician to the likely need of early blood replacement.[33] The classification, while helpful in avoiding

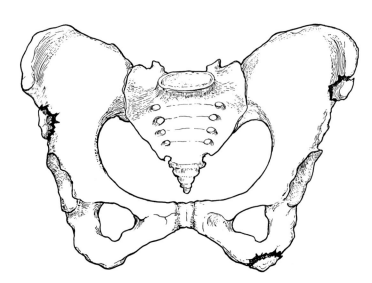

FIG. 25-3. Avulsion fractures. This illustration demonstrates a left anterior superior iliac spine avulsion, a right anterior inferior iliac spine avulsion, and a left ischial tuberosity avulsion. (Kane, W.J.: Fractures of the pelvis. In Rockwood, C.A., Jr., and Green, D.P. [eds.]: Fractures, 2nd. ed., Vol. 2. Philadelphia, J.B. Lippincott, 1984)

the overtreatment of stable fractures and the undertreatment of unstable fractures, cannot be relied on exclusively, since the "most common and catastrophic [pitfall] is to treat an obvious fracture and overlook some associated visceral injury.[57] Even simple and apparently benign pelvic fractures may be associated with serious complicating soft tissue injuries.

Classification of Fractures of the Pelvis[45,46,49,*]

Class I: Fractures of individual bones without a break in the continuity of the pelvic ring
  1. Avulsion fractures
      a. Anterior superior iliac spine
      b. Anterior inferior iliac spine
      c. Ischial tuberosity
  2. Fracture of the pubis or ischium
  3. Fracture of wing of the ilium (Duverney's fracture)
  4. Fracture of sacrum
  5. Fracture or dislocation of the coccyx
Class II: A single break in the pelvic ring
  1. Fracture of two ipsilateral rami
  2. Fracture near or subluxation of the symphysis pubis
  3. Fracture near or subluxation of the sacroiliac joint
Class III: Double breaks in the pelvic ring
  1. Double vertical fractures and/or dislocation of the pubis (straddle fracture)
  2. Double vertical fractures and/or dislocations (Malgaigne's fracture)
  3. Severe multiple fractures

---

* See also Figures 25-3 through 25-8.
(Modified from Key, J.A., and Conwell, H.E.: Management of Fractures, Dislocations and Sprains. St. Louis, C.V. Mosby, 1951)

SPECIFIC COMPLICATIONS AND THEIR MANAGEMENT

Osteoarticular Complications

Osteoarticular complications of pelvic disruptions include delayed union, nonunion, malunion, osteomyelitis, chronic subluxation, and chronic septic arthritis.

For most fractures there are generally accepted periods during which union might

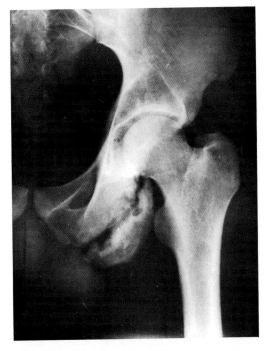

FIG. 25-4. An avulsion of the left ischial tuberosity shows considerable new bone formation 8 weeks after injury. (Kane, W.J.: Fractures of the pelvis. In Rockwood, C.A., Jr., and Green, D.P. [eds.]: Fractures, 2nd. ed., Vol. 2. Philadelphia, J.B. Lippincott, 1984)

be expected to occur, given all of the factors and influences, intrinsic and extrinsic, that were present at the time of injury. (Intrinsic factors include comminution, soft tissue interposition, and whether the fracture is open; extrinsic factors include the patient's age and general health and the presence of associated fractures and injuries.) If a fracture fails to heal during this period, it is then considered a delayed union, but, given further time and additional nonoperative care, such as bedrest or protection from weight bearing, it is expected that a delayed union can heal. If that expectation is not met, the delayed union has become a nonunion, and no further healing will occur without operative intervention. The presence or absence of the potential for healing is the critical factor in determining whether a delayed union or a nonunion is present.

There are two factors that tend to limit the use of the term *delayed union* with respect to pelvic fractures: first, the pelvis,

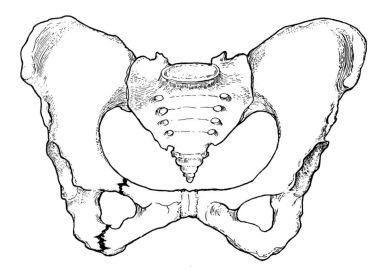

FIG. 25-5. Fractures of the right superior and inferior pubic rami. (Kane, W.J.: Fractures of the pelvis. In Rockwood, C.A., Jr., and Green, D.P. [eds.]: Fractures, 2nd. ed., Vol. 2. Philadelphia, J.B. Lippincott, 1984)

with its lush intraosseous and extraosseous blood supply, usually provides a ready foundation for bony healing, and second, there is no well-defined and widely accepted timetable for the healing of various pelvic fractures, especially the more severe types.

The prevention of delayed union begins with the proper diagnosis and classification of those fractures that have a high potential for slow union owing to their inherent instability. Also important are persistence in pursuing the correct treatment in the face of growing discontent in a patient who may otherwise be feeling well, and appro-

priate reluctance to convert a closed pelvic fracture to an open one without a weighty and otherwise unachievable goal. Although it is important to stress the avoidance of delayed or nonunions, greater emphasis must be given to avoiding prolonged immobilization in the elderly, since their ability to resist the complications of prolonged bedrest must be weighed against their ability to deal with the problems incurred from a potential nonunion.

Nonunion of pelvic fractures has been considered to be uncommon, but Hundley reported 20 symptomatic nonunions among

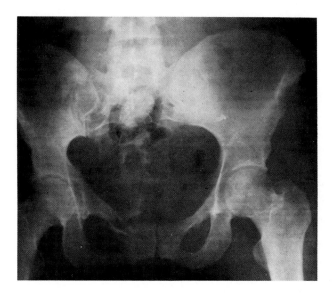

FIG. 25-6. A comminuted fracture of the superior pubic ramus and a fracture of the inferior pubic ramus at its junction with the body of the pubis. (Kane, W.J.: Fractures of the pelvis. In Rockwood, C.A., Jr., and Green, D.P. [eds.]: Fractures, 2nd. ed., Vol. 2. Philadelphia, J.B. Lippincott, 1984)

Fig. 25-7. This Malgaigne fracture consists of a symphyseal separation, fractures of the left superior and left inferior rami, a left sacroiliac dislocation with cephalad displacement of the intervening fragment, and a fracture of the wing of the ilium (Duverney's fracture). (Kane, W.J.: Fractures of the pelvis. In Rockwood, C.A., Jr., and Green, D.P. [eds.]: Fractures, 2nd. ed., Vol. 2. Philadelphia, J.B. Lippincott, 1984)

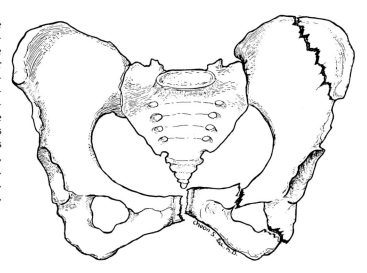

141 pelvic fracture patients.[39] The nonunions occurred only in severe displacement, and 18 of them were Malgaigne fractures (Fig. 25-9). Pennal and Massiah reported 42 patients with pelvic delayed union and nonunion.[71] The average age of the patients was 35, and most were treated nonoperatively with apparently very short periods of immobilization, averaging 8.4 weeks. Tile[96] and Rubash and associates[85] each reported eight patients with nonunion. Only one of Tile's patients required surgical treatment, but in Rubash's series, all were treated surgically and obtained a sound union with general symptomatic relief. It is apparent that there is considerable variation in the treatment of an established nonunion.

The diagnosis of pelvic nonunion is made by a review of the history of pelvic trauma, a critical evaluation of the adequacy of subsequent therapy, and an evaluation of relevant films and the presenting chief complaint, usually pain and discomfort, particularly after stress and activity. Other attendant complaints may include a sense of instability and a limp due to pain or leg-length discrepancy. Physical examination of the pelvic region may reveal palpable

Fig. 25-8. This Malgaigne fracture consists of a symphyseal subluxation, fractures of the left superior and inferior rami, and a dislocation of the left sacroiliac joint. In addition, there is a fracture through the posterior wing of the ilium. (Kane, W.J.: Fractures of the pelvis. In Rockwood, C.A., Jr., and Green, D.P. [eds.]: Fractures, 2nd. ed., Vol. 2. Philadelphia, J.B. Lippincott, 1984)

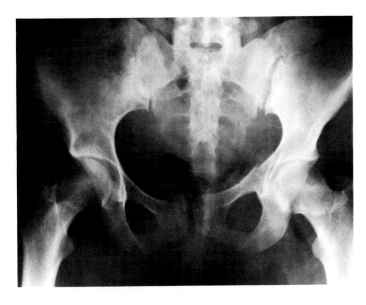

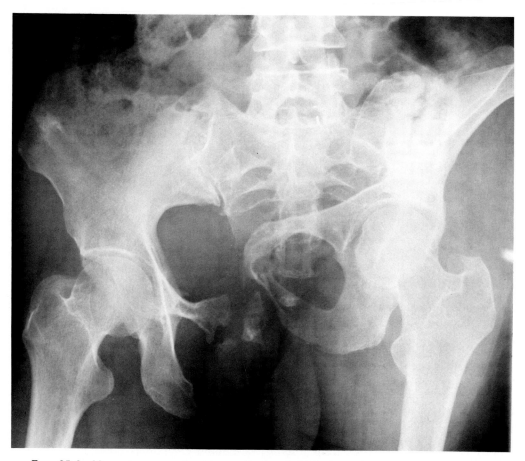

FIG. 25-9. Nonunion secondary to a displaced Malgaigne fracture with established nonunion of the left sacroiliac joint and disruption of the symphysis pubis. Previous attempts at correction included wiring of the symphysis pubis, with no subsequent benefit derived.

instability on compression and during walking in place. Persistent, localized tenderness may be noted, and, on occasion, an audible click or clunk may accompany such maneuvers as iliac crest compression, walking in place, or the FABER test. Plain films, bone scans, and CT scans ordinarily clinch the diagnosis.[91]

The treatment of nonunion of the pelvis should begin with consideration of whether the ununited fragment is the cause of the symptoms, whether the symptoms warrant intervention, and whether the intervention should be directed at repair of the nonunion or excision of the ununited fragment. Since fragments such as those of the distal coccyx and iliac wing or spines do not provide structural stability for the weight-bearing

arches, it is my opinion that, if symptoms warrant, these fragments should be excised.[20,45,101] On the other hand, a painful nonunion through the posterior weight-bearing arch in the vicinity of the sacroiliac joint deserves a vigorous attempt at achieving consolidation of the fragments or arthrodesis of the joint by means of standard orthopaedic approaches to such problems, including bone grafting, decortication, and the use of internal or external splints.[29,31,41,48,53,60,61,64,86,94,95] Hundley was able to treat ten patients for pelvic nonunion with grafting, and all returned to their normal occupation, while none of those who did not undergo surgery did.[39] Of Pennal and Massiah's group of 42 patients, 24 were treated nonoperatively by casts and other devices; ten of these achieved bony union, five returned to their preinjury jobs, seven were rated totally and permanently disabled, and two were rated at a 50% permanent disability. Of the 18 operated on, stabilization and bone grafting were performed in 16; 15 achieved bony union, 11 returned to their preinjury jobs, and none was rated permanently disabled.[71]

What has been said for nonunion applies, in general, for symptomatic subluxation at the symphysis or sacroiliac joint.[9,14,40,55,104] It should be recalled, however, that these joints are especially susceptible to the relaxing characteristics of the hormones elaborated in women just prior to parturition, and consequently, injuries sustained by the woman close to the time of delivery may best be treated by keeping her in a lateral decubitus position in bed. For the same reason, it is theoretically possible that a woman who previously sustained traumatic pelvic joint disruptions might become more symptomatic than the typical third-trimester patient, since her symphyseal and/or sacroiliac ligaments have previously been subject to injury and repair. In such an instance it would be reasonable to anticipate that parturition and bedrest in the full lateral position for a short time postpartum would lead to remission of symptoms.

To achieve union or arthrodesis in a pelvic nonunion or subluxation, stability must be restored to the pelvic ring, and the area should be bone grafted on a bed of decorticated or fish-scaled bone. Since motion in one locus of the pelvic ring betokens motion in another, it is essential to recognize that the major sitting and standing weight-bearing lines of the pelvis run posteriorly and not anteriorly.[13,25,33,55] The symphysis pubis can, for example, in the face of an intact posterior ring, be excised with no effect on the femoroiliosacral or ischiosacral weight-bearing arches. This principle means that the major effort at achieving union should be directed posteriorly. This is not to say, however, that no efforts should be directed anteriorly, but the need is greater posteriorly. The bone stock is bulkier there (and consequently, the likelihood of success is greater), and the complications attendant to a late surgical intervention in the vicinity of the symphysis pubis (*e.g.,* damage to the

urethra, postoperative infection, and failure of internal splinting designed to hold the two pubes together; Fig. 25-10) can be more serious and are more common than those in the posterior structures.

The symphysis pubis can be approached through a low transverse abdominal incision, and after positioning the hemipelves with effective bone clamps, the superior surfaces and the anterior surfaces of the superior pubes can be used for two compression plates applied at right angles to each other.

Iliac nonunions are best approached through an incision over the iliac crest, on each side of the usually vertically oriented nonunion. The gluteus muscles are minimally retracted to allow compression plating after debridement of the pseudarthrosis and autogenous bone grafting.

Sacral nonunions and sacroiliac subluxations are approached through vertical incisions slightly medial to the sacroiliac joints; in nonunion the surgeon will be directly on it, and in subluxation a slightly medial skin incision will allow direct visualization of the sacroiliac joint, which runs from posteromedial to anterolateral. Debridement of the sacroiliac ligamentous remnants can thus be accomplished with a curet or high-speed burr. Because compression of the sacroiliac joint across the interposed cancellous bone graft is desirable, fixation is obtained with various devices. Cancellous lag screws pass through a compression plate that dissipates the force of the screwheads; the screws and plate transfix the joint in a posteromedial to anteromedial direction, perpendicular to the line of the joint, and then pass into the heavy lateral portions of the sacrum. Another method compresses both ilia against the sacrum by means of sharp Leatherman hooks (originally designed for scoliotic spines) inserted into the lateral posterior margins of both ilia and then connected by a $^3/_{16}$-inch compression rod and the necessary nuts; two such sets are used, one superiorly and one inferiorly along the sacroiliac joint. This latter method does require a contralateral incision for insertion of the opposite hooks, and it is advised that the apparatus be removed in a year if mobility of the untraumatized sacroiliac joint is desirable in a premeno-

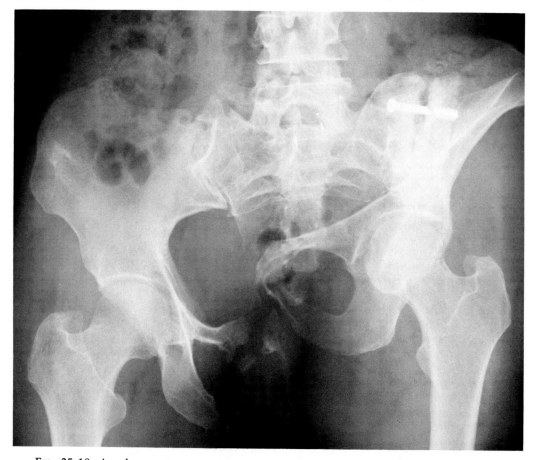

FIG. 25-10. A subsequent repeat attempt at resolution of the pelvic nonunion in the patient shown in Figure 25-9, in which a single screw was used in conjunction with bone grafting, was unsuccessful.

pausal woman who might subsequently become pregnant. In a man or postmenopausal woman, removal of the apparatus is unnecessary.

Whatever the method, sacroiliac fusion is the treatment of choice. Smith-Peterson and Rogers achieved a pain-free state in 89% (23/26) of their patients, and 96% (25/26) returned to their previous occupation (Figs. 25-11 and 25-12).[90]

Malunion of pelvic fragments may be caused by inability to obtain a reduction owing to comminution, inability to achieve reduction short of open surgery, inability to maintain reduction owing to the patient's premature return to activity, or an unjustified estimate of bony stability by the physician. Unstable fractures of the pelvis re-

quire careful and repeated clinical and roentgenographic studies before judgments about increasing activity can be made.

Fortunately, symptomatic malunions tend to be uncommon, and it is unlikely that they would disrupt function to the point where refracture of the pelvis is warranted. Correction of problems of ambulation secondary to pelvic malunion is better handled by surgery and other remedies directed at the lower extremities than those directed at the pelvis.[90] Presumably, overriding of the symphysis pubis could compromise female subsymphyseal dimensions to the extent that sexual activity could be hindered; although I have not personally seen such a complication as the result of trauma, I am aware that it has occurred. It may therefore be necessary in dyspareunia secondary to traumatic alteration of the pubic arch to consider resection of the anterior pelvic ring on one or both sides of the symphysis pubis. In women of child-bearing age, alterations of the pelvis so extensive as to obstruct normal childbirth will necessitate caesarean section. Exostoses secondary to avulsion of tendinous attachments at the pelvis have required excision in rare instances,[20] and the same treatment may be needed in situations in which myositis ossificans disrupts function; careful timing of such surgery on mature myositis ossificans must be exercised to avoid recurrence.

Osteomyelitis or septic arthritis following pelvic fractures is a very serious complication but is apparently uncommon.[13,65,76] Sepsis can occur as a result of open fracture, as a result of violation of the gut by bone fragments, leading to contamination of the fracture hematoma, or, finally, as a result of surgical intervention undertaken to manage a concurrent intra-abdominal surgical emergency, such as visceral disruption or hemorrhage. Missile wounds of the pelvis are particularly susceptible to sepsis, since the missile and its kinetic energy create secondary tissue fragments and cavitation that, in turn, cause sufficient damage to the various viscera that a laparotomy is almost mandatory. In Lucas's series of 20 patients, chronic sepsis, usually with a mixed bacterial flora containing at least one gram-negative organism, occurred in 11.[56] Early preventive steps include laparotomy, diversion of the fecal or urinary stream, and usually drainage of the deep pelvis by coccygectomy. Later therapy includes secondary closure at 7 to 10 days, if possible, or continued open treatment if necessary. Later, debridement and suction-irrigation are used in conjunction with other procedures designed to improve function.

Vascular Complications

Major arterial injury complicates approximately 1% of fractures of the pelvis.* The internal iliac artery is more susceptible to injury than is the external iliac because the internal iliac is less well buffered by muscle

---

* Moore, J.R.: Personal communication.

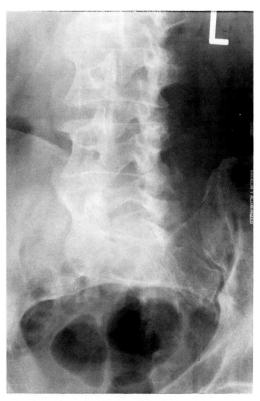

FIG. 25-11. Oblique view of a painful chronic subluxation of the left sacroiliac joint secondary to a displaced Malgaigne fracture sustained 2 years previously.

tissue from the inner wall of the pelvis. The damage to arteries may be due to a laceration, an intimal tear, or an arterial thrombosis, and it is believed that the closed variety of arterial trauma is more common than open laceration. Careful physical examination of the lower extremities should include determinations of distal pulses, temperature, color, capillary filling, and neurologic function. Limb ischemia and generalized hypotension are the typical presenting features of cases with major arterial trauma associated with pelvic fractures.[52] Rothenberger and associates[84] found that patients with open fractures of the pelvis had a fivefold higher mortality rate than did patients with closed pelvic fractures. This was due not only to sepsis, but also to major vascular injury, particularly among pedestrians and motorcyclists, so much so that the authors advocated im-

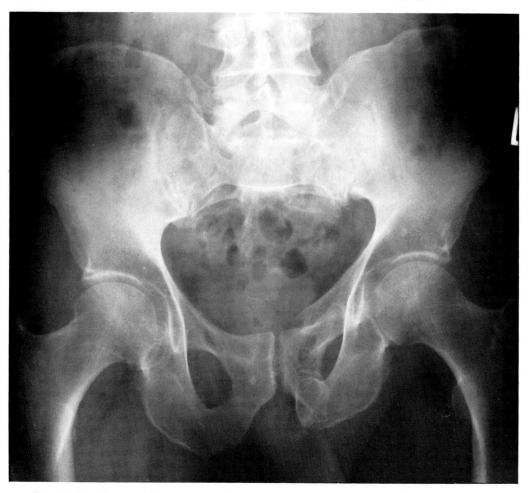

FIG. 25-12. AP view of the pelvis shown in Figure 25-11, 18 months following sacroiliac fusion and successful resolution of symptomatic arthritis.

mediate exploration in pedestrians and motorcyclists who were hypotensive in conjunction with an open pelvic fracture sustained in a motor-vehicle accident.

Once it has been determined that the generalized hypotension has been successfully counteracted, it is imperative not to ascribe hypoperfusion of a limb to "vascular spasm." It is at this point that angiography offers a great opportunity for specific diagnosis of arterial disruptions, and its use should be considered whenever pulses distal to the fracture site diminish or disappear following reduction of the fracture, when a bruit is auscultated, when an extremely large or pulsating hematoma is noted, or when there is severe or recurrent hemorrhage through an open wound.[88]

If arteriography indicates the need for surgical repair, the operative treatment of the injury should follow the standard precepts of anastomosis and grafting. The use of a Fogarty catheter to extract clot material from the distal arterial tree should be followed by irrigation with heparinized saline (5000 units/50 ml saline).[83]

The rich arterial and venous anastomotic network of the pelvis and its viscera is frequently injured, and consequently, retroperitoneal hemorrhage of some degree is an inevitable complication of pelvic fractures. In general, the greater the comminution and displacement of the pelvic fracture, the more massive the local hemorrhage. In addition, fractures through the posterior two thirds of the pelvis are associated with more hemorrhage because more trauma is required to produce a fracture in this area and because the major vessels are situated along the fracture lines. Overall, close to half of all pelvic fracture patients require transfusion.[33,45] The study by Hauser and Perry[32] demonstrated that unstable fractures of the pelvic ring require transfusions 2.5 times more frequently than do the other types of pelvic fractures, and when the transfusions are given, they require 2.5 times as much blood. In a number of series it has been demonstrated that hemorrhage is the most serious complication of pelvic fractures and is directly responsible for approximately 50% of the fatalities in these series.[8,33,70,103] In the series by Conolly and Hedberg,[12] hemorrhagic shock or renal failure secondary to shock was responsible for 75% of the fatalities. The gross mortality for all pelvic fracture patients is approximately 10%, and for major pelvic fractures it is approximately 30%.

Signs and symptoms associated with significant hemorrhage from pelvic fracture can frequently be misinterpreted; associated injuries are blamed for the findings, and the diagnosis of retroperitoneal hemorrhage secondary to pelvic fracture may be temporarily overlooked, especially in the unconscious patient. In other instances there is little doubt as to the cause of the traumatic shock. The diagnosis classically depends on the physical findings of a pale, sweaty, restless patient with a thready, rapid pulse. Contusions about the pelvis, demonstrable pelvic instability on examination of the subcutaneous areas or on compression tests raise the index of suspicion. The arterial pressure is down, as is urinary output, and radiographic studies confirm the extent of the pelvic fractures. The use of contrast agents to determine the integrity of the lower urinary tract may reveal the displacement of these organs secondary to hematoma. Retroperitoneal hemorrhage can mimic intraperitoneal injury with muscle spasm, guarding, rigidity, tenderness, and the hypoactive bowel signs and

distention of ileus. Peritoneal lavage may be needed to discriminate between the two possibilities. Its usefulness and accuracy have been described in a number of reports.[15,19,30,34,36,67,75,81] It has been especially useful in unconscious patients, for whom general anesthesia and laparotomy, unnecessarily undertaken, could be extremely hazardous. It must be emphasized, however, that a laparotomy is well indicated if there is undeniable evidence of intraperitoneal bleeding or visceral perforation. Abdominal CT scans are also useful in diagnosis.[21] Less widely accepted indications for laparotomy include uncontrollable bleeding or the continuing expansion of a suprapubic hematoma.

The usefulness of laparotomy for the direct control of pelvic bleeding is, at the moment, undecided. Undeniably, this heroic measure has saved some patients, but in other instances it has failed. The basis for failure is that ligation of one or more of the named arterial branches after a difficult exposure in a shocky patient may not solve the problem, since there can be "backbleeding" through the rich collateral circulation, and ligation of the arterial system may have little effect if the major bleeding is venous. Another disadvantage of this type of surgical approach is that it causes a loss of the tamponade effect, which the retroperitoneum can usually provide if it is intact.

If surgery is attempted in these circumstances, another critical factor that has been poorly defined is timing. Although some argue that direct control of pelvic bleeding should not be considered until after 20 units of whole blood have been administered,[80] others argue for prompt surgery if a full blood volume replacement in the first hour after arrival at the hospital does not provide sustained circulatory response.[77] Given the lack of consensus,[23,24,33,39,62,63,78,88] I would use this procedure only as a last resort, when all other avenues of therapy have failed.

Fortunately, recent advances in the control of hemorrhage secondary to pelvic fractures have been made. An external counterpressure suit, variously known as an external-counterpressure suit or military antishock trouser (MAST), has been used to help control bleeding and combat shock in patients with pelvic fractures. Counterpressure suits are commercially available; they consist of either wraparound vinyl bags or multiple-compartment trouserlike arrangements that extend from the ankles to the epigastrium and are inflated with air to a pressure of 20 to 25 torr.

Following initial evaluation of the patient's injuries, the counterpressure suit is applied when hypovolemic shock cannot be controlled by whole blood volume replacement. The unit is left in place when retroperitoneal hemorrhage appears to be the problem, or it is applied immediately postoperatively, when abdominal exploration is necessary. All patients have an endotracheal tube in place and are managed with a volume-cycled respirator while the suit is inflated. Ordinarily, this suit is deflated every 6 hours to review the evidence for or against recurrence of the hemorrhage and to inspect the skin. If the counterpressure suit has been applied before the presence or absence of an intraperitoneal problem has been established, more frequent observations in the early postadmission hours will be necessary.

The counterpressure suit is usually left in place from 24 to 48 hours, depending on the patient's clinical response, and then the suit is gradually deflated, or if a multiple-compartment unit is used, the compartments are deflated sequentially, to diminish the impact of any hypotension that might develop as the counterpressure is reduced.

A decrease in vital capacity as a consequence of compression of the abdomen and lower chest by the MAST has been reported. This problem has been minimized by the use of the endotracheal tube with a volume-cycled respirator. An additional benefit of the use of a counterpressure suit is that it does immobilize pelvic fractures and does not seriously complicate lower-extremity fracture care.[5,69]

The physiological effects of the counterpressure suit can be divided into local and systemic ones. The suit increases the extraluminal pressure, thereby reducing the effect of the transmural pressure gradient, which is the effective force expelling blood from a lacerated vessel. As counterpressure reduces transmural pressure, arterial and venous bleeding diminish. External counterpressure also reduces the radii of vessels. According to the Law of Laplace, a decrease in the radius of the vessel will cause a decrease in the tension in the wall of that vessel and, therefore, a decrease in the size of the laceration. It can therefore be seen that the mechanisms by which the counterpressure suit reduces bleeding are by reducing the laceration size and by reducing transmural pressure. This explains why the application of only 20 to 25 torr will arrest massive bleeding from arteries with substantially higher arterial pressures.

The systemic effects of a counterpressure suit are an increase in blood pressure, an increase in central venous pressure, and an increase in cardiac output with no change in circulating plasma volume. These are accomplished by an autotransfusion effect with shunting of blood from those areas under the suit to those areas outside the suit. The volume of this autotransfusion has been estimated to be approximately 1000 ml of blood. Because of these latter effects, the counterpressure suit has been used by rescue squads at accident scenes to provide an emergency autotransfusion (Fig. 25-13).[47]

Another useful development in the control of hemorrhage associated with pelvic fractures is the use of angiography to identify bleeding sites within the pelvis, followed by embolization with autologous blood clots or plugs of Gelfoam. The infusion of vasoconstrictors, which has been used successfully in gastrointestinal tract bleeding, has not been useful in the management of pelvic fractures. The occlusion of torn vessels with inflated intra-arterial balloon catheters is also being investigated.[1,58,80,89] It is obvious that as experience grows in the use of this form of hemorrhage control, it will offer definite advantages over laparotomy, in that it can be performed under local anesthesia without turning the patient or interrupting other therapeutic measures. It should be emphasized, however, that the procedure is not available universally, and its success depends on a great deal of multispecialty expertise and cooperation.[2,3,43,92,98,105]

The management of hemorrhage second-

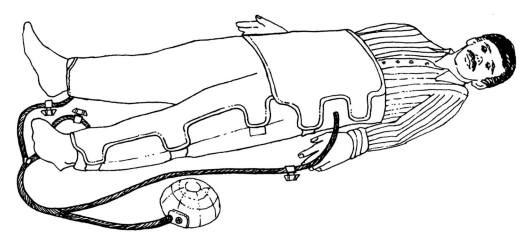

FIG. 25-13. An external-counterpressure suit can be applied to diminish bleeding and to effect the autotransfusion of approximately 2 units of blood from the areas beneath the suit to the core areas that are outside of the suit. (Redrawn from a pamphlet of the David C. Clark Co., Worcester, Mass. 06104)

ary to pelvic fracture should commence with whole blood replacement and the use of a counterpressure suit. Evidence of continuing blood loss and the need for blood replacement would then indicate that consideration be given to angiography and selective embolization with clotting substances if the method is available. Only in the last instance should laparotomy with direct ligation of the bleeding vessel or its proximal source be considered. Another basic in the successful management of hemorrhage associated with pelvic fracture is the early reduction and immobilization of the pelvic fracture.[66,70,82] With the bones in apposition, pressure will be exerted on marrow vessels, and immobilization will augment the benefits derived from the tamponade effect of the retroperitoneum. Overall, serious consideration must be given to the benefits derived from any procedure that requires movement or transportation of the patient, for such benefits must be weighed against the disadvantages occasioned by motion at the fracture sites.

Injuries of the Lower Urinary Tract

Ruptures of the bladder or urethra occur in approximately 13% of patients with pelvic fractures, based on a survey of 4750 cases reported in the literature, but all pelvic fracture patients must be assumed to have urinary tract injuries until proved otherwise, and little or no pathognomonic significance can be ascribed to hematuria or its absence.[6,45,73,102] The inability to void following pelvic trauma may be indicative of serious urologic injury, or it may simply be due to hemorrhage and edema, causing bladder displacement and subsequent urethral stretching and sphincter spasm.

Although there is not absolute correlation between the type of pelvic fracture and the type of urinary trauma, it has been noted that patients with fractures of the anterior pelvis have a higher incidence of urinary tract involvement, particularly those patients with symphyseal separations and fractures of both pubic rami, and most especially those patients with bilateral vertical fractures of the pubis (butterfly fractures).[22,97]

A suggested routine for the evaluation of urologic trauma in association with pelvic fractures should begin with the recognition that a high index of suspicion is essential and that even if the patient has voided grossly clear urine voluntarily, complacency should not be tolerated. Hematuria, whether gross or microscopic, is sufficient indication for a cystogram, and in the male, a urethrogram.

On admission to the emergency room and following resuscitative and diagnostic procedures with greater priority, the patient should be transferred to a proper stretcher that is light, radiolucent, and comfortable.[82]

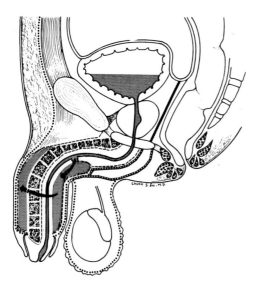

FIG. 25-14. Partial anterior urethral disruption allows extravasation of urine into the penis. The extravasation is limited by Buck's fascia, which is intact. (Kane, W.J.: Fractures of the pelvis. In Rockwood, C.A., Jr., and Green, D.P. [eds.]: Fractures, 2nd. ed., Vol. 2. Philadelphia, J.B. Lippincott, 1984)

A quick history should be obtained, followed by a thorough physical examination, including a rectal examination and possibly an abdominal paracentesis and lavage. Initial radiographic examination of the pelvis defines and focuses attention on a number of sites of concern, and at this point the specific urologic evaluation is undertaken. Urethral catheterization should be performed unless there is significant suspicion of anterior urethral damage based on a history or physical examination that supports the likelihood of a tear of the anterior urethra. A straddle injury with obvious penile or perineal trauma would be an example. In such an instance, a urethrogram should be performed first. The catheterization or urethrogram should be followed by a cystogram and a post-emptying film of the bladder. Intravenous excretory urography should be undertaken when it is indicated by previously obtained information and when it is feasible. In a similar light, cystoscopy and retrograde pyelography may be indicated under certain circumstances.

Rupture of the anterior urethra is uncommonly seen with pelvic fractures in general but may be seen with straddle injuries. The diagnosis is made largely on the basis of the history of the method of injury and signs of perineal or genital injury. In association with the rupture of the anterior urethra, hematuria is commonly seen, and contusions and ecchymoses of the perineum and penis may be noted, as well as signs of extrapelvic extravasation of urine. Under such circumstances, the first diagnostic step after radiographic examination of the pelvis would be to perform a urethrogram (2 ml 30% Renografin) via a bulb syringe. Extraurethral extravasation of the dye confirms the diagnosis. Treatment consists first of a gentle attempt to pass a 5-ml-bag Foley catheter; the diameter of the Foley catheter depends on the diameter of the urethral meatus. If this is unsuccessful, introduction of a soft rubber straight catheter should be attempted—gently—but if this is unsuccessful, no third attempt should be made. If catheterization is successful, the catheter should be left in place for 10 to 14 days if rupture is incomplete or if the extravasation is not extensive, and antibiotic therapy should be instituted. For extensive anterior urethral injury with a considerable amount of extravasation of urine and blood, it will be necessary to perform a urinary diversion by means of a cystostomy and surgical restoration of the continuity of the injured urethra. The complications of this serious injury include infection with abscess formation and necrosis of the urethra, followed by urethral strictures or fistulae (Fig. 25-14).[11]

Rupture of the posterior urethra is the most common lower urinary tract injury seen with pelvic fractures in the male. The membranous urethra is more commonly ruptured than the prostatic urethra. Usually this injury is associated with the severe anterior pelvic displacement seen in transverse pelvic crushes, which result in a lengthened anteroposterior diameter of the pelvis and consequent disruption of the urethra at its entrance into the urogenital diaphragm. The diagnosis is facilitated by the patient's inability to micturate despite a desire to do so and by inability to pass a catheter into the bladder. Bleeding at the external urethral meatus is commonly seen, but this is of variable import in making the diagnosis. Of greatest importance is the rectal examination, which shows a cephalad displacement of the prostate that is pathognomonic for rupture of the posterior urethra. Direct urethrography demonstrates intrapelvic urinary extravasation and confirms the diagnosis.

Briefly, the goals of treatment are to reestablish urethral continuity and to avoid infection. At the outset the patient should be discouraged from attempts to micturate, and adequate urinary diversion should be accomplished by means of a cystostomy. Drainage of urine and blood from the perivesical space is usually considered essential, and the reestablishment of normal urethral alignment and continuity should be handled either by early surgery and the subsequent maintenance of continuity with a traction catheter for 10 to 14 days, or, alternatively, by avoiding early surgery and performing a cystostomy followed by reconstructive urethral surgery 3 months after the injury. A discussion of the merits of each approach to the establishment of urethral continuity is beyond the scope of this chapter. Antibiotic therapy should be initiated and continued for an appropriate period.

The complications of posterior urethral rupture are infection with abscess formation followed by urethral stricture and fistula formation.[16] Less commonly seen is the development of urinary bladder stones. Incontinence and impotence are also complications of this common and serious injury associated with pelvic fracture.[50]

The urinary bladder is ruptured in approximately 4% of pelvic fractures, although the rate seems to be decreasing.[45] The mechanism of disruption may be perforation by bone fragments, or it may be sudden compression of the distended viscus.[44,57] Extraperitoneal ruptures are four times as common as intraperitoneal ruptures and are associated with "butterfly" fractures and the symphyseal disruptions seen in anterior crushing injuries.[74] Diagnosis is frequently delayed and is complicated by the fact that the patient is in severe shock and complains of lower abdominal pain. The patient is unable to void, and there may be bleeding from the meatus. After 12 to 18 hours, signs of peritoneal irritation may be present and further complicate the establishment of the diagnosis. A boggy fullness on palpation and rectal and vaginal examination is found with extraperitoneal ruptures. If the disruption is into the peritoneal cavity, a peritoneal tap and lavage are of considerable diagnostic benefit. The diagnosis can be established decisively by means of a retrograde cystogram and a roentgenogram made after saline washout of the bladder and its contents. Treatment should be started with a gentle attempt to catheterize first with a Foley catheter and second with a straight, soft, rubber catheter. Prompt urinary diversion by means of a suprapubic cystostomy should be accompanied by drainage of extravasated urine and blood from the intraperitoneal or extraperitoneal spaces. Lacerations of the bladder wall should be repaired at surgery and antibiotic therapy instituted. The complications of bladder rupture include sepsis from cellulitis, abscess formation, and bladder neck fibrosis. Rupture of the urinary bladder is accompanied by a significant mortality rate, and in large measure this is due to the problem of making the diagnosis at an early stage in the treatment of a patient with a pelvic fracture (Fig. 25-15).

MISCELLANEOUS COMPLICATIONS

Neurologic injuries occur in approximately 1% of pelvic fractures.[4,10,37,38,42,51,68] These associated injuries may be due to acute stretching, to bony impingement, or, later, to scar or callus exerting pressure in the vicinity of the healing fracture. Cauda equina injuries seen with the frequently overlooked sacral fractures may lead to root paresis at the level of the first and second sacral roots in conjunction with loss of function in calf, hamstring, and buttock muscle groups and sensory changes over the lateral calf and foot.[7] Pain is not a common finding, and bowel and bladder disturbances are not anticipated.

The major point in managing neurologic complications of pelvic fractures is to recognize the degree of disuse atrophy of the lower limbs seen in the patient with pelvic fracture. If one limb has sustained more extensive muscle loss than the opposite side, with paresis of specific muscle groups, there should be little doubt in making the diagnosis of the previously unsuspected

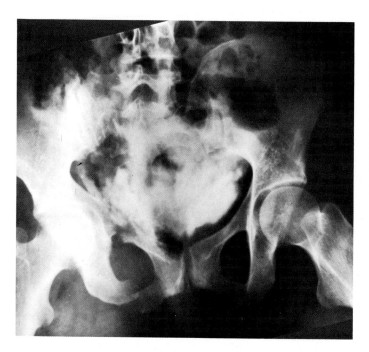

FIG. 25-15. This postvoiding cystogram demonstrates the continued presence of extraperitoneal perivesical contrast material following voiding and saline washout. The rupture was at the inferior portion of the bladder. (Kane, W.J.: Fractures of the pelvis. In Rockwood, C.A., Jr., and Green, D.P. [eds.]: Fractures, 2nd. ed., Vol. 2. Philadelphia, J.B. Lippincott, 1984)

lesion. Sciatic nerve palsy in association with fracture-dislocation of the acetabulum is discussed elsewhere in these volumes.

Other injuries associated with fractures of the pelvis include gynecologic injuries of the uterus and vagina (the latter carries with it a significant morbidity and mortality[70]), as well as testicular and rectal injuries. The accepted management of major rectal wounds has been fecal diversion by colostomy, drainage of the rectal space, closure of the rectal wound, when possible, and the use of systemic antibiotics. Rare injuries associated with pelvic fractures include rupture of the muscles of the abdominal wall and ruptures of the diaphragm. The most important problem in diaphragmatic rupture is the failure to make the diagnosis, as was noted in three of the four cases reported in Peltier's series.[70]

REFERENCES

1. Athanasoulis, C.A.: Angiography to assess pelvic vascular injury. N. Engl. J. Med., 284:1329, 1971.
2. Ayella, R.J., DePriest, R.W., Jr., Khaneja, S.C. et al.: Transcatheter embolization of autologous clot in the management of bleeding associated with fractures of the pelvis. Surg. Gynecol. Obstet., 147:849, 1978.
3. Barlow, B., Rottenberg, R.W., and Santulli, T.V.: Angiographic diagnosis and treatment of bleeding by selective embolization following pelvic fracture in children. J. Pediatr. Surg., 10:939, 1975.
4. Barnett, H.C., and Connolly, E.S.: Lumbosacral nerve root avulsion: Report of a case and review of the literature. J. Trauma, 15:532, 1975.
5. Batalden, D.J., Wickstron, P.H., Ruiz, E., and Gustilo, R.B.: Value of the G suit in patients with severe pelvic fracture. Arch. Surg., 109:326, 1974.
6. Benson, G.S., and Brewer, E.D.: Hematuria: Algorithms for diagnosis: Hematuria in the adult and hematuria secondary to trauma. J.A.M.A., 246:993, 1981.
7. Bonnin, J.G.: Sacral fractures and injuries to the cauda equina. J. Bone Joint Surg., 27:113, 1945.
8. Braunstein, P.W., Skudder, P.A., McCarroll, J.R. et al.: Concealed hemorrhage due to pelvic fracture. J. Trauma, 4:832, 1964.
9. Bucholz, R.W.: The pathological anatomy of Malgaigne fracture-dislocations of the pelvis. J. Bone Joint Surg., 63A:400, 1981.
10. Byrnes, D.P., Russo, G.L., Ducker, T.B., and Cowley, R.A.: Sacrum fractures and neurological damage. J. Neurosurg., 47:459, 1977.
11. Colapinto, V.: Trauma to the pelvis: Urethral injury. Clin. Orthop., 151:46, 1980.
12. Conolly, W.B., and Hedberg, E.A.: Observations on fractures of the pelvis. J. Trauma, 9:104, 1969.
13. Cooke, C.P. III, Levinsohn, E.M., and Baker, B.E.: Septic hip in pelvic fractures with urologic injury: A case report, review of the literature, and discussion of pathophysiology. Clin. Orthop., 147:253, 1980.
14. Day, L.: Open book pelvis: Symphysis pubis diastasis. Orthop. Trans., 2:226, 1978.
15. deVries, J.E., and van der Slikke, W.: False positive peritoneal lavage due to retroperitoneal haematoma. Injury, 12:191, 1980.
16. Diokno, A.C.: Late genitourinary tract complications associated with severe pelvic injury. Surg. Gynecol. Obstet., 150:150, 1980.

17. Dommisse, G.F.: Diametric fractures of the pelvis. J. Bone Joint Surg., 42B:432, 1960.
18. Dorsey, J.S.: Inguinal Aneurism Cured by Tying the External Iliac Artery in the Pelvis. Philadelphia, 820, 1811.
19. Eid, A.M.: Non-urogenital abdominal complications associated with fractures of the pelvis. Arch. Orthop. Trauma Surg., 98:35, 1981.
20. Elton, R.C.: Fracture-dislocation of the pelvis followed by the nonunion of the posterior inferior iliac spine. J. Bone Joint Surg., 54A:648, 1972.
21. Federle, M.P., Crass, R.A., Jeffrey, R. et al.: Computed tomography in blunt abdominal trauma. Arch. Surg., 117:645, 1982.
22. Flaherty, J.J.: Relationship of pelvic bone fracture patterns to injuries of urethra and bladder. J. Urol., 99:297, 1968.
23. Fleming, W.H., and Bowen, J.C. III.: Control of hemorrhage in pelvic crush injuries. J. Trauma, 13:567, 1973.
24. Flint, L.M., Brown, A., Richardson, d J.D., and Polk, H.C.: Definitive control of bleeding from severe pelvic fractures. Ann. Surg., 189:709, 1979.
25. Forsee, G.G.: Clinical observations on pelvic fractures. Am. J. Surg., 38:145, 1924.
26. Froman, C., and Stein, A.: Complicated crushing injuries of the pelvis. J. Bone Joint Surg., 49B:24, 1967.
27. Garcia, A., Jr.: Fractures of the Pelvis. In Bick, E.M. (ed.): Trauma in the Aged, pp. 260–266. New York, McGraw-Hill, 1960.
28. Gilmour, W.R.: Acute fractures of the pelvis. Ann. Surg., 95:161, 1932.
29. Gross, A.: Stabilization of pelvic fractures with Hoffmann external fixation: The French experience. In Brooker, A.F., and Edwards, C.C. (eds.): External Fixation—The Current State of the Art, pp. 123–132. Baltimore, Williams & Wilkins, 1979.
30. Gumbert, J.L., Froderman, S.E., and Mercho, J.P.: Diagnostic peritoneal lavage in blunt abdominal trauma. Ann. Surg., 165:70, 1967.
31. Gunterberg, B., Goldie, I., and Slatis, P.: Fixation of pelvic fractures and dislocations. Acta Orthop. Scand., 49:278, 1978.
32. Hauser, C.W., and Perry, J.F., Jr.: Control of massive hemorrhage from pelvic fractures by hypogastric artery ligation. Surg. Gynecol. Obstet., 121:313, 1965.
33. Hauser, C.W., and Perry, J.F., Jr.: Massive hemorrhage from pelvic fractures. Minn. Med., 49:285, 1966.
34. Hawkins, L., Pomerantz, M., and Eiseman, B.: Laparotomy at the time of pelvic fracture. J. Trauma, 10:619, 1970.
35. Horton, R.E., and Hamilton, S.G.I.: Ligature of the internal iliac artery for massive hemorrhage complicating fracture of the pelvis. J. Bone Joint Surg., 50B:376, 1968.
36. Hubbard, S.G., Bivins, B.A., Sachatello, C.R., and Griffen, W.O., Jr.: Diagnostic errors with peritoneal lavage in patients with pelvic fractures. Arch. Surg., 114:844, 1979.
37. Huittinen, V.M.: Lumbosacral nerve injury in fracture of the pelvis: A postmortem radiographic and patho-anatomical study. Acta. Chir. Scand. [Suppl.], 429:3, 1972.
38. Huittinen, V.M., and Slatis, P.: Nerve injury in double vertical pelvic fractures. Acta. Chir. Scand., 138:571, 1972.
39. Hundley, J.M.: Ununited unstable fractures of the pelvis. J. Bone Joint Surg., 48A:1025, 1966.
40. Jenkins, D.H.R., and Young, M.H.: The operative treatment of sacro-iliac subluxation and disruption of the symphysis pubis. Injury, 10:139, 1978.
41. Johnson, R.: Stabilization of pelvic fractures with Hoffmann external fixation: The Colorado experience. In Brooker, A.F., and Edwards, C.C. (eds.): External Fixation—The Current State of the Art, pp. 133–150. Baltimore, Williams & Wilkins, 1979.
42. Junge, H.: Neurological complications of fractures of the pelvis. Mschr. Unfallh., 55:1, 1952.
43. Kadish, L.J., Stein, J.M., Kotler, S. et al.: Angiographic diagnosis and treatment of bleeding due to pelvic trauma. J. Trauma, 13:1083, 1973.
44. Kaiser, T.F., and Farrow, F.C.: Injury of the bladder and prostatomembranous urethra associated with fracture of the bony pelvis. Surg. Gynecol. Obstet., 120:99, 1965.
45. Kane, W.J.: Fractures of the pelvis. In Rockwood, C.A., Jr., and Green, D.P. (eds.): Fractures. Philadelphia, J.B. Lippincott, 1975.
46. Kane, W.J.: Fractures of the pelvis. In Rockwood, C.A., Jr., and Green, D.P. (eds.): Fractures, 2nd. ed. Philadelphia, J.B. Lippincott, 1984.
47. Kaplan, B.H.: Pneumatic trousers save accident victims' lives. J.A.M.A., 225:686, 1973.
48. Karaharju, E.O., and Slatis, P.: External fixation of double vertical pelvic fractures with a trapezoid compression frame. Injury, 10:142, 1978.
49. Key, J.A., and Conwell, H.E.: Management of Fractures, Dislocations and Sprains, pp. 779–812. St. Louis, C.V. Mosby, 1951.
50. King, J.: Impotence after fractures of the pelvis. J. Bone Joint Surg., 57A:1107, 1975.
51. Lam, C.R.: Nerve injury in fracture of the pelvis. Ann. Surg., 104:945, 1936.
52. Lawson, L.J., and Wainwright, D.: Massive hemorrhage following pelvic fracture: Report of a case. J. Bone Joint Surg., 50B:380, 1968.
53. Letournel, E.: L'osteosynthese des fractures du bassin. In Actualities Orthopediques de l'Hospital Raymond Poincare, Vol. 8. Paris, Masson, 1970.
54. Levine, J.I., and Crampton, R.S.: Major abdominal injuries associated with pelvic fractures. Surg. Gynecol. Obstet., 116:223, 1963.
55. Lewis, M.M., and Arnold, W.D.: Complete anterior dislocation of the sacro-iliac joint. J. Bone Joint Surg., 58A:136, 1976.
56. Lucas, G.L.: Missile wounds of the bony pelvis. J. Trauma, 10:624, 1970.
57. Margolies, M.N., Ring, E.J., Waltman, A.C. et al.: Arteriography in the management of hemorrhage from pelvic fractures. N. Engl. J. Med., 287:317, 1972.
58. McCarroll, J.R. et al.: Fatal pedestrian automotive accidents. J.A.M.A., 180:127, 1962.
59. McLaughlin, H.L.: Fractures of the hips. In Moseley, H.F. (ed.): Accident Surgery. Vol. 1. New York, Appleton-Century-Crofts, 1964.
60. McMurtry, R., Walton, D., Dickinson, D. et al.: Pelvic disruption in the polytraumatized patient. Clin. Orthop., 151:22, 1980.

61. Mears, D.C.: The management of complex pelvic fractures. In Brooker, A.F., and Edwards, C.C. (eds.): External Fixation: The Current State of the Art, pp. 151–177. Baltimore, Williams & Wilkins, 1979.

62. Miller, W.E.: Massive hemorrhage in fractures of the pelvis. South. Med. J., 56:933, 1963.

63. Motsay, G.J., Manlove, C., and Perry, J.F., Jr.: Major venous injury with pelvic fracture. J. Trauma, 9:343, 1969.

64. Müller, J., Bachmann, B., and Berg, H.: Malgaigne fracture of the pelvis: Treatment with percutaneous pin fixation. J. Bone Joint Surg., 60A:992, 1978.

65. O'Keefe, T.J.: Retroperitoneal abscess. J. Bone Joint Surg., 60A:1117, 1978.

66. Orr, H.W.: Osteomyelitis and compound fractures of the pelvis. Surg. Gynecol. Obstet., 54:673, 1932.

67. Pachter, H.L., and Hofstetter, S.R.: Open and percutaneous paracentesis and lavage for abdominal trauma. Arch. Surg., 116:318, 1981.

68. Patterson, F.P., and Morton, K.S.: Neurologic complications of fractures and dislocations of the pelvis. Surg. Gynecol. Obstet., 112:702, 1961.

69. Pelligra, R., and Sandberg, E.C.: Control of intractable abdominal bleeding by external counterpressure. J.A.M.A., 241:708, 1979.

70. Peltier, L.F.: Complications associated with fractures of the pelvis. J. Bone Joint Surg., 47A:1060, 1965.

71. Pennal, G.F., and Massiah, K.A.: Nonunion and delayed union of fractures of the pelvis. Clin. Orthop., 151:124, 1980.

72. Perry, J.F.: Pelvic open fractures. Clin. Orthop., 151:41, 1980.

73. Pokorny, M., Pontes, J.E., and Pierce, J.M., Jr.: Urological injuries associated with pelvic trauma. J. Urol., 121:455, 1979.

74. Prather, G.C., and Kaiser, T.C.: Bladder in fracture of bony pelvis: Significance of "tear drop bladder" as shown by cystogram. J. Urol., 63:1019, 1950.

75. Quinby, W.C., Jr.: Pelvic fractures with hemorrhage. N. Engl. J. Med., 284:668, 1971.

76. Raffa, J., and Christensen, N.M.: Compound fractures of the pelvis. Am. J. Surg., 132:282, 1976.

77. Rankin, L.M.: Fractures of the pelvis. Ann. Surg., 106:266, 1937.

78. Ravitch, M.M.: Hypogastric artery ligation in acute pelvic trauma. Surgery, 56:601, 1964.

79. Redman, H.C.: Computed tomography of the pelvis. Radiol. Clin. North Am., 15:441, 1977.

80. Ring, E.J., Athanasoulis, C., Waltman, A.C. et al.: Arteriographic management of hemorrhage following pelvic fracture. Radiology, 109:65, 1973.

81. Root, H.D., Hauser, C.W., McKinley, C.R. et al.: Diagnostic peritoneal lavage. Surgery, 57:633, 1965.

82. Root, H.D., and VanTyn, R.A.: A device and method for the atraumatic transportation of the injured patient. Surgery, 58:327, 1965.

83. Rothenberger, D.A., Fischer, R.P., and Perry, J.F., Jr.: Major vascular injuries secondary to pelvic fractures: An unsolved clinical problem. Am. J. Surg., 136:660, 1978.

84. Rothenberger, D., Velasco, R., Strate, R. et al.: Open pelvic fracture: A lethal injury. J. Trauma, 18:184, 1978.

85. Rubash, H.E., Nelson, D.D., and Mears, D.C.: Reconstructive surgery of the pelvis. Presented to the American Academy of Orthopaedic Surgeons, New Orleans, 1982.

86. Sahlstrand, T.: Disruption of the pelvic ring treated by external skeletal fixation. J. Bone Joint Surg., 61A:433, 1979.

87. Saletta, J.D., and Freeark, R.J.: Vascular injuries associated with fractures. Orthop. Clin. North Am., 1:93, 1970.

88. Seavers, R., Lynch, J., Ballard, R. et al.: Hypogastric artery ligation for uncontrollable hemorrhage in acute pelvic trauma. Surgery, 55:516, 1964.

89. Sheldon, G.F., and Winestock, D.P.: Hemorrhage from open pelvic fractures controlled intraoperatively with balloon catheter. J. Trauma, 18:68, 1978.

90. Smith-Peterson, M.N., and Rogers, W.A.: End-result study for arthrodesis of the sacro-iliac joint for arthritis—traumatic and non-traumatic. J. Bone Joint Surg., 8:118, 1926.

91. Solonen, K.A.: The sacroiliac joint in the light of anatomical, roentgenological, and clinical studies. Acta. Orthop. Scand. [Suppl.], 27:121, 1957.

92. Stock, J.R., Harris, W.H., and Athanasoulis, C.A.: The role of diagnostic and therapeutic angiography in trauma to the pelvis. Clin. Orthop., 151:31, 1980.

93. Sullivan, C.R.: Fractures of the pelvis. Instr. Course Lect., 18:92, 1961.

94. Tile, M.: Pelvic fractures: Operative versus non-operative treatment. Orthop. Clin. North Am., 11:423, 1980.

95. Tile, M., and Pennal, G.F.: Pelvic disruption: Principles of management. Clin. Orthop., 151:56, 1980.

96. Tile, M.: Fractures of the Pelvis and Acetabulum. Baltimore, Williams & Wilkins, 1984.

97. Trafford, H.S.: Types of fractures of the pelvis with associated urethral ruptures and relative frequency. Postgrad. Med. J., 34:656, 1958.

98. Van Urk, H., Perlberger, R.R., and Muller, H.: Selective arterial embolization for control of traumatic pelvic hemorrhage. Surgery, 83:133, 1978.

99. Wakeley, C.P.G.: Fractures of the pelvis: An analysis of 100 cases. Br. J. Surg., 17:22, 1930.

100. Watson-Jones, R.: Dislocations and fracture-dislocations of the pelvis. Br. J. Surg., 25:773, 1938.

101. ———: Fractures and Joint Injuries. Baltimore, Williams & Wilkins, 1957.

102. Weems, W.L.: Management of genitourinary injuries in patients with pelvic fractures. Ann. Surg., 189:717, 1979.

103. Weil, G.C., Price, E.M., and Rusbridge, H.W.: The diagnosis and treatment of fractures of the pelvis and their complications. Am. J. Surg., 44:108, 1939.

104. Winter, J.E., and Marsh, H.O.: Traumatic separation of the symphysis pubis. Orthop. Trans., 2:221, 1978.

105. Yap, S.N.L.: The management of traumatic pelvic retroperitoneal hemorrhage. Surg. Rounds, 34–44, March 1980.

26 Complications of Treatment of Vascular Injuries to the Extremities

Norman M. Rich

Sixty-five years ago, Bertram Bernheim wrote of combat surgeons in World War I: ". . . he would have been a foolhardy man who would have essayed sutures of arterial or venous trunks in the presence of such infections as were the rule in practically all of the battle wounded."[1] Today, the experience gained from treating the wounded of World War II, Korea, and Vietnam contributes to the current management of vascular trauma and complications that result from attempted vascular repair.

The ultimate complication of vascular injuries to the extremities, gangrene, requires amputation (Fig. 26-1). There are, in addition a variety of associated complications that should be considered. These can range from thrombosis of the distal brachial artery, which may have no associated symptoms because of the extensive collateral circulation around the elbow, to catastrophic exsanguination from disruption of an infected suture line of the common femoral artery.

Complications of peripheral vascular injuries to the extremities can be placed into at least five major categories: (1) Early complications associated with arterial interruption, resulting in varying degrees of ischemia; (2) complications following attempted arterial repair, including thrombosis, stenosis, and infection, with or without hemorrhage; (3) delayed recognition of vascular injuries, including false aneurysms and arteriovenous fistulas; (4) complications associated with concomitant injuries to other structures such as nerves and bone; and (5) complications following venous interruption—acute venous hypertension and chronic venous insufficiency. Thrombophlebitis and pulmonary embolism must also be considered. These major categories are discussed in more detail under specific sections that follow.

Loss of distal viability associated with acute arterial interruption, thrombosis of attempted arterial repair, and infection of arterial repair with subsequent hemorrhage are complications that should be obvious. However, there are many other aspects of complications associated with vascular trauma that must also be considered. These include such important factors as the etiology of the wounding agent (Figs. 26-2 through 26-4), the presence of multiple associated injuries, numerous possible technical problems (Fig. 26-5), and gross structural changes that can occur at the site of the arterial or venous repair or within the conduit that might have been used for the vascular reconstruction. Complications such as thrombophlebitis and pulmonary embolism are more frequently associated with venous injuries than with arterial injuries and are discussed later in a section devoted entirely to problems associated with venous trauma.

It is important to emphasize that many associated complications can be corrected if they are recognized promptly and if the failed arterial repair is reconstructed expeditiously. If unsuccessful arterial repair results in amputation secondary to acute arterial insufficiency, the complication has a final and disastrous result. On the other hand, an amputation is only one method of measuring the success of arterial repair. Thrombosis of the repair can occur, and the degree of development of collateral circulation can help determine the extent of any resulting symptoms that may develop (Fig. 26-6).[23,35]

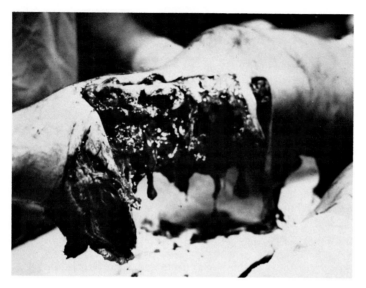

FIG. 26-1. The extent of extremity trauma can contribute to potential complications associated with vascular injury. Massive soft tissue destruction, unstable comminuted fractures (often with missing osseous segments), disruption of nerves, and avulsion of arteries and veins provide challenge for surgical reconstruction. Primary amputation, however, may be the best judgment. (Rich, N.M., Baugh, J.H., and Hughes, C.W.: Popliteal artery injuries in Vietnam. Am. J. Surg., 118:531, 1969)

There are numerous problems associated with attempts to obtain accurate statistics on the management of acute arterial trauma.

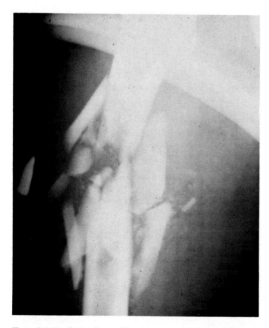

FIG. 26-2. Spicules of bone can penetrate blood vessels. Displaced fractures can impinge on arteries and veins. In this comminuted fracture of the femur, caused by a bullet from an AK-47 assault rifle, the superficial femoral vein was lacerated by the sharp edge of an osseous fragment. (N.M.R., 2nd Surgical Hospital, An Khe, Vietnam, 1966)

DeBakey and Simeone reviewed many of the problems connected with obtaining accurate statistics on the incidence of gangrene after acute traumatic arterial occlusion (Table 26-1).[7] They revealed that Makins' World War I study (1919) was an excellent example of the confusion that results from the inclusion of both acute and nonacute lesions (false aneurysms and arteriovenous fistulas recognized late) in a single series. They found that 49% of Makins' cases were essentially aneurysms. In certain vessels, such as the axillary and subclavian arteries, the proportion of nonacute lesions was greater than 70%. The authors felt that it was difficult to compare the data from Makins' World War I study with their own reviews of American injuries in World War II for the following reasons: (1) The American figures included only the acute lesions, while the British figures included both acute and nonacute lesions; (2) in 85% of the American cases the wounds involved important or critical arteries, while this was true of only 70% of the British cases; and (3) it was felt that some cases of gangrene and amputation were classified as infections rather than as vascular injuries in the World War I study. DeBakey and Simeone also pointed out that it was important to know all of the circumstances about a series of cases of arterial injuries before drawing conclusions from any comparative studies. They emphasized this by showing that the

FIG. 26-3. Blunt trauma can contribute to vascular injury to an extremity. Direct blows, subluxation, displaced fractures, and the temporary cavitational effects of high-velocity missiles can cause contusion, intimal laceration, and thrombosis. This photograph shows contusion with periadventitial hemorrhage of the common femoral artery secondary to direct trauma from a handlebar in a motor scooter accident. (Rich, N.M.: Arterial trauma. In Dale, W.A. [ed.]: The Management of Arterial Occlusive Disease. Chicago, Year Book Medical Publishers, 1971)

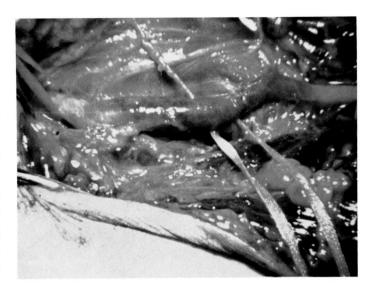

association of concomitant fractures with arterial injuries could increase the amputation rate to approximately 60%, compared to approximately 43% when arterial injuries existed alone.

One finds many disparities in comparing vascular injuries sustained in combat with those found in the civilian community; however, many of these differences are not as great as they were 10 years ago, when injuries by stabbing in the civilian community were compared with high-velocity military gunshot wounds.[56]

Despite all of the limitations of comparing various series involving management of acute arterial trauma, it is important to analyze the published results and to formulate conclusions and specific comparisons

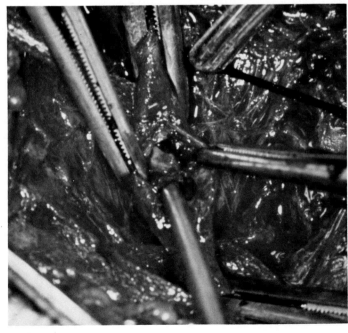

FIG. 26-4. Complications of arterial injury can result from therapeutic and diagnostic procedures. Thrombosis, which developed following percutaneous femoral angiography, is obvious in this common femoral artery. An arteriotomy was performed, followed by removal of the thrombus with a Fogarty balloon catheter. (Rich, N.M., Hobson, R.W. II, Fedde, C.W., and Collins, G.J., Jr.: Common femoral arterial trauma. J. Trauma, 15:628, 1975)

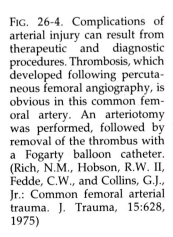

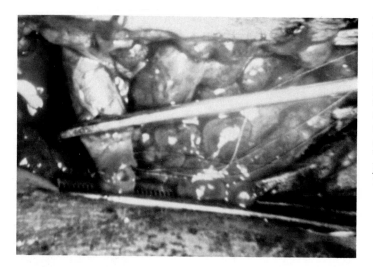

FIG. 26-5. End-to-end anastomosis of an injured artery, as demonstrated here, must be performed without undue tension on the suture line to prevent the complications of stenosis or thrombosis. Atraumatic vascular clamps reduce the possibility of additional arterial injury. (Rich, N.M.: Vascular trauma in Vietnam. J. Cardiovasc. Surg., 11:368, 1970)

where possible. It is particularly important to emphasize that results can be improved only by continuing the evaluation of all

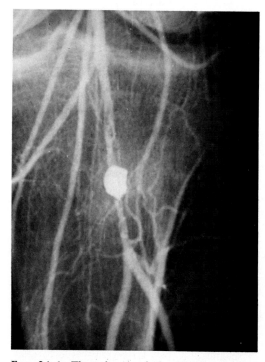

FIG. 26-6. Thrombosis of the distal popliteal artery is demonstrated on this angiogram made approximately 18 months after repair by lateral suture. Note the development of collateral circulation. The offending fragment is adjacent to, but not touching, the artery. (N.M.R., Vietnam Vascular Registry #57)

related material. Attempts should be made to determine the etiology of complications and to establish the most appropriate methods for correcting these complications.

It is necessary to note some of the complications that can result from acute arterial trauma without attempted arterial repair. The most obvious complication is acute distal arterial insufficiency, resulting in a nonviable limb that must be amputated (Fig. 26-7). Nevertheless, emphasis will be placed on complications following attempted arterial reconstructions that were unsuccessful. Early or late thrombosis at the repair site, infection with or without hemorrhage (Fig. 26-8), and early or late stenosis at the repair site are the major complications that can occur. Brief mention will be given to other complications, such as residual distal edema and aneurysmal dilation of vein grafts used as replacement conduits in the arterial system. Amputation rates will be discussed, and mortality rates from representative series will be noted.

There is some confusion in attempting to interpret the actual complication rates associated with attempted arterial repair. In many reports there is no separation from numerous systemic complications specifically related to unsuccessful arterial reconstruction. In the preliminary report from the Vietnam Vascular Registry, Rich and Hughes reported a complication rate of approximately 28% involving major arterial repairs (Table 26-2).[51] The majority of these initial complications, however, were treated

Table 26-1. Amputation Rates Following Arterial Injuries in Combat

ARTERY	BRITISH WORLD WAR I (MAKINS, 1919)*			AMERICAN WORLD WAR II (DEBAKEY AND SIMEONE, 1946)		
	TOTAL LIMBS LOST†	NO. OF CASES	PERCENTAGE	TOTAL LIMBS LOST†	NO. OF CASES	PERCENTAGE
Aorta	5	5	100.0	3	2	66.6
Carotid	128	38	29.6	10	3	30.0
External carotid				3		
Renal				2	2	100.0
Vertebral	3					
Subclavian	45	4	8.8	21	6	28.6
Axillary	108	5	4.6	74	32	43.2
Brachial total	200	12	6.0	601	159	26.5
Above profunda				97	54	5.7
Below profunda				209	54	25.8
Radial-ulnar	59	3	5.0			
Radial				99	5	5.1
Ulnar				69	1	1.5
Radial and ulnar				28	11	39.3
Common iliac	1	1	100.0	13	7	53.8
External iliac	4			30	14	46.7
Internal iliac	1			1		
Femoral total	366	74	20.2	517	275	53.2
Above profunda				106	86	81.1
Below profunda				177	97	54.8
Profunda				27		
Popliteal	144	62	43.1	502	364	72.5
Anterior tibial	26	1	3.8	129	11	8.5
Posterior tibial	97	9	9.2	265	36	13.6
Anterior and posterior tibial	7	2	28.6	91	63	69.2
Peroneal	4	2	50.0	7	1	14.3
Anterior tibial and peroneal	1			5		
Both tibial and peroneal				1	1	100.0
Total	1202	218	18.1	2471	995	40.3

* The figures compiled from Makins' table represent a combination of the totals for gangrene and amputations, so the maximum number was obtained without possible duplication. The numbers represent the minimum number of cases that must have had amputations.
† In the case of aorta, carotids, and renal arteries, the figures indicate the numbers who died or developed cerebral complications.
(Modified from DeBakey, M.E. and Simeone, F.A.: Battle injuries of arteries in World War II: An analysis of 2,471 cases. Ann. Surg., 123:534, 1946.)

successfully by an additional procedure, often during the initial operation. In this report, revisions performed during one operation were counted separately in an attempt to determine the etiology of repair failure. (An example would be thrombosis at the suture line requiring future arterial resection and an additional reconstruction.) Multiple procedures in a single patient were not unusual; some underwent as many as five or six separate procedures. This partly explains the additional number of complications. Also, many patients with a residual complication, such as a thrombosed axillary or brachial arterial repair, remained asymptomatic and did not require additional operations.

In the interim report from the Vietnam Vascular Registry, Rich and associates evaluated the results of 1000 acute major arterial

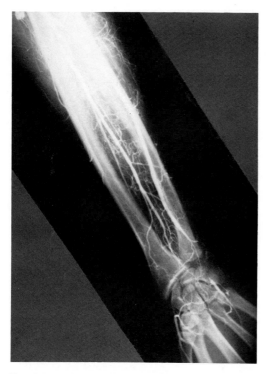

FIG. 26-7. Interruption of smaller-caliber arteries (the radial, ulnar, and tibial arteries are sometimes called "minor" arteries) can result in distal extremity ischemia. This angiogram reveals occlusion of both the radial and ulnar arteries at the wrist with poor distal filling through minimal collateral development. (N.M.R., W.R.A.M.C., 1973)

injuries and found the overall complication rate to be approximately 30% (Table 26-3).[34] Again, many of these complications were managed successfully, either at the time of the initial operation (*e.g.*, a very stenotic lateral suture repair changed to excision of the injured artery with successful end-to-end anastomosis) or in the early postoperative period (*e.g.*, thrombosis of an end-to-end anastomosis done under tension changed to additional debridement with an autogenous saphenous vein graft replacement). In the civilian community, Moore and associates reported 250 arterial injuries and documented a comparable complication rate of 21%.[26]

HISTORICAL NOTES[37,39,40,56]

After Hallowell performed what is generally recognized as the first successful arterial repair in 1759, a lateral repair of a brachial arterial laceration accomplished with a pin and thread, more than 100 years passed before significant progress was made in vascular surgery. The unsuccessful animal experiments by Assman in 1773, in which vascular repairs ended in obliterating endarteritis, undoubtedly had a profound effect on this lack of progress. Eck, a Russian surgeon, was the first to perform a union between two blood vessels when, in 1877,

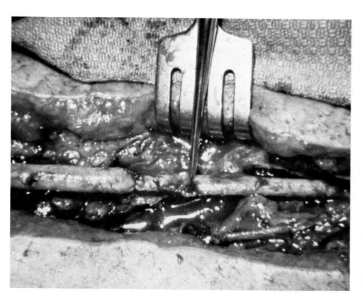

FIG. 26-8. Infection accompanied by profuse hemorrhage is one of the dreaded complications following reconstruction of injured arteries and veins. Disruption of the suture line of this interposition saphenous venous graft, used to repair the superficial femoral vein, resulted in massive bleeding. Ligation of the artery with excision of the graft was necessitated by the associated infection. (N.M.R., Vietnam Vascular Registry #471)

Table 26-2. Initial Complications of Major Arterial Repairs in Vietnam*

ARTERY	DISRUPTION	STENOSIS	THROMBOSIS	AMPUTATION RATE	
				NUMBER	PERCENTAGE
Common carotid		(1†)	4 (1†)		
Axillary	1	2 (1†)	8 (4†)	1	4.5
Brachial	5 (6†)	2 (1†)	16 (6†)	3	2.9
Iliac	(1†)		1 (1†)	0	0.0
Common femoral	2 (5†)	(1†)	4	2	8.3
Superficial femoral	8 (14†)	2	14 (3†)	12	10.3
Popliteal	2 (4†)	1	20 (10†)	25	32.5
Total	18 (30†)	7 (4†)	67 (25†)		

* Many of these initial complications were successfully repaired at the time of the initial operation or during the very early postoperative period.
† These figures represent complications in addition to the complication of initial repair of acute arterial injuries in Vietnam.
(Rich, N.M., and Hughes, C.W., Vietnam Vascular Registry: A preliminary report. Surgery 65:218, 1969)

he created an anastomosis between the portal vein and the inferior vena cava. In Germany, in 1882, Schede successfully performed a lateral closure of a femoral venous laceration and advocated this approach for other such injuries. Murphy performed the first successful end-to-end anastomosis of an artery in man in Chicago in 1896. Many pioneers, including Jassinowsky, in 1889 and Dörfler, in 1899, contributed to the

Table 26-3. Complications Associated With Arterial Repair Management of 1000 Acute Major Arterial Injuries

COMPLICATION(S)	NO. OF PATIENTS (301 TOTAL)	PERCENTAGE (30.1 OVERALL)
Thrombosis	193	
Hemorrhage with or without infection	46	
Massive tissue necrosis, sepsis, venous insufficiency, etc., resulting in amputation	62	
Deaths	17	1.7

(Modified from Rich, N.M., Baugh, J.H., and Hughes, C.W.: Acute arterial injuries in Vietnam. J. Trauma, 10:359, 1970)

clinical and experimental advances in vascular surgery. It was, however, Carrel and Guthrie, in the early part of the 20th century, who made numerous valuable contributions that provided an impetus to vascular transplants with both autografts and homografts. The first clinical application of a vein graft to replace a missing arterial segment was performed by Goyanes in 1906, in Madrid, when he used a segment of the popliteal vein to repair the popliteal artery. The following year in Germany, Lexer performed the first saphenous vein graft of an artery.

As early as 1910 Stich had collected more than 100 reports of arterial repair by lateral suture and 46 by end-to-end anastomosis or vein-graft substitution in man. There was, however, a high failure rate, usually from thrombosis, and few surgeons considered arterial repair worthwhile. The advent of the high-explosive artillery shells and high-velocity bullets in the early part of World War I created relatively massive tissue destruction, which made vascular repair impractical. The lack of antibiotics and blood transfusions, combined with the frequently fatal exsanguination associated with infected vascular repairs, contributed to the continued acceptance (until the early part of the Korean conflict) of ligation as the preferred method.

Thus, complications, particularly throm-

Table 26-4. Representative Reports of Large Series of Patients Sustaining Arterial Trauma

WAR OR CIVILIAN SERIES	AUTHOR	YEAR	NO. OF ARTERIES
World War I	Makins	1919	1202
World War II	DeBakey and Simeone	1946	2471
Korean conflict	Hughes	1958	304
Vietnam war	Rich *et al.*	1970	1000
Houston	Morris *et al.*	1960	220
Atlanta	Ferguson *et al.*	1961	200
Denver	Owens	1963	70
Detroit	Smith *et al.*	1963	61
Dallas	Patman *et al.*	1964	271
Los Angeles	Treiman *et al.*	1966	159
St. Louis	Dillard *et al.*	1968	85
New Orleans	Drapanas *et al.*	1970	226
Dallas	Perry *et al.*	1971	508
Galveston	Moore *et al.*	1971	250
Memphis	Cheek *et al.*	1975	200
Denver	Kelly and Eiseman	1975	116
Jackson	Hardy *et al.*	1975	360
New York	Bole *et al.*	1976	126
Houston	Feliciano *et al.*	1984	221

bosis and infected vascular repairs with associated disruption and hemorrhage, had a profound role in preventing the earlier acceptance and broad application of vascular repair.

In addition to the many reports of various aspects of vascular trauma, there are large series that can be reviewed (Table 26-4).

EARLY COMPLICATIONS ASSOCIATED WITH ARTERIAL INTERRUPTION

Acute arterial thrombosis can have essentially the same effect as acute arterial interruption by ligation. The former can result either from direct arterial injury without repair or from attempted arterial repair. In both situations the significance of the thrombosis is determined, to a great extent, by the availability of collateral circulation.

Acute arterial thrombosis following trauma, for which there has been no arterial repair, may be a difficult diagnosis to make. The diagnosis is more obvious if there is loss of the distal pulses, if pallor and coolness exist, and if there is pain and loss of sensation and motion of the extremity. Any combination of these signs and symptoms, however, may be present, and it may be difficult to ascertain the location and extent of arterial thrombosis. The tragedy associated with this injury is that it may not be recognized until the distal part of the limb has become nonviable. Thrombosis associated with high-velocity missile injuries, fractures, and dislocations may be particularly misleading and difficult to diagnose. An intimal flap or subintimal hematoma may have a delayed progression of several hours before arterial occlusion is completed. The erroneous diagnosis of arterial spasm has been made all too often. Following trauma, nevertheless, this diagnosis should be made only after arterial exploration. The suspicion of probable thrombosis is the safest diagnosis.

COMPLICATIONS FOLLOWING ATTEMPTED ARTERIAL REPAIR

Thrombosis

Various technical errors or difficulties can contribute to thrombosis of an attempted arterial repair. Depending on the availability of collateral circulation, this may or may not result in distal ischemia leading to nonviability of an extremity. The following technical problems are some of the factors that can contribute to thrombosis:

Inadequate arterial debridement
A second adjacent arterial injury
Residual distal arterial thrombus
Severe stenosis at the suture line caused by pulling the suture line too tightly
Severe stenosis at the suture line because there was not sufficient arterial wall remaining for an attempted lateral suture repair
Undue tension on the suture line associated with a significant missing arterial segment
If a graft is used, various problems associated with the graft, such as twisting, making the graft too long, causing a kink, and external compression of the graft
Inability to perform a venous repair when no effective venous return exists.

Inadequate arterial debridement can leave residual ischemic arterial wall, where platelets and thrombin can be deposited to form a thrombus or where an aneurysm can form and rupture. Also, inadequate debridement can leave residual intimal flaps that can cause thrombosis. In the early days of the Korean conflict, the rate of thrombosis was greater than 70% following primary arterial repair as reported by Jahnke.[21] It was felt that this was because the anastomosis of the arterial ends or edges of the wounded artery was performed after merely trimming the loose, fragmented adventitia. Because it was felt that debridement was inadequate and because microscopic changes were seen in the adjacent (grossly) normal-looking artery, it was established that 1 cm of normal-looking artery at each end of the arterial wound should be excised. The success in 1952 and 1953 in Korea was felt to be based in part on this maneuver.[17,18] Nevertheless, it is important to emphasize that in addition to similar impressions gained from the material in the Vietnam Vascular Registry,[34–45,47–51,53–57] Williams[66] and Brisbin and associates[3] reported that they felt that inadequate debridement of the artery and surrounding tissues was a limiting factor in the continued patency of arterial repairs in their Vietnam experience. A surgical and pathological review from the Vietnam experience indicated that success could not be guaranteed by the excision of normal artery adjacent to the injured artery.[54] Perry and associates[33] reported that

in their civilian experience, although there was no persuasive evidence, they felt that inadequate debridement contributed to failures in their studies. Obviously, all devitalized tissue must be excised for optimal results. During the debridement, a thorough knowledge of anatomy is mandatory for proper identification of arteries. Confusion can exist at times, however, particularly when massive tissue destruction has occurred. An example of this problem occurred in Vietnam when surgeons reported that they had ligated a "large" profunda femoris artery. It was not until several days later, when it was noted that there were no palpable distal pulses in the injured extremity, that an arteriogram was obtained to confirm that the proximal right superficial femoral artery, rather than the profunda femoris artery, had been ligated.

Multiple arterial lesions may exist. A second adjacent lesion may cause a persistent failure, despite the fact that the primary arterial repair was technically successful. Intraoperative angiography, including the repair site and the runoff vessels, helps to eliminate this problem. Also, repeated evaluations in the operating room and immediately postoperatively, as well as close postoperative monitoring, help eliminate this problem. Although it is uncommon, three or more arterial lesions may exist in one extremity, particularly in patients who, like those seen in Vietnam, sustained multiple-fragment wounds.

Residual distal thrombus can result in thrombosis of an otherwise technically successful arterial repair. Heparinization during the arterial repair and checking for the quantity and quality of arterial "back-bleeding" can be useful. However, it must be remembered that there can be what is interpreted as adequate back-bleeding in the presence of significant distal thrombus. Careful passage of a Fogarty balloon catheter into the major distal arterial vessels can be useful in retrieving additional distal thrombus. Also, an intraoperative angiogram can be useful in determining whether residual thrombus persists. Cohen and co-workers[6] mentioned that occasionally an apparently simple arterial reconstruction in Vietnam did not function. At reoperation, or during postamputation dissection, extensive thrombosis of the runoff vessels was evident.

Multiple factors can contribute to the failure and compound the difficulty of determining the most significant complicating factor. An example is the case of one Vietnam casualty who had an extensive soft tissue wound of the left lower extremity. A greater saphenous vein graft was used to repair the popliteal artery, and the popliteal vein was repaired end to end. The initial repair was unsuccessful, and a second procedure was performed 5 hours later with the retrieval of some distal thrombus with a Fogarty catheter. There was considerable swelling in the extremity, and fasciotomies were performed. At the time when an above-the-knee amputation was necessary, on the third postoperative day, the vein graft in the popliteal artery appeared to be functioning well. It was felt that there were multiple contributing factors, including the distal thrombus, massive soft tissue destruction, and acute venous hypertension.

Meticulous surgical technique must be used in performing arterial repairs. If a continuous suture line is being created, a "purse-string" effect must not be created by too much pulling on the suture. Interrupted sutures may help prevent this complication in small vessels. Also, a lateral suture repair must not be performed in small vessels or in a large vessel in which a major portion of the artery is missing. This problem can be eliminated by using an autogenous saphenous venous patch graft or by excising the damaged artery, followed by end-to-end anastomosis. Thrombosis at the repair site can also occur if there is undue tension on the suture line. Important collateral branches should not be sacrificed, and joints should not be immobilized in severe flexion in an attempt to perform an end-to-end anastomosis when a significant segment of artery has been removed. On the other hand, the elastic nature of the artery will cause retraction of the ends. Sound surgical judgment must be exercised in determining whether an end-to-end anastomosis can be performed safely or whether an arterial replacement conduit will be necessary to accomplish a successful repair.

If a replacement conduit is needed to effect successful arterial reconstruction, the graft must not be twisted when put into place. Also, leaving the graft too long can result in a kink that can lead to thrombosis. External compression can add to the possibility of thrombosis. Moore and associates[26] mention the problem of a patient with a high-velocity rifle wound in the popliteal space. A saphenous vein graft replacement was necessary to repair the popliteal artery, and a lateral repair of the injured popliteal vein was possible. When the pulses disappeared 8 hours postoperatively, immediate reexploration revealed that the vein graft was redundant and kinked. This was revised following a thrombectomy, and the patient's subsequent course was uneventful. A similar complication was seen in one Vietnam casualty when a vein graft of excessive length, used to repair a popliteal artery, was noted on follow-up arteriogram. Turbulence in the blood flow, caused by grafts that are either too wide or too narrow, can lead to thrombosis. One Vietnam casualty developed thrombosis in a segment of Dacron 10 mm in diameter, which had been used to reconstruct a much smaller axillary-to-proximal-brachial arterial defect.

A number of other factors can contribute to early thrombosis of an arterial repair. If infection occurs in the repair site within the first week, thrombosis may also develop. If the injured artery is arteriosclerotic, additional technical problems can occur. Care must be taken not to embolize arteriosclerotic material into the distal arterial tree or to leave partially elevated arteriosclerotic plaques, which could cause thrombosis. White and associates[65] documented in infants and children some specific problems associated with thrombosis of a major artery that occurred from diagnostic catheterization, either by percutaneous stick or open arteriotomy. They presented the case of a 3-year-old boy who had undergone cardiac catheterization via the left femoral artery. One year later the circumference of his left thigh was 2 cm less than that of the right, and the left calf was 1 cm thinner than the right. The left leg was also 1 cm shorter when measured by scanography. Reduced limb growth can occur following lower-

Table 26-5. Comparison of Treatment and Results in the First 3½ Years and the Last 3½ Years of Acute Arterial Injuries in Houston Prior to July 31, 1956

				RESULTS		
	TOTAL CASES	NO. OF LIGATIONS	NO. OF REPAIRS	NO. WITH PULSES, VIABLE	NO. WITH NO PULSES, VIABLE	NO. OF AMPUTATIONS
First 3½ yr	31	14	13	9	16	5 (16.0%)
Second 3½ yr	105	18	80	76	11	7 (6.6%)

(Modified from Morris, C.G., Jr., Creech, O., Jr., and DeBakey, M.E.: Acute arterial injuries in civilian practice. Am. J. Surg., 93:565, 1957)

extremity arterial occlusions in growing children.

One fairly accurate method of determining whether the arterial repair has been successful and whether the distal arterial tree is patent is to palpate for distal pulses. Even the establishment of a palpable distal pulse does not ensure long-term success of the arterial repair. On the other hand, this can be a fairly accurate method of determining the success of most arterial repairs performed for trauma involving the major arteries of the extremities. In an early major civilian series of 136 acute arterial injuries treated in Houston prior to July 31, 1956, Morris and associates[27] found that pulses were restored immediately in 72 patients and that there was a delayed return of pulses in an additional 27 patients (Table 26-5). The findings of distal pulses in 76 of 80 patients with arterial repair in the second half of their experience emphasizes what has, subsequently, been generally accepted: distal pulses should be easily palpable following arterial repair. It is particularly interesting to note that following arterial ligation, 24 of 32 patients without palpable distal pulses had viable limbs. Drapanas and co-workers[10] reported that pulses were palpable immediately postoperatively in 80% of the patients in their experience who had had repair of arterial injuries in the extremities. Bolasny and Killen[2] reported that they were able to obtain successful restoration of distal pulses in all but two of 33 arteries that were injured secondary to angiographic procedures. Difficulties arise if there are no palpable distal pulses. The

majority of these early complications associated with thrombosis following arterial repair can be corrected. It may be necessary to perform a second operation in the immediate postoperative period if early thrombosis occurs and if the viability of the extremity is in question. However, if the viability is maintained despite thrombotic occlusion of the repair, additional operation can be avoided. This would be particularly imperative in a combat zone or even in a civilian situation in which the patient's general condition would not tolerate an additional procedure. Repeated operations are followed by a higher incidence of infection that may jeopardize life as well as limb. Additional operations can be performed electively if symptoms of arterial insufficiency persist. Collateral circulation, however, may develop to the point where the patient is essentially asymptomatic despite the presence of thrombosis of a major artery, and the patient may not require an additional operation to reestablish arterial patency. The importance of collateral circulation in Vietnam casualties who had thrombosis of arterial repairs was emphasized by Levin, Rich, and Hutton.[23] The Doppler ultrasound device can be used in the early postoperative period to determine the extent of collateral flow distal to the arterial occlusion. Lavenson, Rich, and Strandness[22] emphasized this point from the Vietnam experience, where additional operations in the high-risk group could be successfully delayed.

Confusion, followed by disastrous results, may occur if the physician entertains the diagnosis of arterial spasm rather than accepting the probability that thrombosis has occurred in the artery at the repair site. (In Vietnam[36,56] a widely accepted maxim was that if one thought of spasm, the spelling should be C-L-O-T!) Whenever there is a question of spasm rather than damage to the integrity of an artery, numerous plans have evolved to attempt to relieve the spasm. Employed to differentiate spasm from traumatic arterial injury with occlusion, sympathetic blocks have only confused the problem. The use of sympathetic blocks has only caused unwarranted delays in the majority of patients with arterial injuries. Even under direct vision, diagnosis of arterial spasm has been made when there was actually an intimal rupture or a subintimal hematoma that was not evident from external inspection. Segmental arterial spasm may occur following arterial injury. This may occur adjacent to the recognized trauma. Papavarine hydrochloride, 1% procaine hydrochloride, warm packs applied locally, and hydrostatic dilatation of the involved segment have been employed successfully in the operative field.

The limb that is ischemic after vascular injury often exhibits a contracture. This condition may be reversible if the blood supply is restored within a reasonably short time. Although the best results occur when circulation is restored within 6 hours, there is no definite time beyond 6 hours when restoration of arterial flow should not be attempted. When circulation returns, however, the muscles tend to swell. If fasciotomies, with adequate incisions in the skin and long incisions in the fascia, are not performed promptly, continued edema of the muscle within the closed fascial compartment terminates in ischemia and necrosis.[31,56] Delay in performing adequate fasciotomy in the presence of increasing muscle swelling may result in compression of the vessels with resultant muscle necrosis and nerve damage. These changes are more likely in the anterior compartment in the lower extremity and in the flexor compartment in the forearm. Any degree of muscle necrosis may occur, depending on the severity and period of ischemia. In prolonged ischemia an entire compartment may become necrotic and may be lost. With spotty

necrosis and replacement of fibrous tissue, Volkmann's contracture occurs. The primary ischemia from the vascular injury may not be the only contributing factor. After the blood supply is returned to such areas, the previously ischemic capillaries extravasate fluid to the surrounding tissues. This in turn may obstruct venous return in closed compartments and establish a vicious cycle. Any patient with a vascular injury is a prospective candidate for this complication. The multitude of vascular injuries that occurred in Vietnam prompted numerous suggestions from surgeons for prevention of compartmental ischemic complications. These suggestions have ranged from stabwound fasciotomy to tricompartmental, full-length fasciotomy, to four-compartment decompression through a partial fibulectomy. It has even been suggested by some that a prophylactic fasciotomy should be performed on every patient with a vascular injury in an extremity. In most instances, Volkmann's ischemic contracture can be avoided by early vascular reconstruction, early, adequate fasciotomy, when indicated, and close follow-up observation.

It is difficult to compare the complication rates of various types of arterial repair. A lateral suture repair or an end-to-end anastomosis is usually achieved where there is less general destruction than in a wound that requires an autogenous saphenous vein graft to restore arterial continuity. On the other hand, it is important to determine the complication rate for each specific type of arterial repair. In the short-term follow-up, the results of lateral repair in small lacerated lesions have been excellent. Hughes[17] was able to perform lateral arteriorrhaphy in approximately 10%, or 20 of 211 arterial repairs. Spencer and Grewe[61] reported a higher incidence in performing 13 lateral repairs, nearly 15% of 89 arterial repairs. In these 13 lateral repairs there was only one instance of thrombosis, and only one amputation was necessary. The lateral repair was used when 20% to 30%, or less, of the vessel circumference was lacerated, and this probably contributed to the success. In contrast, however, Jahnke[21] reported a late thrombosis rate of 47% in those cases repaired by lateral suture during the Korean conflict. It is possible that in many of the patients in this latter series, lateral repair was used for lesions in which more than 30% of the circumference of the artery was traumatized. If there was inadequate arterial debridement and inaccurate intimal approximation at the time of repair, leaving an inadequate lumen, thrombosis of the compromised lumen was likely.

Historically, it is warranted to comment briefly on the complications associated with several older types of arterial repairs. DeBakey and Simeone[7] demonstrated that the incidence of amputation was greater, compared with other methods of repair, in 40 arterial injuries in which nonsuture tube vein grafts, as advocated by Blakemore and Lord, were used. When the nonsuture tube vein graft was originally described, it was felt that it would be particularly useful where speed and ease of operation were important, as on the battlefield. DeBakey and Simeone emphasized, however, that the nonsuture anastomosis was neither simple nor as easy to achieve as some of its proponents had claimed. It was recognized that additional experience would make the operation easier. It was pointed out, nevertheless, that a better-than-average surgeon in an evacuation hospital in World War II took 3½ hours to perform the procedure, which was complicated by having the ligature twice slip off the tube. In addition to the technical difficulties involved in the procedure, it was known that in a number of cases, certain difficulties forced abandonment of this method of repair. Another disadvantage of the method involved additional destruction of arterial wall in the course of application of the tube, and the possibility that important collateral branches might be interrupted. Homologous arterial grafts were used as early arterial replacements; however, degenerative changes, with multiple aneurysms developing in the arterial homografts, led to abandonment of this procedure.

In one large civilian series of arterial trauma, Perry and associates[33] had an early occlusion rate of 9.1%, with 19 early occlusions following 207 arterial repairs (Table 26-6). Eight of these occlusions were successfully reoperated, resulting in a corrected 5.2% failure rate. The failures were essentially equally divided between major arteries

Table 26-6. Complications Associated With 207 Arterial Repairs* in a Civilian Series From Dallas

ARTERY	NO. WITH OCCLUSION	REOPERATION SUCCESSFUL	NO. WITH INFECTION
Axillary	2		1
Brachial	4	2	3
Radial-ulnar	4	1	
Renal	1		
Iliac			1
Femoral	5	4	3
Carotid	1		
Popliteal	2	1	
Total	19	8	8

* Initial failure of repair, 9.1%; failure of repair after reoperation, 5.2%
(Modified from Perry, M.O., Thai, E.R., and Shires, G.T.: Management of arterial injuries. Ann. Surg., 173: 403, 1971)

of the upper and lower extremities. The authors found that failures in their series of arterial repairs were equally distributed among the various types of repairs employed. They did not find that the specific technique of arterial repair could be implicated as a factor in the ultimate failure. Failure was due to an anastomosis under tension or stenosis at the anastomotic site, either with end-to-end arterial anastomosis or with arterial tube graft anastomosis.

Ferguson and co-workers,[12] in an earlier civilian report, outlined the relatively early loss of pulses in six of their patients following arterial repair, the type of treatment instituted, and the final results obtained. In two patients in whom thrombectomy of the repair site was performed in the early postoperative period, pulses were restored, and the final result was a normal extremity.

In Vietnam, thrombosis was the most common complication following attempted arterial repair (see Tables 26-2 and 26-3).[35,56] In evaluating 57 patients at Walter Reed General Hospital with complications of arterial repair initially performed in Vietnam, approximately 60% of the complications involved thrombosis (Table 26-7). In this series, thrombosis of brachial arterial repairs constituted nearly half of all of the

Table 26-7. Complications of Arterial Repairs From Vietnam Evaluated at Walter Reed General Hospital

ARTERY	No. With Infection, Hemorrhage, or Both	No. With Thrombosis of Repair	No. With Stenosis of Repair	Total
Carotid	1	4	2	7
Axillary	0	7	3	10
Brachial	1	16	1	18
Femoral	7	2	4	13
Popliteal	2	5	2	9
Total	11	34	12	57

(Rich, N.M., Baugh, J.H., and Hughes, C.W.: Acute arterial injuries in Vietnam. Arch. Surg. 100:646, 1970)

thromboses. Only 20 of the 34 patients required additional arterial reconstruction because of symptoms of arterial insufficiency (Table 26-8).

Infection

Infection is a disastrous complication of arterial repair. Infection causing disruption of an arterial repair can lead to sudden, dramatic, and potentially fatal exsanguination. As in other areas of surgery, prevention is far better than treatment! Prompt diagnosis of arterial injury, use of appropriate antibiotics, adequate wound debridement, restoration of vascular continuity as soon as possible, and adequate systemic nutrition should all help prevent vascular infection.

Table 26-8. Complications of Arterial Repairs in 57 Vietnam Casualties Evaluated at Walter Reed General Hospital

COMPLICATION(S)	No. With Additional Operation	No. With No Operation
Infection, hemorrhage, or both	9	2
Thrombosis	10	24
Stenosis	5	7
Total	24	33

(Rich, N.M., Baugh, J.H., and Hughes, C.W.: Acute arterial injuries in Vietnam. Arch. Surg., 100:646, 1970)

Close observation in the postoperative period of the patient's general status, as well as the character of the local wound, is mandatory. Prompt and aggressive regional treatment of an adjacent infection may prevent a vascular infection. Elimination of as much foreign material as possible is important in contaminated wounds.

Infection in the site of an arterial repair usually results in hemorrhage from disruption of the vascular suture line. Additional repair should not be performed in the infected site. Not only is additional repair usually subjected to an early failure from infection, but the patient's life might be endangered by massive hemorrhage with exsanguination or septicemia. Proximal and distal ligation of the artery in the area of the infected arterial repair is mandatory. Occasionally, it may be necessary to reconstruct the arterial supply from an extra-anatomical location to maintain extremity viability.

There are a number of procedures that may be successful when used in an aggressive approach to the infected wound. This is particularly true if the wound infection is recognized early and if treatment is instituted immediately. Redebridement, muscle flap transposition, instillation of antibiotics into the wound through catheters, continuously or at scheduled intervals, and massive systemic antibiotic therapy have all been successful adjuvants in difficult cases. The problem is magnified if there is a foreign body in the area. This is why the use of Dacron as an arterial substitute in contaminated wounds has been discouraged and why even inert metal used for internal fixation should be avoided in such wounds (Fig. 26-9).

There are few statistics on the incidence of infected arterial repairs following trauma in the civilian community. Drapanas and co-workers[10] reported an infection rate of approximately 5% in their patients with arterial trauma. They noted that infection occurred at the site of injury in extremity wounds and that the majority of these patients subsequently required amputations. Perry and associates[33] found a 3.5% wound infection rate: eight patients among 207 who survived (see Table 26-6). They did not believe that there was any constant

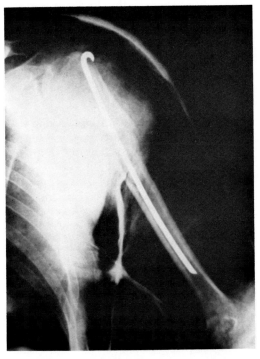

Fig. 26-9. An intramedullary rod was used in an attempt to stabilize the comminuted humeral fracture in this combat casualty, who also had a severed axillary artery. Although this approach has been used successfully in similar civilian injuries, external immobilization of fractures has been the choice in military wounds. (Rich, N.M., Metz, C.W., Jr., Hutton, J.E., Jr. et al.: Internal versus external fixation of fractures with concomitant vascular injuries in Vietnam. J. Trauma, 11:463, 1971)

correlation between the presence of infection and ultimate failure of repair in their series. In only two cases, one brachial arterial repair and one femoral arterial repair, did the infection appear to be significantly involved in delayed postoperative thrombosis.

In Vietnam, infection was the second most common complication following attempted arterial repair (see Table 26-2).[34,35,51,56] Among the 57 patients who were later seen at Walter Reed General Hospital with complications of arterial repairs initially performed in Vietnam, approximately 19%, or 11 of the 57 patients, had infection, with or without hemorrhage (see Table 26-7).[35]

Brisbin and co-authors[3] reviewed the cases of six patients with secondary disruption of arterial repairs that had been performed in Vietnam (Table 26-9). Their stated purpose was to emphasize that in a combat casualty, vessels not critical for limb survival should be ligated and not repaired at the time of initial debridement. They did, however, include one popliteal arterial injury and five injuries to the superficial femoral artery. It would be difficult to establish that these were not critical arteries. Speaking from their experience at Yokosuka Naval Hospital in Japan, where Vietnam battle casualties were received after initial operations had been performed in Vietnam, these authors emphasized the problems encountered in attempts to revise infected vascular repairs. The following case report is a good example:

A 22-year-old Marine received multiple fragment wounds of the left thigh on May 26, 1967, with disruption of the superficial femoral artery. An autogenous saphenous venous graft was used to bridge the arterial defect, and the skin and soft tissues were closed primarily. Approximately 2 weeks later, upon arrival at Yokosuka, a pulsating mass was noted high in the left thigh. Four days later a massive hemorrhage occurred from the proximal vascular anastomosis. Although there was necrotic muscle and an obvious infection, an attempt to revise the anastomosis was made. But approximately 6 days after the second operation, on June 18, 1967, the revision disrupted, and a

Table 26-9. Six Cases of Delayed Rupture of Vascular Repair—Vietnam Experience

Missile	Type of Repair	Days From Repair to Rupture	Vessel Involved	Site of Rupture	Reason for Rupture	Comments
MFW	Vein graft	7	Popliteal	Artery distal to graft	Infection, inadequate debridement	Above-knee amputation due to massive muscle necrosis
MFW	Vein graft	17	Superficial femoral	Proximal anastomosis	Primary wound closure, inadequate debridement	Above-knee amputation due to sciatic nerve palsy
AK-47 bullet	Vein graft	13	Superficial femoral	Body of graft	Primary wound closure infection	Limb survived with bypass graft
MFW	Direct anastomosis	7	Superficial femoral	Artery distal to anastomosis	Inadequate debridement of artery and muscle	Limb survived with ligation
M-14 bullet	Vein graft	25	Superficial femoral	Body of graft	Infection, inadequate debridement exposed graft	Limb survived with ligation
AK-47 bullet	Vein grqaft	6	Superficial femoral	Both anastomoses	Erosion of artery by bone	Limb survived with ligation

(Adapted from Brisbin, R.L., Geib, P.O., and Eiseman, B.: Secondary disruption of vascular repair following war wounds. Arch. Surg., 99:787, 1969)

second massive hemorrhage ensued. It was again obvious that the surrounding soft tissue was infected. An extra-anatomical bypass was then created with a Dacron prosthesis between the external iliac and the superficial femoral arteries. Although the extremity remained viable, an above-the-knee amputation was eventually performed because of muscle contraction and sciatic nerve palsy.

Brisbin and co-workers[3] also emphasized that primary wound closure including the skin was unjustified. Inadequate initial debridement contributed to the complication. Once infection was obvious, repeated attempts to repair the artery should not have been carried out. Ligation of the artery would have been a better choice. If the arterial supply proved critical to the viability of the extremity, an extra-anatomical bypass

could then have been performed. Particularly in the combat zone, the surgeon should resist the temptation to attempt additional vascular reconstruction in such infected wounds. Although there are unusual and isolated instances when this approach has been successful, the numerous serious complications, including a threat to the patient's life, do not warrant the risk.

In their report on secondary disruption of vascular repairs, Brisbin and co-workers[3] outlined the following violations of vascular surgical precepts in the treatment of Vietnam casualties with vascular injuries:

Primary skin closure in a war wound
Placement of a vascular graft in an area of established infection
Inadequate soft tissue debridement in an attempt to conserve tissue for coverage of a vascular repair

Attempted direct repair of a disrupted anastomosis in the presence of infection

Inadequate debridement of a damaged vessel

Suture repair of a lateral arterial laceration in a war wound

Failure to perform fasciotomy

Permitting a vascular graft to remain without soft tissue covering

Detaching the sartorius muscle proximally to cover a vascular graft when the muscle has been deprived of its blood supply by necessary debridement

Records in the Vietnam Vascular Registry are replete with instances in which attempts to perform additional vascular repairs in the presence of infection were followed by subsequent disruption of arterial repairs and various complications.[56] An example is one patient with trauma to the popliteal vessels. A greater saphenous vein graft was utilized to reconstruct the popliteal artery. Approximately 2 weeks later there was massive arterial bleeding from the wound. An attempt was made to repair a hole in the vein graft; however, 3 days later there was recurrent massive arterial hemorrhage, and it was necessary to ligate the distal superficial femoral artery. In one patient managed at Walter Reed General Hospital, infection was not obvious at the time of suture line disruption. Despite an additional repair with all known precautions taken, the suture line disrupted again 4 days later. Arterial ligation and an extra-anatomical bypass through an uninvolved anatomical region, however, are no insurance of complete success. This was established by one patient at Walter Reed General Hospital who had a disrupted common femoral artery repaired. Because without restoration of arterial continuity the patient's lower extremity was obviously doomed, a greater saphenous vein graft was utilized in an extra-anatomical position through the obturator canal. Unfortunately, despite meticulous technique and use of all known precautions, this bypass also became infected and had to be removed. Interestingly, the extremity remained viable after this additional complication, with ligation of the common iliac artery.

If arterial ligation is necessary, it should not be carried out with the artery in conti-

nuity. One patient whose case emphasizes this point was a Vietnam casualty who had an infected wound with disruption of a lateral suture repair of the distal innominate artery. Ligation in continuity of the artery proximal to the area of disruption and distal ligation were elected. There was massive hemorrhage again, with an additional disruption 5 days later. At that time the artery was divided and the ends oversewn. The artery should have been divided at the first operation, ensuring a good, secure ligature control of both ends. It must be remembered, nevertheless, that even suture lines of this type can become infected and can develop subsequent hemorrhage. The problem of repeated attempts to perform a vascular repair in the presence of infection is emphasized in the following Vietnam case review:

The patient initially sustained multiple fragment wounds with transection of the right superficial femoral artery and vein. Among the procedures performed was an end-to-end anastomosis of the greater saphenous vein, proximal to the thigh, near the saphenofemoral junction to the superficial femoral vein (which was more distal in the thigh), and a saphenous vein interposition graft repair of the superficial femoral artery. The following day a tricompartment fasciotomy was carried out, and the vascular repairs were explored. On the fifth postoperative day, when a delayed primary closure of the wound was performed, there was one episode of brisk bleeding from the artery; however, it was stated that no future suture was necessary. Ten days after the injury there was a disruption of the arterial anastomosis. Although it was mentioned that there was edematous tissue with necrosis surrounding the disrupted vein graft, a second greater saphenous vein interposition venous graft was obtained from the opposite extremity and used to reconstitute the arterial flow. Three days after the second vein graft repair, there was another disruption of the proximal anastomosis, and resection and re-anastomosis were carried out. At this time, nearly 2 weeks after the initial injury, a knee disarticulation was necessary because the leg was infected. Approximately 16 days after the initial repair, a third major disruption occurred, and ligation of the superficial femoral artery was carried out. Five days subsequent to this last procedure, disruption of the proximal femoral artery again occurred, and it was necessary to ligate the common femoral artery.

Brisbin and associates[3] based their experience and recommendation that ligation, rather than repair of noncritical arteries, should be carried out at the time of initial debridement partially on statistics from the initial Vietnam Vascular Registry report.[51] They noted the complication rate of approximately 30%. They advocated that the following vessels could usually be ligated in the young without loss of limb: (1) the brachial artery between the profunda and collaterals at the elbow, (2) the ulnar or radial artery alone at any level, (3) the profunda femoris artery, (4) the superficial femoral artery proximal to the genicular collateral, and (5) the posterior tibial, anterior tibial, or peroneal arteries alone at any level. Although there is a place for ligation rather than repair in salvage of life rather than limb, the overall experience would indicate that this recommendation is too general. It is often very difficult to determine at the time of initial debridement which brachial artery, which superficial femoral artery, or which other artery mentioned above, is critical to limb viability. Also, the fairly high complication rate from the Vietnam experience must be considered in proper perspective, particularly noting that many of the complications were those of technique, which were corrected at the time of the initial procedure. It is difficult to appreciate why these authors would recommend superficial femoral arterial ligation when the figures quoted both from World War II by DeBakey and Simeone[7] and from Korea by Inui and associates[19] documented that ligation of the superficial femoral artery in war wounds (presumably in young, healthy males) resulted in a 45% to 75% amputation rate. Ligation of major arteries may be indicated in specific instances, especially if severe soft tissue loss prevents coverage of the repaired artery. In addition, primary amputation may also be indicated in the massively traumatized extremity in which there is extensive damage to major arteries, veins, nerves, bones, and soft tissue (see Fig. 26-1). It is important to exercise sound surgical judgment in making these difficult decisions.

Stenosis

Two major types of stenosis can develop as a complication of attempted arterial repair. The first is purely a technical complication caused by pulling too tightly on the suture during the repair, by attempting to perform a lateral repair without sufficient remaining arterial wall, by suturing arterial wall where residual damage remains, by placing too much tension on the suture line, or by other problems related to the suture line itself. The problem should be readily apparent if an intraoperative arteriogram is obtained. It can be corrected, usually, by performing another repair with more meticulous technique.

The second major type of stenosis usually develops from intimal hyperplasia at the suture line, which manifests itself over a matter of weeks or months. A representative example is one young soldier returning from Vietnam with what appeared clinically to be a successful autogenous interposition venous graft repair of the distal right axillary artery to the proximal right brachial artery. At the time of his initial examination at Walter Reed General Hospital, approximately 1 month after he was wounded, the soldier had bounding radial and ulnar pulses in the right upper extremity, and no bruit was audible along the repair site. Two months later, however, a bruit was heard over the repair site in his right arm, and it was thought that his right radial pulse was somewhat weaker. At 3 months after the initial repair, the patient complained of easy fatigability in his right upper extremity with moderate exercise, he had a loud bruit over the repair site, and his radial pulse was very weak, with no palpable ulnar pulse. Angiography revealed a marked stenosis at the proximal suture line. When this area of the repair was exposed surgically, there was a marked thrill over the stenotic anastomosis; however, the external appearance of the anastomosis did not allow a full appreciation of the degree of stenosis.

It was possible to excise the short segment of marked stenosis and to reconstruct the continuity successfully by new end-to-end anastomosis. Within a 5-year follow-up period there was no clinical evidence of restenosis at the proximal suture line or of stenosis at the distal suture line.

Whether a significantly high number of stenoses will progress to ultimate occlusion might be debatable. We have seen patients in the Vietnam Vascular Registry who have had audible bruit over the repair site. In the past, if there were no associated symptoms, angiography was not performed. However, we are reaching a more aggressive point in the follow-up, and we are attempting to provide further definition of this problem.

Amputation

Although the necessity for amputation is only one gauge of the success of an attempted major artery repair in an extremity, it is a final result. According to DeBakey and Simeone,[7] arterial wounds among American battle casualties in World War II accounted for 20% of all amputations. These authors demonstrated that the results were better in 81 cases in which ligation was performed. The amputation rate was lowered from 49% to 36%, although the group with the lower amputation rate following repair was much smaller than the group that had ligation of major arteries. Suture repair was also considerably better than two nonsuture types of repair: vein graft and tube anastomoses. In the latter two groups of anastomoses, which were also relatively small, the results were even slightly worse than those following ligation. It was pointed out that suture repairs were performed in a selected group of patients with minimal wounds who had no extensive tissue destruction. The amputation rates documented by these authors provide the best statistics on the outcome of arterial ligation (see Table 26-1).

When acute arterial injuries were managed by ligation in World War II, the incidence of gangrene in the lower extremity was twice that in the upper extremity. In reporting some of the experience from the Korean conflict, Ziperman[68] noted that gangrene of the arm required amputation in fewer than 10% of the patients with brachial arterial ligations, compared with a 50% amputation rate with ligation of the femoral artery. From their Korean experience Hughes,[17,18] Jahnke,[21] and Spencer and Grewe[61] also helped demonstrate that the amputation rate could be lowered to approximately 13% following arterial repair, compared with an amputation rate of nearly 50% in World War II, when arterial ligation was practiced. Although the amputation rate remained approximately 13% in Vietnam,[34,51,56] other factors were involved in these statistics (Table 26-10). Attempts were made at limb salvage in Vietnam; this had not been done in other wars. Also, the Vietnam statistics include longer-term follow-up. This is reflected by statistics of both Fisher[13] and Cohen and associates,[6] when they reported an amputation rate of approximately 8% in Vietnam. Rich and Hughes,[51] in the preliminary report from the Vietnam Vascular Registry, recorded that nearly one third of the amputations were performed in the relatively early follow-up period after patients were evacuated from Vietnam. Details of associated injuries, as well as the method of vascular repair, must be available to ensure that adequate and accurate statistical methods are used to evaluate the management of vascular trauma. An example that emphasizes this is one soldier who had a superficial femoral arterial repair in Vietnam. It was noted that he had a below-the-knee amputation on the same side. Initially, this was erroneously attributed to failure of the superficial femoral arterial repair. However, when the detailed records became available, it was evident that the amputation had been necessary at the time of the original debridement, because of massive soft tissue and bone damage. The patient maintained strong femoral and popliteal pulses in his postoperative course, which indicated the success of his arterial repair.

In a large, early series of civilian arterial injuries, Morris and associates[27] documented an overall amputation rate of 8.8%–12 amputations among the 136 arterial injuries (see Table 26-5). In the 93 repairs that were performed, there were seven amputations, an amputation rate of approximately 7.5%. Ferguson and co-authors[12] reported an am-

Table 26-10. Amputation Rate for 950 Acute Major Arterial Injuries in Vietnam (Excluding 50 Carotid Arteries)*

ARTERY	NO. OF INJURIES	NO. OF AMPUTATIONS	PERCENTAGE	PERCENTAGE OF TOTAL
UPPER EXTREMITY				
Axillary	59	3	5.1 ⎫	
Brachial	283	16	5.7 ⎭	2.0
ABDOMEN				
Common iliac	9	1	11.1	0.1
LOWER EXTREMITY				
Common femoral	46	7	15.2 ⎫	
Superficial Femoral	305	37	12.1	11.4
Popliteal	217	64	29.5 ⎭	
Total		128		13.5

* Arteries repaired without subsequent amputations; innominate, subclavian, aorta, and external iliac are not listed in this table.
(Rich, N.M., Baugh, J.H., and Hughes, C.W.: Acute arterial injuries in Vietnam. J. Trauma, 10:359, 1970)

putation rate of 9.8% (17 amputations in 168 patients) where wounds involved extremity arteries. In their series, only restoration of distal pulsations was considered adequate evidence of successful arterial repair. In the group undergoing arterial repair (88 of 200 patients) there were 12 amputations (13.6%). In the 92 patients of 200 in whom acute arterial injuries were managed by ligation of the artery, there were only three amputations (3.3%). However, this cannot be compared to the entire group in which arterial repair was attempted, because ligation was usually used when the injured extremity or visceral artery was small. Smith and co-workers[60] felt that 80% of their 28 patients with acute arterial injuries had either excellent or good results. They mentioned that amputation was necessary in only two cases. In the series of 85 patients with arterial trauma in St. Louis, Dillard and co-workers[9] reported an amputation rate of approximately 3% (2 cases in 67) following arterial injuries to the extremities. Both of these amputations were associated with popliteal artery trauma. Problems associated with popliteal artery injuries were again emphasized, with two amputations required for 10 injuries, a 20% amputation rate for the popliteal artery. Drapanas and associates[10] reported an amputation rate of 7.1% among 181 patients with injuries to arteries of the extremities. Their civilian experience corresponded to the military experience in demonstrating that the location of the arterial injury in an extremity was an important consideration related to the amputation rate. Injuries to the popliteal and combined tibial arteries were followed by a higher incidence of amputation than in injuries of the brachial artery, whether ligation or repair was carried out. Perry and associates[33] reported that amputation was required in only three of 165 patients in whom the vessel injury was ultimately concerned with viability of the extremity, representing an amputation rate of only 1.8%. Patman and associates, in their earlier report from Dallas,[30] reported that eight amputations were required in their series, which involved 221 cases in which extremity arterial injuries ultimately threatened the viability of a limb. This represented a 3.8% true amputation rate in the remaining 209 patients, excluding 12 patients who died (Table 26-11).[4,5,11,20,24,63,67]

Table 26-11. Morbidity and Mortality in 256 Civilian Arterial Injuries*

VESSEL INVOLVED	NO. OF AMPUTATIONS	NO. OF DEATHS
Aorta	0	3
Subclavian	0	1
Axillary	0	3
Hepatic	0	3
Common carotid	0	4
External carotid	0	1
Common iliac	1	3
Hypogastric	0	1
External iliac	0	1
Vertebral	0	1
Common femoral	2	0
Superficial femoral	2	0
Brachial	2	0
Popliteal	1	0
Total	8 (3.8%)	21 (8.2%)

* Dallas, July 1, 1949, to July 1, 1969
(Modified from Patman, R.D., Poulos, E., and Shires, G.T.: The management of civilian arterial injuries. Surg. Gynecol. Obstet., 118:725, 1964)

Death

The exact incidence of death following acute arterial trauma is unknown. Many patients who die of their injuries have an associated massive hemorrhage, which may or may not be recognized. The fact that even after reaching a hospital, patients can bleed to death before an arterial repair can be performed is apparent from the mortality figures of the series reported by Morris and associates,[27] in which seven of the 12 patients who died of their arterial injuries died of blood loss. These included four aortic wounds, two wounds of the carotid artery, and one of the subclavian artery. Particularly in the civilian series evaluating acute arterial injuries, it can be seen that excessive blood loss has been closely associated with many of the deaths. Ferguson and co-authors[12] reported 31 deaths in their series of 200 patients with acute arterial injuries, a mortality rate of 15.5% (Table 26-12). Death was a direct result of blood loss in 84% of the fatal cases. Among those patients in their series with arterial repairs (88 of the 200 patients), there were eight deaths, a mortality rate of 9.1%. Pate and

Wilson[29] noted that there was a mortality rate of nearly 20% (four deaths) in their series of 21 patients with arterial injuries of the base of the neck treated at the City of Memphis Hospitals over a 12-year period. The four deaths resulted from carotid artery injuries in two patients and subclavian artery injuries in the remaining two. Insufficient exposure and inadequate repair were major factors in both patients who had fatal hemorrhages following subclavian artery injuries. A review by Dillard and associates[9] found that there were two operative deaths resulting from 35 arterial injuries caused by knife and glass lacerations. One death was attributed to severe laceration of the left pulmonary artery with massive exsanguination at the time of operation. These authors also presented the interesting and tragic case of a patient whose death was caused by unsuspected massive blood loss from an injury to the superior epigastric artery, which occurred during paracentesis. Saletta and Freeark[58] recorded three deaths, all from early and late effects of excessive blood loss among 57 patients with partially severed arteries, a 5.3% mortality rate.

In addition to the contribution of excessive blood loss to death, it is obvious that the location of the arterial trauma has a significant effect on both morbidity and mortality. In the series reported by Drapanas and co-authors,[10] the majority of deaths

Table 26-12. Causes of Death in 200 Patients With Acute Arterial Injuries*

Hemorrhagic shock	19
Renal failure secondary to shock	6
Secondary hemorrhage	1
Complications of abdominal injuries	3
Tracheal compression due to hemorrhage	1
Pulmonary embolus	1
Total	31 (15.5%)

*Grady Memorial Hospital, Atlanta, Georgia, January 1, 1950, to December 31, 1959
(Modified from Ferguson, I.A., Byrd, W.M., and McAfee, D.K.: Experiences in the management of arterial injuries. Ann. Surg., 153:980, 1961)

Table 26-13. Incidence of Edema Following Repair of Major Arterial Injuries of Extremities

ARTERY REPAIRED	NO. OF REPAIRS	NO. WITH EDEMA*
Subclavian	16	3
Axillary	12	2
Brachial	39	10
Iliac and common iliac	16	9
Superficial femoral	31	11
Popliteal	14	6
Total	128	41

* Factors possibly contributing to the edema: shock (17), severe ischemia (16), vein injury (21)
(Modified from Drapanas, T., Hewitt, R.L., Weichert, R.F., and Smith, A.D.: Civilian vascular injuries: A critical appraisal of three decades of management. Ann. Surg., 172:351, 1970)

occurred in patients whose injuries involved major large arteries, including the thoracic aorta, the abdominal aorta, and the subclavian and iliac arteries. In their New Orleans series of 226 patients with arterial injuries there were 24 deaths, representing a case fatality rate of 10.6%. The majority of deaths involved injury to the aorta, and death occurred in approximately 50% of these injuries (Table 26-13). For the 181 patients with injuries to arteries of the extremities, the case fatality rate was 5.5%.

Perdue and Smith[32] emphasized that the site of arterial injury had an effect on the ultimate outcome, noting that all four of their patients with suprarenal abdominal aortic injuries died, resuscitation being impossible, and that five of the seven patients in their series with trauma to the infrarenal abdominal aorta died in the operating room of exsanguination. Thirty-five of the 90 patients with acute intra-abdominal vascular injury died, a mortality rate of approximately 39%. They also noted in their series that there were only two survivors among 13 patients who received more than 10,000 ml of whole blood.

Other associated injuries can also contribute to the mortality rate. Patman and associates[30] reported an 8.2% mortality rate, with 21 deaths among 256 civilians in Dallas who had arterial injuries. All but one of these patients was admitted in a state of profound shock, and the incidence of associated injuries was also high. In the continuation of this series from Dallas, the mortality rate was noted to be 10.4%, consisting of 27 deaths among 259 patients reported by Perry and associates[33] in 1971. Table 26-14 illustrates the distribution and importance of serious associated injuries that contributed to many of the deaths. In their review of 90 patients with acute abdominal vascular injuries, Perdue and Smith[32] found that the mortality rate increased with the number of associated organ injuries. When there was an isolated intra-abdominal injury, the mortality rate was 17%; this increased to 50% when several other abdominal organs were involved. These authors also found a much higher mortality rate (55%) for multiple-vessel injuries, compared with the 31% mortality for single-vessel injuries. Dillard and associates[9] emphasized the importance of being aware of additional organ trauma, noting that one of their patients who died had an unrecognized laceration of the spleen, which was associated with a left subclavian arterial laceration.

Table 26-14. Mortality Rate Associated With Arterial Injuries

ARTERY	NO. OF DEATHS	ASSOCIATED INJURIES
Aorta	8	Abdominal viscera (8), major vein (4)
Iliac	8	Abdominal viscera (8), major vein (5)
Carotid	4	Stroke (1), intracranial injury (2)
Femoral	3	Multiple injury to chest and head
Axillary	2	Subclavian vein, lung
Subclavian	1	Subclavian, innominate vein, lung
Renal	1	Abdominal viscera, vena cava
Total	27 (10.4%)	

(Modified from Perry, M.O., Thai, E.R., and Shires, G.T.: Management of arterial injuries. Ann. Surg., 173: 403, 1971)

In two recent, large series of civilian arterial injuries, Moore and associates[26] documented a mortality rate of 2.4%, six deaths in their series of 250 vascular injuries in patients treated at the University of Texas Medical Branch Hospitals in Galveston during a 10-year period ending in January 1970. Cohen and associates[6] reported seven deaths among 450 vascular injuries treated in Vietnam during a 6-month period in 1968, a 1.6% mortality rate. The fact that the mortality rate in the combat zone can be compared favorably with that in the civilian community is again emphasized by the interim report from the Vietnam Vascular Registry, in which 1000 patients with acute major arterial injury had a mortality rate of 1.7%, according to Rich and co-workers.[34]

Long-Term Changes

To any scholar interested in vascular trauma, it is readily apparent that there are very few centers that continue to attempt to obtain long-term follow-up of patients who sustained major vascular trauma, owing to the inherent problems of follow-up. Some of the injured patients are not the most reliable, having suffered gunshot wounds in street brawls and similar incidents. Other patients may not reside in the vicinity of the hospital where they were treated. Maintaining current addresses for patients in our changing society, which sees numerous moves for most families, is difficult at best.

The Vietnam Vascular Registry material[34-57] has provided a somewhat unusual opportunity to obtain long-term follow-up on most of nearly 7500 patients in a young, healthy age group, who had sustained arterial trauma. With the combined effort of many individuals and numerous government agencies, an attempt is being made to analyze the information gathered to provide valid statistics and interesting data to be used in the management of civilian arterial injuries. The development of intimal hyperplasia in the relatively short period of less than 1 year has provided valuable information. The long-term follow-up—between 5 and 10 years—is mandatory, to determine the true significance of aneurysmal dilatation that might occur in vein

grafts used as segmental replacements for injured arteries. Anecdotal, individual case reports can be found sporadically in the literature, but the registry records relatively large numbers of patients and will provide some significant statistics.

The complication of aneurysmal dilatation of grafts is diagnosed and documented rather infrequently. It is now believed that the complication occurs more frequently than was previously recognized. Nevertheless, the true significance of generalized fusiform aneurysmal dilatation in an autogenous vein graft used as an interposition replacement to restore arterial continuity is not completely understood at this time. It is well known that aneurysmal dilatation has developed in vein grafts used to replace large arteries, and that this dilatation can be prevented by external support. Although aneurysmal dilatation of a cephalic vein graft replacing a segment of artery was reported by Shaw,[59] Hershey and Spencer[15] did not find in their series that there was any particular dilatation of vein grafts used to repair arterial injuries in extremities. They pointed out that even cephalic and brachial venous comitans, which had very thin walls, also functioned well in their six cases. Hershey and Spencer,[15] documenting their use of autogenous vein grafts, stated that no aneurysms were noted in the ten saphenous vein grafts as long as 6 years after injury. Whelan and Baugh[64] documented the case of a patient at Walter Reed General Hospital who developed aneurysmal dilatation of a popliteal vein used as an autogenous venous graft in the popliteal artery when both the popliteal artery and the vein had been injured. In the Vietnam experience, it was generally recognized that the autogenous greater saphenous vein is the best conduit for segmental arterial replacement. It has been argued that the thinner-walled accompanying vein, such as the popliteal vein, should not be utilized to perform segmental arterial replacement, because there is a greater tendency for dilatation. An example of this is one veteran who had a brachial arterial repair with a segment of brachial vein in Vietnam in 1970. Approximately 4 months later, a follow-up angiogram showed a fusiform aneurysmal dilatation of the vein graft.

Another patient with a high-velocity gunshot wound of the upper thigh had transection of both the superficial femoral artery and vein. After ligation of the superficial femoral vein, a segment of this vessel was used as a substitution graft to restore the continuity of the superficial femoral artery. An arteriogram obtained approximately 3 weeks later showed the 3-cm segment of superficial femoral vein to have a dilatation approximately twice the size of the superficial femoral artery. Within a short time the area became even more aneurysmal, and it was necessary to resect and replace it with a saphenous venous graft.

There are recent reports of diffuse fusiform aneurysmal dilatation in autogenous greater saphenous vein grafts used in aortorenal bypass, and a disturbing finding has occurred in several Vietnam casualties. One patient had had an autogenous greater saphenous vein graft used to bypass his occluded innominate artery, extending from the ascending portion of the arch of the aorta to the innominate bifurcation. Approximately 5 years later, fusiform aneurysmal dilatation was noted in this vein graft, which had remained patent. Another patient had had a left carotid–axillary arterial bypass with an autogenous greater saphenous vein graft in 1970. A follow-up arteriogram in 1974 revealed some fusiform aneurysmal dilatation.

It has been demonstrated, both experimentally and clinically, that trauma can accelerate the local arteriosclerotic process. It is beyond the scope of this chapter to provide a detailed review of this subject, and it is well known that many questions remain to be answered. There are significant medicolegal problems that can develop in the arteriosclerotic patient with minor or major trauma, regardless of whether this condition has previously been diagnosed. DeTakats and Fowler[8] revealed that the relationship of arteriosclerosis of the peripheral vascular tree to trauma may be examined in three categories for medicolegal problems:

Severe blunt or penetrating injuries that rupture, weaken, or close a large vessel. The patient should develop some symptoms, and the evidence of the existing damage should appear within 3 to 4 weeks. It is helpful to have some knowledge of the vascular status before the injury, but this is not always available. Arguments have been marshaled for the vulnerability of a previously diseased vessel, even if it is asymptomatic, such as a thoracic aortic aneurysm after a steering-wheel injury or a sudden thrombosis of an atheromatous popliteal artery after a fall.

Injuries—usually mild, everyday, casual collisions with the environment—that decompensate a previously compensated but precarious peripheral circulation. Although the minor accidents frequently contribute to a natural course of the disease, the circumstances under which they happen and the immediate and early management of the injury have a decisive influence on the extent and duration of the disability, depending on whether the accident occurred at home or at work.

Injuries in which a demonstrable or documented insult affects an arteriosclerotic patient who can produce or exhibit no evidence of a connection between the insult and his peripheral vascular status. Records of previous examinations are extremely important in this situation, for comparison with the objective findings after the injury.

DELAYED RECOGNITION OF VASCULAR INJURIES

If the acute vascular injury initially goes unrecognized, arteriovenous fistulas (Fig. 26-10) and false aneurysms (Fig. 26-11) can develop. This is usually not a true and serious complication, but it does fall into the category of delayed recognition of vascular trauma. Although some of these lesions may be recognized essentially at the time of injury and diagnosed as acute arteriovenous fistula or pulsating hematoma, the majority are recognized days to months following the initial trauma. Successful reconstruction at a later date has usually been possible. Patman and associates[30] noted the development of false aneurysms in 12 patients and arteriovenous fistulas in six patients as late complications in their series of civilians who had sustained arterial trauma. Only one of the patients who de-

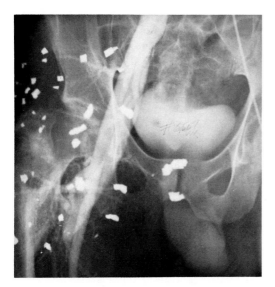

FIG. 26-10. Arteriovenous fistulas may not be clinically recognized at the initial examination. Multiple fragments, as seen here, increase the potential for vascular injuries. This angiogram outlines a profunda femoris arteriovenous fistula. A thrill and bruit were recognized for the first time over the femoral triangle approximately 3 weeks after the patient was wounded. (N.M.R., Vietnam Vascular Registry #6507)

veloped arteriovenous fistula had had an initial exploration of his wound. The fact that the arteriovenous fistula was evident in this patient within 4 hours after injury emphasizes the rapidity with which this complication can develop and demonstrates that arterial trauma did exist but was not recognized. Perry and associates[33] noted in 1971 that there were no late complications of false aneurysms or arteriovenous fistulas among 232 surviving patients in their series from Dallas between 1962 and 1968 (which was a continuation of the series reported by Patman and associates[30] from 1964). Perry and colleagues stressed that this was in contrast to the previous report from Dallas, in which exploration was not performed at the time of initial injury in 17 patients, 12 of whom developed false aneurysms and five of whom developed arteriovenous fistulas. They also found that in 312 patients who had had exploration without the finding of major arterial trauma, there was no mortality, and the only significant morbidity was wound infection

(3.1%). It was pointed out that in many of these operations, vascular exploration was performed in conjunction with debridement of a significant wound of an extremity, and it did not constitute the primary indication for the operation. Rich, Hobson, and Collins[45] reported in 1975 on the Vietnam Vascular Registry evaluation and follow-up of 509 combat casualties with 558 arteriovenous fistulas and false aneurysms. Approximately 50% of these lesions were managed by ligation of the involved vessels, and approximately 50% had vascular reconstruction. From this large series the mortality rate was only 1.8%, and the morbidity associated with the vascular injury was 6.3%. There were eight amputations, for an amputation rate of 1.7%. Potential complications of heart failure, proximal arterial dilatation, and endocarditis were essentially absent.

Thrombus from either the site of arterial injury or the site of arterial repair can

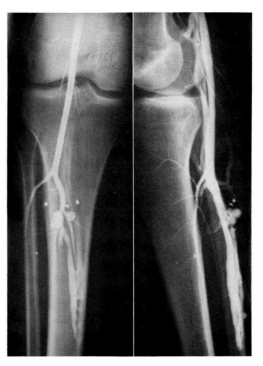

FIG. 26-11. Multiple false aneurysms of the posterior tibial artery, as well as an arteriovenous fistula, are shown on this angiogram. The offending fragments are in close proximity. (N.M.R., Vietnam Vascular Registry #2761)

embolize into the distal arterial branches. This is one of the potential complications associated with false aneurysms. In some unusual situations, such as axillary or brachial arterial trauma caused by prolonged use of crutches, some of the lesions have presented with mural thrombus with distal embolization aneurysm formation with distal embolization. Although available collateral pathways usually assure viability of the upper extremity, some degree of arterial insufficiency may develop and can become disabling. The other complications associated with arteriovenous fistulas include endocarditis, heart failure, and proximal arterial dilatation. These problems have not been reported frequently in the recent literature.

In children there can be increased limb growth associated with vascular trauma, as well as the decreased limb growth that was previously mentioned following arterial thrombosis in children. White and coauthors[65] presented the case of a 9-month-old girl who developed an arteriovenous communication between the right profunda femoris artery and the profunda femoris vein following arterial blood gas sampling, when the needle must have passed through both the artery and the vein, creating a direct communication. Over the next 3 years, the child was constantly in borderline heart failure with a pulse rate of more than 120 beats per minute, and her heart increased in size. When she was 4½ years old, a thrill was noted over her left groin, the left leg was 2 cm longer than the right, and the proximal fibular epiphysis was present on the left and not on the right. Following closure of the arteriovenous fistula, over the next several months the pulse rate gradually returned to normal, and the cardiac failure cleared. Whenever a child is seen with asymmetric increased limb growth, the possibility of an arteriovenous fistula must be considered. Marked improvement or cure can be anticipated with closure of the arteriovenous communications.

COMPLICATIONS ASSOCIATED WITH CONCOMITANT INJURY AND DISEASE

There are numerous other potential and actual complications that can be associated with attempted arterial reconstruction. As with any major operation, injury to other structures can occur. Particular care should be taken to preserve major venous return and to identify and preserve adjacent nerves. The unfortunate mishaps that can occur include the retention of foreign material. One Vietnam casualty had lacerations of the right external iliac artery and vein, among other abdominal wounds. The vein was ligated, and the artery was repaired with end-to-end anastomosis. Postoperatively, the patient complained of occasional abdominal pain, and a roentgenogram of the abdomen revealed a small clamp in the lower abdomen. The vascular bulldog clamp was removed approximately 4 months after the initial operation.

Concomitant injuries to arteries and bone create additional challenge and potential complications. Continuing controversy involves the proper management of a fractured bone with a concomitant arterial injury. In the military experience, immobilization of the fracture by external methods has usually been successful. Attempts at immobilization by intramedullary fixation have generally been avoided in contaminated wounds treated under combat conditions; however, civilian experience with similar injuries has been different (see Fig. 26-9). The failure to recognize arterial trauma associated with fractures has been a particular diagnostic dilemma. Although no arterial repair might have been performed, this must be a complication of the management of patients with concomitant injuries as outlined. If the artery is not explored within a few hours of the time of injury and if, consequently, the arterial obstruction secondary to arterial trauma associated with concomitant fractures and dislocations is not corrected, amputation will almost certainly be necessary. According to Gardner[14] and Miller[25] the amputation rate for such injuries to the lower extremity is nearly 100%. The enigma of the popliteal artery remains, and the amputation rate in both military and civilian experience remains relatively high. Arterial trauma overlooked on the initial examination may present at any time. An example of this is the case of a patient mentioned by Whelan and Baugh[64] in 1967 who had a fracture of the neck of the humerus. There was medial angulation of the distal fragment of the humeral fracture, which lacerated the brachial artery. At the time that open reduction was attempted, a false aneurysm was entered, and arterial ligation was carried out. Although the extremity remained viable, the patient had ischemic symptoms, which were later alleviated by a bypass vein graft.

Injuries to nerves concomitant with arterial injuries have generally been managed by delayed repair of the nerves approximately 3 weeks to 3 months after the initial injury, based on the World War II experience. In the military experience, failure of the primary nerve repair has been a relatively common complication.

Decreased function can be a complication following arterial repair. This may be based partly on the lack of proper physical therapy in the early postoperative period. Drapanas and co-workers[10] found that 20.4% of their patients experienced decreased function— for a long time or permanently—that was not due to any apparent motor nerve or muscle trauma. This occurred in some of their patients who had trauma to major extremity arteries. These authors also documented the fact that 10.2% of their patients with arterial trauma had chronic pain in their salvaged extremities. With or without obvious associated venous trauma, persistent swelling has also been associated with arterial trauma. Again, Drapanas and co-workers[10] emphasized that the development of marked edema was a distressing complication that occurred within a few hours after arterial flow was restored to a previously ischemic limb. Despite the fact that an apparently successful arterial repair was obtained and fasciotomies were performed to decompress the muscle, progressive edema and subsequent necrosis were observed on occasion. Some degree of edema was seen in 41 patients in their series following restoration of arterial flow in an injured extremity (Table 26-15). Factors that were generally believed to be important in the development of edema, including shock, severe ischemia, and concomitant venous injuries, occurred in a fairly large number of patients. However, these authors pointed out that delay in treatment, incidence of venous injury, and presence of shock were not significantly different from the same factors in the group that did

Table 26-15. Deaths due to Civilian Arterial Injuries in 226 Patients in New Orleans: 1942–1969

ARTERY INVOLVED	NO. OF DEATHS
Abdominal aorta	6
Thoracic aorta	5
Subclavian	4
Iliac	4
Superficial femoral	2
Superior mesenteric	1
Renal	1
Carotid	1
Total	24 (10.6%)

(Modified from Drapanas, T., Hewitt, R.L., Weichert, R.F., and Smith, A.D.: Civilian vascular injuries: A critical appraisal of three decades of management. *Ann. Surg.*, 172:351, 1970)

not develop edema. They found that severe ischemia was noted on admission in 40% of the patients who developed edema, as compared with an incidence of 24.1% among patients who did not develop edema.

Although some of the details are not completely understood, numerous clotting defects can be induced by multiple blood transfusions. Disseminated intravascular coagulopathies associated with vascular trauma are being recognized with greater frequency. The hazard of the development of disseminated intravascular coagulopathies increases with each successive unit of blood and can become an appreciable problem, manifested by diffuse, uncontrollable oozing, after approximately 500 ml of blood replacement. The oozing may continue despite all measures, and death can result. Patman and co-workers[30] mentioned that this occurred in two of their 21 patients who died, an incidence of approximately 10% of the total deaths.

Among the assortment of other complications that can be associated with arterial injury and/or arterial repair are unusual complications, such as the development of an aortoenteric fistula. An aortoenteric fistula can develop after repair of a traumatic wound of the aorta or the iliac arteries. However, if a Dacron prosthesis is used in the repair, the incidence could be at least as high as that reported in managing aortoiliac occlusive disease and aneurysmal

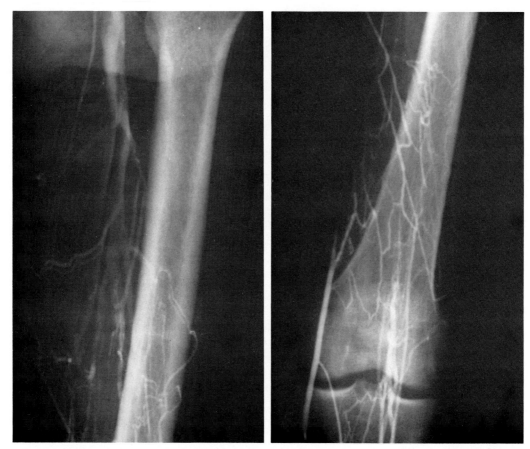

FIG. 26-12. Venous injury, particularly in the lower extremity, can be associated with the complications of acute venous hypertension and/or chronic venous insufficiency. This phlebogram demonstrates interruption of both the greater saphenous vein and the superficial femoral vein. Collateral venous return was poor, and the patient had signs and symptoms similar to those of the postphlebitic syndrome. (Rich, N.M., Hughes, C.W., and Baugh, J.H.: Management of venous injuries. Ann. Surg., 171:724, 1970)

disease of the abdominal aorta. One patient in Vietnam did develop an aortoenteric fistula a short time after a common iliac arterial repair. This patient had sustained multiple fragment wounds in an enemy booby trap. Lateral repairs of the right common iliac artery and left common iliac vein were carried out, as well as repair of several lacerations in the fourth portion of the duodenum. The transverse colon was exteriorized as a loop colostomy because of a perforation. Approximately 2 weeks after he had been wounded, infection and hemorrhage developed, and it was necessary to manage an associated iliac artery–small bowel fistula. The distal aorta was ligated, and the opening in the small bowel was

sutured. One week subsequent to the second operation, the patient developed a small-bowel fistula and pelvic abscess; he died within several days.

COMPLICATIONS ASSOCIATED WITH ACUTE VENOUS TRAUMA

Compared to arterial trauma, there has been relatively little general interest in the management of venous injuries. Concern over the possibility of an increased incidence of thrombophlebitis and pulmonary embolism following attempted repair of injured veins has been a deterrent, even in recent years.[16,42,50,52,56]

If the military experience in Southeast

Asia, from the management of thousands of American wounded, can make a positive contribution in the medical community, it will most likely be in promoting a more aggressive approach toward repair, rather than ligation, of injured veins, particularly in the lower extremities. This was stimulated by the recognition of acute venous insufficiency, which contributed to the relatively high amputation rate following popliteal vascular injuries. Also, in follow-up through the Vietnam Vascular Registry, many Vietnam casualties were seen who had signs and symptoms of chronic venous insufficiency (Fig. 26-12), not unlike those seen in patients with the postphlebitic syndrome.[35]

Based on this clinical experience and the experimental work performed at the Walter Reed Army Institute of Research,[16,42,56] an increased interest has been generated in the past several years for venous repair. A unique opportunity has been afforded by the long-term follow-up in the Vietnam Vascular Registry; one study evaluated the management of 110 injured popliteal veins without associated popliteal arterial trauma.[46] Nearly an equal number of veins were ligated and repaired. Thrombophlebitis and pulmonary embolism were significant complications in this series. The only pulmonary embolus occurred after ligation of the injured vein. However, there was a significant increase in edema of the involved extremity following ligation: 50.9% compared to 13.2% after repair.

REFERENCES

1. Bernheim, B.M.: Blood vessel surgery in war. Surg. Gynecol. Obstet., 30:564, 1920.
2. Bolasny, B.L., and Killen, D.A.: Surgical management of arterial injury secondary to angiography. Ann. Surg., 174:962, 1971.
3. Brisbin, R.L., Geib, P.O., and Eiseman, B.: Secondary disruption of vascular repair following war wounds. Arch. Surg., 99:787, 1969.
4. Burnett, H.F., Parnell, C.L., Williams, G.D., and Campbell, G.S.: Peripheral arterial injuries: A reassessment. Ann. Surg., 183:701, 1976.
5. Cheek, R.C., Pope, J.C., Smith, H.F., and Britt, L.G.: Diagnosis and management of major vascular injuries: A review of two hundred operative cases. Am. Surg., 41:755, 1975.
6. Cohen, A., Baldwin, J.N., and Grant, R.N.: Problems in the management of battlefield vascular injuries. Am. J. Surg., 118:526, 1969.
7. DeBakey, M.E., and Simeone, F.A.: Battle injuries of arteries in World War II: An Analysis of 2,471 cases. Ann. Surg., 123:534, 1946.
8. deTakats, G., and Fowler, E.F.: Trauma to the arteriosclerotic limb. Trauma, 4:47, 1963.
9. Dillard, B.M., Nelson, D.L., and Norman, H.G., Jr.: Review of 85 traumatic arterial injuries. Surgery, 63:391, 1968.
10. Drapanas, T., Hewitt, R.L., Weichert, R.F., and Smith, A.D.: Civilian vascular injuries: A critical appraisal of three decades of management. Ann. Surg., 172:351, 1970.
11. Feliciano, D.V., Bitondo, C.G., Mattox, K.L. et al.: Civilian trauma in the 1980's: A one year experience with 456 vascular and cardiac injuries. Ann. Surg., 199:717, 1984.
12. Ferguson, I.A., Byrd, W.M., and McAfee, D.K.: Experiences in the management of arterial injuries. Ann. Surg., 153:980, 1961.
13. Fisher, G.W.: Acute arterial injuries treated by the United States Army Medical Service in Vietnam, 1965–1966. J. Trauma, 7:844, 1967.
14. Gardner, C.: Traumatic vasospasm and its complications. Am. J. Surg., 83:468, 1952.
15. Hershey, F.B., and Spencer, A.D.: Autogenous vein grafts for repair of arterial injuries. Arch. Surg., 86:836, 1963.
16. Hobson, R.W. II, Rich, N.M., and Wright, C.B.: Venous Trauma: Pathophysiology, Diagnosis and Surgical Management. Mt. Kisko, NY, Futura Publishing, 1983.
17. Hughes, C.W.: The primary repair of wounds of major arteries. Ann. Surg., 141:297, 1955.
18. Hughes, C.W.: Arterial repair during the Korean War. Ann. Surg., 147:555, 1958.
19. Inui, F.K., Shannon, J., and Howard, J.M.: Arterial injuries in the Korean Conflict. Surgery, 37:850, 1955.
20. Jaggers, R.C., Feliciano, D.V., Mattox, K.L. et al.: Injury to popliteal vessels. Arch. Surg., 117:657, 1982.
21. Jahnke, E.J., Jr.: Late structural and functional results of arterial injuries primarily repaired. Surgery, 43:175, 1958.
22. Lavenson, G.S., Jr., Rich, N.M., and Strandness, D.E., Jr.: Ultrasonic flow detector value in the management of combat incurred vascular injuries. Arch. Surg., 102:392, 1971.
23. Levin, P.M., Rich, N.M., and Hutton, J.E., Jr.: The role of collateral circulation in arterial injuries. Arch. Surg., 102:392, 1971.
24. Lim, L.T., Michuda, M.S., Flanigan, D.T., and Pankovich, A.: Popliteal artery trauma: 31 consecutive cases without amputation. Arch. Surg., 115:1307, 1980.
25. Miller, D.S.: Gangrene from arterial injuries associated with fractures and dislocation of the leg in the young and in adults with normal circulation. Am. J. Surg., 93:367, 1957.
26. Moore, C.H., Wolma, F.J., Brown, R.W., and Derrick, J.R.: Vascular trauma, a review of 250 cases. Am. J. Surg., 122:576, 1971.
27. Morris, G.C., Jr., Beall, A.C., Jr., Roof, W.R., and DeBakey, M.E.: Surgical experience with 220 acute arterial injuries in civilian practice. Am. J. Surg., 99:775, 1960.
28. Owens, J.C.: The management of arterial trauma. Surg. Clin. North Am., 43:371, 1963.

29. Pate, J.W., and Wilson, H.: Arterial injuries of the base of the neck. Arch. Surg., 89:1106, 1964.
30. Patman, R.D., Poulos, E., and Shires, G.T.: The management of civilian arterial injuries. Surg. Gynecol. Obstet., 118:725, 1964.
31. Patman, R.D., and Thompson, J.E.: Fasciotomy in peripheral vascular surgery. Arch. Surg., 101:663, 1970.
32. Perdue, G.D., Jr., and Smith, R.B.: Intra-abdominal vascular injury. Surgery, 64:562, 1968.
33. Perry, M.O., Thai, E.R., and Shires, G.T.: Management of arterial injuries. Ann. Surg., 173:403, 1971.
34. Rich, N.M.: Acute arterial injuries in Vietnam: 1,000 cases. J. Trauma, 10:350, 1970.
35. Rich, N.M.: The significance of complications associated with vascular repairs performed in Vietnam. Arch. Surg., 100:646, 1970.
36. Rich, N.M.: Vascular trauma in Vietnam. J. Cardiovasc. Surg., 11:368, 1970.
37. Rich, N.M.: Surgery for arterial trauma. In Dale, W.A. (ed.): Management of Arterial Occlusive Disease, Chap. 14. Chicago, Year Book Medical Publishers, 1971.
38. Rich, N.M.: The fate of prosthetic material used to repair vascular injuries in contaminated wounds. J. Trauma, 12:459, 1972.
39. Rich, N.M.: Fifty years progress in vascular surgery. A.C.S. Bulletin, 57:35, 1972.
40. Rich, N.M.: Vascular trauma. Surg. Clin. North Am., 53:1367, 1973.
41. Rich, N.M.: Elective vascular reconstruction following trauma. Am. J. Surg., 130:712, 1975.
42. Rich, N.M.: Principles in indications for primary venous repair. Surgery, 91:492, 1982.
43. Rich, N.M., Amato, J.J., and Billy, L.J.: Arterial thrombosis secondary to temporary cavitation. Surg. Digest, 6:12, 1971.
44. Rich, N.M., Baugh, J.H., and Hughes, C.W.: Popliteal artery injuries in Vietnam. Am. J. Surg., 118:531, 1969.
45. Rich, N.M., Hobson, R.W. II, and Collins, G.J., Jr.: Traumatic arteriovenous fistulas and false aneurysms: A review of 558 lesions. Surgery, 78:817, 1975.
46. Rich, N.M., Hobson, R.W. II, Collins, G.J., Jr., and Andersen, C.A.: The effect of acute popliteal venous interruption. Ann. Surg., 183:365, 1976.
47. Rich, N.M., Hobson, R.W. II, and Fedde, C.W.: Vascular trauma secondary to diagnostic and therapeutic procedures. Am. J. Surg., 128:715, 1975.
48. Rich, N.M., Hobson, R.W. II, Fedde, C.W., and Collins, G.J., Jr.: Common femoral arterial trauma. J. Trauma, 15:628, 1975.
49. Rich, N., Hobson, R.W. II, Jarstfer, B.S., and Geer, T.M.: Subclavian artery trauma. J. Trauma, 13:485, 1973.
50. Rich, N.M., Hobson, R.W. II, Wright, C.B., Fedde, C.W.: Repair of lower extremity venous trauma: A more aggressive approach required. J. Trauma, 14:639, 1974.
51. Rich, N.M., and Hughes, C.W.: Vietnam Vascular Registry: A preliminary report. Surgery, 65:218, 1969.
52. Rich, N.M., Hughes, C.W., and Baugh, J.H.: Management of venous injuries Ann. Surg., 171:724, 1970.
53. Rich, N.M., Jarstfer, B.S., and Geer, T.M.: Popliteal artery repair failure: Causes and possible prevention. J. Cardiovasc. Surg., 15:340, 1974.
54. Rich, N.M., Manion, W.C., and Hughes, C.W.: Surgical and pathological evaluation of vascular injuries in Vietnam. J. Trauma, 9:279, 1969.
55. Rich, N.M., Metz, C.W., Jr., Hutton, N.E., Jr. et al.: Internal versus external fixation of fractures with concomitant vascular injuries in Vietnam. J. Trauma, 11:463, 1971.
56. Rich, N.M., and Spencer, F.C.: Vascular Trauma. Philadelphia, W.B. Saunders, 1978.
57. Rich, N.M., and Sullivan, W.G.: Clinical recanalization of an autogenous vein graft in the popliteal vein. J. Trauma, 12:919, 1972.
58. Saletta, J.D., and Freeark, R.J.: The partially severed artery. Arch. Surg., 97:198, 1968.
59. Shaw, R.S.: Reconstructive vascular surgery. N. Engl. J. Med. 266:399, 1962.
60. Smith, R.F., Szilagyi, D.E., and Pfeifer, J.R.: A study of arterial trauma. Arch. Surg., 86:825, 1963.
61. Spencer, F.C., and Grewe, R.V.: The management of acute arterial injuries in battle casualties. Ann. Surg., 141:304, 1955.
62. Swan, K.G., Hobson, R.W., Reynolds, D. et al. (eds.): Venous Surgery in the Lower Extremity. St. Louis, Warren H. Green, 1975.
63. Tackett, A.D., and Fale, W.G.: Vascular injuries to the extremities. Am. Surg., 43:488, 1977.
64. Whelan, T.J., and Baugh, J.H.: Non-atherosclerotic arterial lesions and their management. Curr. Probl. Surg., February 1967.
65. White, J.J., Talbert, J.L., and Haller, J.A., Jr.: Peripheral arterial injury in infants and children. Ann. Surg., 167:757, 1968.
66. Williams, G.D.: Peripheral vascular trauma: Report of 90 cases. Am. J. Surg., 116:725, 1968.
67. Youkey, J.R., Clagett, G.P., Rich, N.M. et al.: Vascular trauma secondary to diagnostic and therapeutic procedures: 1974 through 1982, a comparative review. Am. J. Surg., 146:788, 1983.
68. Ziperman, H.H.: Acute arterial injuries in the Korean War. Ann. Surg., 139:1, 1954.

27 Complications in Microvascular Surgery

JAMES R. URBANIAK AND ROBIN R. RICHARDS

Microsurgery has provided the orthopaedic surgeon with an effective means of dealing with many problems previously considered insoluble. The ability to successfully anastomose blood vessels 1 mm in diameter has made digital replantation and free tissue transfer a clinical reality. The first successful digital replantation with microsurgical technique was performed in 1965.[35] Since then, replantation has become commonplace, with most centers reporting viability rates of 80% and greater.[70] Daniel and Taylor described free tissue transfer with microvascular anastomosis in 1973.[14] Many valuable procedures have since been developed, including free vascularized bone transfer,[66] free innervated muscle transfer[39] and toe-to-thumb transfer.[7]

Complications are of particular importance in microvascular surgery. Most replantations and free tissue transfers take many hours of surgery to perform. The success of the procedure may depend on the continued patency of a single arterial and venous anastomosis. Elective reconstructive microsurgery often necessitates the transfer of normal tissue (e.g., a myocutaneous flap, toe, or fibula) to a distant site. If the transfer is not successful, this normal tissue will be lost, the original defect may be greater, and the surgical team will have spent many hours of time and effort.

The prevention of complications is paramount in microvascular surgery, since so much is at stake in each procedure. A successful replantation or free tissue transfer depends on careful preoperative planning, adequate patient preparation, precise intraoperative execution, and continuous postoperative monitoring. Deficiencies at any one of these stages can jeopardize the entire procedure. Few surgical results are as dramatically apparent as the failed replantation or free tissue transfer (Fig. 27-1). Fortunately, effective treatment is available for most complications in microvascular surgery. In this chapter we will discuss complications of microvascular surgery as they relate to anastomotic thrombosis, replantation, and free tissue transfer.

ANASTOMOTIC THROMBOSIS

The most important factor determining anastomotic patency is the technical adequacy of the microvascular repair.[25] Successful microsurgery requires familiarity with the operating microscope, microinstruments, and the handling of small blood vessels.[5] These skills are most appropriately learned in the laboratory. Once the microsurgeon has demonstrated proficiency in this setting, his skills can be transposed to the operating room.[15]

Microvascular anastomosis of small blood vessels is performed with sutures passing through the entire thickness of the vessel wall. Tissue necrosis is produced within the loop of the suture, and a repair process is initiated on each side.[10] Initially, the endothelial surface of the anastomosis is covered by fibrin.[49] By seven days, endothelial regeneration is well underway, crossing the suture line by 14 days. Complete endothelialization of the suture material takes up to 4 weeks.[63] The remaining layers of the vessel wall are repaired by the process of subintimal hyperplasia, which is dependent on the viability of the medial layer. By 4 to 6 weeks the internal elastic lamina of the vessel wall is reconstituted. Anastomotic patency is necessary for any microvascular surgical procedure to be successful. Both local and systemic factors are important in preventing anastomotic thrombosis.

Local Factors

Vessel Damage. Disruption of the intimal layer exposes the subendothelium, which initiates platelet aggregation and

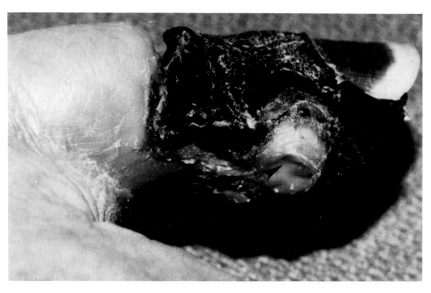

FIG. 27-1. Necrotic toe-to-thumb transfer. This 19-year-old patient was returned to the operating room 48 hours following thumb reconstruction when there was a sudden drop in the temperature of the reconstructed digit. Although the anterior anastomosis, which had thrombosed, was successfully revised, most of the transferred tissue went on to necrosis. A small portion directly over the vascular pedicle survived (*arrowhead*).

thrombus formation. Even small areas of intimal damage can produce sufficient thrombosis to occlude a 1-mm vessel. The intima is delicate and can be damaged enough to produce thrombus formation by merely grasping the full thickness of the vessel wall with a jeweler's forceps.[1] Every effort must be made to avoid intimal damage by careful handling of the vessel by the adventitia. The full thickness of the vessel wall should never be grasped. If mechanical dilation of the vessel is necessary, it must be done gently, preferably with a single pass of the dilator.

Great care must be taken to ensure that the anastomosis is performed between vessels that have been cut back to normal tissue, which is determined by examination under high-power magnification (20× or more). The most common reason for thrombosis of a technically adequate anastomosis in replantation surgery is the failure to appose normal intima to normal intima.[70] Vessel ends should always be inspected under the highest possible magnification to determine that the intima is undamaged. This is particularly important in amputations in which there has been an avulsion component to the injury. Intimal damage may be present at great distance from the site of amputation[20] in such injuries.

During microsurgical anastomosis the vessels must be frequently irrigated. Irrigation prevents desiccation of the tissue, safely removes debris from the vessels, and helps to float apart the vessel walls. A warm solution of heparinized Ringer's lactate (10,000 units per liter) is recommended for irrigation. Heparin helps to prevent the sutures from catching on the tissue, and Ringer's lactate has been shown to cause less endothelial damage than does normal saline.[2]

Suture Material. Nylon suture has consistently produced superior patency rates in experimental studies and is almost universally used clinically.[12,33] The size of the suture material must be appropriate for the vessel being anastomosed, since patency rates are adversely affected by oversized material.[73] In the digit and thumb, 10-0 suture is used, while 9-0 suture is suitable for anastomoses proximal to the wrist. Smaller suture (11-0) is occasionally used for pediatric patients or distal amputations in adults. Cutting needles should never be used to perform a microvascular anastomosis, since they create large holes in the vessel wall and cause thrombosis. In general the least amount of vessel damage is caused by a tapered needle with a diameter similar to that of the suture. A 75-μ needle is used in the digit, a 100-μ needle in the palm, and a 130-μ needle at the level of the wrist. The appropriate selection of suture material minimizes the risk of anastomotic thrombosis.

Anastomotic Technique. The vessel walls in microsurgical anastomoses must be accurately apposed to prevent thrombosis. Gaps between sutures, uneven spacing of sutures, or excessive tension on the knots can all cause thrombosis. Many techniques have been described to anastomose small vessels, including the use of special vascular clamps.[46] Such devices have achieved minimal popularity, and the vast majority of clinical surgeons use the microsuture technique. Continuous suture technique is not used, since it makes it difficult to avoid anastomotic constriction, with resulting lower patency rates.[73] The use of interrupted suture allows adjustments for size discrepancy to be made with relative ease. Such discrepancies are a common problem in free tissue transfer. Both end-to-end and end-to-side anastomoses are possible with the interrupted technique.

The minimum number of sutures necessary should be used to perform the anastomosis. Every suture places an obstruction in the lumen, causes turbulence at the anastomosis, and exposes thrombogenic subintimal tissue. Higher patency rates are achieved with use of the minimum number of sutures necessary to obtain hemostasis. External rings that allow reliable anastomosis of vessels less than 1 mm in diameter with as few as three sutures have been described.[57] In general, we use six to eight sutures to perform a 1-mm arterial anastomosis. Fewer sutures are required for a comparable vein repair, since the blood pressure is less.

Tension. Any anastomosis performed under tension is likely to thrombose. The presence of tension incites spasm, narrows the lumen, and causes tearing of the intima at points of suture entry. When tension is present, there is a tendency to perform an inadequate debridement of the vessel ends in an effort to save length. The surgeon in this situation may be inclined to anastomose vessels that have not been cut back to normal tissue. This invariably leads to thrombosis and failure.

Tension can be avoided by several means. Vessels can be mobilized proximally and distally by division of small side branches. Adequate length can often be gained by this means alone. In replantation surgery, adequate bone shortening is an integral part of the procedure to avoid tension and allow debridement of the vessels as well as tendons, nerves, and skin. It is usually necessary to remove 0.5 cm to 1 cm of bone in the digit and 2 cm to 3 cm of bone in the hand or wrist. More bone can be removed if there has been an avulsion component to the injury.[69] In oblique digital amputations the longer of the two proximal arteries can be mobilized and "shifted" to the opposite (longer) of the two distal vessels. Such shifts can also be performed between fingers. For instance, the radial digital artery of the index finger can be transferred to the thumb when the princeps pollicis artery is irrevocably damaged.

When tension cannot be avoided by other means, vein grafts are necessary. Veins harvested from the volar aspect of the forearm are suitable for use in the hand and digit. The venae comitantes of the radial artery is an excellent donor because of its uniform proximal and distal caliber. The saphenous vein below the knee is suitable for use in the arm proximal to the wrist. Care must be taken to ensure that the vein harvested is not involved by varices or thrombosis. When one is beginning an upper-extremity replantation or revascularization proximal to the hand, it is wise to prepare the leg in case a vein graft is necessary. The vein graft must be carefully marked so that it can be reversed to prevent valves from obstructing flow. Care must be taken not to perform an anastomosis adjacent to a valve, since the increased turbulence may lead to thrombosis. Passage of vein grafts beneath long skin bridges should be avoided, since twisting or kinking of the graft can easily occur. A healthy recipient bed must be prepared for the graft if thrombosis is to be avoided. While awaiting use, the graft should be kept in a suitable environment such as a solution of papaverine and Ringer's lactate to prevent desiccation and spasm.[8]

External Compression.   The patency of any microvascular anastomosis is vulnerable to external compression. This is particularly true of venous anastomoses, since the pressure required for occlusion is relatively low. External compression is minimized by loose closure of the tissues over the anastomosis. Application of split-thickness skin grafts or the use of local rotation flaps may be necessary to prevent compression of the anastomosis. The skin of digital replantations is usually only partially closed; the transverse incisions are closed, and the longitudinal ones are left open. All dressings must allow for postoperative swelling. Plaster splints used as part of the dressing in digital replantations must be applied to the volar surface of the hand to avoid compressing the dorsal veins.

Local Vascular Spasm.   Blood vessels respond to a wide variety of stimuli. These include neurogenic stimulation, circulatory agents such as catecholamines, local metabolites, and trauma.[18] Vascular spasm is a common problem in microvascular surgery and can be produced merely by the dissection necessary to expose the vessel. Gentle dissection of the perivascular tissue and minimal manipulation of the vessels themselves can help to reduce spasm. All irrigation solution should be warmed prior to use in the wound to promote local vasodilation. Once initiated, spasm can be difficult to reverse. The reduction in flow caused by spasm can be of sufficient severity to compromise tissue survival.

Local spasm can be reversed by gentle mechanical dilation of the vessel prior to anastomosis. Papaverine can be used to promote smooth-muscle relaxation, although it tends to form a precipitate when used in the presence of local anesthetic.[59] Reserpine is reported to induce a long-term sympathectomy when administered intra-arterially.[27] Topical anesthetics can also be used to induce sympathetic blockade. Long-acting anesthetics such as bupivacaine

(Marcaine) can produce sympathetic blockade for 7 to 8 hours. When administered intermittently through a catheter placed adjacent to the appropriate peripheral nerve, long-term sympathetic blockade can be obtained in the postoperative period.[51] We use a No. 5 (French) silicone ureteral catheter placed along the peripheral nerve and brought out through the skin adjacent to the incision. The catheter is brought to the outside of the dressing, where bupivacaine can be administered regularly or as necessary.

Systemic Factors

Maintenance of Fluid Balance.   Perfusion of a replanted part or free tissue transfer depends on the maintenance of adequate arterial inflow to the involved tissue. Arterial inflow, in turn, is dependent on adequate cardiac output. Circulating blood volume is important in maintaining the cardiac output. Patients with digital or limb amputations may have lost a significant amount of blood at the time of their injury. This is particularly true of major limb amputations. These patients are often transported over long distances and may not receive adequate fluid replacement. Similarly, free tissue transfer may take many hours, and patients undergoing such procedures may lose large amounts of fluid during operation. The surgeon must carefully assess the patient's preoperative fluid volume status to ensure that blood volume is adequate. During long cases, an accurate record must be kept of blood loss and adequate replacement given. The patient should not be allowed to become hypovolemic, since this will decrease peripheral perfusion and encourage anastomotic thrombosis. Urine output is a good index of tissue perfusion, and a Foley catheter should be placed in the bladder during all long cases and the urine output maintained at least to 50 ml per hour.

Maintenance of Peripheral Vasodilation.   The presence of an adequate cardiac output does not guarantee peripheral perfusion. Peripheral vasoconstriction can cause marked reduction in blood flow to the extremity and jeopardize arterial inflow. Peripheral vasoconstriction occurs as a response to the direct stimulation of peripheral sympathetic nerves and to circulating catecholamines. Patients with digital or limb amputations produce large amounts of catecholamines as a response to trauma, anxiety, and pain. Even patients undergoing elective surgery have greatly elevated norepinephrine and epinephrine levels.[22]

In the preoperative phase, adequate analgesics and sedatives should be given to minimize anxiety and pain. The patient should be kept warm at all times. The injured extremity should be inspected briefly and open wounds dressed with saline-soaked gauze. A compression dressing can then be applied. The limbs should be splinted to reduce painful stimuli.

If possible, regional anesthesia should be used for upper-extremity replantation surgery.[23,64] An effective axillary block induces sympathetic blockade, minimizes the amount of sedation the patient requires, and reduces the possibility of pressure sores during long procedures. Unfortunately, it is not always effective and is not suitable for most pediatric patients. General anesthesia must be used in this situation and for all free tissue transfers. Patients should be placed on a warming blanket to prevent hypothermia during lengthy cases. The patient must be carefully positioned and padded to guard against nerve palsy. The operating room should kept comfortably warm to encourage vasodilation. The maintenance of peripheral vasodilation in the postoperative phase is discussed below.

Maintenance of Acid–Base Balance.
Tissue that is ischemic produces lactic acid. When such tissue is replanted, systemic acidosis can result. This can be a serious problem in major limb replantation. Acidosis can also be caused by inadequate pulmonary ventilation. Acidosis is harmful to both the patient and the revascularized tissue. Systemic acidosis has been shown to decrease the perfusion of the replanted extremity.[16] In major limb replantations, acidosis is minimized by the early placement of an arterial shunt to allow perfusion of the amputated part while bone fixation and debridement is carried out.[47] A Sundt shunt or ventriculoperitoneal shunt is used, depending on the size of the artery. The limb

is allowed to perfuse prior to venous anastomosis. This minimizes the further production of systemic lactic acid, allows the egress of accumulated metabolites, and buys time for definitive bone fixation. Blood must be replaced during this period. Following venous anastomosis, arterial blood gases should be monitored and bicarbonate administered if necessary.

Anticoagulation. Anticoagulants are not necessary to maintain anastomotic patency when normal artery is sewn to normal artery. This is the case in most free tissue transfers. A single bolus of heparin (3000 to 5000 units) is given just prior to performing the anastomosis. This prevents clot formation in the operative field. Continuous anticoagulation is undesirable in this situation, since hematoma formation can result from these wounds, which have usually had extensive dissection. Hematoma formation beneath the flap can compromise flap circulation.

The situation is different in digital replantation. There has often been an element of avulsion to the injury. This can result in undetected areas of intimal damage some distance from the level of amputation. Multiple anastomoses must be performed, and it is often necessary to inflate and deflate the tourniquet a number of times during the procedure. Flow through the dorsal veins is low owing to the small size of the amputated part. The risk of anticoagulation is lower in digital replantations than in free tissue transfer or major limb replantation. We use a continuous heparin infusion for 7 days following digital replantation of avulsed or crushed parts. The partial thromboplastin time is monitored daily and kept at one and one half to two times control. In cases of guillotine-type amputations in which there has been minimal tissue damage, heparinization is not necessary. Heparin should be avoided in major limb replantations in which extensive fasciotomies are required.

Aspirin inhibits platelet aggregation[17] and is useful for all patients who have had microvascular surgery. The initial phase of an arterial thrombosis is caused by platelet aggregation and release of adenosine diphosphate (ADP).[36] Both of these actions are inhibited by aspirin.[45] Patients are given 650 mg of aspirin every 12 hours for 4 weeks following surgery. The evidence for the effectiveness of this regimen in microvascular surgery is empiric.

Dextran is a plasma expander with antiplatelet activity. Low-molecular-weight dextran (dextran 40) is administered intravenously during surgery. A continuous infusion at 7 mg/kg/24 hr is continued for 7 to 10 days postoperatively. Dextran coats platelets and interferes with their aggregation. It also coats erythrocytes and prevents rouleau formation and sludging in the microcirculation.[37,78] Its properties make it suitable for all patients who have had microvascular surgery. As with aspirin, its use in clinical microvascular surgery has been empiric.

COMPLICATIONS OF REPLANTATION

Tissue Preservation.   Preoperative physiologic storage of amputated parts is essential to achieve success in replantation. It is generally felt that replantation should not be attempted if the warm ischemic time of the amputated part exceeds 6 hours.[15] If the amputated part contains muscle, the warm ischemic time is much more critical. Muscle is extremely sensitive to ischemia, compared with tissues such as skin, bone, and tendon.

Cooling reduces metabolic acidosis, muscle autolysis, and bacterial growth. All amputated parts should be cooled during transport to a replantation center. Successful digital replantation with cold ischemic times of 30 to 36 hours have been reported.[3]

Amputated parts can be either wrapped with gauze moistened with Ringer's lactate or saline and placed on ice or immersed in one of these solutions in a plastic bag and the bag placed on ice. Either method results in equal viability rates at 24 hours.[74] The immersion method is preferable for the following reasons: (1) The part is less likely to become frozen ("frostbitten"), (2) the part is less likely to be strangled by the wrappings, (3) the instructions are easier to explain to the primary-care physician, and (4) maceration secondary to immersion is not a problem.

Immediate Postoperative Care.   All re-

plantations are placed in well-padded dressings postoperatively. The patients are kept at bedrest with the extremity elevated to encourage venous drainage. Overhead heaters are often used in the recovery room to warm the patient. The patient's room is kept above 75°F to encourage peripheral vasodilation and improve extremity blood flow.

Every attempt is made to keep the patient relaxed and reduce any stimulus that would promote catecholamine release. Patients are kept in single rooms. Visitors are limited. Smoking is prohibited. Patients receive chlorpromazine 25 mg orally every 8 hours. This helps to reduce anxiety and also promotes peripheral vasodilation. Patients are kept in bed for at least 3 days. Anticoagulation has been discussed previously.

Postoperative Monitoring.   Vascular thrombosis is most common in the first 48 hours following replantation.[43] It becomes less likely as time goes by. The perfusion of replanted digits and extremities must be continuously monitored so that vascular thrombosis can be immediately detected. Color, pulp turgor, capillary refill, and warmth are all useful in assessing the perfusion of replantations. The most useful method of clinical assessment requires a small blunt object such as a ballpoint pen (Fig. 27-2). Pressure is applied to the nail fold, causing blanching of the skin. The pen is then removed and the presence and speed of capillary refill assessed. Sluggish or absent refill indicates arterial thrombosis. Too-rapid refill suggests venous obstruction (Fig. 27-3).

Temperature monitoring provides a practical method of continuous objective measurement of digital perfusion.[33,65] Small temperature probes are taped to the pulps of replanted digits, a control (noninjured) digit, and the dressing. The temperature probes are connected to a YSI Tele Thermometer.* This instrument measures digital temperature, which is then recorded hourly as part of the patient's medical record. Normal digital temperature is from 32°C to 35°C. A temperature drop of greater than 2.5°C in 1 hour or temperature falling

---

* Yellow Springs Instrument Company, Yellow Springs, OH.

FIG. 27-2. Clinical assessment of digital perfusion. A blunt object such as the cap of a ballpoint pen is used to cause blanching of the skin of the nail fold (*arrowhead*). When the blunt object is removed, the presence and speed of capillary refill are assessed. Sluggish or absent refill indicates arterial thrombosis. Too-rapid refill suggests venous obstruction.

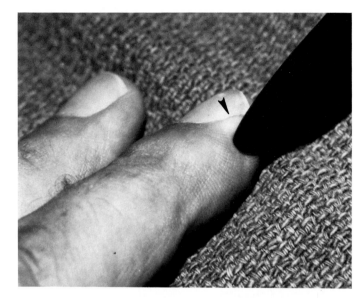

FIG. 27-3. Venous congestion 72 hours following digital replantation. Hyperemia, bluish discoloration, rapid capillary refill, and a drop in the digital temperature suggest venous thrombosis. Anastomotic revision is usually not successful more than 24 hours after replantation. At least two and preferably three veins should be repaired for each digit replanted. Plaster splints should not be applied to the dorsum of the hand. The digit illustrated went on to necrosis.

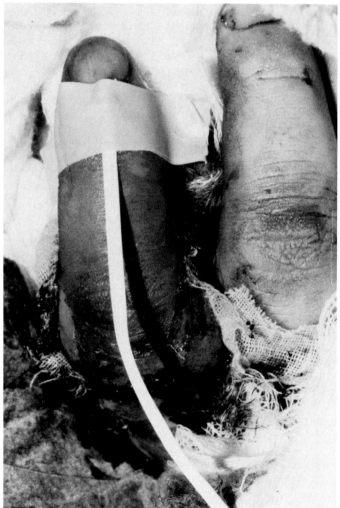

below 30°C is a sign of inadequate perfusion that demands immediate attention.

This method of noninvasive monitoring has the following advantages: (1) nursing personnel perform the hourly measurements and call the physician for significant changes, (2) objective measurements are possible when clinical assessment is difficult (*i.e.*, in a dark-skinned patient), (3) the technique is entirely atraumatic to the digit, (4) the patient is not disturbed by the readings, and (5) the equipment is inexpensive and readily available.

Management of the Failing Replant. When inadequate perfusion of a replanted part is detected, immediate attention is required. The dressing should be removed down to skin to ensure that there is no constriction. Blood may have formed a "cast" around the digit and obstruct flow. Any tight skin sutures should be removed. Depression or elevation of the hand may be helpful, depending on whether the problem is arterial or venous. A stellate block or brachial block (if no regional indwelling catheter is present) should be given to relieve vasospasm.

The status of the patient's anticoagulation should be checked. A bolus of heparin (3000 to 5000 units) often improves perfusion. The patient must be adequately hydrated. The room temperature may have to be elevated. All efforts should be made to calm the patient, especially a child, since pain, fear, and anxiety may instigate unwanted vasospasm.

If these measures fail to restore perfusion, consideration should be given to returning the patient to the operating room. To be effective this must be done within 4 to 6 hours of the loss of perfusion. Reexploration must also be performed within 24 to 48 hours of the replantation if it is to be effective. In the operating room the site of thrombosis must be identified. Thrombectomy, anastomotic revision, or vein grafting of a previously unrecognized damaged vessel segment is sometimes effective in restoring flow. These measures are most effective when acute cessation of arterial inflow is diagnosed and the patient is rapidly returned to the operating room.

Skin Slough. Soft tissue necrosis can expose bone or tendon and cause thrombosis of the underlying vessels. The skin edges of any amputated part have often been crushed at the time of injury. Skin slough is most easily avoided by adequate bone shortening. This allows debridement of the skin edges back to healthy tissue. Closure must be performed without tension to avoid necrosis. In digital replantations, only a few skin sutures are used to approximate the skin edges. The bilateral midlateral incisions used to explore the vessels and nerves are left open to allow for drainage and expansion caused by postoperative swelling and to minimize tension on the skin.[70]

If adequate skin coverage is not present, coverage can be obtained by local rotation flaps or split-thickness skin grafts, which may be meshed. Split skin graft can sometimes be obtained from nonreplantable digits. Inflation of a nonreplantable digit by the subcutaneous injection of saline restores turgor to the digit and makes harvest of a skin graft easier. Local rotational flaps should be used to cover exposed vessels, but vessels will survive and remain patent beneath split-thickness grafts. In major limb replantations in which the patient must be returned to the operating room for wound exploration in 48 hours, temporary wound coverage can be obtained with split-thickness (porcine) xenografts.

Infections. Infection occurs surprisingly infrequently in digital replantation (in 2 of 32 cases in the series of Weiland and colleagues,[77] and in 2% in the series of Morrison and co-workers[43]). The majority of series do not even mention its occurrence. Adequate debridement under magnification, leaving the majority of the wound open, and the routine use of prophylactic antibiotics are factors that contribute to the low infection rate. The treatment of infected replanted digits requires debridement, free drainage, and antibiotic administration. Care must be taken not to injure the arterial or venous anastomoses during drainage procedures. Stiffness is common in replants that have been infected.

Infection is both more common and more serious in major limb replantations. The presence of large amounts of muscle that have been rendered ischemic increases the likelihood of infection. Immediately follow-

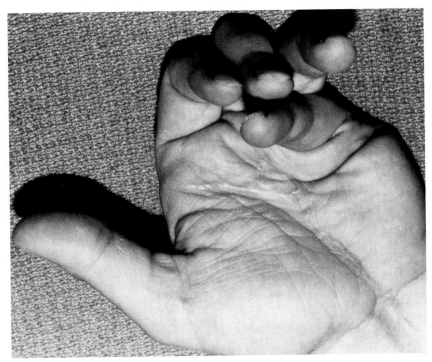

FIG. 27-4. Rotational malunion following transmetacarpal replantation. In flexion, the small finger crosses into the palm. Rotational alignment during replantation should be observed at the time of bone fixation. In flexion, all digits should point toward the scaphoid. A derotational metacarpal osteotomy may be necessary to correct this malunion.

ing revascularization, it is difficult to distinguish contused from necrotic muscle. In addition, some muscle bellies, such as the biceps, may be rendered ischemic owing to damage to their segmental blood supply, even though the limb itself is successfully revascularized. To ensure that muscle debridement is adequate, all major limb replantations must be returned to the operating room within 48 hours of injury for a "second look" procedure. At this time the wound is thoroughly inspected. Muscle necrosis will be apparent at this time, and further debridement can be carried out. Infection is minimized by reducing the presence of necrotic tissue in the wound.

Nonunion. Nonunion rates from 2% to 9% have been noted following digital replantation.[43,71,77] Not all nonunions following digital replantation are symptomatic. For instance, motion at a failed metacarpophalangeal joint arthrodesis site, if painless, may be desirable. Symptomatic nonunions are treated as they would be if the digit had not been replanted.

In contrast to the case in digital replantation, nonunion is common in major limb replantations.[48] Nonunions are more common when the amputation is through diaphyseal bone and when fixation is suboptimal. Stress levels across the fracture site are high, since the extremity is essentially flail until nerve regeneration occurs. The use of vascular shunts (see above) provides for limb perfusion while definitive bone fixation is obtained. Plate fixation is desirable, since it provides rotational stability and allows compression. If delayed union or nonunion develops, bone grafting and revision of fixation should be performed.

Malunion. Malunion is most frequently seen following transmetacarpal replantations. These are complex injuries that require multiple tendon, vessel, and nerve repairs. If care is not taken during bone fixation, rotational malunion may occur (Fig. 27-4).

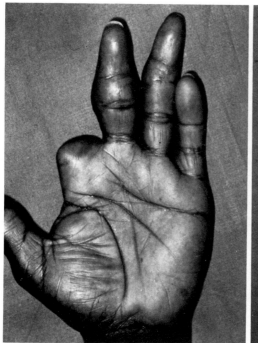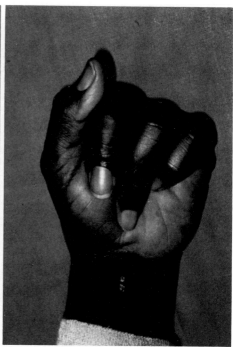

FIG. 27-5. Inadvertent digital exchange. The amputated long finger was transferred to the ring finger and the ring to the long. This did not significantly alter hand function. Digital exchange is therapeutic when an amputated digit is used to reconstruct a nonreplantable thumb.

When the patient flexes the finger of the malunited ray, it crosses the other fingers and may become an obstruction to hand function. This can be avoided if rotational alignment is checked following fixation of each ray. This requires inspecting the volar aspect of the hand and flexing the digit. In flexion all digits should point towards the scaphoid. Additionally, the tips of the finger nail plates must form the proper cascade. A corrective osteotomy has been described for symptomatic rotational metacarpal malunion.[38]

Another form of malunion can occur in multiple digital replantations. It can be difficult to identify the various digits at the time of surgery, and it may become apparent postoperatively that one digit has been "exchanged" for another (Fig. 27-5). This is primarily a cosmetic problem. Digital "exchange" can be deliberate in patients who have a nonreplantable thumb. An amputated digit can be replanted on the thumb rather than to its original position to increase hand function as a whole.

Recovery of Sensibility. Successfully replanted digits and extremities can be expected to recover neurologic function in a fashion similar to other peripheral nerve repairs.[70] The recovery of sensibility following digital replantations has been shown to correlate closely with restored digital vascularity.[19] Younger patients tend to have the best nerve recovery, as do those who have sharp amputations. Amputations occurring distally in the digit have improved sensory recovery. It is preferable to perform nerve repair at the time of replantation, since delayed repair is difficult and lengthens the time required to rehabilitate the extremity. In clean amputations, primary nerve grafts can be used if necessary.

Cold Intolerance. Cold intolerance is an almost universal complaint in patients who have undergone digital replantation.[41,43,58,69,77] However, cold intolerance is not unique to digital replantation. In a study comparing digital amputations with replantations, Jones and associates[28] found an almost equal incidence of cold intoler-

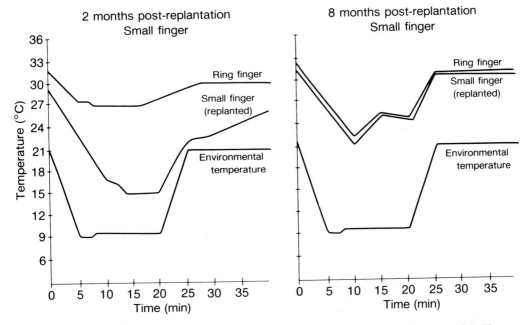

FIG. 27-6. (*Left*) Digital temperature response following replantation at 2 months. The replanted small finger shows an exaggerated temperature drop and a prolonged rewarming time. This type of response is common following digital replantation. (*Right*) Six months later, the temperature response of the replanted digit is similar to that of the normal ring finger. Cold intolerance is also seen in patients with digital amputations. It usually resolves within 2 years of injury.

ance in both groups. Cold intolerance is closely related to the adequacy of digital revascularization.[19] Every effort should be made to maximize the number of arterial repairs in digital replantations. It is desirable to perform two arterial anastomoses even though most digits will survive on one. Cold intolerance improves with time and usually resolves by 2 years (Fig. 27-6).[70]

Pain. Pain is *rare* in successfully replanted limbs. We have not observed causalgia or pain related to a nerve injury or repair in more than 700 attempted replantations. Only one of our patients complained of pain following replantation. This patient had replantation of the hand that had been amputated through the base of the metacarpals. Four weeks after replantation he had pain, swelling, and redness over the dorsal radial aspect of the hand. An arteriogram revealed an arteriovenous fistula (Fig. 27-7). The radial artery had been sutured to a dorsal hand vein. This was corrected by ligation.

Range of Motion. Joint injury, nerve injury, tendon adhesions, and the need for

immobilization can all contribute to joint stiffness following replantation. This is particularly true of digits amputated through the area of the fibro-osseous flexor tendon canal. Soft tissues should be interposed between the fracture site and the tendon repair if they are at the same level. An attempt should be made to repair periosteum as well as capsule and ligaments in the digits to obtain a greater range of motion and good stability. If possible, all tendons should be repaired primarily. Bone fixation should be stable enough to allow active motion to begin at 3 weeks. Most patients begin treatment by a hand therapist at this time.

If excessive stiffness develops, tenolysis can be performed as early as 3 months. If primary flexor tenolysis is not possible, staged tendon reconstruction will be necessary. Most replantations develop approximately 50% of the normal active range of joint motion. There are exceptions to this. For instance, digits replanted distal to the insertion of the superficial sublimis tendon usually develop an excellent range of prox-

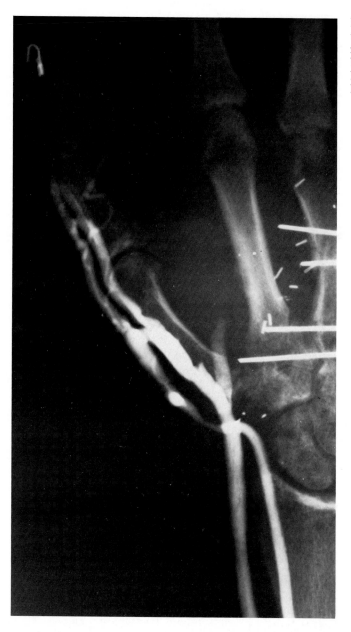

FIG. 27-7. Arteriovenous fistula 4 weeks following transmetacarpal replantation. The radial artery has been anastomosed to a dorsal hand vein. This was corrected by ligation.

imal interphalangeal joint motion (85°).[72] Similarly, hands that have been replanted at the wrist level often develop excellent digital mobility.

COMPLICATIONS OF FREE TISSUE TRANSFER

General Complications

Damaged Recipient Vessels. The two most important factors determining the

success of free tissue transfers are (1) the technical ability of the surgeon and (2) the quality of the vascularity in the recipient bed.[61] Most free tissue transfers in orthopaedic patients are performed for posttraumatic defects. Between injury and the time of free tissue transfers, significant vascular alterations may have occurred in the recipient site. In this situation, preoperative arteriography should always be performed unless an adequate recipient artery has

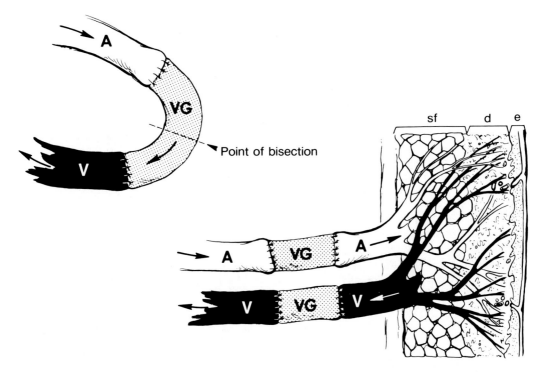

FIG. 27-8. A vein graft (*VG*) can be used to extend the pedicle of a free tissue transfer. An arteriovenous fistula is temporarily created. When the donor tissue is transferred, the pedicle can be divided and the donor vessels anastomosed to the vein graft. Damage to recipient vessels can be avoided by this method. (*A,* artery; *V,* vein; *sf,* subcutaneous fat, *d,* dermis; *e,* epidermis)

been or is to be identified before the tissue transfer.[34]

Arteriography permits assessment of the quality of the vessel that will receive the donor vessel, determines the exact location of the recipient vessel, precisely outlines the vessel's anatomy, and usually shows all collateral circulation. Angiography has not been shown to cause significant intimal damage,[50] and transfer need not be delayed following arteriography.

Damage to recipient vessels can be avoided by the use of vein grafts. As with replantation, the efficacy of vein grafts in free tissue transfer has been well documented.[6] Saphenous vein grafts have been used to extend the pedicle of the latissimus dorsi myocutaneous flap by 28 cm.[56] While donor tissue is being harvested, a second surgical team can obtain a saphenous vein graft. Normal vessels at some distance from the traumatized recipient site can be exposed. The vein graft can then be reversed

and anastomosed to the recipient artery and vein. This creates a temporary arteriovenous shunt (Fig. 27-8). When the donor tissue is transferred, the pedicle can be divided and the donor vessels anastomosed to the vein graft. With this method, discrepancies in the length of the arterial and venous pedicles can be corrected without tension on the anastomoses. Of equal importance, the anastomoses are performed in a normal tissue bed with easier exposure. In addition, the adequacy of the recipient arterial and venous blood flow can be ensured.

The "No-Reflow" Phenomenon. Successful free tissue transfer requires perfusion of the tissue distal to the microvascular anastomosis. An obstruction to blood reflow in peripheral tissue has been termed the *no-reflow phenomenon.* No-reflow is the end result of a combination of intravascular sludging and coagulation, endothelial swelling and desquamation, and perivascular edema—all leading to vessel occlusion and failure of perfusion. Ischemia has been the most consistent cause of the no-reflow phenomenon in the laboratory.[40] Vasospasm may play a role, and ischemic tissue has been shown to be hypersensitive to the effects of circulating catecholamines.[55]

The reversibility of the no-reflow state is time dependent. May and associates found perfusion to fail consistently when tissue had 12 hours of normothermic ischemia.[40] Attempts to prevent the no-reflow phenomenon by the perfusion of tissue with solutions prior to revascularization have been largely unsuccessful.[9,24] Since treatment is ineffective, every effort must be made to avoid no-reflow. Minimization of ischemic time by not dividing the donor vascular pedicle until the recipient vessels are fully prepared is an effective means of prevention. Similarly, anastomotic thrombosis must be promptly recognized and corrected if no-reflow is to be avoided. Prevention of edema or venous engorgement of the transferred tissue is important. This is accomplished by performing the venous anastomosis prior to arterial repair, or by not releasing the arterial clips until venous outflow is established if the artery is repaired first.

Postoperative Monitoring. Effective postoperative monitoring allows the prompt recognition of anastomotic thrombosis and gives time for therapeutic intervention before irreversible ischemic change occurs. Postoperative dressings must be applied so that the skin of cutaneous, myocutaneous, and toe-to-thumb transfers is freely visible. Skin color, warmth, turgor, and the presence of capillary refill are used to assess the perfusion status of the transfer. Nursing personnel are instructed to observe and record the appearance of the flap or transferred digit hourly. Should flap perfusion be in doubt, Daniel and Terzis recommend piercing the skin of the flap with a #11 blade.[15] Bright red bleeding indicates good arterial inflow, oozing of purple blood suggests venous obstruction, and no bleeding suggests arterial thrombosis.

Temperature monitoring provides a convenient and effective method of monitoring toe-to-thumb transfers. Unfortunately, it is not nearly as reliable for cutaneous and myocutaneous flaps. These flaps are relatively thin, and the transmission of heat through the flap from the recipient site makes this method of monitoring unreliable in this situation. Other methods to monitor cutaneous circulation have been described, including administration of intravenous fluorescein,[42] blood gas analysis,[31] use of implantable ultrasonic Doppler probes,[52] transcutaneous PO_2 measurement,[60] and laser Doppler velocimetry.[26] The use of these techniques in the clinical setting is still evolving, and no single method has gained widespread acceptance. There is no satisfactory method of monitoring vascularized bone grafts, although Berggen and co-workers[4] have shown bone scans to be an effective means of assessing perfusion if performed within 7 days of surgery. The problem of monitoring free tissue transfers is being actively researched, and it is likely that effective, reliable methods will eventually evolve. Until this occurs, repeated critical clinical examination of perfusion, when possible, is the most reliable method of detecting anastomotic thrombosis.

Management of the Failing Free Tissue Transfer. When the circulation to a free tissue transfer is observed to be impaired, the patient should be returned to the operating room. Any hematoma that has accumulated beneath the flap should be removed. The anastomoses should be directly inspected and patency tests performed to determine whether arterial or venous thrombosis, or both, is present.

If an arterial thrombosis is diagnosed, the anastomosis is excised. Good proximal inflow must be obtained. This may require the use of a more proximal vessel, in which case a vein graft will probably be needed. The flap artery is irrigated and milked to remove thrombus. The patient should be heparinized. The anastomosis is then revised. The venous anastomosis should be excised to ensure that an outflow of blood is established following revision of an arterial anastomosis. If only a venous thrombosis is present, it should be excised. Bleeding should be allowed for a few minutes to confirm that arterial perfusion is present and to wash out proximal thrombus. The anastomosis is then revised, with a vein graft used if necessary. If possible, a second venous anastomosis should be performed. If anastomotic thrombosis is promptly recognized and the patient is returned to the operating room, many failing free tissue transfers can be salvaged. Ninety percent of failing free tissue transfers can be salvaged if returned to the operating room within 12 hours after the initial procedure. Most of them cannot be salvaged after 24 hours.

A plethora of pharmacologic agents have been described to improve cutaneous circulation and increase flap survival.[30] Most of these have not gained acceptance in the clinical setting. Limited success has been obtained with the use of intra-arterial fibrinolytic agents when surgical thrombectomy is not possible.[29,54] Since the experimental evidence supporting its use is conflicting,[11] we reserve Streptokinase for situations in which surgical thrombectomy is not possible, such as multiple digital artery emboli or thromboses. Small Fogarty catheters can be used down to the level of the superficial palmar arch.

Management of the Failed Free Tissue Transfer. Every microvascular surgeon will eventually be faced with the problem of managing a failed free tissue transfer. Necrosis of a flap does not necessarily mean that it must be removed. As long as infection is not present, cutaneous and myocutaneous flaps can be left in place to serve as biologic dressings. In many cases failed cutaneous flaps can be successful as "crane" flaps. The failed flap is left undisturbed on the recipient bed for 6 to 8 weeks (Fig. 27-9, *A*). At this time the superficial necrotic portion of the flap is carefully resected. The deep portion of the flap may have survived and been revascularized by the process of inosculation (*i.e.,* new vessel ingrowth) (Fig. 27-9, *B*). Split-thickness skin grafts can then be applied to the bed of subcutaneous tissue (Fig. 27-9, *C*). With this technique many cutaneous flaps can be partially salvaged. The coverage obtained by the crane flap is not as desirable as that provided by a successful cutaneous flap but is quite acceptable in many cases.

Failed free bone transfers continue to act as strut grafts, although rapid healing of the graft cannot be expected without an intrinsic blood supply.[75] Since these grafts are harvested with a large cuff of soft tissue, incorporation of the devascularized graft is likely to be delayed. Such grafts should be left in place as long as they serve a mechanical function. Slotting or telescoping of fibular grafts into the bone of the recipient site provides biologic fixation, reduces the need for mechanical devices, and encourages bony union. Union of the devascularized graft may occur at one or both bone anastomoses, in which case further grafting with cancellous bone may encourage healing.

Complications of Specific Free Tissue Transfers

Toe-to-Thumb Transfers. A variety of toe-to-thumb transfers are available, each with its advantages and disadvantages.[37,44] Vasospasm can be a severe problem in these procedures, and particular attention must be paid to hydrating the patient and keeping the patient and the operating room warm. After dissection of the pedicle, the toe is wrapped in warm packs and the tourniquet deflated. If perfusion cannot be established, Lister and associates recommend division of the pedicle and hydrostatic dilatation of the artery.[37] We would recommend *waiting,* maintaining a moist warm environment. If this fails, try application of 1% xylocaine or papaverine. Even with these techniques, reexploration rates greater than 30% for failing perfusion have been reported in these procedures. Since the failure rate is potentially so high continuous postoperative temperature monitoring is necessary. Cold intolerance has also been reported following toe-to-thumb transfers.[37,53]

Complications at the donor site are surprisingly uncommon following toe-to-thumb transfer. Transfer of the second toe causes virtually no alteration in foot mechanics. Transfer of the great toe results in a concentration of weight bearing between the second and third metatarsal heads and slowing of the forward and medial progression of the center of pressure on gait analysis.[53] Weakness of push-off and cutting

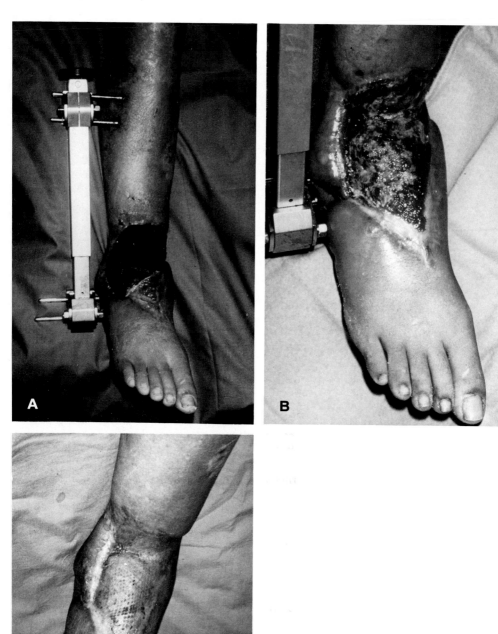

FIG. 27-9. (*A*) Salvage of a free flap by the crane technique. A necrotic scapular flap covers an open fracture of the distal tibia. The flap, which was not infected, was left undisturbed for 8 weeks. (*B*) At 8 weeks the superficial necrotic portion of the flap was resected. The deep portion of the flap was revascularized by inosculation. (*C*) Split-thickness skin grafts were then applied to the bed of subcutaneous tissue. The coverage obtained by this method is not ideal but may be acceptable.

maneuvers has also been reported, although most patients can run on level ground.[53] Partial transfer of the great toe ("wrap-around" technique) theoretically minimizes mechanical alterations in the foot, although this remains to be shown objectively.[44] Greater donor site morbidity is seen when multiple toes are transferred.

Free Fibular Transfer. The fibular diaphysis receives its blood supply from the peroneal artery. Free fibular transfers are harvested on the peroneal artery, thus preserving both the nutrient and periosteal blood supply. The peroneal artery usually arises 1 cm to 2 cm below the lower border of the popliteus muscle. The vascular anatomy is variable, and the peroneal artery may either arise much higher or be absent. Preoperative angiography must be used to determine the artery's presence and its anatomy prior to harvest of the vein graft. If angiography is not performed, it is possible that the posterior tibial artery could inadvertently be sacrificed. When the peroneal artery is absent, the nutrient artery to the fibula arises from the posterior tibial artery. Free fibular transfer is therefore not possible unless the nutrient artery is of sufficient size and length to be safely isolated. The peroneal artery is not always *symmetrically* absent, so bilateral angiograms should be performed prior to free fibular transfers.

Valgus deformity of the ankle can follow resection of the fibula. This tends to occur when large grafts are taken close to the ankle mortise in a growing child, allowing gradual proximal migration of the remaining fibular segment. Weiland and Daniel recommend the use of tibiofibular transfixation screws when a fibula is harvested from a child under the age of 13.[76] The common peroneal nerve must be identified in the proximal part of the wound to avoid injury. In general, patients tolerate partial fibulectomy extremely well and, apart from the valgus deformity in children, have not developed long-term problems.

Free Iliac Crest Transfer. Transfer of the iliac crest based on a vascular pedicle is desirable, since subcutaneous tissue and skin can be included to form an osteocutaneous flap.[68] The successful dissection of the flap is difficult and requires knowledge of the complex anatomy in this region. The flap should be based on the deep (as opposed to the superficial) circumflex iliac artery.[67] Because large, full-thickness portions of the iliac crest are removed, a hernia can occur. Hernias through the donor site can be repaired by supplementation with Marlex or by the technique described by Bosworth. Cowley and Anderson[13] recommend the Bosworth technique, in which the fascia is sewn directly to the ilium.

Cutaneous and Myocutaneous Flaps. Donor site complications are rare following harvest of cutaneous and myocutaneous flaps. Many donor sites can be closed primarily even if large cutaneous flaps have been removed. This includes the donor site of groin, scapular, latissimus dorsi, and tensor fascia lata flaps. Other flaps, such as the dorsalis pedis flap, require skin grafting to obtain closure. It is not unusual for corrugation on the dorsum of the foot to cause a shoeing problem with this flap, so we seldom use it. Suction drains should be used at all donor sites to help prevent hematoma formation, since dead space is usually large.

No functional impairment has been noted following transfer of muscle or myocutaneous flaps such as latissimus dorsi, gracilis, or tensor fascia lata flaps. Other motors usually take over their function, and patients generally do not notice their loss. The only defect at the donor site is the operative scar, which tends to spread because these wounds are often closed with some tension.

Some flaps are more reliable than others. This is particularly true of the latissimus dorsi flap, which has a long pedicle (9 cm) and a sizable artery (2–3 mm). It has been shown to be more reliable than a groin flap, in which the vascular anatomy is variable and the artery much smaller.[62] End-to-side arterial anastomoses are often preferable when revascularizing these flaps. There is often a paucity of arteries owing to trauma at the recipient site. Recipient arteries are not sacrificed with end-to-side anastomoses. Size discrepancies are easily dealt with by this technique, and a mechanism for "runoff" is provided.[21] There are usually enough veins at the recipient site to allow an end-to-end venous anastomosis, but if an end-to-side venous connection is easier, it should be chosen. In summary, we recommend choosing the repair type and sequence that is easier (*i.e.*, end-to-end versus end-to-side and vein first or artery first), depending on the exposure and situation.

REFERENCES

1. Acland, R.: Thrombus formation in microvascular surgery: An experimental study of the effects of surgical trauma. Surgery, 73:766, 1973.
2. Acland, R.D., Lubbers, L.L., Grafton, R.B., and Bensimon, R.: Irrigating solutions for small blood vessel surgery: A histologic comparison. Plast. Reconstr. Surg., 65(4):460, 1980.
3. American Replantation Mission to China: Replantation surgery in China. Plast. Reconstr. Surg., 52:476, 1973.
4. Berggen, A., Weiland, A.J., and Ostrup, L.T.: Bone scintigraphy in evaluating the viability of composite bone grafts revascularized by microvascular anastomoses, conventional autogenous bone grafts, and free non-revascularized periosteal grafts. J. Bone Joint Surg., 64A:799, 1982.
5. Bright, D.S.: Principles of microvascular surgery. In Green, D.P. (ed.): Operative Hand Surgery. New York, Churchill Livingstone, 1982.
6. Buncke, H.J., Alpert, B., and Shah, K.G.: Microvascular grafting. Clin. Plast. Surg., 5:185, 1978.
7. Buncke, H.J., Jr., McLean, D.H., George, P.T. et al.: Thumb replacement: Great toe transplantation by microneurovascular anastomosis. Br. J. Plast. Surg., 26:194, 1973.
8. Catinella, F.P., Cunningham, J.N., Jr., Baumann, F.D. et al.: An ultrastructural comparison of endothelial preservation in vein grafts prepared by various techniques. J. Clin. Surg., 1:393, 1982.
9. Chait, L.A., May, J.W., O'Brien, B.M., and Hurley, J.V.: The effects of the perfusion of various solutions of the no-reflow phenomenon in experimental free flaps. Plast. Reconstr. Surg., 61:421, 1978.
10. Chow, S.P.: The histopathology of microvascular anastomosis: A study of the incidence of various tissue changes. Microsurgery, 4:5, 1983.
11. Cooney, W.P., Wilson, M.R., and Wood, M.D.: Intravascular fibrinolysis of small vessel thrombosis. J. Hand Surg., 8:131, 1983.
12. Corbett, J.: Small vessel anastomosis: A comparison of suture techniques. Br. J. Plast. Surg., 22:16, 1967.
13. Cowley, S.P., and Anderson, L.D.: Hernias through donor sites for iliac bone grafts. J. Bone Joint Surg., 65A:1023, 1983.
14. Daniel, R.K., and Taylor, G.I.: Distant transfer of an island flap by microvascular anastomoses. Plast. Reconstr. Surg., 52:111, 1973.
15. Daniel, R.K., and Terzis, J.K.: Reconstructive Microsurgery. Boston, Little, Brown & Co., 1977.
16. Dell, P.C., Seaber, A.V., and Urbaniak, J.R.: The effect of systemic acidosis on perfusion of replanted extremities. J. Hand Surg., 5:433, 1980.
17. Evans, G., Packham, M.D., and Nishizawa, E.E.: The effect of acetylsalicylic acid on platelet function. J. Exp. Med., 128:877, 1968.
18. Folkow, B., and Neil, E.: Circulation. New York, Oxford University Press, 1971.
19. Gelberman, R.H., Urbaniak, J.R., Bright, D.S., and Levin, L.S.: Digital sensibility following replantation. J. Hand Surg., 3:313, 1978.
20. Glover, M.G., Seaber, A.V., and Urbaniak, J.R.: Intimal damage in avulsion injuries of microsurgical specimens. Trans. Orthop. Res. Soc., 1983.
21. Hurst, L.N., Evans, H.B., and Brown, D.H.: Vasospasm control by intra-arterial reserpine. Plast. Reconstr. Surg., 70:595, 1972.
22. Halme, A., Pekkarinen, A., and Turunen, M.: On the excretion of noradrenaline, adrenaline, 17-hydroxycorticosteroids and 17-ketosteroids during the postoperative stage. Acta Endocrinol. [Suppl.] (Copenh.), 32, 1957.
23. Harmel, M.H., Urbaniak, J.R., and Bright, D.S.: Anesthesia for replantation of severed extremities. In von Herausgegeben, H.J.W., and Zindler, M. (eds.): Anesthesiologie und intensivmedizin, band 138, neue aspekte in der regionalanesthesie 2, pp. 161–166. Berlin, Springer-Verlag, 1981.
24. Harashina, T., and Buncke, H.J.: Study of washout solutions for microvascular replantation and transplantation. Plast. Reconstr. Surg., 56:542, 1975.
25. Hayhurst, J.W., and O'Brien, B.McC.: An experimental study of microvascular technique, patency rates and related factors. Br. J. Plast. Surg., 28:128, 1975.
26. Holloway, G.A., and Watkins, D.W.: Laser Doppler measurement of cutaneous blood flow. J. Invest. Dermatol., 69:306, 1977.
27. Hurst, L.N., Evans, H.B., and Brown, D.H.: Vasospasm control by intra-arterial reserpine. Plast. Reconstr. Surg., 70:595, 1972.
28. Jones, J.M., Schenck, R.R., and Chesney, R.B.: Digital replantation and amputation—Comparison of function. J. Hand Surg., 7:183, 1982.
29. Kartchner, M.M., and Wilcox, W.C.: Thrombolysis of palmar and digital arterial thrombosis by intra-arterial thrombolysis. J. Hand Surg., 1:67, 1976.
30. Kerrigan, C.L., and Daniel, R.K.: Pharmacologic treatment of the failing skin flap. Plast. Reconstr. Surg., 70:541, 1982.
31. Kerrigan, C.L., and Daniel, R.K.: Monitoring acute skin flap failure. Plast. Reconstr. Surg., 71:519, 1983.
32. Kleinert, H.E., Juhala, C.A., Tsai, T., and Van Beek, A.: Digital replantation—selection, technique, and results. Orthop. Clin. North Am., 8:309, 1977.
33. Kleinert, H.E., Kasdan, M.L., and Romero, I.J.: Small blood vessel anastomosis for salvage of severely injured upper extremity. J. Bone Joint Surg., 45A:788, 1963.
34. Koman, L.A., Pospisil, R.F., Nunley, J.A., and Urbaniak, J.R.: Value of contrast arteriography in composite tissue transfer. Clin. Orthop., 172:195, 1983.
35. Komatsu, S., and Tamai, S.: Successful replantation of a completely cut off thumb: Case report. Plast. Reconstr. Surg., 42:374, 1968.

36. Levine, W.G.: Anticoagulant, antithrombotic, and thrombolytic drugs. In Goodman, L.S., and Gilman, A. (eds.): The Pharmacologic Basis of Therapeutics, 5th ed. New York, Macmillan, 1975.

37. Lister, G.D., Kalisman, M., Tsai, T-M.: Reconstruction of the hand with free microneurovascular toe-to-hand transfer: Experience with 54 toe transfers. Plast. Reconstr. Surg., 71:372, 1983.

38. Manktelow, R.T., and Mahoney, J.L.: Step osteotomy: A preuse rotation osteotomy to correct scissoring deformities of the fingers. Plast. Reconstr. Surg., 68:571, 1981.

39. Manktelow, R.T., and McKee, N.H.: Free muscle transplantation to provide active finger flexion. J. Hand Surg., 3:416, 1978.

40. May, J.W., Chait, L.A., O'Brien, B.M., and Hurley, J.V.: The no-reflow phenomenon in experimental free flaps. Plast. Reconstr. Surg., 61:256, 1978.

41. May, J.W., Toth, B.A., and Gardner, M.: Digital replantation distal to the proximal interphalangeal joint. J. Hand Surg., 7:161, 1982.

42. McCraw, J.B., Myers, B., and Shankin, K.D.: The value of fluorescein in predicting the viability of arterialized flaps. Plast. Reconstr. Surg., 60:710, 1977.

43. Morrison, W.A., O'Brien, B.McC., and MacLeod, A.M.: Evaluation of digital replantation—a review of 100 cases. Orthop. Clin. North Am. 8:295, 1977.

44. Morrison, W.A., O'Brien, B.M., and MacLeod, A.M.: Thumb reconstruction with a neurovascular wrap-around from the big toe. J. Hand Surg., 5:575, 1980.

45. Mustard, J.F., and Parkham, M.A.: Thromboembolism: A manifestation of the response of blood to injury. Circulation, 42:1, 1970.

46. Nakayama, K., Tamiya, T., Yamamoto, K., and Akimoto, S.: A simple new apparatus for small vessel anastomosis (free autograft of the sigmoid included). Surgery, 52:918, 1962.

47. Nunley, J.A., Koman, L.A., and Urbaniak, J.R.: Arterial shunting as an adjunct to major limb revascularizations. Ann. Surg., 193:271, 1981.

48. Nunley, J.A., Koman, L.A., and Urbaniak, J.R.: Major upper extremity replantation. Orthop. Trans. 6:512, 1982.

49. O'Brien, B.McC.: Microvascular Reconstructive Surg. Edinburgh, London, and New York, Churchill Livingstone, 1977.

50. Peimer, C.A., and Eckert, B.S.: Microvascular response to angiography. Orthop. Trans., 5:109, 1981.

51. Phelps, D.B., Rutherford, R.B., and Boswick, J.A.: Control of vasospasm following trauma and microsurgery surgery. J. Hand Surg., 4:109, 1979.

52. Pinella, J.A., Spira, M., Erk, Y. et al.: Direct microvascular monitoring with implantable ultrasonic Doppler probes. J. Microsurg., 3:217, 1982.

53. Poppen, N.K., Norris, T.R., and Buncke, H.J.: Evaluation of sensibility and function with microsurgical free tissue transfer of the great toe to the hand for thumb reconstruction. J. Hand Surg., 8:516, 1983.

54. Puckett, C.L., Misholy, H., and Retnisch, J.F.: The effects of streptokinase of ischemic flaps. J. Hand Surg., 8:101, 1983.

55. Richards, R.R., Seaber, A.V., and Urbaniak, J.R.: Chemically induced vasospasm: The effect of ischemia, vessel occlusion and adrenergic blockade. (Submitted for publication)

56. Salibian, A.H., Tesoro, V.R., and Wood, D.L.: Staged transfer of a free microvascular latissimus dorsi myocutaneous flap using saphenous vein grafts. Plast. Reconstr. Surg., 71:543, 1983.

57. Schenck, R.T., Weinrib, H.P., and Labanauskas, I.G.: The external ring technique for microvascular anastomosis. J. Hand Surg., 8:105, 1983.

58. Schlenker, J.D., Kleinert, H.E., and Tsai, T-M.: Methods and results of replantation following traumatic amputation of the thumb in sixty-four patients. J. Hand Surg., 5:63, 1980.

59. Schonwetter, B.S., Seaber, A.V., Urbaniak, J.R., and Bright, D.S.: Use of electromagnetic flowmeters in experimental microvascular surgery. In American Academy of Orthopaedic Surgeons Symposium on Microsurgery: Practical Use in Orthopaedics. St. Louis, C.V. Mosby, 1979.

60. Serafin, D., Lesesne, C.B., Mullen, R.Y., and Georgiade, N.G.: Transcutaneous pO_2 monitoring for assessing viability and predicting survival of skin flaps: Experimental and clinical correlations. J. Microsurg., 2:165, 1981.

61. Serafin, D., Rios, A.V., and Georgiade, N.: Fourteen free groin flap transfers. Plast. Reconstr. Surg., 57:707, 1976.

62. Serafin, D., Sabatier, R.E., Morris, R.L., and Georgiade, N.G.: Reconstruction of the lower extremity with vascularized composite tissue: Improved tissue survival and specific indications. Plast. Reconstr. Surg., 66:230, 1980.

63. Servant, J., Ikuta, Y., and Harada, Y.: A scanning electron microscope study of microvascular anastomoses. Plast. Reconstr. Surg., 57:329, 1976.

64. Shanahan, P.T., and Kleinert, H.E.: Anesthesia management of upper extremity replantation surgery. Anesthesiol. Rev., 10:10, 1983.

65. Stirrat, C.R., Seaber, A.V., Urbaniak, J.R., and Bright, D.S.: Temperature monitoring in digital replantation. J. Hand Surg., 3:342, 1978.

66. Taylor, G.I., Miller, G.D.H., and Ham, F.J.: The free vascularized bone graft: A clinical extension of microvascular techniques. Plast. Reconstr. Surg., 55:533, 1975.

67. Taylor, G.I., Townsend, P., and Corlett, R.: Superiority of the deep circumflex iliac vessels as the supply for free groin flaps: Clinical work. Plast. Reconstr. Surg., 64:745, 1979.

68. Taylor, G.I., and Watson, N.: One-stage repair of compound leg defects with free revascularized flaps of the groin, skin, and the iliac bone. Plast. Reconstr. Surg., 61:494, 1978.

69. Urbaniak, J.R.: Replantation of amputated parts—technique, results, and indications. In American Academy of Orthopaedic Surgeons Symposium on Microsurgery: Practical Use in Orthopaedics. St. Louis, C.V. Mosby, 1979.

70. Urbaniak, J.R.: Replantation. In Green, D.P. (ed.): Operative Hand Surgery. New York, Churchill Livingstone, 1982.

71. Urbaniak, J.R., Hayes, M.G., and Bright, D.S.: Management of bone in digital replantation: Free vascularized and composite bone grafts. Clin. Orthop., 133:184, 1978.

72. Urbaniak, J.R., Roth, J.H., Nunley, J.A. et al.: Should a single amputated digit be replanted. (Submitted for publication)

73. Urbaniak, J.R., Soucacos, P.N., Adelaar, R.S. et al.: Experimental evaluation of microsurgical techniques in small artery anastomoses. Orthop. Clin. North Am., 8:219, 1977.

74. VanGiesen, P.J., Seaber, A.V., and Urbaniak, J.R.: Storage of amputated parts prior to replantation— an experimental study with rabbit ears. J. Hand Surg., 8:60, 1983.

75. Weiland, A.J., and Daniel, R.K.: Microvascular anastomoses for bone grafts in the treatment of massive defects in bone. J. Bone Joint Surg., 61A: 98, 1979.

76. Weiland, A.J., and Daniel, R.K.: Vascularized bone grafts. In Green, D.P. (ed.): Operative Hand Surgery. New York, Churchill Livingstone, 1982.

77. Weiland, A.J., Villarreal-Rios, A., Kleinert, H.E. et al.: Replantation of digits and hands: Analysis of surgical techniques and functional results in 71 patients with 86 replantations. J. Hand Surg., 21: 1, 1977.

78. Winfrey, E.W., and Foster, J.H.: Low molecular weight dextran in small artery surgery. Antithrombogenic effect. Arch. Surg., 88:78, 1964.

28 Complications of Peripheral Nerve Injuries

GEORGE E. OMER, JR.

DEGENERATION AND REGENERATION

Interruption of the structural continuity of a peripheral nerve results in derangement of the involved nerve cells, connective-tissue elements, lymphatic vessels, blood vessels, and ectodermally derived specialized supportive cells. The functional unit is a neuron, which consists of the nerve cell nucleus and cytoplasm (soma or perikaryon) in the anterior column of the spinal cord (motor) or the dorsal root ganglia (sensory), the nerve cell cytoplasm in the dendrites (receiving) and the axon (efferent), and the anatomical unit at the synaptic terminal (such as the extrafusal fibers of muscles or Meissner's corpuscles). If the central cell body (perikaryon) were the height of an average man, its axon would be 1 to 2 inches in diameter and would extend more than 2 miles.[31] Proteins migrate from the perikaryon into the axon, and metabolic products flow from the axon to the perikaryon, so that the volume of the axon may be as much as 300 times that of the central cell body.[144] The number of neurons is constant after birth, and there is no replacement when a nerve cell is destroyed. Nerve regeneration after peripheral trunk injury is reconstitution of nerve cells that were deranged but survived.

The anatomy of a peripheral nerve is shown in Figure 28-1. A nerve fiber is composed of the axon and the Schwann cell sheath. All axons are surrounded by Schwann cells, which are of neuroectodermal origin. Unmyelinated fibers consist of several axons in furrows on the surface of the Schwann cell. The axons pass through chains of longitudinally aligned Schwann cells. Myelinated fibers are within a sheath composed of concentrically arranged lamellae consisting of alternating layers of lipid and protein, which are wrappings of Schwann cell plasma membrane around the axon. The nodes of Ranvier are the segments of the axon that are devoid of a myelin sheath.

Nerve fibers are usually grouped into a bundle called a funiculus. The terms *funiculus, fasciculus,* and *fascicle* are synonymous. Each funiculus usually contains motor, sensory, and sympathetic nerve fibers of varying proportions. Funiculi are often cross-linked with other groups of funiculi and form the funicular plexus within the peripheral nerve. The amount of crosslinking is varied according to the particular peripheral nerve and the level in the extremity.[55]

Connective-tissue elements include three supporting envelopes: the epineurium, the perineurium, and the endoneurium. The superficial layers of the peripheral nerve are termed the *epineurium.* The outer condensed layer is termed *circumferential epineurium* and is continuous with the *mesoneurium,* the suspending mesentery of the peripheral nerve. The groups of funiculi lie in a loose areolar tissue sheath called the *intraneurial epineurium.* The epineurium contains lymphatic vessels and blood vessels. The epineurium can occupy 25% to 75% of the cross-sectional area of a peripheral nerve.[155] Over a joint, the epineurium may be condensed. The funiculus is surrounded by a connective-tissue condensation termed the *perineurium.* The perineurium appears to be a prolongation of the membranes that cover the central nervous system. The endoneurium is the extracellular compartment that surrounds Schwann cells and their axons.

Traumatic injuries to peripheral nerves disrupt the continuity of the nerve fibers. The central body (perikaryon) responds with greatly increased metabolic activity and associated hypertrophy. The hypertrophy be-

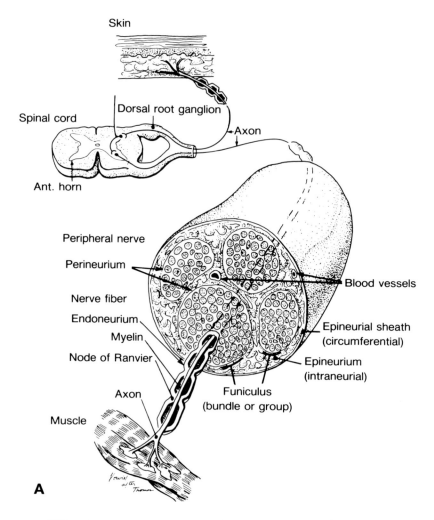

Skin

Spinal cord

Dorsal root ganglion

Axon

Ant. horn

Peripheral nerve

Perineurium

Blood vessels

Nerve fiber

Endoneurium

Myelin

Node of Ranvier

Epineurial sheath
(circumferential)

Epineurium
(intraneural)

Axon

Muscle

Funiculus
(bundle or group)

A

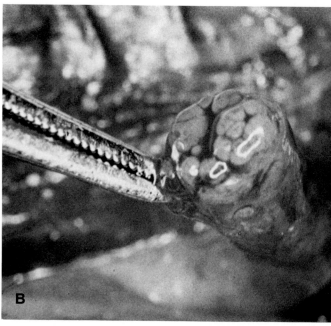

B

FIG. 28-1. (*A*) Schematic diagram of the anatomy of a peripheral nerve. (*B*) Cross section of a peripheral nerve. (*A*, after Grabb, W.C.: Management of nerve injuries in the forearm and hand. Orthop. Clin. North Am., 1[2]:419, 1970)

gins approximately the fourth day after injury and increases until approximately the twentieth day, but the increased metabolism continues as long as anabolic proteosynthetic activity is sustained. These metabolic changes within the perikaryon reflect a phase of neuronal survival (hypertrophy), followed by a phase of neuronal regeneration (axon sprouting). The more proximal the extremity injury and the greater the violence to the axon, the more severe the reaction within the perikaryon. Estimates of cell death during the third to ninth week following section of a nerve trunk range from 16% to 83%.[155] Even when the nerve cell survives, the volume (length) of axon that must be regenerated may exceed the metabolic capacity of the perikaryon. A child has a greater regeneration potential than an adult and a shorter axon distance between the spinal cord and functional end organs. Although axon regeneration appears to be more effective in the young, cortical reorientation may be a more important factor.

In the severed axon, both the proximal and distal stumps immediately develop marked edema. The distal stump of the nerve fiber, separated from its source of nourishment, undergoes several events termed *Wallerian degeneration*. The axon and myelin sheath degenerate, and Schwann cells and macrophages remove the debris. Morphologic changes occur within 24 hours after injury, and all unmyelinated axons degenerate within 1 week.[125] There is progressive decrease in the funicular cross-sectional area, and the endoneurial shrinkage may reach a maximum as early as 3 months after injury.[168] Wallerian degeneration occurs for a variable distance within the proximal stump.

Axon sprouting may begin by 96 hours after injury if the transsection was distal with minimal concomitant injury.[155] In a severe injury, such as a high-velocity gunshot wound, the axonal sprouting may begin 3 cm proximal to the actual severed stump, and it may be 3 weeks before axonal regeneration is prominent.[155,168] It is important to note that (1) the response of the supporting structures is immediate, and (2) the response of axonal sprouting at the site of

injury is delayed through the phase of neuronal survival.

In the distal stump the Schwann cells form tubules for regenerating axons. Those derived from myelinated nerve fibers are sometimes termed the *bands of Bünger* or *Schwann tubes*. Most new fibers, whether myelinated or unmyelinated, pass down new endoneurial tubules, thus precluding perfect end-organ specificity because the regenerating axons seldom use old endoneurial tubules.[17] In a mixed nerve, perhaps 50% of the regenerating motor axons will grow down sensory pathways. In like manner, sympathetic and cutaneous sensory axons regenerating through endoneurial tubes destined for muscle form no functional end-organ connections and deny the entry of motor axons to the end-organ.[43] Only slight rotation of either end of a severed nerve would produce misdirected axons or oppose the majority of axons to an impervious epineurium and perineurium. Problems related to axon misdirection are strong arguments in favor of microscopic control of funicular alignment when a severed nerve is sutured.

Denervation of skeletal muscle results in muscle fiber atrophy and derangement, with progressive distortion of the motor end-plate by proliferating connective tissue. Although the muscle will persist for at least 1 year, the destruction of the motor end-plate begins by the third month after denervation.[144,168] The clinical impression that electrical stimulation of denervated muscle delays motor end-plate destruction has not been supported by human microscopic studies or measured work capacity of the muscle before and after denervation. Sensory receptor end-organs (Meissner's corpuscles) that are denervated undergo progressive degeneration over several months.[54] Clinical results for sensibility depend on reinnervated cutaneous mechanoreceptors.[30]

There are three periods of delay in axonal regeneration: neuronal survival, crossing the area of trunk disruption (repair site), and end-organ connection. Neuronal survival requires 4 to 20 days, depending on the level and severity of the axonal injury. The axon requires 3 to 50 days to traverse the scar at the site of nerve suture.[44] The axon then proceeds down the distal endoneurial tube at a rate of approximately 1 mm to 3 mm per day, a rate of growth that gradually slows as the length of the axon increases. The time phase of neural regeneration may continue for a period of 300 days in a major nerve with a proximal injury. The final delay occurs during the reorganization of a connection with the muscle or sensory end-organ. The patient's age and the tissue homeostasis of the involved extremity are important factors. For practical purposes, a rate of 1 mm per day is accurate over the entire period of axon regeneration.[144,155]

In the clinical situation, there are three basic regeneration patterns following injury:[140] Minimal injury is termed *neurapraxia*, in which the nerve is intact but conduction is impaired. Moderate injury, termed *axonotmesis*, is characterized by interruption of the axons and their myelin sheaths (nerve fiber); however, the endoneurium remains intact and guides the regenerating axons to their appropriate peripheral connections. Severe injury, termed *neurotmesis*, describes a nerve that has either been completely severed or is so seriously disorganized that spontaneous regeneration is impossible. Most traumatic accidents, including fractures, dislocations, and gunshot wounds, can result in any one of these three types of injury. Lacerations usually result in neurotmesis.

RESULTS OF UNTREATED INJURIES

The incidence of nerve injuries associated with fractures is unknown. A humeral fracture is the most likely fracture to have an associated nerve injury.[113] The radial nerve is involved in 60%, the ulnar nerve in 18%, the common peroneal nerve in 15%, and the median nerve in 6% of all neuropathies resulting from fractures. Nerve problems occur in 18% of knee dislocations, usually traction injuries that vary from neurapraxia to neurotmesis. The sciatic nerve or its peroneal component is injured in approximately 13% of posterior dislocations of the hip or posterior acetabular fractures. Shoulder dislocations have associated axillary nerve stretch injuries in 5% of cases. The prognosis is different for closed and open fracture injuries, and is related to the severity of damage to the extremity. Seddon[141] reported 83.5% spontaneous recovery in 109 cases of closed fracture of the upper extremity with associated nerve injury, but only 65% in 37 cases of open fractures with neuropathy.

Nerve injury associated with traction has a poorer prognosis than does neuropathy related to fractures. During World War II,[22] only 58% of patients with traction injuries at the knee and continuity of the peroneal nerve had functional motor recovery, and the prognosis of traction injuries was unaffected by surgical exploration. Dorsiflexion against gravity returned in only 36% of patients with traction to the peroneal nerve.

High-velocity gunshot wounds often produce a pressure disturbance in the tissues that results in loss of function without disruption of peripheral nerves. Foerster[36] reported retrospectively on 2915 cases of motor paralysis during World War I, of which 1980 (67%) improved with conservative treatment. Sunderland[155] studied a series of military patients during World War II and documented spontaneous recovery in 68% of the cases. In a prospective study of 595 gunshot wounds during the Vietnam War, Omer[93] determined that spontaneous recovery occurred in 227 of 331 (69%) low-velocity gunshot wounds and 183 of 264 (69%) high-velocity gunshot wounds. Neurapraxia and axonotmesis injuries are approximately equal in gunshot wounds, with the clinical time scale for spontaneous recovery being 1 to 4 months for neurapraxia and 4 to 9 months for axonotmesis.[93] Rakolta and Omer[131] noted that spontaneous regeneration may be delayed up to 11 months without excluding the possibility of complete recovery.

Low-velocity gunshot wounds result in a higher percentage of peripheral nerve disruption (neurotmesis) than do high-velocity missile wounds. Civilian handgun injuries are usually low-velocity wounds with a smaller shock wave and temporary cavitation and therefore may not require extensive debridement and delayed primary closure.[73] Shotgun wounds have a higher percentage of peripheral nerve injuries and require thorough debridement, early exploration of the wound tract and related neurovascular structures, and delayed primary closure.

Spontaneous recovery of peripheral nerve injuries resulting from shotgun wounds has been reported as only 45%.[128]

Lacerations are low-velocity injuries that do not demonstrate significant spontaneous recovery. The major problem is that the minimal nerve involvement is not diagnosed because most of the nerve's function can be demonstrated.[105] Lacerations with associated loss of peripheral nerve function should be diagnosed clinically as severed-nerve lesions (neurotmesis) until proven otherwise by intraoperative examination.

It is appropriate at 3 to 4 months to explore the clinically complete nerve lesion in missile and shotgun wounds above the elbow or knee, stretch injuries from dislocated joints, severely comminuted fractures, and fractures adjacent to joints.[105] However, approximately 60% of these nerves will have a neuroma-in-continuity,[60] and a decision about resection of the neuroma may require special equipment for recording a nerve action potential. Lacerations require exploration and suture of disrupted nerves at the time of injury.

SURGICAL MANAGEMENT

Technique of Evaluating Nerve Action Potentials for Neuroma-in-Continuity

Most nerve injuries undergoing regeneration require 3 or more months before either sufficient axons reach motor terminals or adequate motor end-plate reconstruction occurs to permit either stimulation or electromyographic testing to show significant reversal of denervation changes. Recording directly from a peripheral nerve has been used since the 1930s and is the best method for evaluating a lesion in continuity. The nerve is dissected free from its bed for 6 cm to 8 cm on each side of the suture line or neuroma-in-continuity. The exposed nerve is then suspended on bipolar platinum electrodes proximally and a recording electrode distally, as described by Kline.[59] The electrodes are connected to shielded lead wires, and both may be heat sterilized. The recording wires are directed through a standard amplifier and then to an oscilloscope. The potentials traced on the oscilloscope screen are recorded by a camera. Stimuli

are delivered to the proximal electrodes by a battery-powered stimulator. The lowest threshold necessary to obtain a distal potential is determined, and the stimulus voltage is then increased until potentials of maximum amplitude and complexity are obtained. The recording electrode is then moved distally, and potentials at multiple points along the course of the regenerating nerve are obtained. Use of a tourniquet may result in ischemic changes that interfere with the response of the nerve to the electrical stimulus. The tourniquet should be deflated 15 to 20 minutes before recording is attempted.

Nerve action potentials provided reliable information for or against regeneration when done 12 or more weeks after suture or injury. Kline reported his experience with 213 major nerve injuries[61] and recorded that recovery did not occur in any patient in whom a nerve action potential was absent across the lesion 8 or more weeks following injury.

External Neurolysis

In external neurolysis the scar tissue is resected at the mesoneurium and immediate subcircumferential epineurial levels, but the intraneurial epineurial layers are not dissected to separate the funiculi. External neurolysis has an undeserved reputation as an effective operation to restore function in a nerve found to be in continuity.

Most nerve injuries that retain continuity will result in spontaneous recovery. Omer followed 648 nerve lesions that were the result of either closed injuries or open injuries, with the involved nerve shown to be in continuity at the time that the extremity wound was debrided.[93] Spontaneous recovery occurred in 454 lesions (70%). The time scale for spontaneous recovery of nerve lesions resulting from fractures and dislocations or crush injuries was 1 to 4 months. The time scale for spontaneous recovery of nerve lesions resulting from gunshot wounds was 3 to 9 months. These results suggest that neurapraxia recovers in 1 to 4 months and axonotmesis recovers at 3 to 9 months. There is doubt as to the success of external neurolysis if function of the extremity returns during the time scale for spontaneous recovery after injury; the intact nerve, in that case, might have recovered without surgery. It is unlikely that external scarring contributes to nerve dysfunction because a partial nerve function level seldom regresses, and microscopic studies of nerve lesions-in-continuity reveal that the lack of distal regeneration correlates with the degree of intrinsic nerve disruption. In a series of 59 cases in which external neurolysis was performed, we recorded only 18 (30%) that did not recover function during the projected time scale for spontaneous recovery. The surgery associated with nerve action potential study is an effective external neurolysis.

All normal nerves have mesoneurium that, much like the mesentery of the bowel, supports the segmental blood supply within the nerve. When stripped of this mesoneurium, the nerve may lose its longitudinal blood supply and function solely as an *in situ* nerve graft. As little as 6 cm to 8 cm of nerve divested of mesoneurium may constitute a loss of segmental blood supply sufficient to produce necrosis of that segment of the nerve.[147]

Internal Neurolysis

Internal neurolysis produces a separation of funiculi (nerve bundles) by splitting or dissecting intraneurial epineurial tissue layers. This must be done under magnification (3.5×–6×), or the procedure will increase scar and decrease internal circulation. Internal neurolysis should be considered only in repeated compression lesions, such as a carpal tunnel syndrome with median nerve pain, or for an acute injection injury.[171] The epineurium is opened with sharp dissection, and the funiculi are teased apart by placing the points of fine scissors between the funiculi and opening the blades parallel to the funiculi. Magnification is required to identify the crossover of a funiculus from one nerve bundle group to another, and these funiculi must be left intact. The longitudinal incision in the epineurium should not expose the freed funiculi to pressure or traction. For example, I prefer a lateral incision at the carpal level to avoid compression from volar flexion and traction caused by dorsal tendon motion over the freed funiculi. Saline injection into a nerve for internal neurolysis is a harmful procedure, since one does not release thickened epineurium by such a technique, and there may be some damage to individual funiculi.

Nerve Suture

Bjorkesten quotes Guret that, "at the end of the 18th century, the surgeon Gabriele Ferrara of Milan sutured the great sciatic nerve, using as material tortoise tendons softened in wine." This may be the first recorded nerve suture in man, but the result was not documented.[3]

There are only two principles in the techniques for suture repair: (1) align the funiculi, and (2) avoid tension in all suture lines. The technique used for nerve suture is the only factor affecting the return of function that is fully under the control of the attending surgeon.

Magnification is essential to distinguish the epineurium from the perineurium. Ocular loupes (2.5×–6×) have been used in operating rooms for many years. Operating microscopes are available with 40× magnification, but 20× is adequate for suture of almost all nerves. The nerve stumps must be debrided to normal tissue that demonstrates funicular patterns free of scar. A neurectotome or miter box can be helpful in squaring the nerve stumps, especially when one is performing a secondary repair and a large neuroma and distal fibroma have formed.

Suture material should be nonreactive to body tissues and small in diameter. Nylon provokes the least tissue reaction, followed by stainless steel, Ethiflex, and silk. However, nylon is brittle and springy and requires multiple knots. Nylon sutures of size 10-0 are readily obtainable for use with needles that can split a human hair. The use of silicone rubber (Silastic) cuffs about a suture line has been recommended for minimal neuroma formation.[32] The Silastic cuff may result in local tissue reaction with potential slough of soft tissue and is not indicated in most cases.

Instruments are available to handle the small needles and fine suture material. Spring-loaded needle holders with fine jaws can hold 3-mm to 4-mm needles. No. 5 and No. 7 jeweler's pickup and atraumatic forceps should be used. Special 10-0 tying forceps are available. It is important that these stainless steel microscopic instruments be nonmagnetic. These instruments are difficult to use with precision, and continuous practice for improved dexterity with instruments and magnification is essential for an appropriate suture in a reasonable period.

At the University of New Mexico, cats have been placed in pulsed electromagnetic fields following transection and repair of the common peroneal nerve. Horseradish peroxidase enzyme studies were used to localize the residual cell bodies in the anterior horns of the spinal cord.[13] The ratio of labeled cell bodies to unlabeled cell bodies in the anterior horn is improved when the pulsed electromagnetic field is used.[126] However, it has not been determined that the pulsed electromagnetic field stimulates neuron survival, nor has the appropriate wave form been identified for nerve regeneration. There is extensive reorganization within the regenerating nerve. Present surgical techniques that coapt endoneurial tubes in the proximal and distal stumps of the disrupted nerve really offer little hope that appropriate matching will be accomplished. There should be additional techniques developed to promote control between central and peripheral connections.

Epineurial Suture. Flourens (1828) and Baudens (1836) are credited with first utilizing the epineurial suture technique for nerve repair (Fig. 28-2).[120] The wound must be debrided and the nerve inspected for orientation. Surface markings within the circumferential epineurium, such as longitudinal blood vessels, are commonly used to align the proximal and distal nerve stumps and prevent malrotation of the funiculi. The most difficult technical step is the transection of the nerve to achieve a flat stump for the nerve end and to obtain a flush joint for the anastomosis. The nerve may be wrapped or fitted into a neurotome, then cut with a knife or scissors to obtain a transverse matched surface between the nerve stumps. If a significant amount of scar is found within the nerve, the transection procedure is repeated until fasciculi are easily identified. The funicular pattern on both sides of the divided nerve should be compared to confirm the rotational orientation. The marked branching and intermingling of the funiculi in a peripheral nerve trunk make it difficult to match the proximal and distal funicular pattern if a segment of nerve has been removed. Most cleanly severed peripheral nerves may be repaired by the epineurial suture technique, especially proximal (high) lesions in which there are many funiculi that cannot be easily identified or matched.

The epineurial suture is performed with fine nylon suture (8-0 to 10-0) to coapt the nerve stumps. Initial sutures are placed 180° around the circumference (9 and 3 o'clock), and the aligned anterior arc of epineurium is repaired with interrupted sutures. The nerve is then rotated 180° by passing one of the initial coaptation sutures posteriorly and turning the unrepaired posterior epineurium into view. The posterior epineurium is then repaired with interrupted sutures. A running suture is not used because a tight knot at the end of the repair would constrict the circumference of the nerve. The tourniquet should be released prior to the final sutures to evacuate any hematoma between the nerve stumps. The operative field should be moistened frequently with normal saline or Ringer's solution.

Histologic examination of epineurial repairs done without magnification or fine suture material has demonstrated funicular malalignment with gaps, overriding, buckling, and straddling.[33,44] The amount of tension used in suturing a nerve is directly related to the resulting connective-tissue proliferation at the anastomosis.[160] Circumferential tension, with a decrease in the cross-sectional area, causes deflection of the funicular alignment, with many regenerating axons ending blindly in the epineurium. Longitudinal tension may result in subepineurial and intrafunicular hemorrhages with fibrosis. Bora and associates have utilized a combined circumferential epineurial–intraneurial epineurial interrupted suture that would accurately align the funiculi and close the epineurium with a single stitch.[7] Snyder uses a long, single intraneurial stay suture in small nerves.[148]

Funicular (Fascicular, Bundle) Suture (Fig. 28-3). Langley (1917) recommended funicular sutures to obtain a better clinical result for sensory and motor function.[66] Sunderland advocated funicular sutures

A

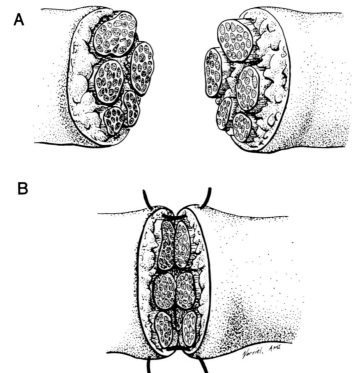

B

FIG. 28-2. (*A* and *B*) Epineurial circumferential closure technique for nerve suture. (*C*) Lacerated peripheral nerve. (*D*) Surface match for epineurial closure.

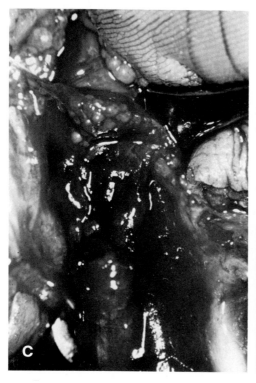

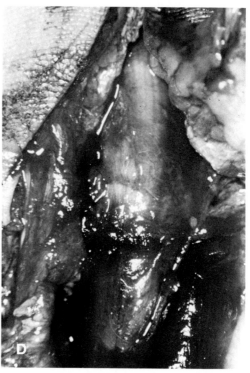

FIG. 28-3. (*A*) Nerve laceration with identification of fascicular bundles for matching. (*B*) Fascicular bundle repair technique with sutures through the intraneurial epineurium.

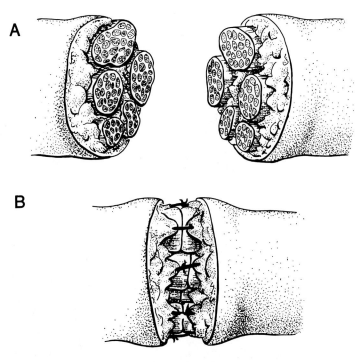

following his anatomic studies of the funicular patterns in peripheral nerves.[154] Accurate alignment and approximation of funiculi are critical for maximum neuronal regeneration. It is important to realign proximal sensory funiculi with distal sensory funiculi and proximal motor funiculi with distal motor funiculi. Precise electrical stimulation can be used to identify appropriate funiculi,[64,159] but without sophisticated equipment, one can use the size and grouping of proximal funiculi to match the distal funiculi. In acute injuries the visual method of identification and alignment is excellent and is useful in secondary repairs in which less than 1 cm of nerve tissue has been excised. A rapid radiochemical assay for choline acetyltransferase activity can be determined for fascicles.[34] Mixed motor-sensory fascicles have a fivefold increase in activity, and pure motor fascicles have a tenfold increase in activity compared with pure sensory nerves. The results can be obtained within 1 hour.

Suture of the intraneurial epineurium (the condensed connective tissue about groups of funiculi) is performed with 9-0 or 10-0 suture material, and magnification is essential for accurate alignment of the funiculi and placement of the sutures. A minimal number of interrupted sutures are used to approximate the selected funiculi. The neurorrhaphy should be accomplished without longitudinal or circumferential tension, a principle equally important for either epineurial or funicular approximation. The tourniquet should be released prior to the final sutures to evacuate any hematoma. The epineurium need not be repaired and can be excised for a centimeter proximal and distal from the suture line to ensure that this outer layer does not interpose between the approximated funiculi. Technically, the funicular repair is similar to the epineurial repair but is performed with small structures.

Controlled studies of epineurial and funicular neurorrhaphies have been done in animals.[7,16] Critical comparison of the clinical results, with objective measurements and statistical analysis, has not demonstrated significant differences between the two techniques when appropriate suture, instruments, and magnification are used.[164]

Nerve Gap Closure. A delayed nerve suture is often required in a complicated peripheral nerve injury. The nerve gap is a significant problem in delayed nerve suture because nerves tend to retract, and the neuroma and fibroma must be excised. There should be minimal tension at the suture line, and failures have been reported when stretching is as little as 5% of the length.[69] In our experience, a nerve gap of 7.5 cm is the maximum that can be approximated without requiring rigid immobilization of the extremity in flexion.[98]

There are several methods of closing a nerve gap.

Mobilization of the nerve. If the nerve is mobilized, it must then survive on the internal longitudinal circulation. Stripping more than 14 cm to 15 cm of mesoneurium deprives the nerve of its segmental blood supply, so that the nerve functions only as a graft *in situ*.[147]

Transposition and rerouting. An example is transferring the ulnar nerve from the extensor to the flexor surface at the elbow.

Flexion of joints. The elbow or knee should not flex beyond 90°, or the wrist beyond 30°. After the initial healing period of 3 to 6 weeks, joints should be extended only 10° per week to prevent intrinsic ischemia.[52]

Shortening the skeleton. This procedure is potentially dangerous because all soft tissue structures, such as muscle–tendon units, are relatively lengthened and weakened. (Another unacceptable method is use of a bulb suture, with subsequent acute stretching of the nerve.)

Nerve grafting. Autogenous material is preferred for nerve grafts; the sural nerve and the medial or lateral antebrachial cutaneous nerves are the best sources of graft material. Irradiated nerve homografts have been recommended, but they have not demonstrated consistent clinical value.

Nerve Grafts and Pedicles. The first documented nerve graft was performed by J. J. Philipeaux and A. Vulpian in 1870.[77] A nerve graft provides a scaffold that assists the regenerating axons to find their way into the distal nerve stump and restore the original pattern of innervation. The nerve graft must be acceptable to the body without producing an inflammatory response or

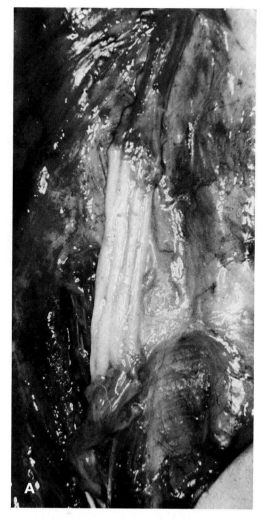

FIG. 28-4. (*A*) Sural nerve cables placed between fascicular groups as the technique for autogenous nerve grafts. (*B*) Two 10-0 or 11-0 sutures are enough to anchor each end of the sural cable.

constrictive fibrosis, it should be of small enough diameter to revascularize readily, and it should have a funicular (fascicular) pattern similar to that of selected funiculi in the proximal and distal suture lines.

The donor nerve should be visualized for atraumatic removal. For example, the sural nerve is usually removed from the leg through a Z-step longitudinal incision, although multiple transverse incisions can be used. The initial incision is just distal and posterior to the lateral malleolus, where the

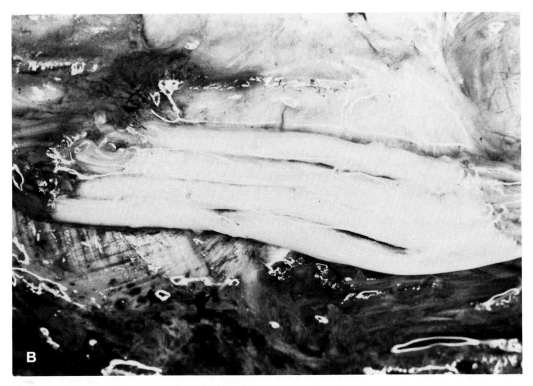

FIG. 28-4. (*Continued*)

sural nerve usually has two branches. Both branches must be identified, and the nerve is then removed from the leg. In the calf the sural nerve is deep to the investing fascia in a longitudinal groove in the posterior aspect of the gastrocnemius muscle adjacent to the short saphenous vein. The communicating branch of the peroneal nerve frequently joins the sural nerve in the proximal calf and must be severed to obtain the full length of the sural nerve. In an adult, 35 cm of sural nerve should be obtained from each leg.

Seddon[142,144] popularized the multiple cable graft. The technique includes suturing multiple nerve segments together to equal the diameter of the disrupted nerve, thus forming a multiple-segment cable. The cable graft is superior to a large-diameter nerve graft because the multiple cables develop an adequate intergraft circulation, while the large-diameter nerve will undergo central necrosis. The multiple cable graft is sutured proximally and distally to bridge the gap in the disrupted nerve.

Millesi[80,81] has improved the multiple cable graft by developing an interfunicular (fascicular) technique that emphasizes no tension at suture lines, accurate funicular alignment, and excision of the epineurium (Fig. 28-4). The healthy epineurium is opened longitudinally, both proximal to the neuroma and distal to the fibroma. Groups of funiculi (fascicles) that have the approximate cross-sectional area of the donor nerve are cut at different levels in both the proximal and distal stumps. The local epineurium, which has been opened, is excised. A sketch of the funicular pattern of the nerve ends is made to plan the connecting multiple cable graft. The donor nerve graft is sectioned to fit the gap in the disrupted nerve. Each segment of donor nerve should be without either tension or redundancy. An operating microscope is most useful because 10-0 material should be used for the suture. One suture connects the intraneurial epineurium of the selected funiculus to the circumferential epineurium of the donor nerve at both proximal and distal ends. Occasionally, as determined under magnification, an additional 10-0 suture is necessary to establish optimal alignment and contact. Within 20 minutes, natural fibrin clotting provides sufficient tensile strength to prevent disruption if the graft is long enough to neutralize any tension in the longitudinal direction.[80]

Sometimes a funiculus to be grafted is smaller in cross-sectional area than the donor nerve, and the donor nerve can be split longitudinally to remove one of the funiculi. If indicated, a tourniquet should be used in nerve grafting, but the pressure is released and meticulous hemostasis obtained prior to wound closure. The involved limb is immobilized in comfortable extension for 21 days, and then activity is commenced. In contrast, nerve suture under tension requires 3 to 6 weeks of postoperative immobilization and then gradual extension of flexed joints at 10° per week.

After the nerve graft has been performed, the axons cross the proximal suture site and regenerate toward the distal suture site. In a long nerve graft the distal site may scar and block before the axons reach that level. Clinically, this becomes apparent as the advancing Tinel sign stops and does not proceed. If there is more than a 30-day delay at this point, one should expose the distal suture site and use electrodiagnostic techniques (nerve action potentials) to evaluate the neuroma-in-continuity. If there is no distal electrical conduction, the distal suture site should be resected and a second neurorrhaphy performed.

Interfunicular grafts allow the separation of critical function on an anatomical basis. For example, in one patient at the University of New Mexico, a laceration of the ulnar nerve at the wrist involved both the main trunk of the nerve and the dorsal cutaneous branch. The dorsal cutaneous branch was isolated from both the proximal and distal nerve segments and used as the donor nerve.[86] After 10 months, the patient had minimal clawing and good recovery of hypothenar muscle function.

A large gap involving both the median and ulnar nerves in one extremity can be bridged by a nerve pedicle.[153] The proximal median nerve is sutured to the proximal ulnar nerve to form a U above the combined

nerve gap. The ulnar nerve is measured retrograde from this suture line to determine the length required to close the gap in the median nerve. The ulnar nerve is severed at that point so that the distal segment will degenerate and allow axons from the median nerve to cross the U suture line and grow in retrograde fashion up the proximal ulnar nerve. One should remove a short section of the proximal ulnar nerve to be certain that it will not regenerate distally and block the retrograde growth of median nerve axons. After an appropriate interval to allow the median nerve to grow around the U loop (1 mm per day), the loop pedicle can be transferred and sutured to the distal stump of the median nerve. On occasion, the loop pedicle can be sutured to the distal stumps of both the median and ulnar nerves.

A similar pedicle graft of U loop can be dissected between the tibial and peroneal segments of the sciatic nerve to bridge a gap proximal to the knee. Distal to the knee, the tibial and peroneal nerves can be sutured in a fashion similar to that for the median and ulnar nerves in the forearm. One should sketch the funicular pattern of the pedicle end and the distal nerve stump and attempt to match patterns for funicular alignment. An interfunicular graft suture technique can be used. Pedicle U-loop nerve grafts have not been uniformly successful in adults,[93] although the procedure has given good clinical results in children.

Prognostic Factors for Functional Recovery After Nerve Suture

Age is the most significant single factor in recovery following nerve suture. Almost all patients up to the age of puberty have good clinical results following nerve suture. The young patient has a greater intrinsic capacity for sensory reeducation and motor adaptability than does the older patient.

The more extensive and severe the injury to the involved extremity, the longer the time required for tissue homeostasis. Nerves are only as functional as the pertinent sensory receptors and muscle–tendon motors. Multiple nerve involvement is a more serious problem for functional recovery of the entire extremity than is an isolated nerve injury. Severe vascular deficiency or chronic osteomyelitis each contributes to fibrotic infiltration and delayed healing.

The more proximal the injury to the nerve, the longer the tissues will be denervated and the slower the recovery of function. One can expect axon regeneration to be vigorous for the first year after injury in an adult,[155] but if the interval between injury and end-organ reinnervation is longer than 1 year, functional recovery will be limited. The poor prognosis for functional recovery related to anatomical level is emphasized in a very proximal injury of the ulnar or sciatic nerve, where it may be 20 cm to 30 cm to the most proximal end-organ. The interval between injury and nerve suture is important in all injuries, but it becomes critical in these very proximal nerve lesions when extremity complications have delayed anastomosis until 12 or more weeks after injury. In these cases the surgeon must determine early that the nerve suture has been successful and that axons have crossed into the distal nerve stump, or prepare to resuture the nerve. A periodic series of nerve evaluation tests performed 12 weeks after suture of a very proximal injury of the sciatic nerve would be of minimal value if the regenerating axons could not reach end-organs to demonstrate motor, sudomotor, or sensory activity. A delay of 36 to 48 weeks before the periodic nerve evaluation tests could demonstrate that the sutured nerve was not regenerating and would ensure inadequate reinnervation of far distal end-organs, even with resuture of the nerve. The concept of a second operation after 12 to 16 weeks to evaluate the nerve action potential should be applied in many delayed sutures, as well as the very proximal nerve injury.

EVALUATION OF FUNCTIONAL LOSS

A common complication of peripheral nerve injury is functional loss following initial nerve suture. The timing of further operative intervention depends on the total response of the extremity and the extent of nerve regeneration. The prognosis for regeneration cannot be assessed without testing functional loss and recovery. Assessment of the established peripheral neuropathy requires multiple quantitative tests that are repeated at regular intervals. Rehabilitation of the patient includes a coordinated program of evaluation, surgery, reeducation, reevaluation, and reconstruction.

Surgical Procedure

To evaluate the clinical result, it is important to know the technique of nerve repair, and most current descriptions are inadequate. The surgical repair should be defined by the description of four steps in technique:

1. Stump preparation, including description of the fascicular pattern of the nerve segment
2. Approximation of the nerve ends, including the amount of tension and translocation of the nerve stumps
3. Coaptation, either direct (neurorrhaphy) or indirect (nerve graft), and including the specific tissues sutured
4. Technique used to maintain the coaptation, such as stitching or fibrin clotting

In addition, one should know the exact site of the lesion, the damage to adjacent tissues, the interval between injury and repair, the state of the musculature, the use of a tourniquet, and the position and duration of immobilization.[117]

Assessment of Individual Nerve Loss and Recovery

The motor strength of individual re-innervated muscles and the sensibility level of the individual peripheral nerve are the most important assessments. Assessment of the established peripheral neuropathy requires multiple quantitative tests that are repeated at regular intervals of approximately 12 weeks.

Sensation. Sensation is the activation of impulses in the afferents of the nervous system and the subjective appreciation of the physical stimulus.[94] Protective sensation is the recognition of pressure, pain, cold, or warmth before tissue damage results from the stimulus. The pinprick test will demonstrate protective sensation. A more reliable technique to estimate loss of protective sensation is to ask the patient to map the area with normal sensibility with his finger.[111]

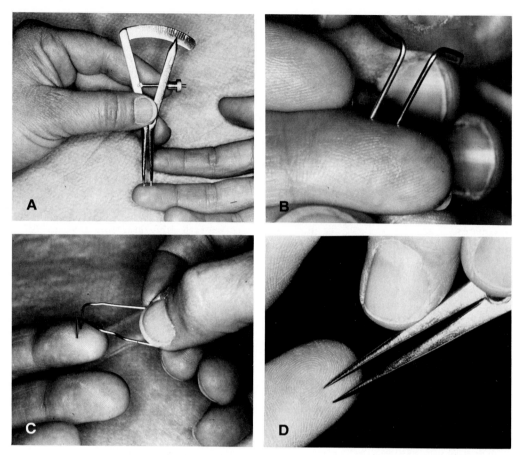

Fig. 28-5. Techniques for testing light touch in the hand. (*A*) Static two-point discrimination distance. The line of application is over the digital nerve in the longitudinal axis of the finger. (*B*) A paper clip is an acceptable instrument for the static two-point discrimination test. (*C*) Moving two-point discrimination distance. The pressure from the instrument should not produce an ischemic blanching of the skin. (*D*) An eye caliper used as testing instrument for the moving two-point discrimination test.

Tinel's Sign. Sensation perceived in the distal cutaneous distribution could appear by 4 to 6 weeks after injury. We initiate percussion with the stem of a tuning fork (30 cps) over the trunk of the involved nerve, beginning at the distal portion of the extremity to delay the patient's potential discomfort until the final point of the test.[120] An advancing (distal) level of response does not guarantee that there is a sufficient quantity of axons for clinical function. In addition, there is no measurement of quality, so the response may indicate hyperesthesia rather than normal sensation.

Body Position/Movement Recognition. The patient with normal sensation can identify the passive position and directional change in a joint. In the shoulder joint, 1° of passive movement can be recognized, and a given position can be reproduced within 2°, whereas an interphalangeal joint requires 5° to 10° of passive movement for recognition. The recognition of two-point discrimination for light touch is in reverse ratio to recognition of joint movement and is more acute distally on the extremity.

Sensibility. Sensibility is the capacity for precise interpretation of sensation.[169] For example, two-point discrimination distance is more a judgment of than the recognition of pressure sensation (Fig. 28-5).[109] All current tests to examine the degree of

Table 28-1. Interpretation of the Von Frey Test of Sensibility

AESTHESIOMETER PROBE NUMBER	CALCULATED PRESSURE (g/mm²)	INTERPRETATION
2.44–2.83	3.25–4.86	Normal light touch
3.22–4.56	11.1–47.3	Diminished light touch; point localization* intact
4.74–6.10	68.0–243.0	Minimal light touch; area localization† intact
6.10–6.65	243.0–439.0	Sensation, but without localization sensibility

* Point localization: the dowel is in contact with the skin point stimulated.
† Area localization: the dowel is in contact with any point inside the zone of the area being tested (in the hand or foot).

functional loss of sensibility are related to cutaneous touch/pressure sensation and should be compared with test results from the contralateral extremity. Normal cutaneous sensation provides normal-quality sensibility, termed *tactile gnosis* by Moberg.[82]

Von Frey Test (Table 28-1). Weinstein[169] utilized 20 nylon monofilaments marked 1.65 to 6.65. Normal sensibility localizes pressure at the hand between probes marked 2.44 to 2.83. The probe number represents the logarithm of 10 times the force in milligrams required to bow the monofilament. The monofilament is applied perpendicular to the body surface, and pressure is increased until the monofilament bends. If the patient feels the pressure, he localizes the touch point. The monofilament should be applied 3 times; if the patient does not localize the same monofilament twice in the same area, a larger monofilament is selected for testing.[170]

Weber/Moberg Two-Point Discrimination Test (Table 28-2). The Weber/Moberg Two-Point Discrimination Test determines whether the patient can discriminate between being touched with one or two points and the minimal distance at which two points touching the skin are recognized. The testing instrument can be a Boley gauge, a blunt eye caliper, or an ordinary paper clip (see Fig. 28-5).[83] The perpendicular pressure from the testing instrument should not blanch the skin. When two points are applied, they should make simultaneous contact in the longitudinal axis of the finger over either the radial or ulnar digital nerve. We use a series of one or two points applied in random sequence but done at least three times for each selected distance.[90] The normal threshold for the volar surface of the hand varies from 2 mm to 5 mm at the fingertip to 7 mm to 10 mm at the base of the palm. The threshold for the dorsal

Table 28-2. Static Two-Point Discrimination Distance in the Volar Surface of the Hand

	HAND ZONE	DISTANCE (mm)		
		NORMAL	DIMINISHED	ABSENT
Between fingertip and DIP* joint	7	2–5	6–10	10+
Between DIP joint and PIP* joint	6	3–6	7–10	10+
Between PIP joint and finger web	5	4–7	8–10	10+
Between finger web and distal palmar crease	4	5–8	9–20	20+
Between distal palmar crease and central palm	3	6–9	10–20	20+
Base of palm and wrist	1–2	7–10	11–20	20+

* DIP, distal interphalangeal; PIP, proximal interphalangeal.

Table 28-3. Moberg and British Research Council Systems for Evaluating Sensibility

MOBERG SCALE	BRITISH CODE	SENSIBILITY DESCRIPTION
Good	S4	Normal sensibility
		Two-point discrimination distance of 12 mm or less—tactile gnosis
Fair		Two-point discrimination distance of 12 mm to 15 mm
Poor	S3+	Some recovery of two-point discrimination within the autonomous area of the nerve
Bad	S3	Return of superficial cutaneous pain and tactile sensibility throughout the autonomous area with disappearance of any previous overreaction
	S2	Return of some degree of superficial cutaneous pain and tactile sensibility within the autonomous area of the nerve
	S1	Recovery of deep cutaneous pain sensibility within the autonomous area of the nerve
	S0	Absence of sensibility in the autonomous area of the nerve

surface is higher in all zones: normal is 7 mm to 12 mm, diminished is 13 mm to 20 mm, and absent is greater than 20 mm. All test results should be compared with findings on the contralateral extremity.

Weber/Dellon Two-Point Discrimination Test. Although the static two-point discrimination distance correlates with constant touch, such as various pinch positions, it does not assess tactile gnosis, which requires movement.[178] The moving two-point discrimination test is performed with an ordinary paper clip. The paper clip is moved along the volar surface of the pulp tip of the finger. The stimulus of one or two points is applied in random sequence, while 7 of 10 responses must be correct before proceeding to the next lower value. Distance recognition in normal discrimination is 2 mm in the distal finger tip, which is the only area tested.[26]

Ridge Sensitometer Test. A progressively higher ridge passed over a smooth finger or toe pulp surface has been used to evaluate "depth sense." The ridge will normally be identified at a height between 0.15 mm and 0.30 mm.[129]

Sensibility is more difficult to evaluate than motor strength and amplitude. Voluntary movement is an essential component of precise sensibility, and the moving finger should identify textured fabrics, geometric shapes, and three-dimensional letters. Moberg[85] believes that the sensibility system adopted by the British Research Council in 1954 is inadequate to rate functional loss. However, this is the system generally used for evaluation (Table 28-3).[143]

Motor Function (Table 28-4). The voluntary muscle test to examine muscle strength is based on the use of gravity and resistance, as first devised by Lovett in 1912

Table 28-4. Interpretation of Tests of Motor Function

GRADE				DESCRIPTION
100%	5	N	Normal	Complete range of motion against gravity with full resistance
75%	4	G	Good	Complete range of motion against gravity with some resistance
50%	3	F	Fair	Complete range of motion against gravity
25%	2	P	Poor	Complete range of motion with gravity eliminated
10%	1	T	Trace	Evidence of slight contractility; no joint motion
0%	0	0	Zero	No evidence of contractility

FIG. 28-6. Voluntary muscle tests. (*A*) Strength is graded by resistance to movement. The muscle–tendon unit should be palpated to determine function. (*B*) The active range of motion should be measured.

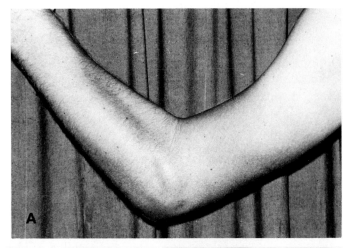

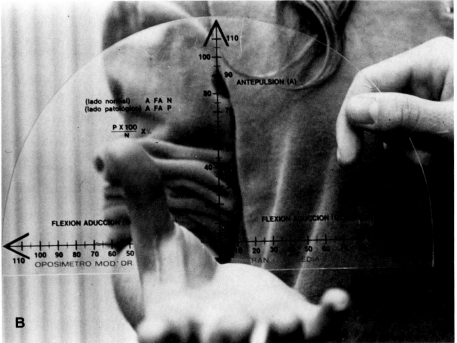

(Fig. 28-6, *A*).[103] The examiner grades muscle strength by palpation of the involved muscle–tendon unit, and resisting movement of a bone–joint lever arm motored by the involved muscle. Trick movements must be detected, and if there is a questionable motor activity, a local anesthetic is indicated to block competing or anomalous innervation.

The active range of motion can be quantified with a goniometer across an appropriate joint (Fig. 28-6, *B*). Strength can be quantified with the aid of resistance instruments, such as grip and pinch meters. The contralateral extremity (if normal) should be used for comparison.

Sudomotor Function. Moberg's[82] Ninhydrin printing test is the most accurate test of sudomotor function. The o-phthalaldehyde-in-xylene test is also precise.[56] Other dyes used for sudomotor function tests include Minor's iodine and starch

Table 28-5. British Medical Research Council System for Grading Peripheral Nerve Motor Recovery

GRADE	DESCRIPTION
M5	Complete recovery
M4	All synergic and independent movements are possible.
M3	All important muscles act against resistance.
M2	Return of perceptible contraction in both proximal and distal muscles
M1	Return of perceptible contraction in proximal muscles
M0	No contraction

in oil, cobalt chloride, and quinizarin. O'Riain[127] noted the phenomenon of skin wrinkling in warm water, which is related to sympathetic activity and is a useful test in children. Sudomotor tests provide useful information on the progress of recovery but are irrelevant in end-result evaluation.

Electrodiagnostic Studies. Electromyography. Denervation potentials do not develop immediately in a denervated muscle but are usually associated with Wallerian degeneration, occurring 1 to 3 weeks following injury. Electromyography cannot be used to predict the quality or quantity of reinnervation.

Nerve Conduction. Velocities of nerve conduction in the upper extremity range from 45 to 80 meters per second.[2] Axons of larger diameter conduct at a faster rate, and newborn infants have a conduction time that is one-half that of adults. Determination of the conduction velocity of sensory nerves is the only objective study to measure sensation.

Evaluation of Total Extremity Functional Result

Motor Function Grading (Table 28-5). The British Medical Research Council[143] introduced a system that attempts to assess the motor recovery of a peripheral nerve in relation to the resulting action from combined muscles. This is most useful in proximal (high) lesions.

To use the British Research Council grading system, "proximal" and "distal" muscles must be defined for each nerve (Table 28-6).

Extremity Coordination. Coordination is the end product of motor and sensory coordination. Grasp and pinch can be measured with dynamometers, which should be adjusted to fit the finger span of the patient. The best comparison is the grasp

Table 28-6. Proximal and Distal Muscles Innervated by the Peripheral Nerves

PROXIMAL MUSCLE	DISTAL MUSCLE
RADIAL NERVE	
Brachioradialis	Abductor pollicis longus
Extensor carpi radialis longus	Extensor pollicis longus
Extensor digitorum communis	Extensor pollicis
Extensor carpi ulnaris	
MEDIAN NERVE	
Pronator teres	Abductor pollicis brevis
Flexor carpi radialis	
Flexor digitorum superficialis	
Flexor pollicis longus	
ULNAR NERVE	
Flexor carpi ulnaris	Abductor digiti quinti
Flexor digitorum profundus (ring and little)	Interossei
COMMON PERONEAL NERVE	
Tibialis anterior	Extensor digitorum brevis
Extensor digitorum longus	
Extensor hallucis longus	
Peronei	
TIBIAL NERVE	
Gastrocnemius and soleus	Abductor hallucis
Tibialis posterior	Intrinsic muscles of the sole of the foot
Flexor digitorum longus	
Flexor hallucis longus	

Table 28-7. Grading System for Combined Findings of Motor and Sensibility Function

| | | | SENSIBILITY FUNCTION | |
NERVE	GRADE	MOTOR FUNCTION (SEDDON[144])	SEDDON[144]	MOBERG[85]
Median	Good	M3	S3+ or S4	2 pt. < 12 mm
	Fair	M2	S3	2 pt. < 15 mm
	Bad	M0 or M1	S1 or S2	2 pt. < 20 mm
Ulnar	Good	M4	S3	2 pt. < 15 mm
	Fair	M3	S2	Lost
	Bad	M1 or M2	S0 or S1	Lost
Radial	Good	M4		
	Fair	M3		
	Bad	M1 or M2		
Common peroneal	Good	M4		
	Fair	M3		
	Bad	M1 or M2		
Tibial	Good	M3	S3 or S4	2 pt. < 12 mm
	Fair	M2	S3	2 pt. < 15 mm
	Bad	M0 or M1	S1 or S2	Lost
Digital	Good		S3+ or S4	2 pt. < 12 mm
	Fair		S3	2 pt. < 15 mm
	Bad		S1 or S2	2 pt. < 20 mm

or pinch strength of the contralateral hand.[92] In the weak hand, Swanson uses a rolled tourniquet cuff, and grip is expressed in terms of changing tourniquet pressure, such as 135/50 torr.[156]

Moberg's Picking-up Test. We have the patient gather nine small objects from a tabletop and put them into a container while his eyes are closed. The objects may include a key, marble, nut, bolt, paper clip, coin, safety pin, chalk, or similar items. The patient attempts to identify the objects. The patient is timed, and a comparison of periodic tests indicates the changing status of coordination.[106]

Tactile gnosis can also be tested by writing numbers on a digit, identifying a coin, or palpating arrows or type; in all tests the patient closes his eyes.

Grading Clinical Recovery (Table 28-7). Appropriate multiple tests should be repeated at intervals of approximately 12 weeks.[92] The result is an evaluation of motor function, sensibility, and coordination of the extremity. The appropriate time to attain maximum clinical recovery depends on the level and severity of the nerve lesion. Evaluation studies should demonstrate the definitive clinical recovery in 3 to 5 years after nerve repair.

Any grading system must be flexible enough to combine motor and sensory findings to demonstrate a "good" clinical recovery.

Ratings should be based on comparison with corresponding function on the contralateral side. A good clinical result is one with good protective sensation, good tactile discrimination for precise sensibility, restoration of fine digital movements, and restoration of motor function to a degree that makes corrective devices and surgical reconstruction unnecessary.

PAIN

Pain can be totally incapacitating following traumatic injuries to and iatrogenic procedures on the peripheral nerves. Pain is an unpleasant sensory and emotional experience associated with actual or potential tissue damage, or described in terms of such damage.[79] There is no objective method to measure pain. The recognition of pain is subjective and depends on the intensity of the peripheral stimulus, central summation, and the personality of the patient.

The pain threshold is the least stimulus at which a subject perceives pain.[79] The pain tolerance level is the greatest stimulus intensity causing pain that a subject is prepared to tolerate.[79] Age, sex, race, ethnic group, religion, and other factors influence pain tolerance.[137] A number of traits are characteristic facets of personality, such as: anxiety, expressiveness, depression, or hypochondriasis.[67] In the experimental setting, pain threshold and tolerance can be determined by several techniques and show high reliability. Clinicians may believe that the patient who complains about pain more than "average" has a low threshold, but this is an error. The readiness to communicate the pain is a function of expressiveness, and this in turn is associated with a degree of extraversion.[151] In experimental studies, Lynn and Eysenck[71] found that pain tolerance of college students was negatively correlated with neuroticism and positively correlated with extraversion. In clinical situations, anxiety is associated with acute pain and the anticipation of body harm, while depression is associated with chronic pain and intropunitive anger. Sternbach and associates[152] found that patients with low back pain of less than 6 months' duration obtained Minnesota Multiphasic Personality Index (MMPI) profiles within normal limits, while those patients with low back pain of longer duration had markedly elevated scores for depression, hypochondriasis, and hysteria.

Experienced surgeons who spend time with their patients and make thoughtful decisions based on objective findings plus clinical impressions usually obtain good results with elective surgery, even with patients who have abnormal MMPI scales. However, the MMPI aids in confirming clinical impressions of a patient's psychological status and serves as a useful diagnostic device when the clinician is insecure about his decision for surgery. In a practical sense, the attending surgeon must learn to identify the unstable emotional personality. These patients will require much more time and explanation to cope with their pain.[39]

Chronic pain is defined as pain that persists or recurs at intervals for months or years.[6] Chronic pain is caused not only by pathologic processes in the nervous system, but also by psychopathology and environmental influences. Chronic pain is a wicked energy that imposes excessive psychological, social, and economic stresses on the patient. More than 40 million Americans are either partially or totally disabled by chronic pain, and as a result nearly 700 million work days are lost annually, which together with health care costs and compensation total approximately $50 billion each year.[6] The pattern for development of a chronic pain syndrome follows a sequence: nociceptive stimulus, to sensation of pain, to suffering, to pain behavior—which may continue in the absence of tissue damage. It is important to emphasize that pain, along with the associated suffering, is actually an emotional phenomenon.[21] It is important to delineate psychosocial factors, and some characteristics of an established pain syndrome include

Symptoms lasting longer than 6 months
Minimal objective physical findings
Evidence of medication abuse
Somatic preoccupation, with poor appetite, loss of energy, insomnia, and diminished ability to concentrate
Attempts to manipulate the surgeon, family, and environment

For elective surgical procedures, an important concept is the prevention of pain.[102] If a cutaneous nerve, such as the superficial radial nerve, is partially cut, the appropriate procedure is prompt suture of the laceration. In extensive injuries, venous repair is important for the prevention of edema. Surgical release of fascial sheaths is performed when indicated. During the early postoperative period one should attempt to abort edema. Early motion must be initiated, such as shoulder exercises when the fingers should not move. Early motion is essential to prevent joint contractures and muscle atrophy, and active motion is begun before pain is appreciated by the patient. Medications during the early postoperative period should include aspirin and perhaps a tranquilizer. Aspirin blocks the metabolic pathway from injured cells to the formation of prostaglandins and thromboxanes.[45] A mild tranquilizer, such as hydroxyzine pamoate, reduces the incidence of analgesic side-effects, including nausea and vomiting, and promotes the inhibition of anxiety.[74] These medications are most effective during the first 24 to 72 hours after surgery. Postoperative pain should be evaluated promptly; one should never wait for the full development of an established pain syndrome before initiating aggressive treatment. For example, the osteoporosis of Sudek's atrophy is not evident by x-ray for 5 to 8 weeks postinjury, but the patient has pain from the time of injury.

Differential Diagnosis

It is necessary to evaluate the potential etiology of pain from the pain site to the spinal cord. A detailed history and a thorough physical examination should be obtained. The history is obviously important in such problems as brachial plexus neuropathy, diabetes, or paresthesia of the hand following radiation therapy for lung cancer.[63] Routine laboratory studies, such as sedimentation rate, are useful. Roentgenographic evaluation may require plain radiographs in multiple planes, computed tomography, cinefluoroscopy, arthrography, discography, and computed tomographic metrizamide myelography. Technetium and gallium radionuclide scanning are used to confirm clinical observations. It is impossible to separate the functional activity of the nervous system from the vascular system; the Dopper examination[5] is a flow detector, while plethysmography is a volumetric analysis of flow.[176] Thermography can be employed to identify sensory root involvement.[62] Nerve conduction testing is useful to localize the level of dysfunction, to distinguish partial and complete lesions, and to differentiate muscle from nerve pathology.[25] Diagnostic confusion lies in the numerous sources from which painful symptoms may arise, with massive overlap and similarities in the clinical picture. For example, hypertrophic osteoarthritis of the cervical spine may produce pain in several ways: (1) direct nerve compression, of either the nerve roots or the spinal cord, which results in muscle weakness and sensory abnormalities over specific dermatomes, (2) vertebral artery insufficiency and compression of the posterior cervical sympathetic plexus by osteophytes from the zygapophyseal joints or the uncovertebral articulations, resulting in potential cervical migraine, neck, or arm pain, (3) thoracic outlet compression

from spasm of the scalene muscles, (4) irritation of the joint capsules with their intrinsic innervation, which may result in paresthesia in the neck, the tip of the shoulder, the lateral aspect of the arm, or the hand.

It is useful to divide the pattern of subjective symptoms into categories, such as (1) nociceptive peripheral increased stimulus, (2) summation of the reflex sympathetic overflow, (3) inflammatory or systemic pain, which may be generalized, (4) central pain, (5) cancer pain, and (6) personality dysfunction.[99]

There are only two principles in the treatment of an established pain syndrome involving the upper extremity: (1) relieve the subjective pain experience, and (2) institute active function of the involved extremity.[120]

Subjective Relief Techniques

Peripheral Nociceptive Stimulus. Pain may develop after local trauma for many reasons. The damaged portion of the nerve may develop intraneural fibrosis, or external adhesions may transfix the nerve to its bed. Friction on a nerve will result in inflammatory changes and further fibrosis. The compressed nerve will have venous stasis, capillary leakage, and perineurial edema.[136] Decreased blood flow can be associated with pain, as in any compression syndrome.[38] Any procedure producing vasodilatation may relieve this pain.

The peripheral nociceptive stimulus is often associated with trigger points. A trigger point or area is a small, hypersensitive region from which impulses bombard the central nervous system and give rise to referred pain. The termination of pain by either local injection of an anesthetic or hyperstimulation will normalize function and help prevent recurrence of abnormal neural activity.[78] Methods of hyperstimulation analgesia have included intense cold, intense heat, chemical irritation, dry needling, or acupuncture. Moxa, or moxibustion, has a purpose similar to acupuncture and consists of the application to the skin of combustible cones of powdered leaves of *artemisia vulgaris*. The cones are placed in charted spots and set on fire; they are extinguished after a blister is formed. There are special charts for moxa points, but the cones can also be applied to the acupuncture points. Many a Korean patient in U.S. 8th Army hospitals during the 1950s had the complication of a series of small round burns from initial Korean Han–Yak (Chinese: Yin–Yang) therapy. Western authors have recommended massage and stretching of the underlying muscles after trigger-point injection.[135]

A peripheral nerve responds to injury, whether partial or complete, with proliferation of connective tissue and regeneration of damaged axons to form a neuroma. The neuroma becomes symptomatic depending on the quality of regeneration and is influenced by the extent of fibrosis, vascularity, infection, foreign material, and other local factors. Neuromas with inadequate numbers of large myelinated axons or outer fibrous layers develop hyperpathia. Hyperpathia is a painful syndrome characterized by over-reaction and aftersensation to stimuli.[79] The patient characteristically has extreme sensitivity directly over the neuroma, altered sensibility in at least part of the area supplied by the nerve, and sustained, widely distributed, poorly localized pain.[177]

Percutaneous injection about the painful neuroma should provide local anesthesia. Bupivacaine hydrochloride has a longer duration of anesthesia than does lidocaine hydrochloride. Percutaneous injection of triamcinolone acetonide about the neuroma after a cutaneous block with 2% lidocaine hydrochloride has been reported to relieve the pain symptoms in 50% of patients after one injection and in 80% of patients after multiple injections.[146]

Percussion or massage of painful neuromas has been a clinical procedure in amputees since the First World War. Rubber mallets, mechanical vibrators, or ultrasonic treatments provide the repetitious percussion. Anesthesia may be necessary over a trigger area at the onset of treatment, but later the percussion or massage should be done without local anesthesia.

A peripheral chemical sympathetic block may be performed on the ward (Fig. 28-7, *A* and *B*).[121,122] A 16-gauge needle is inserted just proximal to the "trigger point," and a flexible 18-gauge polyethylene intravenous catheter is inserted through the needle. The needle is removed, leaving the catheter in place. A solution of 0.5 ml of lidocaine hydrochloride, 0.5%, is injected. If the pain is relieved, the catheter is capped and taped in place, allowing exercise activity. Additional periodic injections of lidocaine solution are based on the duration of pain-free activity. The periodic infusion has been continued from a few days up to 2 weeks. If there is more than one "trigger point," separate catheters should be used. This method has not been effective in patients in whom the pain has been untreated for 3 or more months.

A neuroma can be classified as a terminal bulb or a neuroma-in-continuity. A painful partial nerve disruption may benefit from internal neurolysis and graft repair of some fascicular groups.[150] If there is no useful distal sensory or motor function, an end-to-end anastomosis should be performed after removal of the neuroma-in-continuity.[114] Terminal bulb neuromas typically occur in amputation stumps.[110,115] Although many procedures have been reported, present methods include simple resection of the neuroma, capping of the terminal portion with silicone, or transposing the entire neuroma to a new site.[51,161] The most reliable procedure is transfer of the neuroma, attached to the proximal nerve stump, to a new site where compression is unlikely and traction is minimal. The neuroma should be placed in an area of good circulation with a thick subcutaneous layer that is free of scar.[65] Success has been reported in 82% of patients treated with this technique.

Summation of Reflex Sympathetic Overflow. Many clinical syndromes have been described that include burning pain, abnormal vasomotor response, and dystrophy. Classic causalgia may have variants termed *Leriche's posttraumatic pain syndrome* (minor causalgia), *Sudek's atrophy,* or *shoulder–arm–hand syndrome.*[67] Phantom pain is identical to reflex sympathetic dystrophy but adds postural cramping or squeezing. Reflex sympathetic dystrophy may not develop immediately but gradually increases to dominate the clinical picture.

The loss of control of vascular, sudomotor, pilomotor, and muscle tone will result in profound nutritional (trophic) changes. There is atrophy of subcutaneous tissue,

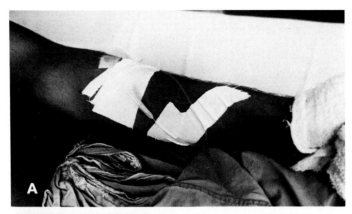

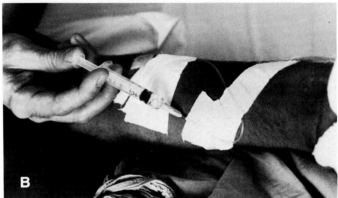

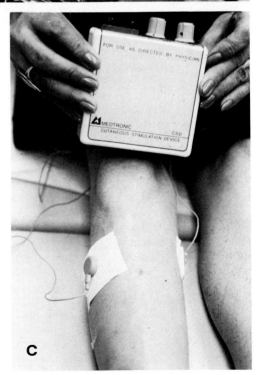

FIG. 28-7. Techniques for relief of chronic pain. (A) Peripheral chemical sympathetic block with the local anesthetic introduced through a flexible 18-gauge polyethylene intravenous catheter. (B) Additional periodic injections are based on the time of pain-free activity. (C) A transcutaneous electrical nerve stimulator. The intensity should be controlled by the patient.

skin, muscle, and bone. In the early stages the residual limb is markedly swollen and warm. There is hyperesthesia to light touch and sensitivity to cold. After 2 to 3 months, there is fibrotic brawny edema. Contractures become fixed owing to lack of active motion. Roentgenograms of the distal bones show patchy osteopenia. A bone scan (technetium-99m etidronate sodium) will be positive before the bone resorption is visible on plain films. Six to nine months after the onset of pain, the extremity becomes pale and cool with either hyperhidrosis or dryness. Pain may dominate, or the extremity may be absolutely rejected by the patient.

In those patients with vasospastic disorders or Raynaud's symptoms associated with pain, it is important to measure digital blood flow. We follow Porter's[130] method: the patient sits quietly for 30 minutes in a warm room with the temperature approximately 24°C. The digital pulp temperature is determined with an electronic telethermometer. The patient's hands are then immersed in an ice water mixture for 20 seconds, and the digital pulp temperature is measured until the temperature returns to the baseline value for 45 minutes. Normal temperature recovery time is 10 minutes, with a range from 5 to 20 minutes. The digital temperature test can be supplemented with arteriography to differentiate arterial spasm from organic obstructive disease. The arteriovenous communications and the precapillary arterioles of the extremities are sympathetically innervated, and a variety of drugs that decrease sympathetic activity should be beneficial for the patient with painful Raynaud's symptoms. A variety of drugs have been proposed for intra-arterial injection, including the alpha receptor–blocking drugs tolazoline hydrochloride (Priscoline) and phenoxybenzamine hydrochloride, the beta-adrenergic receptor–blocking drug propranolol hydrochloride, and the neuronal norepinephrine depletors reserpine, methyldopa, and quanethidine. Griseofulvin has also been used because it has a direct vasodilator action exclusive of the sympathetic innervation. Acevedo and co-workers inject 1.25 mg reserpine in 10 ml normal saline into the brachial artery over 1 minute[1] and report beneficial results both in patients

with no surgical treatment and in those previously submitted to preganglionic sympathectomy. Porter obtained excellent response in patients with Raynaud's symptoms with repeated brachial artery injections of reserpine (0.25 mg) at approximately 2- to 3-week-intervals.[130] Porter also treated 23 patients with oral quanethidine, 10 mg daily, and then increased the level by 10 mg each week until there was hypotension or symptomatic improvement. Two patients could not tolerate quanethidine even at the minimal dose of 10 mg daily because of hypotension and were changed to phenoxybenzamine 10 mg daily. After an average follow-up of 12 months, 19 of the 23 patients had significant reduction in the frequency and severity of Raynaud's attacks.

Chronic small-vessel digital ischemia associated with pain, severe cold intolerance, and occasional finger tip ulceration is often found in frostbite, posttraumatic crush injuries, and chronic vascular disease. A residual group of these patients are not improved with direct injection of intra-arterial vasodilators, tobacco abstinence, and central ganglionic blocking agents. Digital sympathectomy consists of isolating the terminal branches of the sympathetic nerves that travel with the peripheral nerves, dividing these branches, and stripping the adventitia of the digital arteries.[35] Several millimeters of adventitia should be removed from pertinent arteries, such as the common digital vessels in the palm. These patients should be evaluated first with radioisotope imaging of the distal circulation, peripheral pulse volume recordings, cold stress testing, and distal chemical sympathetic blockade of the digital nerves.[175]

Chuinard and associates[20] have reported the use of reserpine administered intravenously to relieve pain in large-vessel spasm and sympathetic overflow. The technique is the same as that used for intravenous regional anesthesia. One milligram of reserpine diluted in 50 ml of normal saline solution is injected, and the tourniquet is released after 15 minutes. The authors reported that 21 of 25 patients obtained pain relief.

Hannington-Kiff introduced the regional intravenous sympathetic block technique with quanethidine.[47] Under tourniquet control, 20 mg of quanethidine in 20 ml of normal saline is injected slowly into a vein. The tourniquet is deflated in 20 minutes.

Most patients do not have localized distal vascular involvement, and early treatment includes chemical central interruption of the abnormal sympathetic reflex, and a cervical sympathetic block should be performed as a diagnostic test as well as a therapeutic procedure. We use 1% lidocaine hydrochloride to produce peripheral warming and loss of sweating, as well as relief of pain. The anterior approach is preferred for the isolated stellate block, using the technique described by Kleinert and associates.[58] A series of four or five blocks should be given on consecutive days; one placebo of normal saline solution given during the series will confirm the value of the sympathetic block. Leffert and colleagues at the Massachusetts General Hospital have developed a technique for continuous sympathetic blockade that employs an indwelling catheter for injection about the stellate ganglion.

Surgery should be performed when the burning pain completely responds to central chemical sympathectomy but requires repeated blocks for the long-term relief of pain. The effectiveness of sympathectomy is not related to interrupting a sensory pathway from the extremity, but to eliminating the sympathetic efferent discharge to the peripheral arteries and sweat glands. Surgical sympathectomy will relieve only burning pain; associated painful neuromata or arthritic pain will not be altered. We favor the transaxillary approach over the posterior transcostal approach, with removal of the sympathetic chain from the fourth thoracic level superior to include the lower half of the stellate ganglion. Horner's syndrome is often not present after the transaxillary approach, which permits removal of only the lower half of the stellate ganglion, but it is more often present following the supraclavicular approach and can be most annoying to the patient. Postoperative sudomotor function tests should demonstrate complete sympathetic denervation of the involved extremity.

Transcutaneous electrical nerve stimulation should be considered for those patients whose pain persists after chemical central sympathetic block (Fig. 28-7, C). Three sites of electrode placement are used: (1) over a large nerve trunk proximal to the pain site, (2) at the periphery of a painful area if the lesion appears primarily cutaneous, or (3) directly over a pain site if proximal nerve trunks are not readily stimulated.[42] The intensity should be varied by the patient because stimuli that are too intense overcome the inhibition mechanism and produce additional pain. Pain relief is complete in fewer than one third of patients,[40] and the best results are obtained when the transcutaneous electrical stimulation is initiated within 3 months of the onset of pain.

In 1967, Sweet and Wall[171] implanted electrodes directly on the median and ulnar nerves of a patient with traumatic hyperpathia. At Duke University, Nashold and associates[88] reported 38 peripheral nerves in 35 patients stimulated with electrodes over periods of 4 to 9 years. There was successful relief of pain in 53% of patients with upper-extremity pain. Direct stimulation of the peripheral nerves is more effective in the upper extremity than in the lower extremity.

Acupuncture is an ancient technique involving the use of point pressure to relieve pain.[78] Traditional teaching identifies 365 to 400 acupuncture points along the 12 meridian channels that contain the Yin–Yang forces controlling the energy of life.[165] Modern laboratory studies imply that acupuncture analgesia is transmitted by the nervous system and requires an intact functional nervous system to be successful.[163] If an intact dynamic interaction (control gate) among large and small afferent neurons is required, then acupuncture should be ineffective in the disrupted nerve, such as a terminal bulb neuroma, and should be more effective in reflex sympathetic summation than in peripheral nociceptive stimulus.

An additional neurophysiologic explanation of acupuncture is that some humeral agent may be responsible, and this may explain the generalized alterations in pain threshold that have been reported in humans. Naloxone, an opiate antagonist, reverses the analgesia of acupuncture-like transcutaneous electrical nerve stimulation, but not that of traditional transcutaneous electrical nerve stimulation.[19,145] Acupuncture-like TENS has a frequency of 2 Hz, while traditional TENS has a frequency of 50 Hz to 100 Hz. Acupuncture or low-frequency transcutaneous electrical nerve stimulation is associated with gradual onset of both analgesia and elevation of pain threshold, which may last for hours after the stimulation has stopped.[149]

Inflammatory or Systemic Pain. Rheumatoid arthritis, diabetes, and other systemic conditions may result in stiffness and pain. This can be a serious complication of appropriate rehabilitation for a peripheral nerve injury. One may use a tourniquet and intravenous regional block with 30 ml of 1% lidocaine hydrochloride and 40 mg of methylprednisolone sodium succinate.[174] During the 20 to 30 minutes of analgesia, one can manipulate stiff joints and stretch contracted web spaces.

Central Pain. Severe pain is frequently cited by patients as the most incapacitating characteristic of their central nervous system postinjury (stroke or trauma) syndrome. Pain of central origin is generally hyperpathic, paroxysmal, and spontaneous—descriptions used by patients including burning, searing, crawling, crushing, and gripping. This monstrous agony may command all of the patient's attention and thus seriously interfere with all attempts for rehabilitation. The pain from nerve root avulsion is severe, having the characteristics of causalgia. Arachnoiditis may follow iophendylate myelography in the presence of nerve root avulsion, with a very poor prognosis. Central pain is not often resolved by any singular treatment program, and a multifaceted approach has the best result.

Beneficial medical treatment has come from the use of anticonvulsants, principally phenytoin sodium (Dilantin) and carbamazepine (Tegretol), or tricyclic antidepressant drugs such as amitriptyline hydrochloride (Elavil) or doxepin hydrochloride (Sinequan).[174] Dilantin may be given up to 300 mg to 500 mg daily in divided or single doses taken with food. Elavil may be given 25 mg at bedtime and at intervals during the day, up to 150 mg maximum daily dosage. Dilantin and Elavil may be used together.[167] Elavil and Sinequan facilitate serotonin utilization in the central nervous system, a process involved in the transmis-

sion of pain-suppressing signals. Benson advises a phenothiazine such as fluphenazine hydrochloride (Prolixin), which potentiates any narcotic, possesses an analgesic property of its own, and depresses the response to peripheral stimuli. The recommended dosage is 1 mg three times daily; this may be increased to a total of 10 mg per day.[177] Tegretol is the more effective drug but is prone to cause toxic symptoms such as nausea, vomiting, or unsteady gait. Because it is more often toxic, Tegretol should be increased slowly from a starting dose to 200 mg a day, gradually increasing up to a maximum of 1500 mg in divided doses. In the event that toxic symptoms occur, the increasing dose should be temporarily postponed, the dosage "plateaued" for a few days at previously tolerated levels, and then gradually increased again until pain is relieved or toxic symptoms appear again.[45] Because of hemopoietic suppression, it is appropriate to follow patients on Tegretol with monthly hemoglobin and white cell count studies. An occasional sedative hypnotic for a particular situation may be effective. Hydroxyzine pamoate (Vistaril) in doses of 25 mg to 50 mg four times a day does not produce dependencies or withdrawal effects. Narcotics are not indicated for chronic pain syndromes.

In addition to medication, electrical stimulation and psychotherapy have been effective in carefully selected cases. A neurostimulator may be inserted into the medial or lateral thalamus for pain that is diffuse, highly agonizing, and of the highest central origin. Electrical stimulation may reduce the pain by 50% or more in approximately half of the patients with stroke, trauma, or quadriplegia.[132]

Cancer Pain. Patients should be considered for an invasive operation when their pain is proven to be intractable to more conservative pain relief techniques. Spinal dorsal sensory root rhizotomy through laminectomy is indicated in patients who have unilateral pain involving the brachial plexus if the involved extremity is functionally useless. Reports of rhizotomy have indicated limited success and disappointing long-term results.[124] Cordotomy is indicated when the pain is diffuse and involves areas innervated by many roots in a functioning upper extremity. Destructive lesions in the thalamus, brain stem, and frontal lobes have been employed for many years. Cingulumotomy is the one technique that is still used for patients in whom anxiety and depression are major factors. None of these procedures provides long-lasting pain relief,[70] and they are most useful in patients who are expected to live no more than 1 year. The return of pain after surgery is related to the increased activity of polysynaptic systems (paleospinothalamic or spinoreticulothalamic) that are widespread in the brain stem and thalamus. These polysynaptic systems are infinitely complex and diffuse and eventually frustrate any ablation procedure.

Personality Dysfunction. Personality dysfunction is a component of all of the pain symptom categories, yet may become the primary stimulus for chronic pain. There are a number of clinical conditions that demonstrate personality dysfunction, such as: (1) clenched fist syndrome, (2) factitious lymphedema, or (3) S-H-A-F-T syndrome.[166] When the patient with a very unstable personality acquires a chronic pain syndrome, the result is often medication abuse and psychosis before treatment can be undertaken. The general physical condition of these patients may have deteriorated owing to inadequate sleep, improper diet and exercise, medication abuse, or other complications. Depression may progress to the point that these patients develop an attitude of hopelessness. Often these patients become narcotic addicts, with these symptoms: (1) increased dose tolerance, (2) psychic craving, (3) withdrawal syndrome, and (4) inability to abstain from narcotics. These patients may be placed on an inpatient status for 48 hours to establish a "drug profile" whereby their medications are accurately recorded by close nursing supervision. Gradual reduction of the narcotics and/or sedative hypnotics by 10% per day permits elimination of the dependency-producing drugs.[45]

Electromyographic biofeedback may be used to relieve tension. To be effective, this modality must be given with maximal therapist support. In the latter part of the 18th century, the German physician Franz Anton Mesmer developed modern techniques for hypnosis. Experiments in hypnosis have shown that subjects can distort perception as well as motor movements, and through hypnosis one can produce partial to total anesthesia. Successful acupuncture and hypnosis both require the cerebral cortex to activate complex conditioned reflexes that raise pain thresholds, remove anxiety and tension, and relieve depression.

When pain dominates the clinical situation, a simple medical impairment classification would be as follows:[157]

100%	P4	Severe enough to prevent all activity
75%	P3	Prevents some activity
50%	P2	Interferes with activity
25%	P1	Annoying
0%	P0	Normal

Functional Activity

The second principle in the treatment program of an established pain syndrome is functional activity. Passive modalities will improve circulation, decrease edema, and prepare the patient for voluntary participation in active modalities such as athletics.

Passive modalities include massage, vibrators, stump wrapping, faradic muscle stimulation, ice packs, hot packs, paraffin packs, microwaves, ultrasound, and inflatable splints with positive–negative pressure. In the apprehensive patient, use of these modalities may have to be preceded by very delicate techniques, such as stroking the skin with a feather. Our desensitization techniques include handling foam rubber chips, jelly beans, navy beans, and rice to provide progressively greater contact pressure. Some passive modalities may be contraindicated, such as the whirlpool bath, because its dependent heat may increase edema. The passive program should maintain joint motion, prevent contracture, and desensitize hyperesthetic areas.

The more important phase is voluntary functional activity. Special care should be directed toward warming-up key areas of circulation such as the rotator cuff muscles in a shoulder–arm–hand syndrome. Total body conditioning is important, and the patient should be ambulatory if possible. Function can be developed with diversional games, athletics, assigned work, and activities of daily living. It is important that the health-care team be compassionate, yet obtain maximal effort from the patient. The best functional activity occurs when the patient returns to his or her usual work. With the continued use of functional activity, patients ultimately "cure" themselves.

REHABILITATION PROCEDURES FOR EXTREMITIES WITH PERIPHERAL NERVE DEFECTS

Reeducation of Motor Function

Many factors influence the final function of an extremity with a peripheral nerve loss. The patient will alter motor patterns to obtain the best available function for each situation. For example, patients with loss of volar pulp sensibility to the index finger will adapt by "divorcing" the index finger and extending it out of the pinch pattern, which will be altered to a chuck between the thumb and the middle or ring finger. The abnormal motor habit will continue, even with return of normal sensibility to the index finger, unless the patient is reeducated first to observe and then to use the index finger deliberately for pinch. Careful instruction must be given to the patient with a nerve-deficient extremity and reinforced at regular intervals. Visual control of motor reeducation prevents abnormal motor habits that lead to distorted sensibility patterns.

In addition to the problem of altered functional patterns, the patient may have a structural block of motor function. For example, in the footdrop problem secondary to peroneal palsy, the patient may be unable to position the foot to use the normal plantar flexor muscles for gait. "Clawed fingers" secondary to ulnar palsy will prevent effective grasp of large objects. The blocked motor pattern is treated best in the lower extremity with orthoses to position the extremity and special shoes to prevent repetitive trauma or infection. Dynamic splints can be used in the upper extremity to place the hand in position to use the remaining functional muscle–tendon units. Splints should be fabricated for each patient and changed whenever there is a change in nerve status. Problems in splinting the

forearm, wrist, and hand are the maintenance of the transverse palmar arch and the thenar web space, adequate lumbrical and thenar stops to maintain the functional position, and excessive tissue tension caused by dynamic traction.

Selected early tendon transfers may be used to support the extremity internally in position to make optimal use of the remaining active muscle–tendon units.[95] These early tendon transfers should be internal splints to enhance function while the patient awaits the return of nerve control and total muscle activity. The muscle–tendon units used for an early transfer for internal support should be synergistic with the muscle–tendon unit to be replaced, such as a wrist flexor for a finger extensor. A synergistic tendon will be able to call on spinal reflex arcs and other feedback mechanisms to enhance proper patterns of motion. Two principles should be followed: (1) Use as few muscle–tendon transfers as possible, since any active muscle–tendon unit used to restore a useful extremity position will weaken the strength and coordination of the residual active function. (2) The tendon transfers used must not cause deformity when nerve recovery is obtained. For example, it would be foolish to transfer the flexor carpi ulnaris, the palmaris longus, and the flexor carpi radialis to produce thumb and finger extension in a case of radial palsy and then have spontaneous recovery of the radial nerve; active wrist flexion would be impossible.

Selected early tendon transfers to improve coordination and stimulate sensibility are best used in the upper extremity.[101] The pronator teres transferred to the extensor carpi radialis brevis will produce active wrist extension and allow intrinsic muscle finger extension in radial palsy (Fig. 28-8). Transfer of the flexor digitorum superficialis of the ring finger to the abductor pollicis brevis and extensor mechanism of the thumb will produce active opposition in distal (low) median palsy (Fig. 28-9). Dynamic internal splinting in distal (low) ulnar palsy can be done by splitting the flexor digitorum superficialis of the middle finger into three slips; the radial half of the tendon is directed across the adductor pollicis and beneath the index flexor tendons into the

FIG. 28-8. Transfer of the pronator teres tendon (*PT*) to the tendon of the extensor carpi radialis brevis muscle (*ECRB*) to obtain active wrist extension in radial palsy. (*BR*, Brachioradial muscle; *ECRL*, extensor carpi radialis longus tendon) (After Omer, G.E., Jr.: Evaluation and reconstruction of the forearm and hand after acute traumatic peripheral nerve injuries. J. Bone Joint Surg. 50A:1454, 1968)

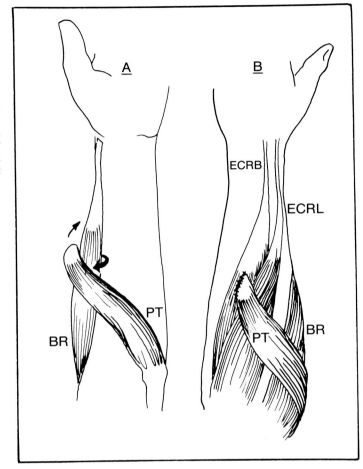

FIG. 28-9. Transfer of the extensor indicis proprius tendon (*EIP*) around the wrist, with the pisiform used as a pulley point, to the tendon insertion of the abductor pollicis brevis muscle (*APB*) to obtain active abduction (opposition function) of the thumb in median palsy. (*EDC*, extensor digitorum communis; *EPL*, extensor pollicis longus muscle) (After Omer, G.E., Jr.: Tendon transfers for reconstruction of the forearm and hand following peripheral nerve injuries. In Omer, G.E., and Spinner, M. [eds.]: Management of Peripheral Nerve Problems. Philadelphia, W.B. Saunders, 1980)

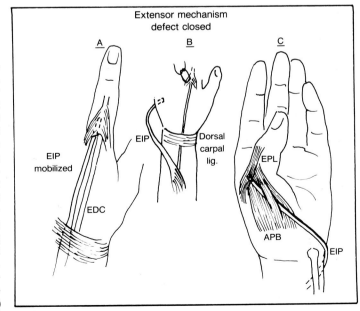

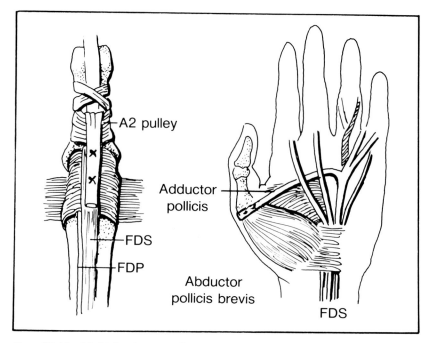

FIG. 28-10. Multiple-slip transfer of the tendon of the flexor digitorum superficialis of the ring finger (*FDS*) to the abductor tubercle of the first metacarpal and to the A2 portion of the flexor sheath of the ring and little fingers to prevent clawing and to increase thumb–index pinch in low ulnar palsy. (*FDP*, flexor digitorum profundus) (After Omer, G.E., Jr.: Ulnar nerve palsy. In Green, D.P. [ed.]: Operative Hand Surgery. New York, Churchill Livingstone, 1982. Reprinted by permission of the artist, Elizabeth Roselius)

tendon of the abductor pollicis brevis for improved pinch, and the two slips of the ulnar half of the tendon are directed volar to the intermetacarpal ligament into the central slip of the extensor mechanism insertion of the middle phalanx for correction of clawing.[91,96]

An alternate insertion for the two ulnar slips is the A2 pulley to provide additional power for grasp (Fig. 28-10).[116,118] Only one tendon is used to support the extremity in position internally for optimal use of the remaining active muscle–tendon units. Isolated tendon transfers in the lower extremity usually cannot support the limb against gravity and the force of residual active muscle–tendon units.

Motor reeducation includes careful visual supervision of all extremity activity and periodic monitoring of habit patterns to avoid abnormal function. External splints or early tendon transfers as internal splints may be indicated to position the extremity to obtain optimal use of the active muscles while one awaits the return of nerve functional control of inactive muscles. Daily use of the remaining muscle–tendon units will stimulate sensation and improve coordination.

Tendon Transfers

The objective of tendon transfers is to achieve a limited but balanced functional performance by means of redistributing assets rather than creating new motor and sensory units.

Patient motivation must be factored into the decision about reconstructive procedures. The patient must have developed the cerebral imprint for the function to be reconstructed, be able to comprehend what is to be done, and be prepared to accept the postoperative discipline. Homeostasis of the involved extremity must be established prior to reconstructive surgery. There should be stable skeletal alignment with adequate passive motion across joints. Soft tissues should be free of scar contracture and have adequate circulation.

After complete evaluation of the patient, all possible surgical solutions should be considered. Nerve suture is the basic approach to a nerve palsy, but tendon transfers or joint arthrodeses may be acceptable alternatives. Inasmuch as each patient has special problems, reconstruction must be individualized.

The motor muscles selected must be more than strong enough because they will need to pull free of the healing scar and in the process will usually lose one grade of muscle strength on Lovett's clinical scale of strength. The presurgical action of the selected motor muscle should be synergistic with the anticipated new action, or at least retrainable by conscious control. Paralyzed muscles that have regained function following nerve suture usually lack the individualized control and strength desirable for successful transfer.[90]

The motor muscle should be carefully mobilized to protect the neurovascular bundle, which usually enters the proximal third of the muscle. The direction of pull for the transferred tendon should be in as near a straight line as possible. The transferred tendon should not cross raw bone. Muscle–tendon units that must move through fascial planes, such as an interosseous membrane, should have a large opening with the muscle placed in the fascial window; the exterior muscle fibers will "freeze," but the interior muscle fibers will retain motion. If the tendon is placed in the fascial window, it will bind fast, and motion will be lost.[95] The angle of approach between the transferred tendon and its insertion should be small. A pulley is required for a large angle of approach. When the angle is larger than 45°, the result is actually a loss of force secondary to friction. The more distal to the axis of joint motion that a tendon is anchored, the more force the muscle can exert across the joint, but also the more excursion required of the tendon to provide

a normal range of motion for the joint. Suture material for tendon fixation should be monofilament steel or synthetic material likely to cause minimal tissue reaction.

The tension of a tendon transfer is judged best while the extremity is placed in the position it will assume when the transferred tendon contracts. For extensor transfers, the resting tension should be strong enough to hold the extremity passively in functional position against gravity. Flexor tendons often cross more than one joint and should be fixed at greater than normal tension against gravity. It is appropriate to attach the transferred tendon under greater than normal tension. This brings perception of the new muscle motion more readily into consciousness, because stretch reflexes and other feedback mechanisms are stimulated when opposing muscles restore the neutral position of the extremity.[123]

For an extremity to function, stability must be provided by the contraction of balanced and coordinated muscles in tendon transfers. Synergistic muscles are preferred for the correction of motor dysfunction because they are quickly used and provide coordination. Instability of a proximal joint will result in dysfunction of more-distal joints. Stability for weight bearing is of great importance in the lower extremity, while precise mobility is essential in the upper extremity.

Axillary Palsy. Loss of axillary (circumflex) nerve function may occur as an isolated injury, for example, a shoulder dislocation, but is usually associated with an injury to other nerves of the brachial plexus. The axillary nerve motors the deltoid muscle, and neuropathy is recognized by the loss of humeral abduction. There is associated weakness of external rotation of the humerus, which is severe if the suprascapular nerve is also injured.

Goldner[41] releases the trapezius muscle from the scapula and clavicle and elongates the muscle with fascia lata to the greater tuberosity of the humerus and the shoulder cuff. The humerus is held at 90° from the body and 10° flexion. This position is maintained for 6 weeks. In addition, the biceps brevis muscle is detached from the coracoid and transferred to the acromion. The pectoralis major is elongated with fascia and transferred to the anterolateral shoulder cuff. The long head of the triceps muscle is detached from the scapula and transferred to the acromion. The latissmus dorsi and teres major are transferred from the medial aspect of the humeral shaft to the anterolateral aspect of the humeral shaft to provide external rotation.

Because the results of shoulder arthrodesis are predictable, it remains a technique of choice. The position of shoulder fusion is very important. Rowe[134] recommends 15° to 20° of humeral abduction from the scapular vertebral border, 25° to 30° of humeral forward flexion from the plane of the scapula, and 40° to 50° of humeral internal rotation. Leffert[68] notes that patients with pectoral transfers for elbow flexion should have as much as 30° of humeral abduction to improve the line of pull of the transfer. Patients with a fixed or anticipated flexion contracture of the elbow should have less internal rotation and forward flexion for the humerus. Unless there is good scapular control, function will be inadequate.

Musculocutaneous Palsy.   Isolated loss of musculocutaneous nerve function results in weakness of elbow flexion. If the flexor-pronator muscles are intact, the patient may evidence weak elbow flexion. All reconstructive procedures to restore elbow flexion require shoulder stability or control.

Transfer of the latissimus dorsi is our technique of choice.[139] While the neurovascular pedicle is preserved, the muscle is mobilized and fixed to the coracoid process of the scapula and to the biceps tendon at the elbow. If the shoulder is arthrodesed, only the thoracic attachment of the muscle need be changed to the biceps tendon. The paralyzed biceps muscle may require resection to provide room for the transferred latissimus dorsi. Fixation of the transfer is commenced at its distal end when the entire muscle is mobilized.

The pectoralis major may be used to replace a paralyzed biceps muscle.[18] The pectoralis muscle is changed to a two-joint muscle with attachment to the coracoid process and the distal biceps tendon and radial tubercle.

After tendon transfers, the elbow should be maintained in 90° to 100° of flexion for 6 weeks before guarded exercises are begun. It is then kept in a sling between exercise periods for 3 additional months to encourage a permanent flexion contracture of 20° to 30°. This will provide mechanical advantage when flexion is initiated.

Radial Palsy.   There is loss of gross grip strength related to radial nerve loss because wrist extension is necessary for stabilization and full excursion of the digital flexors. When the base of the thumb is unstable owing to paralysis of the abductor pollicis longus muscle, precision pinch is weak. Furthermore, the digits cannot be extended to surround objects. Inasmuch as all these functions must be restored, active flexion of the wrist should also be retained.[172]

Wrist extension is obtained by transferring the insertion of the pronator teres muscle to the extensor carpi radialis brevis tendon. The pronator teres should be released from the radius and passed subcutaneously over the brachioradialis and extensor carpi radialis longus to its new insertion.

Stability of the proximal thumb is obtained by splitting the flexor carpi radialis tendon at its insertion and transferring the radial half of the split tendon into the abductor pollicis longus tendon. An alternative measure is to remove the extensor pollicis brevis tendon from the first dorsal compartment, bringing it across the volar side of the distal forearm and suturing it side-to-side to the palmaris longus tendon.

One of the oldest transfers for radial palsy is the flexor carpi ulnaris to the extensor digitorum communis.[107] The flexor carpi ulnaris should be released to the proximal third of the forearm and directed subcutaneously around the ulna and superficial to the tendons of the extensor digitorum communis, so that from the little finger to the index finger the transferred tendon is attached in a progressively more distal line of sutures, yet the suture line is proximal to the dorsal retinaculum. A suture is placed both proximally and distally at the site of attachment to each slip of the extensor digitorum communis. Tension on the extensor digitorum communis tendons is increased across the wrist from the little finger to the index finger so that the fingers are held in functional extension against gravity. After the tension is set for the extensor digitorum communis, the extensor pollicis longus tendon is added as the final insertion of the flexor carpi ulnaris transfer. This transfer often results in a radial deviation of the hand. After a few months, the patient can usually extend one finger or all fingers at will, by way of selective flexor power coupled with mass extension.

Finger extension can also be obtained by transfer of the flexor digitorum superficialis tendons of the long and ring fingers.[8] The tendons are placed through large windows in the interosseous membrane just proximal to the pronator quadratus. It is important to release the tourniquet before passing the tendons through the windows to prevent damage to the central vessels volar to the interosseous membrane window; bare tendons will stick, with resulting loss of motion. The superficialis of the long finger is attached to the extensor digitorum communis tendons. The superficialis of the ring finger is attached to the extensor pollicis longus and the extensor indicis proprius. A passive fist is formed with the wrist held in 45° of extension, and the tendons are sutured at normal tension.

Postoperatively, the forearm is maintained in 30° pronation, the wrist in 40° to 45° extension, the metacarpophalangeal joints in 0° extension, and the interphalangeal joints in 15° flexion. Six weeks postsurgery, rigid immobilization is discontinued, and a spring-action cock-up splint is positioned to obtain independent action for wrist and finger extension.

Median Palsy. Synchronism, the quality of grace and fluidity, involves simultaneous flexion and extension of joints.[172] The deletion of flexor digitorum sublimis function lessens the degree of flexor domination over the combined extensor–intrinsic complex and the synchronous action of normal flexion for the distal and middle phalanges of the fingers. This cannot be reconstructed. In a high (proximal) palsy, flexion and opposition of the thumb and flexion of the long and index fingers can be reconstructed. There is also weakness of wrist flexion and forearm pronation.

Thumb flexion is obtained by adequate release of the brachioradialis muscle from the radius and by transferring its tendon to the flexor pollicis longus. This transfer converts the brachioradialis from a one-joint to a multiple-joint muscle, with a different tension for grasp when the elbow is moved from extension to flexion.

Thumb opposition does not require power as much as adequate motion; thus, transfer of the extensor indicis proprius is our technique of choice. The extensor indicis proprius is transferred subcutaneously around the ulnar border of the wrist, with the pisiform used as a pulley, then across the palm and metacarpophalangeal joint into the abductor pollicis brevis and extensor pollicis longus.[14,116] The extensor digiti minimi transfer has the same advantages as the extensor indicis proprius transfer.[138] A wrist extensor prolonged with a free tendon graft can be used with a pisiform pulley.[49] The advantage of using extensor muscle–tendon transfers is that new strength is introduced into the power train for flexion, whereas flexor muscle–tendon transfers represent a rearrangement of strength already decreased by the median nerve palsy.

Flexion of the long and index fingers is obtained by suturing the tendons of the index and long flexor digitorum profundus side-to-side with the ring and little tendons of the flexor digitorum profundus. The ulnar-innervated portion of the muscle will then pull the tendons of the median-innervated portion of the muscle through a functional range of motion. A double line of sutures is important to prevent "whipsawing" of the tendons with a power grip. The profundus tendons to the index and long fingers can be tenodesed across the distal interphalangeal joint to increase the mechanical advantage at the proximal interphalangeal joint.[90]

After operation, a circular plaster cast is applied to hold the thumb in full opposition with flexion of the interphalangeal joint. The dorsal immobilization extends through the distal interphalangeal joints and holds the elbow at a right angle to protect the brachioradialis transfer. After 3 weeks, the plaster cast is shortened for elbow motion. Guarded motion of the wrist is instituted approximately 5 weeks after reconstruction.

Ulnar Palsy. The hand with ulnar palsy has a profound weakness. There is loss of (1) flexion of the proximal phalanges of the fingers (if the extrinsic muscle function is intact, the ring and little fingers will claw), (2) synchronism for metacarpophalangeal and interphalangeal joint flexion, and the fingers curl into the palm; objects are pushed away instead of grasped; (3) powerful key pinch for the thumb and weakness of thumb–index tip pinch; and (4) active lateral mobility of the fingers in extension (inability to adduct the extended little finger to the extended ring finger). In a high (proximal) ulnar palsy there is also inability to flex the distal phalanges of the ring and little fingers and partial loss of wrist flexion. The impairment for power grip is greater than the loss of power for precise grip. Ulnar palsy results in a hand with so many functional problems that there is no accepted program for reconstruction.[116,118]

The residual strength for palmar adduction of the thumb (key pinch) is diminished as much as 75% to 85% in ulnar palsy.[72] The brachioradialis muscle or a wrist extensor can be extended with a free tendon graft that passes volar between the third and fourth metacarpal and inserts on the abductor tubercle of the thumb.[9] Hamlin and Littler[46] recommended a long or ring flexor digitorum superficialis transfer in low (distal) palsy. The superficialis tendon is detached in the finger, tunneled across the volar surface of the adductor pollicis, and sutured to the adductor pollicis tendon at its insertion.

The abducted little finger is corrected by transfer of the ulnar half of the tendon of the extensor digiti minimi.[4] The ulnar half of the tendon is inserted into the flexor tendon sheath just distal to the A1 pulley if the little finger is clawed. If the little finger is not clawed, the tendon slip is passed beneath the deep transverse metacarpal ligament and sutured into the phalangeal attachment of the radial collateral ligament of the metacarpophalangeal joint of the little finger. This procedure also improves the stability of the transverse metacarpal arch.

We have utilized a long or ring flexor digitorum superficialis tendon to improve synchronism for metacarpophalangeal and interphalangeal joint flexion and key pinch for the thumb, and for the flattened unstable metacarpal arch. The ring superficialis tendon is used only if the flexor digitorum profundus is not paralyzed. This procedure does not increase power for gross grip because it does not increase the number of muscle–tendon units in the power train.[112]

The best method to increase power for gross grip is to add an extensor muscle–tendon unit to the power train for flexion of the proximal phalanx. Burkhalter and Strait[15] use a free tendon graft, palmaris longus or plantaris, to prolong the extensor carpi radialis longus muscle–tendon unit. The free graft is split into two slips, which are passed through the intermetacarpal spaces between the long–ring and ring–little fingers. Each tendon slip is passed volar to the deep transverse metacarpal ligament and attached to the proximal phalanx. If there is a flexion contracture of the wrist, the flexor carpi radialis is detached and used as the motor muscle.[133]

Thumb–index tip pinch is improved when the metacarpophalangeal joint of the thumb is arthrodesed.[90,107] Neviaser and associates[89] recommend the transfer of a slip of the abductor pollicis longus elongated with a free tendon graft, palmaris longus or plantaris, into the tendon of the first dorsal interosseous. The extensor pollicis brevis has been transferred to the tendon of the first dorsal interosseous.[12]

Common Peroneal Palsy. The common peroneal division of the sciatic nerve is injured more often than the tibial division. The common peroneal division is relatively fixed at both the sciatic notch and the neck of the fibula and is subject to more internal stretching by high-velocity injuries. The common peroneal division also has less connective-tissue volume than the tibial division, and its axons are more vulnerable to mechanical injury.[155]

Common peroneal palsy results in loss of dorsiflexion of the foot with associated loss of eversion of the foot. If there is a fixed equinus deformity, it must be corrected. Serial short leg casts, applied with the knee flexed and the foot in maximum dorsiflexion, are usually successful. Plantar fascia stripping, tendocalcaneus lengthening, or posterior capsulotomy may be necessary.

Reconstruction of the equinovarus deformity usually includes a bony stabilization as well as tendon transfers. A triple arthrodesis, combined with a posterior bone block, is more effective than an isolated bone block or a Lambrinudi arthrodesis. Even with stabilization of the foot, the ankle will dislocate without tendon transfers or an orthosis.[108] In addition, unless the influence of the posterior tibialis muscle is removed, varus deformity will occur at the ankle joint.

Anterior transfer of the tibialis posterior tendon can be either through the interosseous membrane or around the medial side of the tibia.[23] If the transfer is through the interosseous membrane, a large hole should be made. The tibialis posterior muscle–tendon unit is passed through the generous opening until the muscle belly is wedged between the tibia and the fibula; the tendon alone in the opening will fibrose to the interosseous membrane, with loss of motion. The transfer is protected for at least 6 months by an orthosis that maintains a dorsiflexed position. Full active dorsiflexion is rarely restored by this transfer alone; the extremity requires reeducation. In the chronic problem, it may take months to revise compensatory movements, such as lifting and flexing the leg to step forward.

Tibial Palsy. The foot with tibial palsy has a marked deformity. The tendocalcaneus becomes elongated, the calcaneus is rotated into dorsiflexion by the intrinsic muscles, and the plantar fascia is contracted.

In the skeletally mature foot, the initial surgery is a foot stabilization procedure with a plantar fasciotomy if there is a cavus deformity. The Hoke procedure[53] is more effective than a standard triple arthrodesis. The foot stabilization should displace the foot as far posteriorly as possible to lengthen the bony lever arm and lessen the power required to plantar flex the foot.

The tibialis anterior muscle is the only isolated tendon with sufficient strength to produce active plantar flexion when the triceps sura is paralyzed.[50,173] The tibialis anterior transfer should be done through the interosseous membrane. The transfer should be protected for at least 6 months by an orthosis with a reverse calcaneal stop.

If the great toe has persistent clawing, the interphalangeal joint of the toe is arthrodesed, and the extensor hallucis longus tendon is transferred to the flexor hallucis longus tendon.[108]

Femoral Palsy. The muscles innervated by the femoral nerve are not critical for an upright stature or locomotion on an even surface. Quadriceps loss is most evident while climbing stairs or an inclined plane.

Correction of quadriceps paralysis may be done by anterior transfer of the biceps femoris muscle through a lateral approach.[50,108] The tensor fascia and the intermuscular septum are excised for 10 cm to allow free excursion of the biceps femoris tendon and to prevent flexion contracture of the knee. The biceps femoris tendon is anchored to the anterior surface of the patella. The extremity is immobilized for 12 weeks, and the knee is protected until phase conversion has been achieved.

Reeducation of Sensibility

Attempts have been made to examine sensibility in quantitative terms, but the response is subjective and not objective. For example, there is no correlation between sensory nerve conduction velocity and two-point discrimination distance after the surgical repair of peripheral nerves.[2] Sensibility for light touch pressure usually returns in the young patient after nerve suture, while sensory nerve conduction velocity does not recover. There is a pattern to each patient's sensibility, and the pattern can be observed by variations in functional ability. For example, the volar finger pulp two-point discrimination distance in nondiabetic blind persons who have been trained to read Braille has been recorded at 1.5 mm, in contrast to the normal two-point discrimination distance of 3 mm to 5 mm.[48]

Dellon[27,28] has demonstrated the graded or progressive recovery of sensibility in the hand after peripheral nerve injury. An evaluation series demonstrated the usual order for recovery: (1) pain perception (pinprick), (2) low-frequency flutter (tuning fork at 30 cps), (3) moving touch (finger stroke), (4) constant touch (two-point discrimination distance), and (5) high-frequency vibration (tuning fork at 256 cps). The patient's ability to interpret the testing stimulus correctly improved with experience.

A sensibility education program should assist the patient to (1) exploit the full potential of any sensory return and (2) recognize and interpret an altered profile of sensory impulses. Curtis and Dellon[24] have developed a sensibility reeducation program for the upper extremity that is based on stimulation of the appropriate group-A-beta axons for the perception of touch. A patient can enter this reeducation program at any time after perception of 30 cps flutter and after moving-touch stimuli are regained in a previously numb area. During the early phase of the program the patient strokes the anesthetic area with a finger from the other (normal) hand or with the eraser end of a pencil, and then firmly touches the anesthetic area with a normal finger or the eraser end of a pencil. This early phase aids in the perception of moving touch and constant touch. The late phase of the program consists of holding, moving, and discriminating the size difference between square and hexagonal nuts and small or large cap nuts. Each exercise is performed with the patient first observing the stimulus and focusing his attention on how it "feels" as he is watching the exercise. Then, with his eyes closed, he must concentrate on associating whatever (altered) profile of impulses he is receiving centrally with what he knows is happening at his fingertip. He must learn what this altered perception means and reassociate the new sensation with the old action. The exercise time should be 10 to 15 minutes per session, with the exercises performed in a quiet room with the patient rested and prepared to concentrate. The exercise should be repeated three to four times each day. When perception of moving touch and constant touch has progressed to the volar pulp tip of the involved finger, a quantitative study of functional sensibility is begun, using the Weber two-point discrimination test. We use this study only once each day. In addition, a tuning fork with high-frequency vibration (256 cps) can determine daily the position of sensibility for vibratory touch. If the vibratory touch is perceived more distally than is constant touch, the reeducation program is not meeting its potential because constant touch should return before vibratory touch. Therefore, the patient should increase his exercise periods and work with greater concentration. Dellon[29] recorded the recovery of normal two-point discrimination distance within 2 to 6 weeks of entering this program.

Patients with sciatic nerve loss often submit the sole of the foot to excessive pressure, with resulting blisters and ulcers. Brand[11] has utilized special microcapsules that break and release dye on a variety of pressures. A group of microcapsules comprising a range of shell (pressure) strength and containing different-colored dyes are impregnated into a thin (0.050-inch) sheet of polyurethane foam that becomes the sole of a sock. Use of the sock for several hours will identify areas of excessive pressure and aid in the fitting of special shoes to avoid localized excessive pressure. A second technique is the use of electronic pressure-sensitive discs[11] that identify the first time excessive pressure is applied to any given area of the foot. We recommend that these patients walk barefoot in their home; this moving-touch stimulus is a useful reeducation technique when there is dysesthesia secondary to a qualitative change in sensibility.[10]

Reconstruction of Sensibility

Tactile gnosis is very important as a "sensory feedback" for precise function,[84] but voluntary motor activity is an essential component of tactile gnosis.[119] Tendon transfers should be done before sensory reconstruction is undertaken, because abnormal patterns of motor activity enhance the distortion of sensibility that accompanies a peripheral nerve deficit.

Island Pedicle Flaps. Neurovascular cutaneous island pedical flaps for the reconstruction of peripheral nerve defects have been used primarily to restore median nerve sensation.[97] If the ulnar nerve is to be the donor, only the common digital nerve between the ring and little fingers is available, since sensibility along the ulnar aspect of the ltitle finger is essential in total median nerve loss. The usual technique is to transfer a cutaneous island, with its neurovascular pedicle, from the ulnar aspect of the ring finger to the ulnar-volar aspect of the thumb pulp.[104,112] A large island should be dissected from the ulnar-volar aspect of the ring finger. The superficial vascular arch may have to be interrupted and the radial portion freed to swing with the cutaneous island. A double island along the ulnar border of the ring finger, across the distal edge of the palm and along the radial border of the little finger, has been transferred to the thumb–index web space.[96,104,119] A radial-innervated cross-finger flap from the index to the thumb pulp will provide a critical area with sensation.[37]

Omer[104] reported his findings in 15 patients with high (proximal) median nerve loss who were followed with evaluation tests of sensibility. There was a gradual reduction from normal sensation to merely protective sensation. This loss of sensibility was related to the associated motor loss for the radial side of the hand; without adequate motion and power for precise prehension, sensibility for precise prehension is lost.

In the patient with a neurotrophic ulcer of the heel related to tibial palsy, a cutaneous island can be constructed from the plantar skin overlying the phalanges and the metatarsophalangeal joint of the big toe.[57] The cutaneous island, with its neurovascular pedicle, is then rotated into the heel defect. The big toe is filleted through the metatarsophalangeal joint, and the dorsal skin provides the necessary flap to cover the donor defect. These cutaneous islands remain well vascularized, and sensation is appreciated. The entire dorsum of the foot has been elevated as a flap and has been used to resurface defects in both malleoli and the tendocalcaneal area.[75,76]

There is disorientation of sensitivity in all neurovascular island pedicle flaps.[100] For several months after transplant the patient recognizes stimulation in the island as originating from the original donor site. Later, sensation is interpreted in both the recipient and donor sites. In an emergency, such as flame burn, the patient loses the ability of interpretation and first moves the original donor site. There is also a high incidence of cold intolerance, and paresthesia is common at the margin of these flaps.

Microsurgical free flaps should include donor skin that approximates the quality of the recipient skin, with a sensory pattern that is predictable for precise sensibility.

Morrison and colleagues[87] have described a modification of the toe-to-thumb transfer that is a free neurovascular wraparound flap from the big toe. The trimmed nail and nail bed are included to prevent pulp swivel. The thumb skeleton is sculptured from the iliac crest and grafted to the proximal thumb. The dorsalis pedis and long saphenous vein are left long and are anastomosed to the radial artery and the cephalic vein at the level of the snuffbox of the wrist. The deep peroneal nerve is joined to the superficial radial nerve, and the plantar digital nerves are joined to the thumb digital nerves.

Free vascularized nerve grafts have been developed to increase the survival of a long or thick nerve graft.[158] These techniques may be used when the graft bed is ischemic or scarred, when the free transfer of a thick nerve is desired, or when there is a great gap in the nerve required for distal function. There are a great number of new techniques involving composite free transfer of nerves.

Combined Nerve Palsies

Low median–ulnar palsy is the most common combined nerve palsy. The complete loss of palmar sensation and intrinsic muscles produces a severe claw hand. Reconstruction of the thumb is extremely important. Adduction contracture must be avoided. The patient flexes the wrist to obtain greater finger extension, but with prolonged use this results in a fixed flexion contracture of the wrist. Following individualized transfers, the residual loss of sensibility should be a greater functional problem than should basic patterns for motion (Table 28-8).

High Median–Ulnar Palsy. The hand will rarely be used for precision activity following high median–ulnar palsy, and it is best to direct surgical endeavors toward a key pinch and a simple grasp. Sensation can be transferred to the radial-volar aspect of the hand, but this will not provide precise sensibility.[96,107] The skeleton of the index finger is removed distal to the proximal third of the second metacarpal. The insensitive distal index skin is discarded. The fillet index finger flap is then fitted into an additional volar defect created in the insensitive palmar skin. This broad-based finger flap is innervated by the superficial radial nerve and provides protective sensibility for key pinch (Table 28-9).

High Radial–Ulnar Palsy. Patients with high radial–ulnar palsy retain radial-volar sensibility, and reconstruction is a useful investment to improve function (Table 28-10).

Table 28-8. Surgical Correction of Combined Low (Distal) Median–Ulnar Palsy

NEEDED FUNCTION	PREFERRED TRANSFER
Thumb adduction (key pinch)	Brachioradialis with free tendon graft between the third and fourth metacarpals to the abductor tubercle of the first metacarpal
Thumb abduction (opposition)	Extensor indicis proprius to the tendons of the abductor pollicis brevis and extensor pollicis longus
Thumb–index tip pinch	Abductor pollicis longus slip with free tendon graft to the tendon of the first dorsal interosseous; arthrodesis, MCP joint of the thumb
Restoration of the metacarpal (palmar) transverse arch and adduction for the little finger	Extensor digiti minimi to the deep transverse metacarpal ligament (the extensor digitorum communis to the little finger must be active)
Power flexion of the proximal phalanx; integration of MCP and IP motion	Extensor carpi radialis longus to all four fingers with a four-tailed free graft and flexor sheath (A2 pulley) insertion; or use the flexor carpi radialis if the wrist is in flexion contracture
Volar sensibility	Free neurovascular cutaneous island flap

MCP, metacarpophalangeal; IP, interphalangeal

Table 28-9. Surgical Correction of Combined High (Proximal) Median–Ulnar Palsy

NEEDED FUNCTION	PREFERRED TRANSFER
Thumb adduction (key pinch)	Extensor carpi radialis longus with free tendon graft between the third and fourth metacarpals to the abductor tubercle of the first metacarpal
Thumb flexion (position)	Extensor indicis proprius to flexor pollicis longus
Thumb abduction (opposition)	Extensor pollicis brevis rerouted around the tendon of the flexor carpi radialis (the thumb MCP joint is fused)
Thumb–long (index) pinch (tip pinch)	Arthrodesis, MCP joint of thumb; abductor pollicis longus slip with a free tendon graft to the tendon of the first dorsal interosseous tendon
Finger flexion (gross grip)	Brachioradialis to the tendons of the flexor digitorum profundus; tenodesis of the DIP joint, three ulnar fingers
Integration of MCP and IP motion for finger flexion	Tenodesis of all three digits with a free tendon graft from the dorsal apparatus to the deep transverse metacarpal ligament
Restoration of the metacarpal (palmar) transverse arch and adduction for the little finger	Extensor digiti minimi volar to the deep transverse metacarpal ligament into the proximal phalanx or dorsal apparatus (the extensor digitorum communis to the little finger must be active)
Wrist flexion	Extensor carpi ulnaris to the insertion of the flexor carpi ulnaris
Radial-volar sensibility	Superficial radial innervated index fillet flap to the palm

MCP, metacarpophalangeal; DIP, distal interphalangeal; IP, interphalangeal

Table 28-10. Surgical Correction of Combined High (Proximal) Radial–Ulnar Palsy

NEEDED FUNCTION	PREFERRED TRANSFER
Thumb adduction (key pinch)	Half of the flexor digitorum superficialis (middle) as a split transfer to the abductor tubercle of the first metacarpal
Clawed fingers	Half of the flexor digitorum superficialis (middle) in two slips as a flexor sheath (A2) insertion to the ring and little fingers; later, if indicated: arthrodesis, PIP joint, if the patient is unable to extend the ring and little fingers fully
Proximal thumb stability and wrist flexion (radial)	Flexor carpi radialis (yoke insertion) to the abductor pollicis longus and extensor pollicis brevis
Wrist flexion (ulnar)	Palmaris longus to the insertion of the flexor carpi ulnaris
Thumb–index tip pinch	Arthrodesis, MCP joint of the thumb
Wrist extension	Pronator teres (yoke insertion) to the extensor carpi radialis longus and extensor carpi ulnaris
Finger and thumb extension	Flexor digitorum superficialis (index and long) through the interosseous membrane to the extensor digitorum communis and extensor pollicis longus
Finger flexion (ring and little only)	Tenodesis of the flexor digitorum profundus index and long (active motors) to the ring and little flexor digitorum profundus; tenodesis, DIP joint, ring and little fingers, using the flexor digitorum profundus
Volar sensibility (ring and little fingers)	Free neurovascular cutaneous island flap

PIP, proximal interphalangeal; MCP, metacarpophalangeal; DIP, distal interphalangeal

The loss of balanced power across the proximal interphalangeal joints may ultimately result in deformity. An arthrodesis can be done after the onset of deformity at this level.

High Radial–Median Palsy. Reconstruction in high radial–median palsy will give a hand that functions only slightly more effectively than a prosthesis. Carpal arthrodesis is indicated because all wrist motors are lost except the flexor carpi ulnaris. Finger flexion is obtained by tenodesis of the flexor digitorum profundus. Finger and thumb extension is obtained by transfer of the flexor carpi ulnaris. Tenodesis of the flexor pollicis longus and the abductor pollicis longus provides minimal stability for the thumb. The transfer of intrinsic muscles for thumb abduction should not be attempted until the wrist is stabilized and there is good adduction power.

Surgeons who undertake reconstruction of extremities with peripheral nerve loss should be experienced enough to select the appropriate procedures for the individual patient. To gain adequate strength for a specific function, a new muscle–tendon unit is usually added to the power train rather than redistributing muscles that have related function. Precise sensibility requires precise motion, which is very difficult to achieve following peripheral nerve loss.

REFERENCES

1. Acevedo, A., Reginato, A.J., and Schnell, A.M.: Effect of intraarterial reserpine in patients suffering from Raynaud's phenomenon. J. Cardiovasc. Surg., 19:77, 1978.
2. Almquist, E., and Eeg-Olofsson, O.: Sensory-nerve-conduction velocity and two-point discrimination in sutured nerves. J. Bone Joint Surg., 52A:791, 1970.
3. Bjorkesten, G.: Suture of war injuries to peripheral nerves: Clinical studies of results. Acta. Chir. Scand. [Suppl. 119], 95:1, 1947.
4. Blacker, G.J., Lister, G.D., and Kleinert, H.E.: The abducted little finger in low ulnar palsy. J. Hand Surg., 1:190, 1976.
5. Blair, W.F., Greene, E.R., and Omer, G.E., Jr.: A

method for the calculation of blood flow in human digital arteries. J. Hand Surg., 6:90, 1981.

6. Bonica, J.J.: Current status of pain therapy. In The Interagency Committee on New Therapies for Pain and Discomfort: Report to the White House, pp. 111–114, May 1979. U.S. Department of Health, Education, and Welfare, Public Health Service, National Institutes of Health. Seymour Perry, M.D., Chairman.

7. Bora, W.F., Pleasure, D.E., and Didizian, N.A.: A study of nerve regeneration and neuroma formation after nerve suture by various techniques. J. Hand Surg., 1:138, 1976.

8. Boyes, J.H.: Tendon transfers for radial palsy. Bull. Hosp. Jt. Dis., 15:97, 1954.

9. Boyes, J.H.: Bunnell's Surgery of the Hand, 4th ed., pp. 12–17, 514. Philadelphia, J.B. Lippincott, 1964.

10. Brand, P.W.: Management of sensory loss in the extremities. In Omer, G.E., Jr., and Spinner, M. (eds.): Management of Peripheral Nerve Problems, pp. 862–872. Philadelphia, W.B. Saunders, 1980.

11. Brand, P.W., and Ebner, J.D.: Pressure sensitive devices for denervated hands and feet, a preliminary communication. J. Bone Joint Surg., 51A: 109, 1969

12. Bruner, J.M.: Tendon transfer to restore abduction of the index finger using the extensor pollicis brevis. Plast. Reconstr. Surg., 3:197, 1948.

13. Brushart, T., Tarlov, E.C., Mesulam, M.-M.: Specificity of muscle reinnervation after epineurial and individual fascicular suture of the rat sciatic nerve. J. Hand Surg., 8:248, 1983.

14. Burkhalter, W.E., Christensen, R.C., and Brown, P.: Extensor indicis proprius opponensplasty. J. Bone Joint Surg., 55A:725, 1973.

15. Burkhalter, W.E., and Strait, J.L.: Metacarpophalangeal flexor replacement for intrinsic paralysis. J. Bone Joint Surg., 55A:1667, 1973.

16. Cabaud, H.E., Rodkey, W.G., McCarroll, H.R., Jr. et al.: Epineural and perineural fascicular nerve repairs: A critical comparison. J. Hand Surg., 1:131, 1976.

17. Cabaud, H.E., Rodkey, W.G., and Nemeth, T.J.: Progressive ultrastructural changes after peripheral nerve transection and repair. J. Hand Surg., 7:353, 1982.

18. Carroll, R.E., and Kleinmann, W.B.: Pectoralis major transplantation to restore elbow flexion to the paralytic limb. J. Hand Surg., 4:501, 1979.

19. Chapman, C.R., and Benedetti, C.: Analgesia following transcutaneous electrical stimulation and its partial reversal by a narcotic antagonist. Life Sci., 21:1645, 1977.

20. Chuinard, R.G., Dabezies, E.J., Gould, J.S. et al.: Intravenous reserpine for treatment of reflex sympathetic dystrophy. ASSH proceedings. J. Hand Surg., 5:289, 1980.

21. Clawson, D.K., Bonica, J.J., and Fordyce, W.E.: Management of chronic pain problems. Instr. Course Lect., 21:8, 1972.

22. Clawson, D.K., and Seddon, H.J.: The later consequences of sciatic nerve injury. J. Bone Joint Surg., 42B:213, 1960.

23. Cozen, L.: Management of foot drop in adults after permanent peroneal nerve loss. Clin. Orthop., 67:151, 1969.

24. Curtis, R.M., and Dellon, A.L.: Sensory re-education after peripheral nerve injury. In Omer, G.E., Jr., and Spinner, M. (eds.): Management of Peripheral Nerve Problems, pp. 769–778. Philadephia, W.B. Saunders, 1980.

25. Delagi, E.F.: Electrodiagnosis in peripheral nerve lesions. In Omer, G.E., Jr., and Spinner, M. (eds): Management of Peripheral Nerve Problems, pp. 30–43. Philadelphia, W.B. Saunders, 1980.

26. Dellon, A.L.: The moving two-point discrimination test: Clinical evaluation of the quickly adapting fiber/receptor system. J. Hand Surg., 3:474, 1978.

27. Dellon, A.L.: Evaluation of Sensibility and Reeducation of Sensation in the Hand. Baltimore, Williams and Wilkins, 1981, 263 pp.

28. Dellon, A.L.: Reeducation of sensation in the hand following nerve suture. Clin. Orthop., 163: 75, 1982.

29. Dellon, A.L., Curtis, R.M., and Edgerton, M.T.: Re-education of sensation in the hand after nerve injury and repair. Plast. Reconstr. Surg., 53:297, 1974.

30. Dellon, A.L., and Munger, B.L.: Correlation of histology and sensibility after nerve repair. J. Hand Surg., 8:871, 1983.

31. Ducker, T.B.: Metabolic consequences of axotomy and regrowth. In Jewett, D.L., and McCarroll, H.R., Jr. (eds.): Nerve Repair and Regeneration: Its Clinical and Experimental Basis, pp. 99–104. St. Louis, C.V. Mosby, 1980.

32. Ducker, T.B., and Hayes, G.J.: Experimental improvements in the use of Silastic cuff for peripheral nerve repair. J. Neurosurg., 28:582, 1968.

33. Edshage, S.: Peripheral nerve suture, a technique for improved intraneural topography, evaluation of some suture materials. Acta. Chir. Scand. [Suppl. 331], 1964.

34. Engel, J., Ganel, A., Melamed, R. et al.: Choline acetyltransferase for differentiation between human motor and sensory nerve fibers. Ann. Plast. Surg., 4:376, 1979.

35. Flatt, A.E.: Digital artery sympathectomy. J. Hand Surg., 5:550, 1980.

36. Foerster, O.: Handbuch der Neurologie, Part 2. Berlin, Julius Springer, 1929.

37. Gaul, J.S.: Radial-innervated cross finger flap from index to provide sensory pulp to injured thumb. J. Bone Joint Surg., 51A:1257, 1969.

38. Gelberman, R.H., Hergenroeder, P.T., Hargens, A.R. et al.: The carpal tunnel syndrome: A study of carpal tunnel pressure. J. Bone Joint Surg., 63A:380, 1981.

39. Geldard, F.A.: The Human Senses, 2nd ed. New York, John Wiley & Sons, 1972.

40. Goldner, J.L.: Pain: Extremities and spine—evaluation and differential diagnosis. In Omer, G.E., Jr., and Spinner, M. (eds.): Management of Peripheral Nerve Problems, pp. 119–175. Philadelphia, W.B. Saunders, 1980.

41. Goldner, J.L.: Muscle–tendon transfers for partial paralysis of the shoulder girdle. In Evarts, C.Mc. (ed.): Surgery of the Musculoskeletal System, Vol. 3, pp. 167–183. New York, Churchill Livingstone, 1983.

42. Goldner, J.L., Nashold, B.S., and Hendrix, P.C.: Peripheral nerve electrical stimulation. Clin. Orthop., 163:33, 1982.

43. Grabb, W.C.: Management of nerve injuries in the forearm and hand. Orthop. Clin. North Am., 1:419, 1970.

44. Grabb, W.C., Bement, S.L., Koepke, G.H., and Green, R.A.: Comparison of methods of peripheral nerve suturing in monkeys. Plast. Reconstr. Surg., 46:31, 1970.

45. Halpern, L.M.: Analgesic drugs in the management of pain. Arch. Surg., 112:861, 1977.

46. Hamlin, C., and Littler, J.W.: Restoration of power pinch. J. Hand Surg., 5:396, 1980.

47. Hannington-Kiff, J.G.: Intravenous regional sympathetic block with quanethidine. Lancet, 1:1019, 1974.

48. Heinrichs, R.W., and Moorehouse, J.A.: Touch perception in blind diabetic subjects in relation to the reading of Braille type. N. Engl. J. Med., 280:72, 1969.

49. Henderson, E.D.: Transfer of wrist extensors and brachioradialis to restore opposition of the thumb. J. Bone Joint Surg., 44A:513, 1962.

50. Herndon, C.H.: Tendon transplantation at the knee and foot. Instr. Course Lect., 18:145, 1961.

51. Herndon, J.H., Eaton, R.G., and Littler, J.W.: Management of painful neuromas in the hand. J. Bone Joint Surg., 58A:369, 1976.

52. Highet, W.B., and Sanders, F.K.: Effects of stretching nerves after suture. Br. J. Surg., 30:355, 1943.

53. Hoke, M.: An operation for stabilizing posterior feet. J. Orthop. Surg., 3:494, 1921.

54. Jabaley, M.E., Burns, J.E., Orcutt, B.S., and Bryant, W.M.: Comparison of histologic and functional recovery after peripheral nerve repair. J. Hand Surg., 1:119, 1976.

55. Jabaley, M.E., Wallace, W.H., and Heckler, F.R.: Internal topography of major nerves of the forearm and hand: A current review. J. Hand Surg., 5:1, 1980.

56. Juhlin, L., and Shelley, W.B.: A stain for sweat pores. Nature, 213:408, 1967.

57. Kaplan, I.: Neurovascular island flap in the treatment of trophic ulceration of the heel. Br. J. Plast. Surg., 22:143, 1969.

58. Kleinert, H.E., Cole, N.M., and Wayne, L.: Posttraumatic sympathetic dystrophy. Orthop. Clin. North Am., 4:917, 1973.

59. Kline, D.G.: Early evaluation of peripheral nerve lesions in continuity with a note on nerve recording. Am. Surg., 34:77, 1968.

60. Kline, D.G.: Evaluation of the neuroma in continuity. In Omer, G.E., Jr., and Spinner, M. (eds.): Management of Peripheral Nerve Problems, pp. 450–461. Philadelphia, W.B. Saunders, 1980.

61. Kline, D.G., and Hackett, E.R.: Reappraisal of timing for exploration of civilian peripheral nerve injuries. Surgery, 78:54, 1975.

62. Koob, S.: Thermography in hand surgery. Hand, 4:64, 1972.

63. Kori, S.H., Foley, K.M., and Posner, J.B.: Brachial plexus lesions in patients with cancer: 100 cases. Neurology, 31:45, 1981.

64. Kutz, J.E., Shealy, G., and Lubbers, L.: Interfas-cicular nerve repair. Orthop. Clin. North Am., 12:277, 1981.

65. Laborde, K.J., Kalisman, M., and Tsi, T.-M.: Results of surgical treatment of painful neuromas of the hand. J. Hand Surg., 7:190, 1982.

66. Langley, J.N.: Observations on degenerated and on regenerating muscle. J. Physiol., 51:377, 1917.

67. Lankford, L.L.: Reflex sympathetic dystrophy. In Omer, G.E., Jr., and Spinner, M. (eds.): Management of Peripheral Nerve Problems, pp. 216–244. Philadelphia, W.B. Saunders, 1980.

68. Leffert, R.D.: Reconstruction of the shoulder and elbow following brachial plexus injury. In Omer, G.E., Jr., and Spinner, M. (eds.): Management of Peripheral Nerve Problems, pp. 805–816. Philadelphia, W.B. Saunders, 1980.

69. Liu, C.T., Benda, C.E., and Lewey, F.H.: Tensile strength of human nerves—experimental, physiologic, and histologic study. Arch. Neurol. Psychiatr., 59:332, 1948.

70. Long, D.M.: Relief of cancer pain by surgical and nerve blocking procedures. J.A.M.A., 244:2759, 1980.

71. Lynn, R., and Eysenck, H.J.: Tolerance for pain, extraversion and neuroticism. Percept. Mot. Skills, 12:161, 1961.

72. Mannerfelt, L.: Studies on the hand in ulnar nerve paralysis: A clinical–experimental investigation in normal and anomalous innervation. Acta Orthop. Scand. [Suppl. 87], 1966.

73. Marcus, N.A., Blair, W.F., Shuck, J.M., and Omer, G.E., Jr.: Low-velocity gunshot wounds to the extremities. J. Trauma, 20:1061, 1980.

74. Mayer, D.J., and Hayes, R.: Stimulation-produced analgesia: Development of tolerance and cross-tolerance to morphine. Science, 188:941, 1975.

75. McCraw, J.B., and Furlow, L.T., Jr.: The dorsalis pedis arterial flap. In Grabb, W.C., and Myers, M.D. (eds.): Skin Flaps, pp. 517–524. Boston, Little, Brown & Co., 1975.

76. McCraw, J.B., and Furlow, L.T., Jr.: The dorsalis pedis arterialized flap: A clinical study. Plast. Reconstr. Surg., 55:177, 1975.

77. McFarlane, R.M., and Mayer, J.R.: Digital nerve grafts with the lateral antebrachial cutaneous nerve. J. Hand Surg., 1:169, 1976.

78. Melzack, R.: Myofascial trigger points: Relation to acupuncture and mechanisms of pain. Arch. Phys. Med. Rehabil., 62:114, 1981.

79. Mersky, H.: Pain terms: A list with definitions and notes on usage. International Association for the Study of Pain (IASP), Subcommittee on Taxonomy. Pain, 6:249, 1979.

80. Millesi, H.: Fascicular peripheral nerve repair using cutaneous nerve grafts. In Daniller, A.I., and Strauch, B. (eds.): Educational Foundation of the American Society of Plastic and Reconstructive Surgeons Symposium on Microsurgery, Vol. 14, pp. 154–160. St. Louis, C.V. Mosby, 1976.

81. Millesi, H.: Interfascicular nerve grafting. Orthop. Clin. North Am., 12:287, 1981.

82. Moberg, E.: Objective methods for determining the functional value of sensibility in the hand. J. Bone Joint Surg., 40B:454, 1958.

83. Moberg, E.: Relation of touch and deep sensation

to hand reconstruction. Am. J. Surg., 109:353, 1965.

84. Moberg, E.: Reconstructive hand surgery in tetraplegia, stroke, and cerebral palsy: Some basic concepts in physiology and neurology. J. Hand Surg., 1:29, 1976.

85. Moberg, E.: Sensibility in reconstructive limb surgery. In: Fredericks, S., and Brody, G.S. (eds.): Educational Foundation of the American Society of Plastic and Reconstructive Surgeons Symposium on the Neurologic Aspects of Plastic Surgery, Vol. 17, pp. 30–35. St. Louis, C.V. Mosby, 1978.

86. Moneim, M.S.: Interfascicular nerve grafting. Clin. Orthop., 163:65, 1982.

87. Morrison, W.A., O'Brien, B.McC., and MacLeod, A.M.: Thumb reconstruction with a free neurovascular wrap-around flap from the great toe. J. Hand Surg., 5:575, 1980.

88. Nashold, B.S., Goldner, J.L., Mullen, J.B., and Bright, D.S.: Long-term pain control by direct peripheral-nerve stimulation. J. Bone Joint Surg., 64A:1, 1982.

89. Neviaser, R.J., Wilson, J.N., and Gardner, M.M.: Abductor pollicis longus transfer for replacement of the first dorsal interosseous. J. Hand Surg., 5: 53, 1980.

90. Omer, G.E., Jr.: Evaluation and reconstruction of the forearm and hand after acute traumatic peripheral nerve injuries. J. Bone Joint Surg., 50A: 1454, 1968.

91. Omer, G.E., Jr.: Restoring power grip in ulnar palsy. J. Bone Joint Surg., 53A:814, 1971.

92. Omer, G.E., Jr.: Assessment of peripheral nerve injuries. In Cramer, L.M., and Chase, R.A. (eds.): Educational Foundation of the American Society of Plastic and Reconstructive Surgeons Symposium on the Hand, Vol. 3, pp. 1–11. St. Louis, C.V. Mosby, 1971.

93. Omer, G.E., Jr.: Injuries to nerves of the upper extremity. J. Bone Joint Surg., 56A:1615, 1974.

94. Omer, G.E., Jr.: Sensation and sensibility in the upper extremity. Clin. Orthop., 104:30, 1974.

95. Omer, G.E., Jr.: The technique and timing of tendon transfers. Orthop. Clin. North Am., 5: 243, 1974.

96. Omer, G.E., Jr.: Tendon transfers in combined nerve lesions. Orthop. Clin. North Am., 5:377, 1974.

97. Omer, G.E., Jr.: Neurovascular island flaps and fillet of finger. In Grabb, W.C., and Myers, M.B. (eds.): Skin Flaps, pp. 371–480. Boston, Little, Brown, & Co., 1975.

98. Omer, G.E., Jr.: Nerve injuries: Primary vs. secondary suture vs. nerve grafts. Dallas Med. J., 62:401, 1976.

99. Omer, G.E., Jr.: Management of pain syndromes in the upper extremity. In Hunter, J.M., Schneider, L.H., Mackin, E.J. and Bell, J.A. (eds.): Rehabilitation of the Hand, pp. 341–349. St. Louis, C.V. Mosby, 1978.

100. Omer, G.E., Jr.: Neurovascular sensory island transplants. In Fredericks, S., and Brody, G.S. (eds.): Educational Foundation of the American Society of Plastic and Reconstructive Surgery Symposium on the Neurological Aspects of Plastic

Surgery, Vol. 17, pp. 52–60. St. Louis, C.V. Mosby, 1978.

101. Omer, G.E., Jr.: Tendon transfers as early internal splints following peripheral nerve injury in the upper extremity. In Hunter, J.M., Schneider, L.H., Mackin, E.J., and Bell, J.A. (eds.): Rehabilitation of the Hand, pp. 292–296. St. Louis, C.V. Mosby, 1978.

102. Omer, G.E., Jr.: Management of the painful extremity. In Ahstrom, J.P. (ed.): Current Practice in Orthopaedic Surgery, Vol. 8, pp. 86–98. St. Louis, C.V. Mosby, 1979.

103. Omer, G.E., Jr.: The evaluation of clinical results following peripheral nerve suture. In Omer, G.E., Jr., and Spinner, M. (eds.): Management of Peripheral Nerve Problems, pp. 431–442. Philadelphia, W.B. Saunders, 1980.

104. Omer, G.E., Jr.: Neurovascular cutaneous island pedicle flaps. In Omer, G.E., Jr., and Spinner, M. (eds.): Management of Peripheral Nerve Problems, pp. 779–790. Philadelphia, W.B. Saunders, 1980.

105. Omer, G.E., Jr.: The results of untreated traumatic injuries. In Omer, G.E., Jr., and Spinner, M. (eds.): Management of Peripheral Nerve Problems, pp. 502–506. Philadelphia, W.B. Saunders, 1980.

106. Omer, G.E., Jr.: Sensory evaluation by the pick-up test. In Jewett, D.L., and McCarroll, H.R., Jr. (eds.): Nerve Repair and Regeneration: Its Clinical and Experimental Basis, pp. 250–251. St. Louis, C.V. Mosby, 1980.

107. Omer, G.E., Jr.: Tendon transfers for reconstruction of the forearm and hand following peripheral nerve injuries. In Omer, G.E., Jr., and Spinner, M. (eds.): Management of Peripheral Nerve Problems, pp. 817–846. Philadelphia, W.B. Saunders, 1980.

108. Omer, G.E., Jr.: Tendon transfers as reconstructive procedures in the leg and foot. In Omer, G.E., Jr., and Spinner, M. (eds.): Management of Peripheral Nerve Problems, pp. 873–880. Philadelphia, W.B. Saunders, 1980.

109. Omer, G.E., Jr.: Methods of assessment of injury and recovery of peripheral nerves. Surg. Clin. North Am., 61:303, 1981.

110. Omer, G.E., Jr.: Nerve, neuroma, and pain problems related to upper limb amputations. Orthop. Clin. North Am., 12:751, 1981.

111. Omer, G.E., Jr.: Physical diagnosis of peripheral nerve injuries. Orthop. Clin. North Am., 12:207, 1981.

112. Omer, G.E., Jr.: Reconstructive procedures for extremities with peripheral nerve defects. Clin. Orthop., 163:80, 1982.

113. Omer, G.E., Jr.: Results of untreated peripheral nerve injuries. Clin. Orthop., 163:15, 1982.

114. Omer, G.E., Jr.: The neuroma-in-continuity. In Strickland, J.W., and Steichen, J.B. (eds.): Difficult Problems in Hand Surgery, pp. 369–373. St. Louis, C.V. Mosby, 1982.

115. Omer, G.E., Jr.: The painful neuroma. In Strickland, J.W., and Steichen, J.B. (eds.): Difficult Problems in Hand Surgery, pp. 319–323. St. Louis, C.V. Mosby, 1982.

116. Omer, G.E., Jr.: Ulnar nerve palsy. In Green, D.P. (ed.): Operative Hand Surgery, pp. 1061–1080. New York, Churchill Livingstone, 1982.

117. Omer, G.E., Jr.: Report of the committee for evaluation of the clinical result in peripheral nerve injury. II. J. Hand Surg., 8:754, 1983.

118. Omer, G.E., Jr.: The palsied hand. In Evarts, C.McC. (ed.): Surgery of the Musculoskeletal System, Vol. 2, pp. 407–438. New York, Churchill Livingstone, 1983.

119. Omer, G.E., Jr., Day, D.J., Ratliff, H., and Lambert, P.: Neurovascular cutaneous island pedicles for deficient median nerve sensibility. J. Bone Joint Surg., 52A:1181, 1970.

120. Omer, G.E., Jr., and Spinner, M.: Peripheral nerve testing and suture techniques. Instr. Course Lect., 24:122, 1975.

121. Omer, G.E., Jr., and Thomas, S.R.: Treatment of causalgia: Review of cases at Brooke General Hospital. Tex. Med., 67:93, 1971.

122. Omer, G.E., Jr., and Thomas, S.R.: The management of chronic pain syndromes in the upper extremity. Clin. Orthop., 104:37, 1974.

123. Omer, G.E., Jr., and Vogel, J.A.: Determination of physiological length of a reconstructed muscle–tendon unit through muscle stimulation. J. Bone Joint Surg., 47A:304, 1965.

124. Onofrio, B.M., and Campa, H.K.: Evaluation of rhizotomy: Review of 12 years experience. J. Neurosurg., 36:751, 1972.

125. Orgel, M.G.: Experimental studies with clinical application to peripheral nerve injury: A review of the past decade. Clin. Orthop., 163:98, 1982.

126. Orgel, M.G., O'Brien, W.J., and Murray, H.M.: Pulsing electromagnetic field therapy in nerve regeneration. Plast. Reconstr. Surg., 73:173, 1984.

127. O'Riain, S.: New and simple test of nerve function in the hand. Br. Med. J., 3:615, 1973.

128. Paradies, L.H., and Gregory, C.F.: The early treatment of close-range shotgun wounds to the extremities. J. Bone Joint Surg., 48A:425, 1966.

129. Poppen, N.K.: Clinical evaluation of the von Frey and two-point discrimination tests—correlation with a dynamic test of sensibility. In Jewett, D.L., and McCarroll, H.R., Jr. (eds.): Nerve Repair and Regeneration: Its Clinical and Experimental Basis, pp. 421–434. St. Louis, C.V. Mosby, 1980.

130. Porter, J.M., Snider, R.L., Bardana, E.J. et al.: The diagnosis and treatment of Raynaud's phenomenon. Surgery, 77:11, 1975.

131. Rakolta, G.G., and Omer, G.E., Jr.: Combat-sustained femoral nerve injuries. Surg. Gynecol. Obstet., 128:813, 1969.

132. Ray, C.D.: Spinal epidural electrical stimulation for pain control: Practical details and results. Appl. Neurophysiol., 44:194, 1981.

133. Riordan, D.C.: Tendon transfers for nerve paralysis of the hand and wrist. Curr. Prac. Orthop. Surg., 2:17, 1964.

134. Rowe, C.R.: Reevaluation of the position of the arm in arthrodesis of the shoulder in the adult. J. Bone Joint Surg., 56A:913, 1974.

135. Rubin, D.: Myofascial trigger point syndromes: An approach to management. Arch. Phys. Med. Rehabil., 62:107, 1981.

136. Rydevik, B., Lundborg, G.H., and Bagge, U.: Effects of graded compression on intraneural blood flow. J. Hand Surg., 6:3, 1981.

137. Schachtel, H.J.: Pain and religion. Cancer Bull., 33:84, 1981.

138. Schneider, L.H.: Opponensplasty using the extensor digiti minimi. J. Bone Joint Surg., 51A:1297, 1969.

139. Schottstaedt, E.R., Larsen, L.L., and Bost, F.C.: Complete muscle transposition. J. Bone Joint Surg., 37A:897, 1955.

140. Seddon, H.J.: Three types of nerve injury. Brain, 66:237, 1943.

141. Seddon, H.J.: Nerve lesions complicating certain closed bone injuries. J.A.M.A., 135:691, 1947.

142. Seddon, H.J.: The use of autogenous grafts for the repair of large gaps in peripheral nerves. Br. J. Surg., 35:151, 1947.

143. Seddon, H.J. (ed.): Peripheral Nerve Injuries. Medical Research Council, Special Series, No. 282. London, Her Majesty's Stationery Office, 1954.

144. Seddon, H.J.: Surgical Disorders of the Peripheral Nerves, 2nd ed. Edinburgh, Churchill Livingstone, 1975.

145. Sjolund, B., Terenius, L., and Eriksson, M.: Increased cerebrospinal fluid levels of endorphins after electro-acupuncture. Acta Physiol. Scand., 100:382, 1977.

146. Smith, J.R., and Gomez, N.H.: Local injection therapy of neuromata of the hand with triamcinolone acetonide, a preliminary study of twenty-two patients. J. Bone Joint Surg., 52A:71, 1970.

147. Smith, J.W.: Factors influencing nerve repair. I. Blood supply of peripheral nerves. II. Collateral circulation of peripheral nerves. Arch. Surg., 93: a, 335, b, 433, 1966.

148. Snyder, C.C.: Epineurial repair. Orthop. Clin. North Am., 12:267, 1981.

149. Snyder, S.H.: Opiate receptors and internal opiates. Sci. Am., 236 (March):44, 1977.

150. Spinner, M.: Injuries to the Major Branches of Peripheral Nerves of the Forearm, 2nd ed., pp. 54–63. Philadelphia, W.B. Saunders, 1978.

151. Sternbach, R.A.: Modern concepts of pain. In Dalessio, D.J. (ed.): Wolff's Headache and Other Head Pain, 4th ed. New York, Oxford University Press, 1980.

152. Sternbach, R.A., Wolf, S.R., Murphy, R.W., and Akeson, W.H.: Traits of pain patients: The low-back "loser." Psychosomatics, 14:226, 1973.

153. Strange, F.G.St.C.: An operation for nerve pedicle grafting. Br. J. Surg., 34:423, 1947.

154. Sunderland, S.: The intraneural topography of the radial, median, and ulnar nerves. Brain, 68:243, 1945.

155. Sunderland, S.: Nerves and Nerve Injuries, 2nd ed. Edinburgh, Churchill Livingstone, 1978.

156. Swanson, A.B.: Evaluation of impairment of function in the hand. Surg. Clin. North Am., 44:925, 1964.

157. Swanson, A.B., Goran-Hagert, C., Swanson, G.deG.: Evaluation of impairment in hand func-

tion. In Hunter, J.M., Schneider, L.H., Mackin, E.J., and Bell, J.A. (eds.): Rehabilitation of the Hand, pp. 31–69. St. Louis, C.V. Mosby, 1978.

158. Taylor, G.I.: Nerve grafting with simultaneous microvascular reconstruction. Clin. Orthop., 133: 56, 1978.

159. Terzis, J.K., Dykes, R.W., and Hakstian, R.W.: Electrophysiological recordings in peripheral nerve surgery: A review. J. Hand Surg., 1:52, 1976.

160. Terzis, J., and Williams, H.B.: Functional evaluation of free nerve grafts. In Daniller, A.I., and Strauch, B. (eds.): Educational Foundation of the American Society of Plastic and Reconstructive Surgeons Symposium on Microsurgery, Vol. 14, pp. 140–146. St. Louis, C.V. Mosby, 1976.

161. Tupper, J.W., and Booth, D.M.: Treatment of painful neuromas of sensory nerves in the hand: A comparison of traditional and newer methods. J. Hand Surg., 1:144, 1976.

162. Tursky, B., and O'Connell, D.: Reliability and interjudgment predictability of subjective judgments of electrocutaneous stimulation. Psychophysiology, 9:290, 1972.

163. Ulett, G.H.: Acupuncture treatments for pain relief. J.A.M.A., 245:768, 1981.

164. Urbaniak, J.R.: Fascicular nerve suture. Clin. Orthop., 163:57, 1982.

165. Veith, I.: Acupuncture in traditional Chinese medicine. Calif. Med., 118:70, 1973.

166. Wallace, P.F., and Fitzmorris, C.S., Jr.: The S-H-A-F-T syndrome in the upper extremity. J. Hand Surg., 3:492, 1978.

167. Ward, N.G., Bloom, V.L., and Friedel, R.D.: The effectiveness of tricyclic antidepressants in the treatment of co-existing pain and depression. Pain, 7:331, 1979.

168. Weeks, P.M., and Wray, R.C.: Management of Acute Hand Injuries: A Biological Approach, 2nd ed. St. Louis, C.V. Mosby, 1978.

169. Weinstein, S.: Tactile sensitivity of the phalanges. Percept. Mot. Skills, 14:351, 1962.

170. Werner, J.L., and Omer, G.E., Jr.: Procedures evaluating cutaneous pressure sensation of the hand. Am. J. Occup. Ther., 24:347, 1970.

171. White, J.C., and Sweet, W.H.: Pain and the Neurosurgeon: A Forty-year Experience. Springfield, Ill.: Charles C. Thomas, 1969.

172. White, W.L.: Restoration of function and balance of the wrist and hand by tendon transfers. Surg. Clin. North. Am., 40:427, 1960.

173. Wiesseman, G.J.: Tendon transfers for peripheral nerve injuries of the lower extremity. Orthop. Clin. North Am., 12:459, 1981.

174. Wiley, A.M., Poplawski, Z.B., and Murray, J.: Post-traumatic dystrophy of the hand. Orthop. Rev., 6:59, 1977.

175. Wilgis, E.F.S.: Evaluation and treatment of chronic digital ischemia. Ann. Surg., 193:693, 1981.

176. Wilgis, E.F.S.: Techniques for diagnosis of peripheral nerve loss. Clin. Orthop., 163:8, 1982.

177. Wilson, R.L.: Management of pain following peripheral nerve injuries. Orthop. Clin. North Am., 12:343, 1981.

178. Wynn Parry, C.B.: Rehabilitation of the Hand, 3rd ed. London, Butterworths, 1973.

29 Complications of Multiple Trauma

Sigvard T. Hansen, Jr.

The terms *multiply injured* and *severely injured patient* have been defined in various ways.[15] The following synthesis of current definitions has been used in this chapter: The multiply injured or severely injured patient is one in whom two or more systems have been affected by injuries or in whom severe or multiple fractures are a potential cause of secondary organ failure. Injuries are severe enough to be life threatening if timely and appropriate intervention is not provided.

The ultimate complication in the multiply injured patient is, of course, death, but the spectrum of complications short of death is extremely broad. Most, if not all, of these complications are mentioned individually in Dr. David Murray's comprehensive introductory chapter to this text (see Chap. 1). It is my belief that rapid intervention and proper timing of treatment are of the essence in managing the multiply injured patient. In this chapter, therefore, the complex of complications, both actual and potential, will be examined chronologically from the time of injury.

EMERGENCY RESPONSE AND PATIENT RESUSCITATION

An initial cause of complications can be a significant delay in resuscitation of the victim because of delayed reporting of the accident or the delayed arrival of well-trained ambulance or paramedic teams. Thus, the first requirement for avoiding major complications is an efficient system for reporting accidents and for informing citizens of the proper procedure for notifying authorities of an accident and beginning resuscitation of the victim. The reporting system might consist of a simple, uniform telephone number such as 911; the report should be received instantly by a well-trained operator who obtains accurate information on the patient's status and location and immediately transmits this information to trained emergency medical technicians (EMTs). Citizen training should include a knowledge of cardiopulmonary resuscitation (CPR) and basic first aid. The local government or community must take responsibility for this citizen training and for developing and maintaining adequate reporting and response systems.

The emergency response system must consist of two levels of support: (1) ambulances or aid cars manned by attendants trained as EMTs who arrive quickly at the scene of the accident and (2) paramedics with further training who arrive shortly thereafter. The EMTs and the first-response vehicles should be associated with local fire departments, which are located in such a way as to provide a 2- to 5-minute response to any area of the community. The more highly trained paramedics could be based at hospitals and could arrive at the scene of the accident within 10 to 15 minutes to back up the EMTs.

Quick response and adequate resuscitation are extremely important for avoiding complications. Respiratory obstruction can cause death in minutes, and rapid reversal of this condition by a CPR-trained citizen, an EMT, or a paramedic on site can save not only the patient's life but also his brain function. Injuries causing major bleeding and hypovolemic shock create fewer and less severe complications when the shock is reversed within 30 minutes. In fact, the severity of general complications is proportionally related to the time in excess of 30 minutes required for reversal of shock.[14]

Rib fractures can occur if CPR with manual sternal compression is used. Fractured ribs pose a potential threat to the lungs from pneumothorax and to the liver from major hemorrhage. These complications are very dangerous but are treatable if recognized early.

AIRWAY AND FLUID RESTORATION AND MAINTENANCE

Since establishing and maintaining a free airway is the first priority in treating the multiply injured patient, it is also the first area in which complications may arise. Occasionally, intubation or tracheotomy is necessary; either procedure must be performed accurately, by well-trained personnel, to avoid damaging the airway. By working with anesthesiologists during their training, paramedics become expert at performing an intubation, and this procedure is generally safe when carried out by them.

To reverse the serious consequences of prolonged shock, fluid replacement should begin at the site of the accident whenever blood loss is suspected or confirmed. At times, fluid replacement should be started even before the patient is evacuated from the accident site, but it is certainly the next priority after establishment and maintenance of respiration and an airway.

In addition to administration of fluids, blood may be drawn on site and taken by police car or other emergency vehicle to the local blood bank. The blood can be typed within 10 minutes, and thus appropriate supplies can be available in the emergency room of the trauma center by the time the patient has been resuscitated, extricated, stabilized, and transported to the hospital. The request for blood supplies is normally made by the back-up physician at the trauma center.

Fluid administration procedures are not usually complicated when peripheral sites on the body are used to gain access to the veins. In the event that access to the subclavian vein is attempted, care must be taken to avoid vein wall injury and significant intrathoracic bleeding. In our institution, the subclavian site is used infrequently for administering intravenous fluids because of the potential for these serious complications. Peripheral veins, or even external jugular veins, are used more commonly. On rare occasions septic phlebitis can occur even with careful handling of these central veins if sterile technique is not used, or if catheters are not exceptionally well taken care of and are not changed frequently. Septic phlebitis can be a virtually fatal complication if it reaches the central venous system.

Evacuation of the patient from the site of the accident is the next period during which complications can be created. The evacuation process can be extremely complex if the patient is at the bottom of a crevasse or an elevator shaft, or is trapped in a crushed vehicle. Care must be taken that torches, saws, ropes, hooks, or other equipment do not further injure the patient. Moreover, the ever-present possibility of spine instability dictates that in many of these patients spinal alignment and traction must be maintained while the patient is moved. So-called log rolling must be done until the patient has been transported to the trauma center or emergency room and appropriate films have been obtained. Long-bone fractures, especially of the femur and tibia, must also be aligned and the limb kept in traction during all moves to prevent further damage to the soft tissues. Spine boards, leg traction devices, and other equipment for skeletal stabilization should be part of the EMT's armamentarium. Otherwise, a satisfactory substitute must be devised on site. In our experience, paraplegia or quadriplegia is rarely caused, or even aggravated, by moving an injured patient. The possibility is always present, however, and the consequences of such an event are devastating.

DIAGNOSIS AND EMERGENCY TREATMENT

Once the multiply injured patient is brought to the emergency room of the local hospital or to the trauma center, the potential is created for numerous further complications during attempts to diagnose and treat his or her injuries. Because many accidents occur at night, when the regular hospital staff is not present, potentially dangerous diagnostic and therapeutic procedures may have to be carried out quickly by personnel with less than ideal experience in performing them.

Instability of the spine must always be

considered a possibility until ruled out, and thus the care taken in moving the patient at the site of the accident must be continued in the emergency room. At the same time, maintenance of the airway and circulation must be continued while diagnostic and therapeutic procedures are initiated. Potentially lethal problems requiring the most rapid intervention must be ruled out first. These include intracranial bleeding (extradural hemorrhage),[2] major vascular rupture (of the thoracic aorta or other major vessels),[1,8] pneumothorax,[12] and visceral laceration or rupture (*e.g.*, of the liver or spleen).[16]

Invasive diagnostic and therapeutic measures such as the insertion of chest tubes, abdominal lavage, and angiographic studies all carry a certain risk of complications. These include vascular injury, nerve injury, infection, and false-negative or false-positive results.

The solution for minimizing complications related to diagnosis is adequate training of emergency-room physicians and all paramedical personnel and the establishment of regional trauma centers.[3] The worst complications arise when the necessary diagnostic procedures are not performed and a lethal or treatable lesion is missed or left untreated. For example, without the use of adequate diagnostic techniques, a widening mediastinum may go unrecognized, and a resultant aortic rupture may lead to fatal hemorrhage.[20]

CONTROL OF MASSIVE HEMORRHAGE

One of the most common and most serious life-threatening problems in the multiply injured patient is massive bleeding (defined as a loss of more than 15 units of blood). In the orthopaedic area this problem frequently occurs when an unstable pelvic fracture is part of the injury complex or when splenic, liver, or even kidney rupture accompanies long-bone fractures. Isolated long-bone fractures are not commonly associated with massive bleeding. Femoral fractures and other open fractures may be accompanied by arterial injury and very significant bleeding, but this is a rare occurrence.

Modern blood-bank techniques make the benefits of blood transfusion far greater in general than the risks, particularly when only a few units of blood are given. Recent fractionation techniques used by most blood banks provide for the removal of platelets, albumin, and cryoprecipitates, and thus the blood available for transfusion in trauma centers is modified or occasionally provided in the form of packed red cells. An advantage of the fractionation techniques is that special components of blood are available for use in certain circumstances, but a disadvantage is that complications of massive transfusion are somewhat increased by the use of this modified blood.[11]

The general risks of blood transfusion, such as disease transmission, immunologic reactions, and allergic reactions, are multiplied by the number of units given. Hepatitis has been the most feared transfusion-related disease in the past and continues to be a major problem, but a new and even more feared problem has recently arisen—that of acquired immune deficiency syndrome (AIDS). Less significant viral diseases are rarely transmitted through blood transfusions; in the United States, malaria and brucellosis are also very rare complications. Immunologic reactions can occur even when good matching techniques have been used. The risk of this complication is increasing in the current population because patients may have received transfusions previously and may have developed special antibodies. Also, human clerical errors are inevitable, and their likelihood is increased with the rapid transfusion of many units of blood.

Multiple transfusions present their own risks. Coagulopathy and bleeding problems, most commonly caused by dilutional thrombocytopenia, may arise after 12 to 15 units of blood have been administered. Monitoring for this complication consists of beginning platelet counts after 8 to 10 units have been given. Also, the surgeon must watch for evidence of pathologic bleeding from wound edges, needle stick sites, and other areas of skin penetration.

Considerable thought has been given to prophylactic platelet administration for reducing the risk of thrombocytopenia.[5] There is evidence that this measure is wasteful, however, and should be used only when a

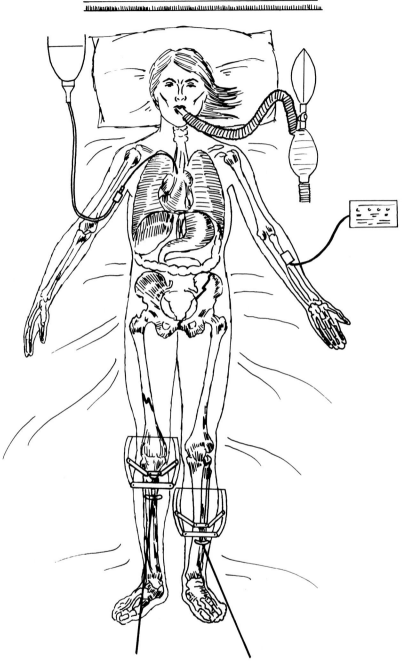

FIG. 29-1. The horizontal crucifixion syndrome. A typical multiply injured patient has a variety of orthopaedic injuries, including fractures of the femur, proximal tibia, and pelvis. The patient is placed supine in traction and requires positive end-expiratory pressure (PEEP) for his pulmonary problems. Cardiac monitoring is carried out via a Swan-Ganz catheter. Arterial line monitors enter one arm, and intravenous hyperalimentation lines enter the other. With the patient in this "horizontal crucifixion" position, the abdominal contents push against the diaphragm, compromising aeration of the lower lung. The combination of sedatives to promote tolerance of the PEEP and narcotics to control pain suppresses the normal diurnal physiology, thereby hindering normal periodic increases in pulse rate, peristalsis, urinary drainage, and muscle movement to promote circulation.
(Continued)

platelet count of less than 100,000 is documented and pathologic bleeding is noted.*

Disseminated intravascular coagulation (DIC) from consumption coagulopathy may also occur in multiply traumatized patients, along with its multifactorial causes, which include tissue injury, hypothermia, central nervous system injury, and hypotension. Hypothermia in particular may be a problem in the multiply injured and transfused patient unless a concerted effort is made to keep both the patient and the transfused blood warm. Hypothermia also increases the effect of other toxic by-products of massive transfusion, such as citrate and lactate. Citrate may bind ionized calcium and increase the hypothermia-induced myocardial depression.

Finally, microembolization of debris in the transfused blood is cumulative with the administration of many units. This problem, along with hypotension and hypothermia, may cause sludging and localized abnormality in various areas such as the lungs, consequently causing or aggravating adult respiratory distress syndrome (ARDS) and DIC.

The key element in avoiding all of these problems is timing. Multiply injured patients must be retrieved, resuscitated, diagnosed, stabilized, and treated in an expeditious manner so that massive bleeding is prevented. For the orthopaedist, expeditious treatment often means very early reduction and immobilization of long-bone and pelvic fractures by external fixation, internal fixation, or even a specialized spica cast.

---

* Heimbach, D.M.: Personal communication, 1985.

REPAIR AND RESTORATION OF INJURED SYSTEMS

The next phase of management of the multiply injured patient is repair and restoration of organ systems and skeletal structures. Timing is a key factor at this stage, and complications increase with a delay in definitive treatment. Ruptures of major vessels and visceral organs (*e.g.,* liver, spleen, pancreas) need early, if not immediate, attention. It is well established that healing of open fractures is enhanced, and complications from infection are reduced, if these fractures are thoroughly cleansed and debrided within 10 hours of injury. It has been recognized only recently, however, that early, if not immediate, stabilization of fractures of the long bones and spine may also have a great effect on reducing general complications such as fat embolism, ARDS, failure of organs other than the lungs, nutritional depletion, and negative nitrogen balance.[19]

The Nijmegen study[7] and studies by Meek and colleagues,[13] Riska and associates,[17,18] Johnson and co-workers,[9] and LaDuca and associates[10] have all shown fewer complications and a decreased mortality rate with early stabilization of fractures and have proved that early surgery is of greater benefit than risk. This has certainly been my experience, although I have not conducted a randomized study to document these observations. Immediate skeletal fixation also appears to facilitate soft tissue healing and to decrease the severity, if not the incidence, of infection in open fractures.[4,6]

Clinical observation reveals that revascularization or restoration of normal circulation is facilitated immeasurably by initial

---

FIG. 29-1. (*cont.*) Normal nutrition becomes impossible, and a negative nitrogen balance commonly develops. The supine position may also cause an increase in intracranial pressure. The primary visual input to the brain is of the ceiling, and the main auditory input is the beeping of the equipment. Continuation of these conditions may bring about a downward spiraling of the patient's status, with incumbent problems such as malnutrition, constipation, urinary stasis and infection, pulmonary infection and dependence on respiratory assistance, vascular sludging with thromboembolism, bedsores, and depression. The orthopaedic traumatologist could reverse much of the potential risk of these problems by immediately restoring the skeleton. Skeletal stabilization would permit the patient to be nursed with the chest upright and thus would allow respiratory assistance to be removed much earlier than otherwise. Other advantages would be the return of normal alimentation, decreased intracranial pressure, a decreased need for narcotics (and, therefore, enhanced alertness), and much earlier rehabilitation.

stabilization of the skeleton. To appreciate this fact, one need only contemplate the problems of managing a grade V open fracture or a traumatic amputation, or of undertaking reimplantation, in a limb that has not been skeletally stabilized. Of all of the long bones, stabilization of the femur is the most important for facilitating patient care.[19] If the femur is not fixed, the patient is doomed to the so-called horizontal crucifixion position in the surgical intensive care unit and will suffer such attendant problems as compromised pulmonary function, probable increased CSF pressure, and delayed gastric emptying (Fig. 29-1).

An unstable fracture of the spine or pelvis entails even more compromise, but traditionally these fractures are not often stabilized in the immediate postoperative period. In addition to restricting the patient to the supine position, these fractures cause pain and necessitate the administration of narcotic or other depressive medication. These medications inhibit normal vital functions and, when the patient must remain supine, they promote atelectasis and pneumonia, depressed peristalsis and constipation, urinary stasis and infection, vascular sludging with thrombosis and thromboembolism, pressure necrosis and ulceration of the skin, and occasionally pulmonary embolism. In addition, food intake and nutrition are suppressed, with the development of a negative nitrogen balance, and subsequently the patient experiences poor tissue healing. Finally, the patient may become seriously depressed even if he was not already experiencing depression before injury; it is our observation that depression and other psychiatric abnormalities are common preinjury conditions in the multiply traumatized patient and may cause or contribute to the patient's accident. For these reasons we now encourage immediate fixation in selected cases of spinal, pelvic, and acetabular fractures in our trauma center when definition of the fracture is clear enough in the acute phase to allow us to determine the pathologic anatomy and we are able to stabilize the fractures quickly and efficiently.

We virtually always perform immediate stabilization of all femoral fractures and any open fractures in the multiply injured patient, and we generally achieve excellent results with this approach. The use of this protocol is exemplified in the following case study.

Case One

A 28-year-old man was injured when his motorcycle struck a tree and then a fence at high speed. Paramedics who stabilized his condition at the scene of the accident noted an unstable pelvic fracture and externally rotated lower extremities but no significant injury to the head, chest, or abdomen. He had a blood pressure reading of 130/90, a pulse rate of 102, and a respiration rate of 20 on initial examination, and only on arrival at the hospital, within an hour after the accident, did the paramedics note the beginning of abdominal distention.

On his arrival at the emergency room the patient was alert; his vital signs were fairly stable, his peripheral pulses were intact, and he had no neurologic deficit. The hematocrit count, which was 45 in the field, dropped to 32 in the emergency room after some crystalloids and 1 unit of blood had been given. The patient's urine showed gross blood, and peritoneal dialysis showed microscopic blood. Roentgenograms of the chest and spine were normal, but a comminuted subtrochanteric fracture of the left femur was noted (Fig. 29-2), and a comminuted fracture of the proximal third of the right femur was detected (Fig. 29-3). Also noted were a pubic diastasis of 6 cm and a very displaced transverse fracture of the right acetabulum with widening of both sacroiliac joints (Fig. 29-4). Bilateral x-ray films of the tibia and fibula were normal, and IVP was reported as normal.

A provisional diagnosis in the emergency room included pelvic and acetabular fractures, probable renal contusion, bilateral upper femoral fractures, and potential massive internal blood loss secondary to all of these injuries. The patient's condition was stabilized over approximately 4 hours in the trauma center by means of splinting of the extremities and administration of approximately 3000 ml of lactated Ringer's solution accompanied by 3 units of whole blood. All of

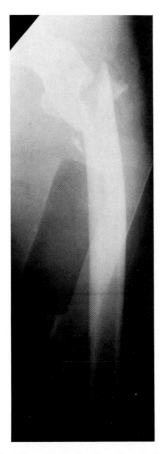

FIG. 29-2. Comminuted subtrochanteric fracture of the proximal third of the left femur.

rhage and comminution, as well as the patient's very heavy musculature, made the anatomic reduction difficult, but excellent stability was accomplished nevertheless.

Then with one major move the patient was shifted onto his left side and placed on a fracture extension table (Maquet) appropriate for closed intramedullary nailing. With the patient in this position, the transverse acetabular fracture was reduced and plated through a single posterolateral incision, and an interlocking (Klemm) nail was placed in the intramedullary canal of the comminuted right femur.

Because there were some technical difficulties, the total time of surgery extended to approximately 8 hours. The patient was managed with volume res-

the diagnostic tests were carried out during this time, and intra-abdominal bleeding was ruled out. Appropriate films were taken as aids in planning the restorative skeletal surgery.

Approximately 5 hours after the accident, the patient was taken to the operating room. The following plan was instituted for stabilization of each fracture with minimal movement of the patient. The patient was placed supine on a fracture table, and a two-hole plate was used to close the pubic diastasis through a short vertical incision. Then, with minimal movement, the patient was eased distally onto a fracture extension table while still in the supine position, and his left subtrochanteric fracture was fixed with an AO condylar blade plate through a standard lateral incision. Extensive hemor-

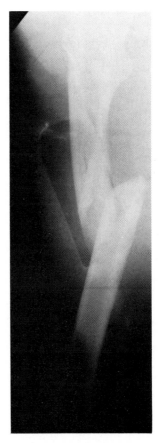

FIG. 29-3. Comminuted fracture of the proximal third of the right femur immediately after injury.

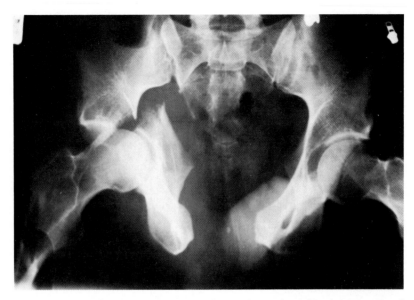

FIG. 29-4. Initial film of the patient's pelvis shows the wide pubic diastasis, the displaced transverse fracture of the right acetabulum, and the widening of the sacroiliac joints, particularly on the right side.

piration and appropriate fluids throughout surgery and remained stable. He required 15 liters of ½ normal saline and 13 units of whole blood, and he was also given 12 units of platelets secondary to transfusion thrombocytopenia. Because of the large amount of fluid and blood administered, and because the patient's final platelet count was only 75,000, we elected to use a bilateral hip spica cast at the end of the operation to give maximum support to the soft tissues and minimize the chance of further bleeding (Fig. 29-5).

Over the next few days, which the patient spent in the intensive care unit, he remained physiologically stable with no major bleeding, pulmonary dysfunction, or febrile response. He was disoriented, however, and occasionally became hallucinatory and combative. Nevertheless, his condition improved rapidly, and he was transferred from the intensive care unit on the fourth day after injury. By this time he required no pain medication, and his mental status was improved. By the sixth day after injury, extra postoperative nutritional support was given, but the patient had some gastritis and a poor appetite and assimilated the extra nutrients poorly for several more days. The patient's intermittent confusion, particularly at night, persisted for almost 10 days.

Ten days after operation, the spica cast was removed. Assisted motion of the hips and knees was begun, and the patient gradually began sitting. The patient's Foley catheter was removed after about a week, but for another 10 days he had intermittent difficulties with urination, including burning. These difficulties, which were related to the local damage from the pubic diastasis, resolved during the patient's hospitalization.

The patient required antacid medications throughout the course of treatment for gastritis and had some difficulty with adequate nutritional intake during the first 3 weeks. In addition, he was constipated intermittently during these 3 weeks but responded to standard measures.

The patient was actually ready for mobilization and discharge planning by about 2½ weeks after injury, but he remained in the hospital for a total of 26 days because his need to remain non–weight bearing for an additional 6 weeks required that he make the arrangements and gain the skills necessary for wheelchair use at home.

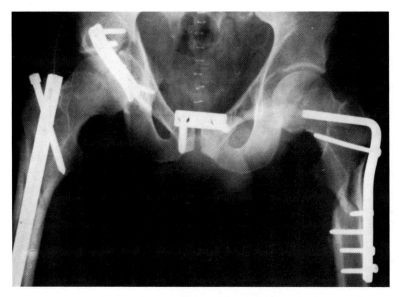

FIG. 29-5. Approximately 13 hours after injury and just before application of the postoperative hip spica cast, all fractures have been anatomically stabilized except for the left subtrochanteric fracture, which is very stable, even though it displays some slight varus angulation and rotation.

During his last week in the hospital he experienced no complications and was involved with physical therapy and with preparing his home for hospital bed and wheelchair use. On discharge from the hospital he was able to transfer independently from the bed to the wheelchair and back and had achieved a 90° range of motion in the knees and hips bilaterally (Fig. 29-6).

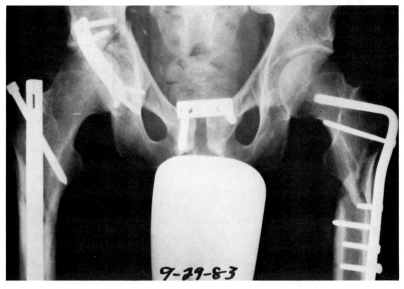

FIG. 29-6. One month later, the pubis has widened slightly. The patient is stable and is nearly asymptomatic but still uses the wheelchair and performs active-assisted exercises for his hips and knees.

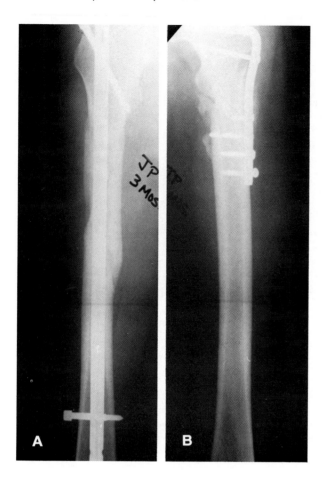

FIG. 29-7. (*A*) At 3 months the distal interlocking screw in the right femur has been removed. The patient has begun full weight bearing on that side but still requires some protection on the left side. (*B*) No further films were taken, since the patient proceeded to clinically normal healing and function.

On follow-up in the outpatient clinic, the patient was allowed to bear full weight on the right side after removal of the distal interlocking screw 3 months after injury (Fig. 29-7). Full weight bearing on the left side was begun 3½ months after injury. By 5 months the patient was walking with a virtually normal gait and was allowed to return to his work as an auto mechanic. By 8 months after injury the patient stated that he saw no reason to continue regular follow-up visits and would return only if he had symptoms. Hardware removal was planned to take place approximately 1½ years after injury at a mutually convenient time.

Long bones other than the femur, and in particular the tibia and the humerus, may occasionally need stabilization to enhance general patient mobilization and to reduce pain and the need for narcotics. More often, however, the rationale for stabilization should be to prevent local soft tissue damage from open or intra-articular fractures. Well-executed repair with careful attention to preserving and restoring blood supply aids soft tissue healing in addition to restoring normal anatomy. In intra-articular fractures, early anatomic and stable internal fixation allows early motion and maintenance of functional, if not normal, joint motion.

In the case of open injuries, failure to carry out this technically demanding accurate repair process early may lead to osteomyelitis, pyarthrosis, joint incongruity, stiffness, and atrophy. Even in closed fractures the term *fracture disease* describes the syndrome of local complications that arises when prolonged rest is prescribed for treatment of these fractures. Disuse leads to osteoporosis, atrophy of muscle and other soft tissues, adhesions and stiffness in joints, and loss of articular cartilage.

Finally, serious consideration must be given to any crush injuries sustained by a polytraumatized patient, particularly an older patient. A crush injury to one or more extremities in combination with other injuries may raise the total injury, reflected in the injury severity score (ISS),[7] to such an extent that we can predict that the patient's organ systems will be unable to process the total volume of injury breakdown products. A patient with such extensive injuries rarely survives the trip to the hospital in an area not served by excellent paramedics. When highly trained paramedics have provided initial care, however, the trauma team is usually able to manage patients with multiple extremity fractures and other visceral injuries, including one or more crushed limbs.

In the postinjury period, the crush injury patient may not be able to generate the nutrients or the healing potential necessary for handling the entire complex of injuries because of decreased protein and caloric intake. In such instances we have found that it is frequently necessary to sacrifice one or more limbs to save the patient's life. Although this situation occurs most often in patients more than 40 years of age, it occasionally arises in a younger patient. The most severely damaged or least salvageable limb, which has usually sustained a crush or vascular injury, should be amputated immediately above the site of major damage. The amputation not only accelerates the overall repair effort significantly, but also decreases markedly the load on the organ systems. At this point the amputated limb becomes a valuable source of vessels, skin, and bone for use in repair of the patient's other injuries. Specifically, the talus and os calcis make outstanding bone graft material, and saphenous veins and uncontused skin salvaged from the amputated extremity may be of significant value in vascular repair and skin grafting procedures. If an early amputation is not performed, a patient may suffer severe pulmonary, liver, kidney, and nutritional failure and may ultimately lose the limb, provided that he survives the other injuries. Such a

situation is illustrated in the following case study.

Case Two

A 45-year-old man was injured in a high-speed motorcycle accident while intoxicated. He sustained no significant head, chest, or abdominal injuries. His orthopaedic evaluation on presentation revealed a closed midshaft fracture of the left humerus (Fig. 29-8) and ipsilateral grade I open fractures of the radius and ulna (Fig. 29-9). The extremity was pulseless and without sensorimotor function below the axilla (Fig. 29-10). The patient also had a grade II open segmental fracture in the middle third and distal third of the left femur, which extended

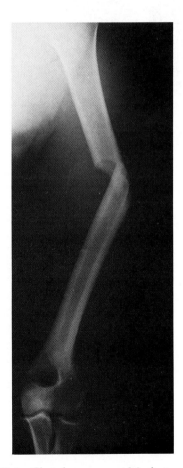

FIG. 29-8. Closed upper midshaft transverse fracture of the left humerus.

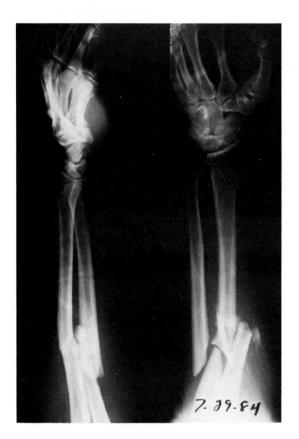

FIG. 29-9. Comminuted proximal fractures of both bones of the left forearm.

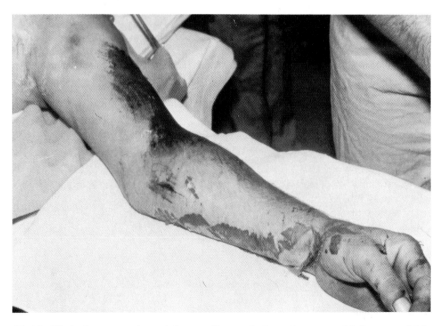

FIG. 29-10. Clinical presentation of the swollen, pulseless, denervated left arm, which was found to have a complete brachial plexus avulsion.

FIG. 29-11. Comminuted and segmental fracture of the left femoral shaft.

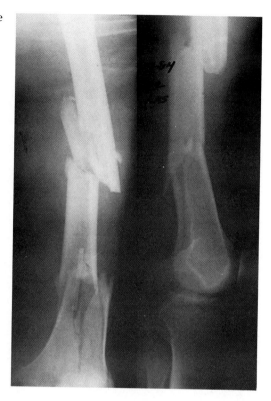

into the intracondylar region (Fig. 29-11); a comminuted grade II open fracture of the left patella; a grade IV open fracture in the distal third of the left tibia with a pulseless hypoesthetic foot (Fig. 29-12); and a closed, comminuted pilon fracture of the right ankle, which was neuromuscularly intact (Fig. 29-13).

After initial evaluation and fluid resuscitation, the patient was rushed to the operating room, where the vascular and orthopaedic surgeons jointly approached the multiple injuries. Vascular flow to the left upper extremity was reinstituted with a vascular shunt while the distal fracture of the left tibia was debrided and rigidly stabilized with a plate. A vascular shunt was then used to reconstitute blood flow to the left foot while the left humeral (Fig. 29-14) and forearm fractures (Fig. 29-15) were rigidly stabilized with plates. The brachial plexus was found to be completely disrupted at the level of the shoulder. Intraoperative arteriography revealed an injury to the left popliteal

artery. The intra-articular components of the fractures of the left femur and patella were anatomically restored (Fig. 29-16).

The surgical procedure had to be discontinued before completion of rigid stabilization of all fractures because of excessive blood loss (more than 35 units) and the onset of a dilutional coagulopathy refractory to appropriate platelet and factor transfusions. The vascular shunts were replaced with saphenous vein grafts, and the popliteal artery injury was temporized with a Gortex graft. The segmental femoral fracture was stabilized with an external fixation device, and the tibial fracture was splinted.

The patient was returned to the operating room 5 days after injury for fixation of the femoral fracture with a long blade plate, skin grafting on the left upper extremity, and an ipsilateral below-knee amputation necessitated by ischemia refractory to extensive attempts at vascular salvage (Fig. 29-17). Ten days after injury, open reduction and internal fixation of

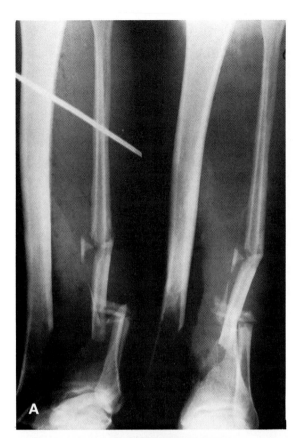

FIG. 29-12. (*A* and *B*) Initial presentation of the grade IV open fracture of the left tibia, which was rendered pulseless by a popliteal artery injury.

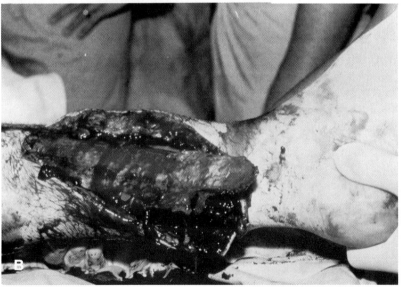

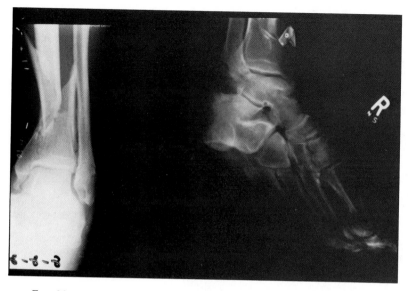

FIG. 29-13. Closed, comminuted pilon fracture of the right ankle.

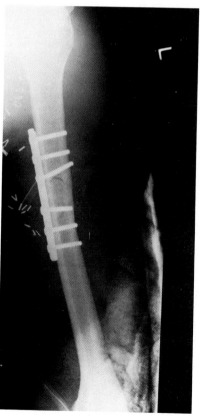

the right pilon fracture (Fig. 29-18) and revision of the left below-knee amputation were performed. Because the function of the insensate, flail upper extremity was expected to be nil, and because retention of this injured limb would have provided a further metabolic burden to this multiply traumatized patient, an above-elbow amputation was performed 12 days after injury (Fig. 29-19). At 3 weeks postinjury the patient experienced a septic rupture of the popliteal Gortex graft. An emergency revision of the above-knee amputation was required, but the proximal two thirds of the femur, including the plate, were left intact (Fig. 29-20).

The patient's hospital course was further complicated by infection of his right pilon fracture when attempted coverage with an abductor hallucis flap failed,

FIG. 29-14. The plate was applied to the medial side of the left humerus through the open wound after vascular repair of the brachial plexus.

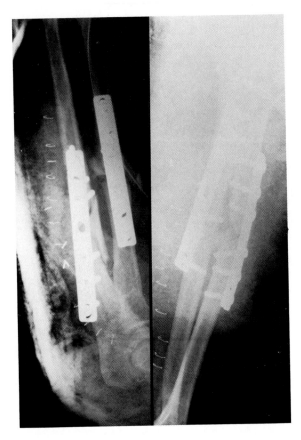

FIG. 29-15. Double-plate stabilization of the proximal fractures of the radius and ulna on the same side as the humeral fracture and the vascular injury. By this time it was known that the brachial plexus was completely disrupted at the level of the shoulder.

because of multiple amputation debridements of the left arm and leg, and because of the nutritional depletion of the patient, who required tube feedings.

The patient was discharged from the hospital and returned home three months after injury, having received nearly 75 units of blood and having undergone 12 separate surgical procedures that left him with a left above-elbow amputation and an ipsilateral above-knee amputation.

SUMMARY

It is important to note that all of the complications mentioned in Dr. Murray's opening chapter may occur in the multiply injured patient. The special problems associated with injuries to other systems make complications infinitely more likely to arise in the multiply injured patient than in either the patient with an individual injury or the well-prepared patient undergoing elective surgery. The effective management of the multiply injured patient requires teamwork on the part of community members, hospital staffs, and physicians. Community facilities must develop systems for efficient accident reporting and a rapid emergency response, hospitals must be committed to providing skilled support services, and physicians in the multiple specialties must provide care in a coordinated manner. Optimally, the multiply injured patient should arrive at the hospital having already been managed promptly and efficiently with emergency stabilization. Once the patient reaches the hospital, efficient triage, diagnosis, and treatment should lead to repair and rehabilitation of injured systems with few, if any, complications.

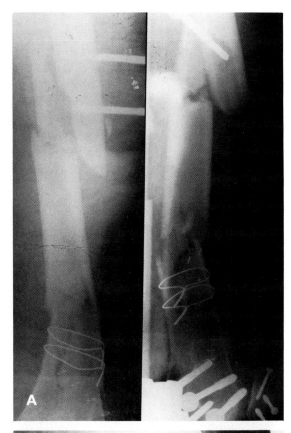

Fig. 29-16. (A) Restoration of the fractured patella and the intracondylar region of the fractured femur, where a popliteal artery lesion also existed. (B) The rest of the femur was initially stabilized with an external fixation device.

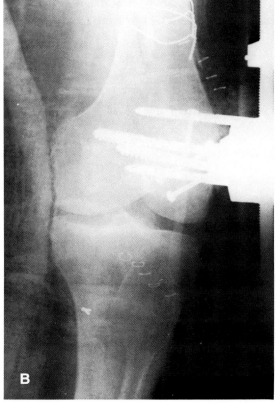

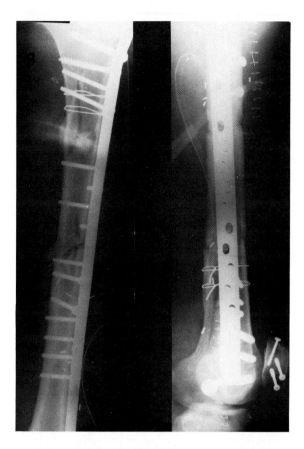

FIG. 29-17. Definitive stabilization of the entire femur 5 days after injury. At this time it was noted that the lower leg had become ischemic from the popliteal artery injury and was becoming necrotic. An amputation was subsequently performed.

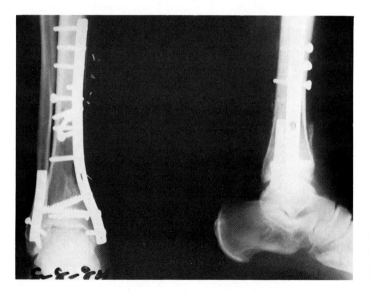

FIG. 29-18. The pilon fracture of the right ankle, the only injury to this limb, was stabilized 10 days after injury.

FIG. 29-19. Twelve days after injury, an above-elbow amputation of the insensate and vascularly deprived left upper extremity was performed because of distal necrosis.

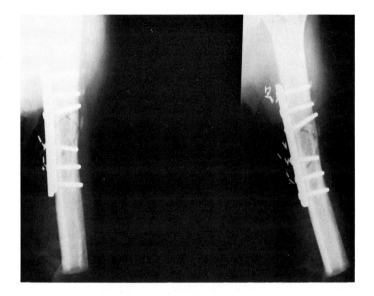

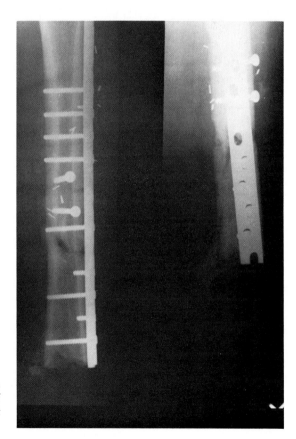

FIG. 29-20. An above-knee amputation was required 3 weeks after injury because of septic rupture of the popliteal Gortex graft above the below-knee amputation site.

REFERENCES

1. Ayella, R.J., Hankins, J.R., Turney, S.Z., and Cowley, R.A.: Ruptured thoracic aorta due to blunt trauma. J. Bone Joint Surg., 17A:199, 1977.
2. Bakay, L.: Brain injuries in polytrauma. World J. Surg., 7:42, 1983.
3. Boyd, D.R., and Cowley, R.A.: Comprehensive regional trauma/emergency medical services (EMS) delivery systems: The United States experience. World J. Surg., 7:149, 1983.
4. Chapman, M.W., and Mahoney, M.: The role of early internal fixation in the management of open fractures. Clin. Orthop., 138:120, 1979.
5. Counts, R.B., Haisch, C., Simon, T.L., et al.: Hemostasis in massively transfused trauma patients. Ann. Surg., 190:91, 1979.
6. Franklin, J.L., Johnson, K.D., and Hansen, S.T.: Immediate internal fixation of open ankle fractures. J. Bone Joint Surg., 66A:1349, 1984.
7. Goris, R.J.A.: The injury severity score. World J. Surg., 7:12, 1983.
8. Heberer, G., Becker, H.M., Dittmer, H., and Stelter, W.J.: Vascular injuries in polytrauma. World J. Surg., 7:68, 1983.
9. Johnson, K.D., Cadambi, A.J., and Seibert, B.: Incidence of A.R.D.S. in patients with multiple musculoskeletal injuries: Effect of early operative stabilization of fractures. J. Trauma (in press).
10. LaDuca, J.N., Bone, L.L., Steibel, R.W., and Border, J.R.: Primary open reduction and internal fixation of open fractures. J. Trauma, 20:580, 1980.
11. Maier, R.V.: The consequences of massive blood transfusion. Surg. Rounds, August 1984, p. 57.
12. Mattox, K.L.: Thoracic injury requiring surgery. World J. Surg., 7:49, 1983.
13. Meek, R.N., Vivoda, E., Crichton, A., and Pirani, S.: Comparison of mortality of patients with multiple injuries according to method of fracture treatment. In Proceedings of the Canadian Orthopaedic Association Annual Meeting, June 8–12, 1980, Calgary, Alberta. J. Bone Joint Surg., 63B: 456, 1981.
14. Messmer, K.F.W.: Traumatic shock in polytrauma: Circulatory parameters, biochemistry, and resuscitation. World J. Surg., 7:26, 1983.
15. Olerud, S., and Allgöwer, M.: Evaluation and management of the polytraumatized patient in various centers. World J. Surg., 7:143, 1983.
16. Polk, H.C., and Flint, L.M.: Intra-abdominal injuries in polytrauma. World J. Surg., 7:56, 1983.
17. Riska, E.B., von Bonsdorff, H., Hakkinen, S., et al.: Prevention of fat embolism in early internal fixation of fractures with multiple injuries. Injury, 8:110, 1976.
18. ———: Primary operative fixation of long bone fractures in patients with multiple injuries. J. Trauma, 17:111, 1977.
19. Tscherne, H., Oestern, H.J., and Sturm, J.: Osteosynthesis of major fractures in polytrauma. World J. Surg., 7:80, 1983.
20. West, J.G., Trunkey, D.D., and Lim, R.C.: Systems of trauma care. Arch. Surg., 114:455, 1979.

30 Orthopaedic Complications of Athletic Injuries and Their Treatment

JOSEPH S. TORG

Sports medicine may best be described as a multidisciplinary effort to provide total health care for athletes. People from the various medical specialities, the allied health professions, and the fields of physical education and exercise physiology are involved in injury prevention, physical conditioning, and the diagnosis, treatment, and rehabilitation of injuries and diseases. Because most of the problems that arise in the pursuit of recreational and competitive athletics involve the various structures of the musculoskeletal system, the orthopaedic surgeon has assumed a position of prominence in this area of medicine. Specifically, it is the orthopaedic surgeon who is responsible for managing the "battle wounds" of the athlete (Fig. 30-1). In this role he has developed new principles for managing musculoskeletal injuries that aim to return the injured athlete to his activity in the shortest period at the highest level of proficiency, with the least degree of risk. To achieve this goal is not to compromise old principles but rather to develop new ones that will meet the needs of the high-performance athlete and yet not jeopardize his physical well-being. Complications in this area of medicine can be divided into three categories: temporary failure to achieve this goal, permanent failure, and complications that result in disability in areas of activity other than athletics.

The causes of poor results and complications in the management of problems affecting the athlete are numerous. Failure to diagnose a condition accurately or treat it correctly is an obvious cause. A common reason for treatment failure is undue haste in getting the athlete to return to his activity. A common and probably unappreciated source of problems is the failure of the physician to rehabilitate the injured part adequately, despite appropriate definitive management. Complications and poor results can occur if a patient does not understand his role in achieving a desired result or does not cooperate. Complications of athletic injuries, like any others, are better avoided before they occur.

Most important, however, both the physician and the athlete must realize that many of the problems encountered in sports medicine are not entirely solvable. The natural course of many injury states that affect the athlete are such that expectation for complete resolution of the problem is unrealistic. Osteochondritis dissecans of the humeral capitellum in a juvenile pitcher and irreparable disruption of the anterior cruciate ligament in a high-performance amateur or professional athlete are such situations. In such instances, however, it is equally important that the responsible physician recognize the inevitable course of an unsolvable problem and set realistic goals and expectations for the athlete from the beginning.

Chronologically, the "playing life" of an athlete can be divided into three phases: juvenile, adult, and middle age. The juvenile category encompasses both preadolescence and adolescence. Preadolescence is that period from childhood to the onset of secondary sex characteristics, which occurs between 12 and 14 years of age in females and between 14 and 16 years of age in males. Significant is the fact that prior to puberty and the increase in muscle mass, the injury rates in the preadolescent group are quite low. Adolescence is marked by the onset of secondary sex characteristics,

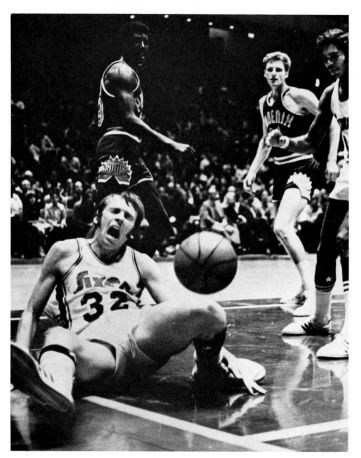

FIG. 30-1. The goal of the orthopaedic surgeon involved in sports medicine is to return the injured athlete to his activity in the shortest period, at the highest level of proficiency, with the least degree of risk. Successful management of the athlete's problems requires that accurate diagnosis be followed by implementation of appropriate treatment and rehabilitation. In addition, understanding and cooperation on the part of the patient are essential. Of paramount importance is that both the physician and the athlete must realize that not all problems are entirely solvable, and realistic goals for end results must be established from the beginning. (Photo by W. R. Everly III, Philadelphia Daily News)

increase in muscle mass, and closure of the epiphyses and the epiphyseal plates. Injury rates and their problems increase precipitously during this period. Problems encountered during the juvenile period are frequently related to aberrations in the process of endochondral ossification or trauma to the various epiphyseal growth plates.

With the closure of the growth areas and full development of the other structures of the musculoskeletal system, the young adult athlete encounters a different group of injuries, with their associated problems and, in addition, a higher injury rate. This period of life is characterized by strains, sprains, subluxations, dislocations, fractures, and their sequelae. The middle-aged athlete, on the other hand, experiencing the somewhat poorer physical condition associated with the normal processes of tissue deterioration, faces yet another group of problems—those associated with attritional and degenerative musculoskeletal changes.

COMPLICATIONS OF ATHLETIC INJURIES IN JUVENILES

Injury rates are low during the juvenile period, and even tackle football presents no greater danger for the participant than do other daily activities. The significant problems that do occur, however, usually involve the components of the skeletal system responsible for the growth and development of bone.

Endochondral ossification is the mechanism by which longitudinal and configurational bone growth is effected by the orderly transformation of hyaline cartilage to mature cancellous bone. It can best be described in terms of specific areas of growth, each having its own peculiarities that make it susceptible to injury (Fig. 30-2).

The epiphysis is the secondary center of ossification at each end of the long bones. It develops from a cartilage anlage by endochondral ossification but actually contributes little, if anything, to longitudinal growth. With a few exceptions, the epiphysis is bounded on one end by articular cartilage and on the other by the growth plate. From the standpoint of blood supply, it is isolated from the shaft of the bone by the growth plate. If the epiphyseal vessels are injured, the epiphysis undergoes avascular necrosis. Also, these relatively fragile secondary centers of ossification are prone to avascular changes from compressive forces. Such localized avascular changes are called *osteochondrosis.*

The growth plate is the component of endochondral ossification responsible for longitudinal growth. Siffert divided the plate into three functional zones: the growth zone, the zone of cartilage transformation, and the zone of ossification.[61] It is recognized that compression of the plate retards growth, probably at the growth zone. Conversely, distracting forces stimulate germinal cell proliferation. The zone of ossification is the area most susceptible to stress in the growth plate. Here, shearing forces separate the plate between the last layer of cartilage cells and the zone of provisional calcification. This is the mechanism responsible for the vast majority of growth plate injuries.

Adjacent to the growth plate lies the metaphysis, and next, the diaphysis. Aberrations in the growth plate may become manifest in these areas.

An apophysis is a secondary center of ossification responsible for configurational, rather than longitudinal, growth. Also, it is neither covered by articular cartilage nor involved in a joint but, rather, serves as a site for muscle attachment. Apophyses and

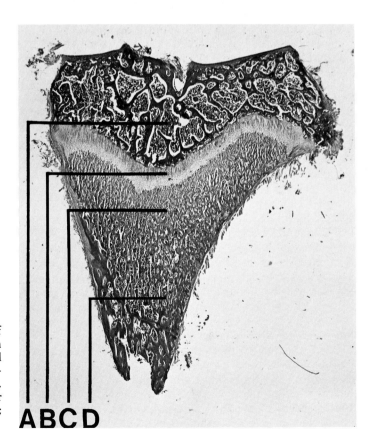

FIG. 30-2. Photomicrograph of a segment of a proximial tibia demonstrates the essential structures involved in endochondral ossification: *A,* epiphysis; *B,* epiphyseal or growth plate; *C,* metaphysis; *D,* diaphysis.

ABCD

their growth plates react to physiologic and pathologic stresses in the same manner as epiphyses.

Disorders of the Throwing Arm

Repeated stresses of throwing on the various elements of endochondral ossification about the shoulder and elbow may result in a variety of lesions that have been attributed to, but are certainly not limited to, Little League pitching. These lesions may occur from a variety of activities such as gymnastics, wrestling, tennis, or any sort of throwing action. Although the repeated microtrauma that a given activity inflicts on the various growth areas occurs during the more vulnerable period of 8 through 12 years of age, it is not until the child reaches adolescence that clinical problems (and roentgenographic manifestations) appear.

Little League shoulder is a term used to identify two roentgenographically distinct lesions involving the proximal humerus.[3,22] *Little League elbow*, on the other hand, refers to a group of disorders affecting the growth elements of the radius, ulna, and humerus in the elbow joint.

Little League shoulder may present either as an abnormal radiolucency involving the proximal humeral metaphysis adjacent to the epiphyseal plate (Fig. 30-3) or as an area of mottled radiolucency involving a circumscribed segment of the proximal humeral epiphysis (Fig. 30-4). Both lesions present with shoulder pain on throwing, and the roentgenographic manifestations are believed to represent an area of aseptic necrosis. When there is widening, demineralization, and fragmentation of the proximal humeral metaphysis, the process is self-limited, although it may take from 9 to 12 months for reossification to present a normal roentgenographic appearance. In this instance, treatment consists of limiting activity during the symptomatic phase and prohibiting pitching or any similar activity until roentgenograms are normal. A circumscribed area of osteochondrosis involving the humeral head, may go on to loose-body formation, requiring arthrotomy to remove the fragment.[45]

Little League elbow is a term used to refer to several different problems.[13] *Medial epicondylar apophysitis*, a vague term, can

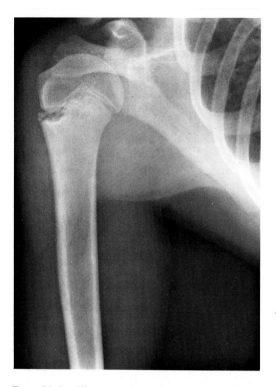

FIG. 30-3. This roentgenogram demonstrates mottled radiolucency involving the proximal humeral metaphysis adjacent to the epiphyseal plate, which is characteristic of one form of Little League shoulder called osteochondrosis of the proximal humeral metaphysis. The process appears to be self-limiting, and treatment is simply to have the youngster refrain from pitching until roentgenograms are normal. The lesion requires 8 to 12 months for roentgenographic demonstration of reossification.

be manifest as one of three different clinical and roentgenographic entities.[2,63,71]

Accelerated medial apophyseal growth with delayed closure of the medial epicondylar growth plate is seen in Little Leaguers who have been allowed to pitch repeatedly. Generally, the symptoms are minimal, and the diagnosis is made on the basis of the roentgenogram. This condition does not cause significant disability. If symptoms warrant treatment, simply resting the arm is sufficient.

Traction apophysitis likewise has a classic roentgenographic picture. Again, the cause is repeated pitching, which can produce pain, swelling, and tenderness over the medial humeral epicondylar apophysis. If

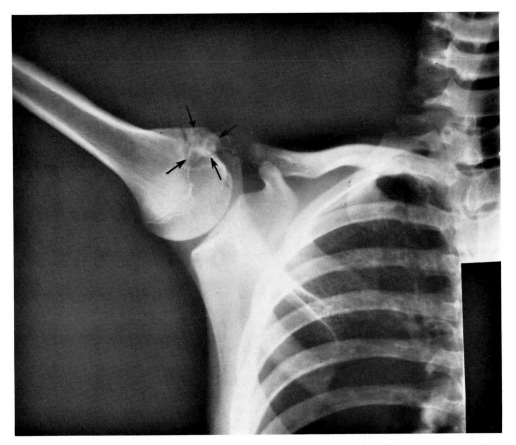

FIG. 30-4. A second form of Little League shoulder, osteochondrosis of the proximal humeral epiphysis, is demonstrated roentgenographically by a circumscribed area of mottled radiolucency (*arrows*). This lesion may result in loose bodies being ejected into the joint, requiring surgical removal.

symptoms are significant, the arm should be rested.

Complete avulsion of the medial epicondylar apophysis occurs acutely with attempts to throw as hard as possible. Pain, swelling, and tenderness are present over the apophysis. If separation of the apophysis is less than 5 mm, the extremity should be immobilized in plaster for 3 weeks. If the separation is 5 mm or more, open reduction and pin fixation are indicated.

Osteochondrosis of the radial head is a relatively rare lesion, although Ellman has documented five cases,[23] Adams two,[2] and Tullos and King one each,[40,73] all in preadolescent pitchers. Characteristically, pain develops in the elbow of the pitching arm and increases with throwing. Clinically, swelling and tenderness are localized over the radial head, and there is limitation of extension (Fig. 30-5). Ellman found roentgenographic and histologic changes in the radial head similar to those seen in the capital femoral epiphysis in Legg-Calvé-Perthes disease—that is, condensation, fragmentation, and bony restoration with deformity, articular incongruity, and subsequent arthritic changes. Initial treatment consists of immobilization until the acute symptoms subside. Any further pitching is prohibited. If the radial head becomes markedly deformed (Fig. 30-6), excision may be considered after growth has been completed (Fig. 30-7).

Osteochondrosis of the humeral capitellum is a disease process involving the

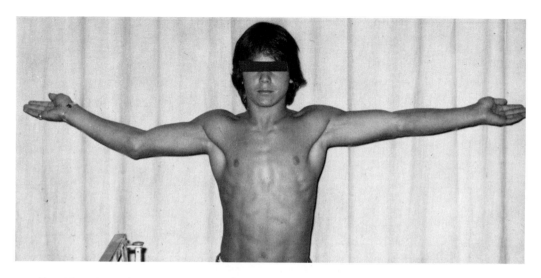

FIG. 30-5. Osteochondrosis of the radial head can result in limitation of elbow motion in all planes: flexion, extension, supination, and pronation. Despite removal of the radial head, flexion contracture may persist.

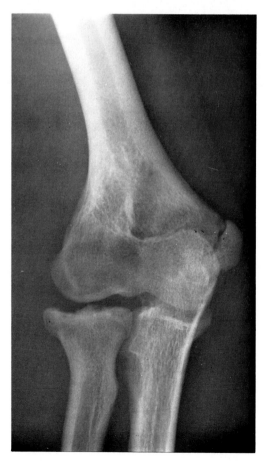

elbow of the adolescent athlete who is engaged in pitching or other activities in which repeated compressive forces have been exerted at the radiocapitellar joint. Although most cases reported in the literature are attributed to pitching, we have seen the disorder in a wrestler and a gymnast. The clinical course is predictable. Initial symptoms of pain and stiffness in the involved elbow are accompanied by roentgenograms demonstrating cystic changes in the humeral capitellum (Fig. 30-8). Conservative management (immobilization and rest) does not appear to retard the development of erosive changes on the capitellar joint surface (Fig. 30-9), ejection of loose bodies into the joint, and subsequent hypertrophy and deformity of the radial head. Surgical intervention directed at removing the loose bodies, shaving the irregular capitellar surface, and drilling the capitellum results in relief of pain and some increase in motion.[67] However, few if any athletes return to successful throwing, and most

FIG. 30-6. Roentgenographic demonstration of the terminal phase of osteochondrosis of the radial head reveals irregular hypertrophy of the radial head with radiocapitellar incongruity.

FIG. 30-7. The surgical findings of osteochondrosis of the radial head are deformity and articular cartilage destruction.

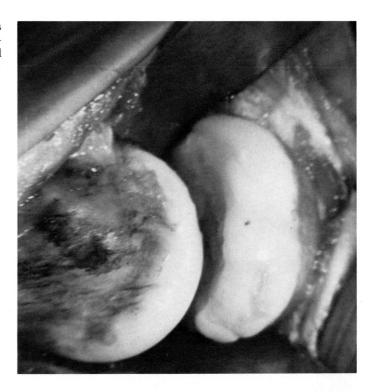

develop irreversible degenerative changes in the joint.[14]

Nonunion through a stress fracture of the olecranon epiphyseal plate has been observed in the pitching elbow of an adolescent baseball player.[70] The mechanics of the act of pitching have been described by King as consisting of four phases: (1) windup, (2) cocking, (3) acceleration, and (4) release and follow through.[40] Whipping the elbow from its flexed position in the acceleration phase involves forceful contraction of the triceps muscle. As a result of repeated forceful pitching, traction to the olecranon epiphysis is exerted on the adjacent olecranon epiphyseal plate. This can result in a stress fracture that, with continued pitching, has resulted in a nonunion through this area (Fig. 30-10). An inlaid autogenous bone graft will effect a satisfactory healing of the lesion.

Lesions of the Apophysis of the Ischial Tuberosity

Avulsion of the apophysis of the ischial tuberosity rarely occurs in adolescents. It is generally recognized that the acute lesion should be treated conservatively. Despite treatment, hypertrophic callus formation associated with a painful nonunion can develop (Fig. 30-11). The patient has discomfort with activity and also while sitting. Depending on the degree of discomfort and disability, *en bloc* resection of the avulsed fragment and hypertrophic callus is indicated. With the patient supine on the table, the hip is flexed to 90° and an incision is made proximal and parallel to the gluteal crease. This position brings the lesion closer to the skin surface. The gluteus maximus is reflected up and laterally; care is taken to protect the sciatic nerve, which lies between the ischium and the greater trochanter, and the lesion is carefully dissected subperiosteally from the origin of the hamstring muscles. The periosteum is then sutured into the soft tissue attachments of the ischium, and the wound is closed.

Lesions of the Knee

Traction apophysitis of the tibial tuberosity, commonly referred to as Osgood-Schlatter's disease, occasionally eventuates

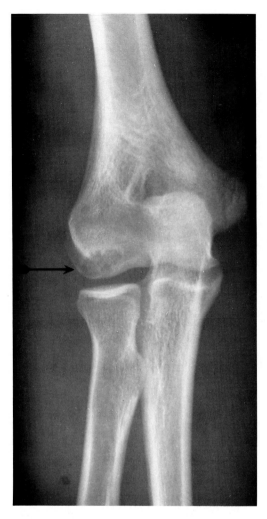

FIG. 30-8. Osteochondrosis of the humeral capitellum is manifested roentgenographically by irregular, radiolucent cyst formation in the involved area (*arrow*).

in the development of a bony ossicle within the substance of the infrapatellar tendon in the vicinity of its insertion (Fig. 30-12). The development of a fibrous nonunion or bursa between the ossicle and the tibial tuberosity may cause pain with activity or kneeling. Usually, such a lesion responds to conservative management with application of cold and protective padding. When the patient's activities are limited because of discomfort, excision of the ossicle may be indicated. The lesion is simply shelled out of the

tendon through an incision, with the tendon split in line with the long axis of its fibers.

Osteochondritis dissecans involving the femoral condyle is actually three separate and distinct entities. Variations in the ossification pattern of the distal femoral epiphysis may result in radiolucent roentgenographic defects in the knees of the preadolescent, which may well be bilaterally symmetrical in appearance (Fig. 30-13). An incidental roentgenographic finding, this "abnormality" is usually discovered when roentgenograms are taken to investigate other complaints. With continued growth and development of the epiphysis, the appearance becomes more nearly normal. No treatment or limitation of activity is indicated. The osteosclerotic form of osteochondritis dissecans of the femoral condyle presents a well-circumscribed radiodense lesion (Fig. 30-14) that may or may not be symptomatic and may or may not heal *in situ.* The radiolucent form of osteochondritis dissecans presents roentgenographically as a large radiolucent defect involving most of the articular surface of the involved condyle (Fig. 30-15). This lesion also may or may not heal *in situ.*

It has been our experience with both the osteosclerotic and radiolucent lesions that the clinical course is difficult to predict on the basis of roentgenographic appearance. When either lesion is not associated with objective findings such as quadriceps atrophy or fusion, careful observation suffices. When objective findings are associated with the lesion, arthroscopic examination of the joint is indicated. If the articular cartilage is unaffected, drilling the lesion, with subsequent immobilization and no weight bearing, often effects healing.

Despite appropriately employed conservative and surgical approaches, the lesion can separate partially or completely and become a free-floating loose body. In osteosclerotic lesions, in which the defect is usually less than one third of the width of the articulating surface of the condyle, simple excision of the lesion achieves a satisfactory result. However, for separation of an osteolytic lesion, which is usually quite large and encompasses more than half of the joint surface, the fragment must be

FIG. 30-9. Findings at surgery reveal a circumscribed area of articular cartilage necrosis involving the capitellar surface. This disease process will eventually produce ejection of osteochondral loose bodies into the joint, requiring surgical removal.

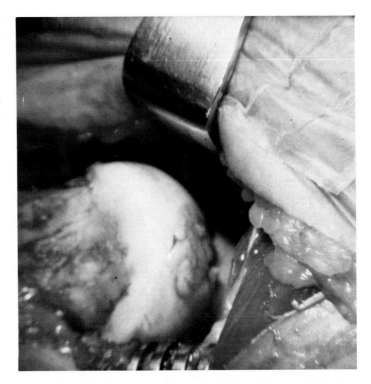

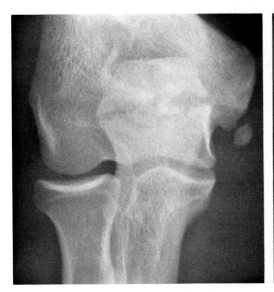
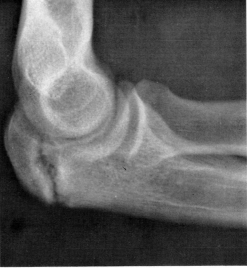

FIG. 30-10. Anteroposterior and lateral roentgenograms of the pitching-arm elbow of a 16-year-old boy demonstrate a stress fracture through the olecranon epiphyseal plate. The transverse, irregular radiolucency with sclerotic borders is observed across the proximal part of the olecranon. The lesion involves the site of a former epiphyseal plate of the olecranon. The roentgenographic picture is consistent with that of a fracture nonunion. Also noted on the anteroposterior view is a small, oval radiopacity that represents a residuum of the fragmentation of the medial epicondylar apophysis.

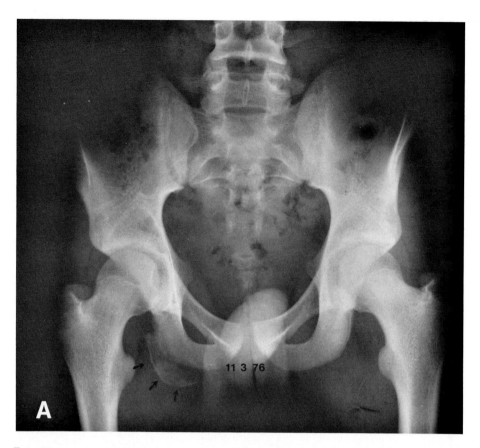

Fig. 30-11. (*A*) Anteroposterior roentgenogram of the pelvis of a 16-year-old boy demonstrates an avulsion of the right ischial apophysis (*arrows*). (*B*) Roentgenogram obtained 5 months after the injury demonstrates incomplete healing of the avulsed fragment. The patient complained of pain on activity or sitting. At surgery there was a fibrous union of the fragment. Removal of the fragment resolved the complaints.

reattached in its bed. The bed should be meticulously denuded of all fibrous tissue before the fragment is reinserted and fixed with either Smillie nails or cross-threaded Steinmann pins that can be withdrawn percutaneously.

Lesions of the Growth Plate. The epiphyseal plate, or growth plate, is the weakest link in the musculoskeletal chain of a juvenile athlete. Whereas in a skeletally mature person, a force exerted on a joint in a plane other than that of its normal motion will cause disruption of a ligament or fracture, in the juvenile athlete it will cause an injury to the epiphyseal plate. Salter has classified these injuries and has called attention to the fact that when a

fracture crosses the epiphyseal plate or compressive forces destroy the germinal cell layer, angular deformities can occur.[63] Attention should be called, also, to the fact that in fractures through but not across the plate, inadequate reduction or loss of reduction can also result in malunion.

Angular deformities at the knee may result from injury to the distal femoral or proximal tibial epiphyseal plates. A genu varum or genu valgum deformity exceeding 10° is unacceptable and should be corrected (Fig. 30-16). We have found the Moore osteotomy–osteoclasis technique to be well suited for correcting these problems.[55] The femur is exposed at the metaphyseal–diaphyseal junction. With care taken to pre-

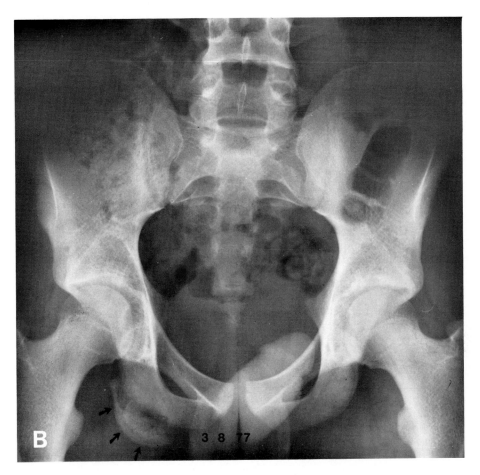

FIG. 30-11. (*Continued*)

serve the periosteum, an incomplete oste-otomy is performed, and a wedge of bone three quarters of the diameter of the part is removed, with its base directed toward the concavity of the deformity. The wedge is then reduced to small fragments and placed back in the defect, and the perios-teum is carefully closed. The extremity is immobilized in a hip spica cast. After 3 weeks a wedge of plaster is removed from the cast, and a manual osteoclasis is per-formed under radiographic guidance. At this point the osteotomy site will have a "lead-pipe" malleability, and enough an-gulation is taken to achieve the desired result (Fig. 30-17). The cast is sealed, and the patient may walk on crutches without bearing weight. When the osteotomy is stable, the cast is removed, and the patient is placed on a non-weight-bearing, crutch-

walking rehabilitation program. Actual weight bearing is not permitted for 4 months.

Injury to the knee of the juvenile with a patent epiphysis may well be an undis-placed fracture through the growth plate. "Unstable" knees in this age group should be examined under anesthesia with stress films to demonstrate whether the apparent instability is due to ligamentous disruption or an undisplaced fracture through the growth plate (Fig. 30-18). Needless to say, undisplaced epiphyseal fractures do not warrant surgical intervention for either di-agnosis or treatment.

The Value of Roentgenography

Evaluation of knee complaints in a ju-venile patient should always include roent-genographic examination. Although lesions

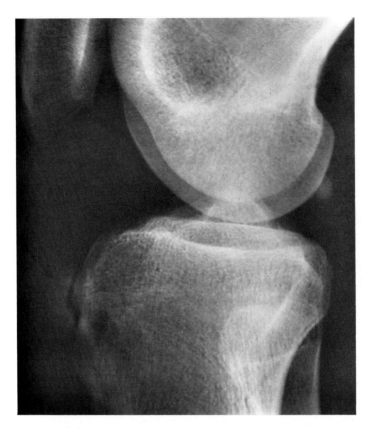

FIG. 30-12. Lateral roentgenogram of the knee demonstrates a large bony ossicle within the substance of the infrapatellar tendon. This lesion, which is a sequela of Osgood-Schlatter's disease, may require surgical excision if it is painful.

common in adults (ligamentous and meniscal derangements) are rarely demonstrable by x-ray, in juveniles roentgenograms are frequently diagnostic. The relative frequency with which benign and malignant tumors occur in the vicinity of the knee joint in juveniles emphasizes the necessity of a thorough diagnostic workup.

COMPLICATIONS OF ATHLETIC INJURIES IN YOUNG ADULTS

Myositis Ossificans

Traumatic myositis ossificans can occur as a complication of a direct-blow injury to muscle.[35,66] Heterotopic bone and cartilage formation ocurs in the substance of moderately and severely contused muscle tissue for reasons yet undetermined.[58,73] The problem does not occur in instances of pure muscle strain injury. Propensity for the development of myositis ossificans is related to the severity of the initial injury and to reinjury during recovery. Aegerter and Kirkpatrick[4] and Gilmer and Anderson[28]

have described the histologic sequence of the process. Examination of the involved muscle tissue reveals an edematous inflammatory reaction, with an exudative cellular infiltration the initial response to hemorrhage. Collagen formation then occurs, and this collagen undergoes dystrophic calcification. This is followed by metaplasia of the collagenoblasts into osteoblasts and chondroblasts. The vigorous osteoblastic activity that follows produces many immature and hyperchromatic osteoblasts that form irregular, crude osteoid. Aegerter and Kirkpatrick caution that it may be impossible to distinguish myositis ossificans from osteosarcoma solely on the basis of histologic findings.[4]

Clinically, within 24 hours of the injury, the involved thigh becomes significantly enlarged and painful, with associated warmth of the involved area. Joint motion becomes significantly limited, and there is usually an associated effusion. The key to clinical recognition of an incipient myositis ossificans is the remarkable warmth of the

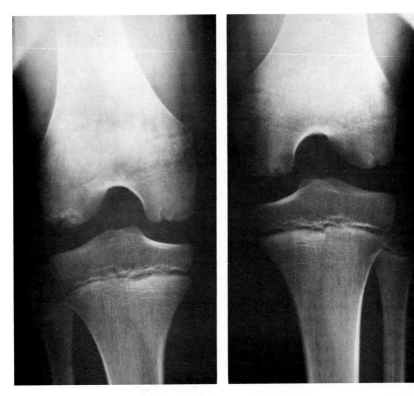

FIG. 30-13. Anteroposterior roentgenograms of both knees demonstrate symmetrical defects in both the medial and lateral femoral condyles, anomalies of ossification. These normal variations of ossification of the distal femoral epiphysis are uncommon in preadolescents. Treatment is contraindicated.

lesion and the associated decrease in joint motion.

Roentgenographic changes occur 2 to 4 weeks after the injury and initially consist of a "cotton candy" appearance of the lesion. As the lesion matures, it becomes more "osseous" in appearance. In the milder forms the lesion may be reabsorbed. With repeated insult, massive projection of bone may form (Fig. 30-19).

Initial management entails recognition of the problem; simply, a warm contusion is an incipient myositis ossificans. Jackson and Feagin have divided the treatment program

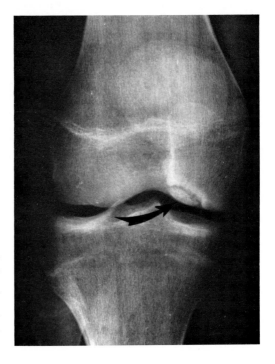

FIG. 30-14. Anteroposterior roentgenogram of the knee demonstrates an osteosclerotic form of osteochondritis dissecans involving the lateral portion of the medial femoral condyle (*arrow*). When associated with clinical signs and symptoms, if the articular cartilage is intact, this lesion should be drilled to stimulate healing.

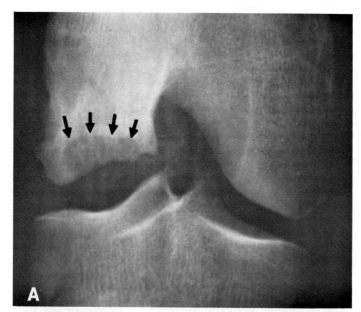

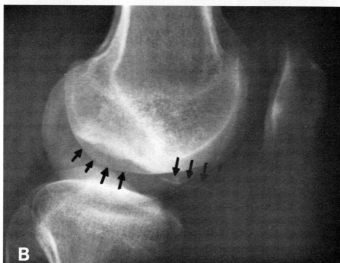

FIG. 30-15. Anteroposterior (*A*) and lateral (*B*) projections of the knee demonstrate a large, osteolytic osteochondritis dissecans lesion of the lateral femoral condyle (*arrows*). Anterior displacement of the fragment is evident on the lateral view. Such a lesion should be replaced in its bed and fixed internally.

into three phases, each dealing with a specific aspect of the problem: hemorrhage and inflammation, restricted knee motion, and muscle weakness.[37]

Phase I of treatment is directed toward minimizing hemorrhage and inflammation and consists of rest, elevation, and compression of the part. Ice should be applied to the lesion. There is absolutely no place for the use of heat, in any form, in the management of this or the later phases. Massage and range-of-motion exercises should also be avoided.

Phase II begins when the warmth of the lesion has abated and active control of the muscle has been regained. Active range-of-motion exercises are initiated. When the quadriceps is involved, primary emphasis is on regaining full knee extension. When full extension and 90° of knee flexion are reached, the patient moves into the next phase. This part of the program must be carefully supervised by a physical therapist or an athletic trainer experienced in the management of sports injuries.

During phase III, progressive resistance

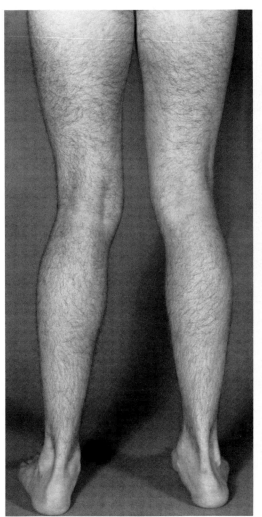 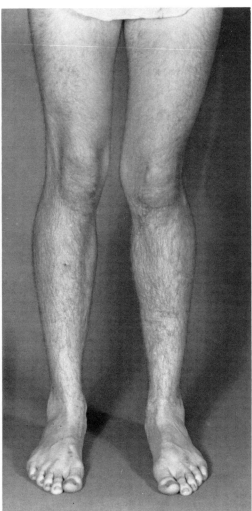

FIG. 30-16. The lower extremities of a 16-year-old youngster who sustained a Salter class V distal femoral epiphyseal injury playing football. A 17° valgus deformity resulted.

exercises are added to restore full strength as well as motion. Also, during this phase the patient may begin conditioning and agility exercises and may participate in non-contact activities.

Depending on the severity of the initial injury, delays in the institution of appropriate treatment, and episodes of reinjury, myositis ossificans may run a protracted course. In the best of circumstances, in severe cases, disability may last 3 to 6 months.

Surgery has a limited place in the management of myositis ossificans. A satisfac-

tory result can be achieved with carefully supervised nonsurgical measures. Lipscomb and co-workers believe that surgery is indicated in instances in which a large mass of mature lamellar bone is associated with pain, muscle weakness, and a significant loss of joint motion.[46]

Stress Fracture

Repeated deformation of a relatively inelastic material in alternating compression and tension can result in fatigue failure of the material. Earlier reports described march fractures, which occurred in military re-

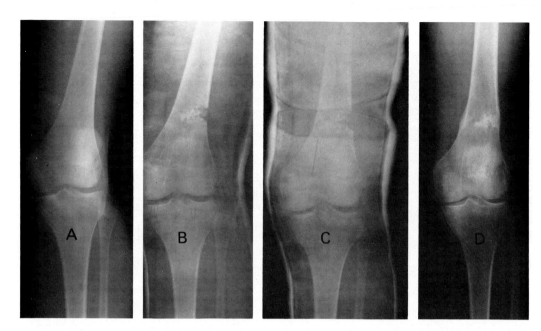

FIG. 30-17. Roentgenograms demonstrate the sequential steps of the Moore osteotomy–osteoclasis technique to correct angular deformity of long bones. (*A*) Preoperatively there was a 17° genu valgum deformity. (*B*) A roentgenogram was taken following incomplete osteotomy of the distal femur; the osteotomy site was protected by a plaster-of-paris cast. (*C*) Roentgenogram taken after osteoclasis demonstrates correction of the angular deformity. (*D*) Roentgenogram made 4 months after the initial osteotomy demonstrates correction of the angular deformity and healing at the osteotomy site.

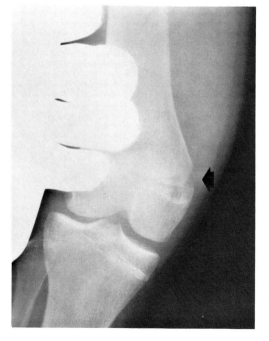

cruits, fresh from civilian life, who were taken on forced marches during basic training.[42,44,50,57] More recently, the more appropriate term *stress fracture* has been adopted, and these lesions have become commonplace among distance runners and other athletes, such as basketball and soccer players, who do a great deal of running.[21,62] The history is characterized by a vague discomfort, usually prevalent while sprinting or after activity, roentgenograms that are negative for 2 to 4 weeks after the onset of the complaints, and involvement primarily of the bones of the lower extremities. The incidence of the various involved bones

FIG. 30-18. Stress roentgenogram of the knee obtained with the benefit of general anesthesia reveals that the apparent medial instability is due to a nondisplaced fracture (*arrow*) through the distal femoral epiphysis.

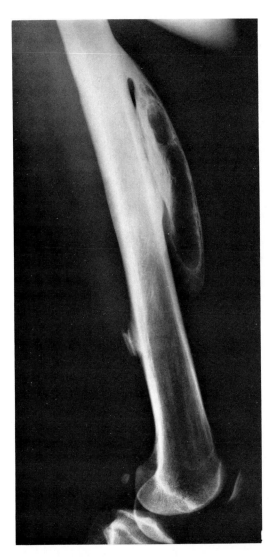

FIG. 30-19. Lateral roentgenogram of the femur and soft tissues of the thigh shows a massive myositis ossificans. This lesion was demonstrated in a 34-year-old athlete who had successfully completed twelve seasons as a professional basketball player.

When the lesion occurs in the tibia or fibula, it should be differentiated from shin splints and anterior compartment syndrome. In any bone, the stress fracture may be confused with a benign reactive process such as osteoid osteoma or with a malignant tumor. Because of the onion-skin appearance of the periosteal elevation, the roent-

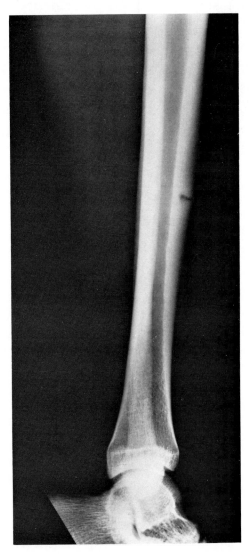

is as follows: fibula 25%, metatarsals 20%, tibia 20%, os calcis 15%, femur 10%, and others 10%.[47] When roentgenograms eventually demonstrate change, it is usually secondary to periosteal elevation that may present an onion-skin appearance. Defects to all or part of one cortex may be visualized, but not always (Fig. 30-20).

FIG. 30-20. Lateral roentgenogram of the tibia of a 20-year-old college football player demonstrates a stress fracture involving the anterior cortex at mid-shaft. There is no evidence of periosteal new bone, but characteristic involvement of one cortex is clearly demonstrated.

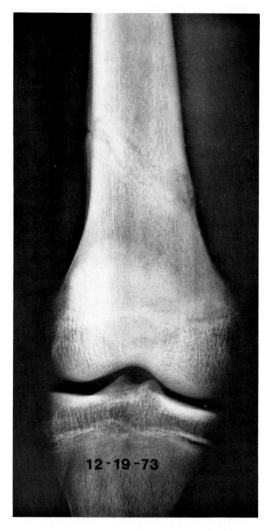

12-19-73

FIG. 30-21. Anteroposterior roentgenogram of the distal femur of a 16-year-old cross-country runner demonstrates a stress fracture complicated by a superimposed traumatic fracture. Periosteal new bone formation associated with a full-thickness lytic defect raised suspicions of a malignant tumor. However, patience and plaster casting resulted in uncomplicated healing.

genogram may be erroneously interpreted as representing an osteogenic sarcoma (Fig. 30-21). The histologic appearance of reactive new bone formation may also be similar to that observed in osteogenic sarcoma. Obviously, amputation of the limb because of mistaken diagnosis must be avoided. A high index of suspicion of the possibility of a stress fracture in a person engaged in excessive activity associated with a characteristic roentgenographic picture should establish the proper diagnosis.

Treatment of stress fractures consists of resting and protecting the involved bone. Plaster immobilization is not necessary. However, the patient should not be exposed to direct impact trauma until the lesion is symptom free and roentgenographically healed. Direct impact to the area of stress fracture can convert the lesion to a complete break through the entire bone. Should this occur, the basic principles of fracture management should be employed, consisting of accurate reduction and plaster-of-paris or another appropriate form of immobilization, until the lesion heals.

Drug Treatment in Athletic Injuries

Therapeutic agents used to counteract the local inflammatory response to injury include the corticosteroids and phenylbutazone. The rationale for their use is that with acute trauma or chronic irritation to muscles, tendons, ligaments, bursae, and synovia, local hyperemia, interstitial hemorrhage, edema, and transudates that impede healing and cause pain occur. Presumably, these agents act to impede this inflammatory response and thus facilitate healing and earlier return to function. However, it must be understood that their use in this manner is entirely a matter of personal choice and totally unsubstantiated by any acceptable clinical or laboratory evidence. Also, the use of the corticosteroids and phenylbutazone in this area involves both theoretical and real risks.

The natural and synthetic corticosteroids have numerous pharmacologic actions. The effect sought when they are used in sports medicine is the modification of the inflammatory response by stabilization of lysosomes. There is also, however, an associated inhibition of fibroblast proliferation and an increase in collagen breakdown. Those particular derivatives whose relative potencies are greatest in this respect are triamcinolone, paramethasone, betamethasone, and dexamethasone. In that it is accepted that a single dose of corticosteroid is virtually without harmful systemic effects, it appears reasonable that these drugs should be used in certain instances in which trauma has induced an inflammatory response but in which subsequent tissue repair is not anticipated. Conditions meeting these criteria are acute and chronic tenosynovitis and bursitis, tennis elbow, chronic rotator cuff strains, hemarthrosis without ligamentous injury, synovitis secondary to degenerative changes, and mild ligament sprains. In any situation in which there is disruption of normal tissue stability, such as an incomplete or complete muscle or ligament tear, corticosteroids are contraindicated because of their adverse effect on the reparative processes.

Because of their pronounced anti-inflammatory effect, hydrocortisone (Compound E) and its derivatives have been injected directly into tendon sheaths and tendon substance itself in the treatment of tenosynovitis. Acute rupture of the Achilles, peroneal, and suprapatellar tendons has been reported in the literature following repeated local injections of insoluble corticosteroid.[8,9,18,36,43] Unverferth postulated that rupture occurred because the symptoms of tenosynovitis were masked by the corticosteroids.[74] In addition, he was able to demonstrate in a controlled study that frequent, repeated corticosteroid injections into the Achilles tendon of a rabbit resulted in an average difference of 35% in the modulus of elasticity when compared to tendons injected with saline. Thus, in addition to masking symptoms, it appears that the corticosteroid actually causes a decrease in tensile strength and contributes to tendon destruction, particularly when the injection enters the tendon itself.[38]

Phenylbutazone (Butazolidin), an oral, nonhormonal anti-inflammatory agent, is effective in diminishing the inflammatory response to acute and chronic trauma. A decision to use this agent in an otherwise young, healthy adult must be weighed against the known toxic effects on the gastrointestinal tract and hematopoietic system. Specifically, adverse reactions may include ulcerative esophagitis, acute and reactive gastric and duodenal ulceration with perforation and hemorrhage, ulceration and perforation of the large bowel, occult gastrointestinal bleeding with anemia, and gastritis. Phenylbutazone has been reported to cause agranulocytosis, aplastic anemia, hemolytic anemia, thrombocytopenia, pancytopenia, and general bone marrow depression. In addition, the drug may be responsible for allergic dermatologic reactions. Because of the unpredictability and severity of the potential side-effects of phenylbutazone, each patient should be forewarned of them, and a complete blood count should be performed every 2 weeks. The manufacturer recommends that the therapeutic goal be short-term relief of severe symptoms with the smallest possible doses. The effect of the drug is usually manifest by the third or fourth day of treatment. If a favorable clinical response does not occur by this time, use of the drug should be discontinued. The dosage should be reduced when improvement of symptoms occurs, and use of the drug should be discontinued as soon as possible. To minimize gastric upset, phenylbutazone should be taken with meals. Its use is absolutely contraindicated in children 14 years or younger.

Complications in the Shoulder

Acromioclavicular Joint Injury.   Injury to the acromioclavicular joint is not an uncommon problem in sports medicine. The mechanism of injury is basically impact to the point of the shoulder, which depresses the acromion in relation to the clavicle. Injury to the joint, its capsule, and the other supporting structures, namely the coracoclavicular ligament and the attachments of the trapezius and deltoid muscles, may occur in various degrees of severity. First-degree sprain of the acromioclavicular joint occurs when the capsule is stretched but structural stability is not lost. However, there is a meniscus in this joint, and in first- and second-degree sprains this structure can be deranged. Second-degree sprains involve rupture of the joint capsule without disruption of the coracoclavicular ligament. Third-degree sprains of the acromioclavicular joint involve disruption of both the joint capsule and the coracoclavicular ligament. Fourth-degree sprains are those in which there is also disruption of the supporting attachments of the trapezius and deltoid muscles. As a general guide, first- and second-degree sprains are treated conservatively, third-degree sprains may be treated either conservatively or by open methods, and fourth-degree sprains generally require open reduction and fixation.

Bergfeld has demonstrated that in the athlete it is generally first- and second-degree sprains that leave the patient with residual problems.[10] Reviewing 128 first- and second-degree injuries treated by conservative methods, including symptomatic, simple sling, acromioclavicular splints, and injection with lidocaine (Xylocaine) and cortisone, Bergfeld carried out a follow-up consisting of both clinical and roentgenographic examination. Of the patients with first-degree sprains, 39% had residual symptoms; 9% were judged to be significant. Of 31 patients with second-degree sprains, 65% were symptomatic; 20% of these were considered significant. Residual abnormal physical findings—cosmetic deformity, swelling, decreased mobility, pain with stress or palpation, and crepitus—were present in 43% of the first-degree sprains. Roentgenographic changes, consisting of resorption of the distal clavicle with periarticular calcification and deformity, occurred in 29% of the first-degree sprains and 48% of the second-degree sprains (Fig. 30-22). Thus, it is evident that in the athlete, management of first- and second-degree acromioclavicular sprains by currently accepted methods results in residual complaints and abnormal physical and roentgenographic findings in a significant number of patients. Bergfeld concluded that "when subjected to critical analysis, the first- and second-degree sprain of the AC joint is a more significant problem than commonly believed."[10]

Nuisance complaints resulting from first- and second-degree sprains may be treated with ice, analgesics, and judicious use of intra-articular corticosteroids. However, when there is significant disability accompanied by roentgenograms demonstrating changes involving the distal end of the clavicle, resection may be indicated. To be emphasized is the fact that resection of the distal end as described by Mumford should not be performed if the coracoclavicular ligament has been disrupted. Also, resection of the segment of the clavicle should include all of the clavicle to the outermost insertion of the coracoclavicular ligament. Under no circumstances should the supporting structures be violated. If too short a segment is removed, a painful, deformed pseudojoint may result.

Complications following treatment of third- and fourth-degree acromioclavicular joint disruption in athletes do not appear to be a problem. However, if the athlete is disabled after treatment for this injury, it must be kept in mind that simple resection of the distal end of the clavicle with disruption of the coracoclavicular ligament will result in elevation of the distal end of the clavicle and loss of its strutting effect. A procedure that combines resection of the distal end of the clavicle with a reconstruction of the coracoacromial ligament as described by Weaver and Dunn is indicated.[75] It must be emphasized, however, that normal roentgenograms or cosmetic deformity alone are not indications for these procedures; rather, they should be reserved for those patients who have significant pain and disability.

Clavicle Fractures. Fractures of the shaft of the clavicle may occur to the inner, middle, or outer thirds. With the exception of that occurring at the distal tip, nonunion should be treated by bone graft with the Phemister technique (Fig. 30-23).

Nonunion of fractures to the lateral tip of the clavicle in which there is integrity of the coracoclavicular ligament may be treated by simple excision of the fragment (Fig. 30-24). If, however, the attachment of the coracoclavicular ligament is involved in the site of nonunion, bone grafting is mandatory (Fig. 30-25).

Glenohumeral Joint Dislocation. Recurrent anterior dislocation or subluxation of the glenohumeral joint is a predictable sequela of abduction-external rotation injuries that result in separation of the cartilaginous labyrinth or fracture of the bony glenoid (Fig. 30-26). Rarely does the defect heal, regardless of the period of immobilization. A young, active athlete will again disengage the humeral head from the glenoid whenever he repeats, with force, the movement that caused the initial injury.

Those who experience recurrent anterior dislocation only while participating in their activity and not otherwise, may solve the problem by wearing a shoulder harness of

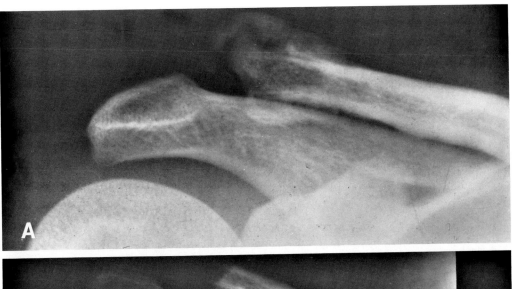

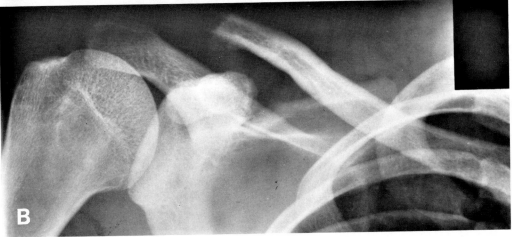

FIG. 30-22. (*A*) Roentgenogram of a first-degree acromioclavicular sprain complicated by resorption of the distal clavicle associated with periarticular calcification and deformity. (*B*) In the presence of an intact coracoclavicular ligament, resection of the distal end of the clavicle removes the source of the patient's complaint yet does not disrupt the strutting effect of the clavicle on the scapula.

the Dennison-Wyre type, which prevents abduction of the humerus. For those whose activity precludes the use of a harness or who experience difficulty in everyday activities, surgical intervention should be considered. We tend to agree with Allman[6] and other proponents of the modified Bristow procedure as the operation of choice for recurrent subluxation or dislocation.[17,31,52]

Incidence of recurrence following the Bristow procedure is low, on the order of 2% to 3% (Fig. 30-27). The major problem following the procedure occurs in the throwing athlete because of limitation of external humeral rotation. Lombardo and colleagues reported the average limitation to be 11° of external rotation, and in their series of 51 cases, no patient regained his preinjury throwing ability following surgery.[47]

Posterior glenohumeral joint dislocation occurs infrequently. The mechanism is the opposite of that which produces anterior dislocation, that is, adduction and internal rotation of the humerus. Because of the

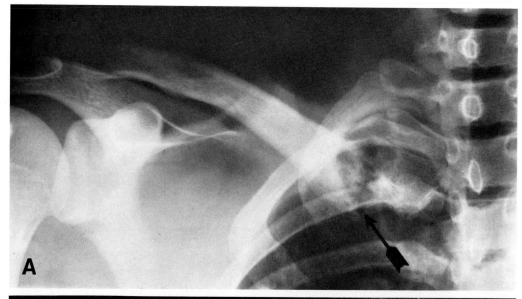

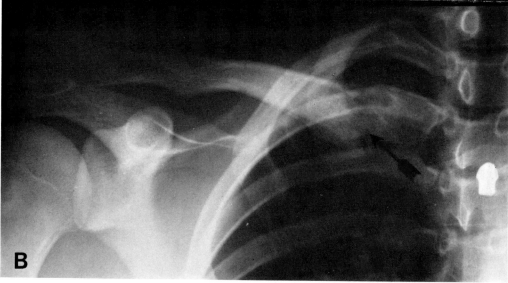

FIG. 30-23. (*A*) Roentgenogram demonstrates a fracture of the inner third of the clavicle (*arrow*) that failed to unite despite 6 weeks of figure-eight immobilization. The patient was a college quarterback who complained of pain and weakness on attempting to throw the football. (*B*) A Phemister onlay graft and 8 weeks' immobilization in a shoulder spica cast produced union across the fracture site (*arrow*).

relatively normal attitude of the involved extremity and the deceptive roentgenographic appearance of the lesion in the anteroposterior projection (Fig. 30-28, *A*), a posterior glenohumeral dislocation may be overlooked by the unwary examiner. A key to diagnosis is the inability of the patient to rotate the humerus externally past neutral. Axillary-projection roentgenograms will not have the deceptive appearance of standard anteroposterior views (Fig. 30-28, *B*). Reduction of a missed glenohumeral dislo-

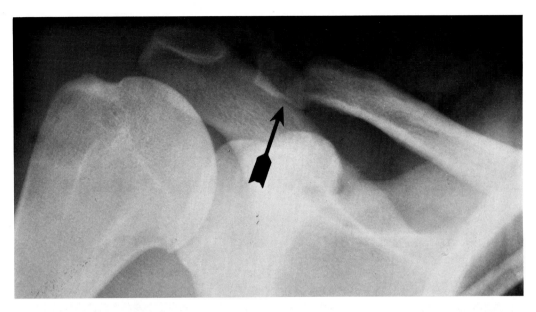

FIG. 30-24. A 24-year-old professional football quarterback experienced delayed union of a fracture involving the distal tip of the clavicle (*arrow*). The fracture was not diagnosed when it first occurred, and the patient subsequently felt pain and weakness when throwing. Because the lesion is distal to the attachment of the coracoclavicular ligament, simple resection of the fragment resolved the problem.

cation should first be attempted by closed manipulation performed under general anesthesia. If this is unsuccessful, open reduction is indicated. There is no single clearly superior procedure for definitive surgical correction of recurrent posterior dislocation of the shoulder. The literature describes shortening of the infraspinatus muscle to prevent internal rotation, posterior bone block, and scapular osteotomy.

Complications in the Hand

The most common injuries to the hands of athletes are those involving the proximal interphalangeal (PIP) joints. Because coaches and players alike tend to treat PIP injuries as inconsequential, significant problems are frequently compounded by neglect. McCue and co-workers have described a group of lesions that, when undiagnosed and mistreated for several months, develop into painful, stiff, deformed fingers that they call *coach's fingers.*[49] Included in this group are neglected collateral ligament injuries, articular fractures, fracture-dislocations, boutonnière deformities, and "pseudo-boutonnière" deformities.

Complete collateral ligament ruptures commonly involve the vulnerable radial collateral ligament of the middle joint. The injuries may be divided into two groups: acute (those treated within 3 months of injury) and chronic (those treated more than 3 months after injury). Operative repair is indicated for all complete lesions. Chronic lesions are reconstructed by transferring the adjacent sublimis slip to the proximal end of the collateral ligament.

Articular fractures involving the interphalangeal joints in which there is condylar displacement or an oblique fracture involving more than one quarter of the articular surface are best treated by open reduction and internal fixation (Fig. 30-29). Also, displaced volar lip fractures may go on to dorsal subluxation and are likewise treated surgically (Fig. 30-30).

Interphalangeal dislocations are frequently, and perhaps appropriately, reduced by the coach or trainer. If treatment stops

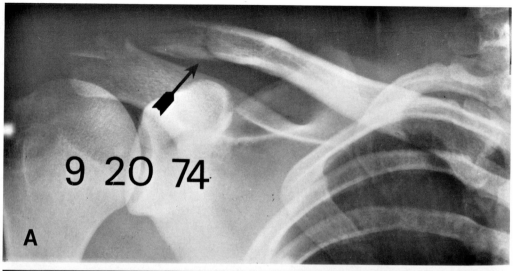

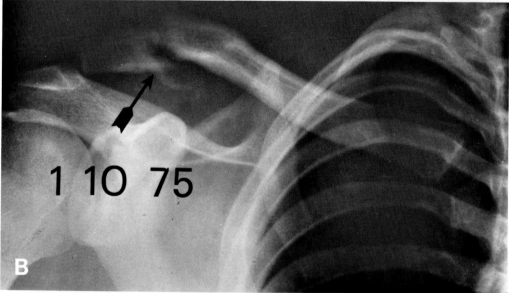

FIG. 30-25. (*A*) Because of inadequate immobilization, this fracture of the distal third of the clavicle proximal to the insertion of the coracoclavicular ligament (*arrow*) subsequently became displaced, and delayed union occurred. (*B*) Elevation of the fragments is due to the loss of the restraining effect of the coracoclavicular ligament. Simple excision of the distal fragment is contraindicated. This particular problem was rectified by a Phemister onlay bone graft and adequate immobilization in a shoulder spica cast (*arrow*).

here and if there is a fracture involving the volar lip of the base of the middle phalanx with an associated dorsal subluxation of the joint, a stiff and painful finger is inevitable. All dislocations should be x-rayed. In addition, examination of joint stability under metacarpal block is also indicated. In the event of an unstable fracture-dislocation or dislocation, operative stabilization of the joint is indicated.

Boutonnière Deformity. Traumatic disruption of the central slip from the dorsal

FIG. 30-26. Fracture of the anterior bony glenoid (*arrow*) is often associated with subluxation or dislocation of the glenohumeral joint. However, in most instances, the defect is separation of the cartilaginous labrum from the glenoid, a situation not discernible on roentgenograms.

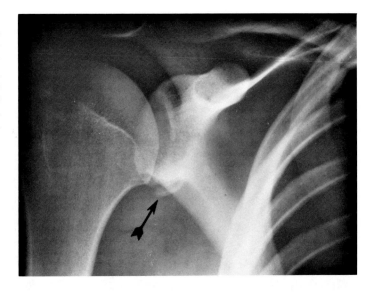

lip of the middle phalanx, if untreated, will lead to a boutonnière deformity with hyperextension of the proximal and distal joints and flexion of the middle joint. When there is point tenderness over the dorsal lip of the middle phalanx, this joint should be immobilized in full extension in such a way that active and passive flexion of the distal joint is permitted. With this form of immobilization, an athlete may continue his

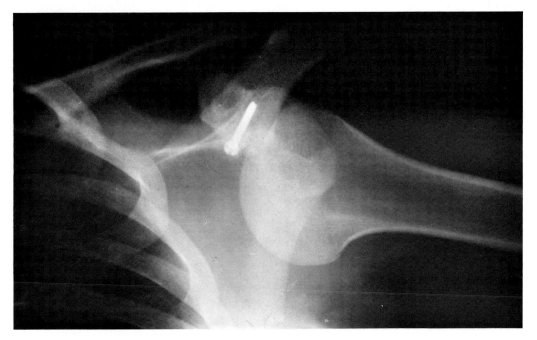

FIG. 30-27. A rare complication following a Bristow procedure for recurrent dislocation of the shoulder is redislocation. The probable cause, in this instance, is that the transplanted coracoid was placed too high, as indicated by the position of the coracoid screw.

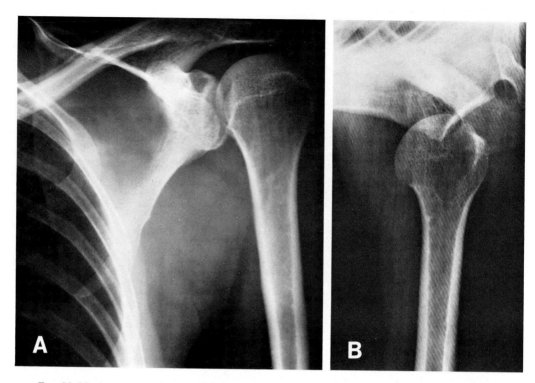

FIG. 30-28. Anteroposterior (*A*) and axillary (*B*) views of the glenohumeral joint demonstrate posterior dislocation of the humeral head in relation to the glenoid. The appearance in the anteroposterior view is somewhat deceptive, but there is no question as to the nature of the lesion in the axillary projection.

activity without interruption. In cases seen late or in which splinting has failed, surgical intervention is indicated.

"Pseudo-boutonnière" deformity can result from a hyperextension injury to the middle joint. McCue and associates describe four diagnostic features: (1) flexion contracture of the middle joint, (2) slight hyperextension of the distal joint, (3) roentgenographic evidence of calcification, and (4) a history of hyperextension injuries to the middle joint.[49] He also identifies mild and severe forms. A mild "pseudo-boutonnière" deformity is a flexion deformity of less than 40° and responds to prolonged splinting. The severe deformity has more than 45° of flexion in the middle joint and cannot be controlled by splinting. Surgical intervention is necessary for the severe form.

Complications in the Knee

Problems related to the management of knee injuries in athletes remain among the most vexing to the orthopaedist. Complications may result from surgical and nonsurgical methods of treatment. For example, conservative management of a traumatic insult to the knee may be followed by recurrent effusion, buckling, instability, and general deterioration of the joint, but the same sequence of events may be observed after treatment by surgical intervention. In either instance, an exact diagnosis of the specific anatomical derangement or structural deficiency is necessary if appropriate measures are to be taken to solve the problem.

Anterior Cruciate Instability. Failure of the acutely traumatized knee of an athlete to respond to the basic conservative modalities of rest and rehabilitation of the involved joint can, in most instances, be attributed to inaccurate diagnosis of the nature of the injury. The most frequently overlooked problem is a twisting injury to the knee in which no instability can be

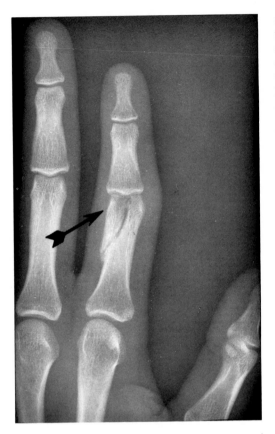

69% of knees operated on for various derangements. Also, the anterior cruciate ligament was torn in 79% of those operated on for lesions of the medial meniscus. We would certainly concur with Allman, who has stated that "isolated tear of the anterior cruciate ligament is the beginning of the end for the athlete."[6] The instability created by anterior cruciate ligament deficiency results in posterior subluxation of the medial femoral condyle on the tibia with tearing and/or posterior peripheral separation of the posterior horn of the medial meniscus. Once the stabilizing effect of the medial meniscus is disrupted, there is tearing and subsequent laxity of the medial capsular and posterior medial corner. Subsequently, there is disruption of the integrity of the lateral meniscus and its attachments with increasing instability and disability.

FIG. 30-29. Anteroposterior roentgenogram of the index finger of a 16-year-old football player demonstrates malunion of an intercondylar, intra-articular spiral fracture involving the proximal interphalangeal joint (*arrow*). There is disruption of the joint surface as well as angular deformity of the digit. The patient would have benefited from open reduction and internal fixation of this lesion.

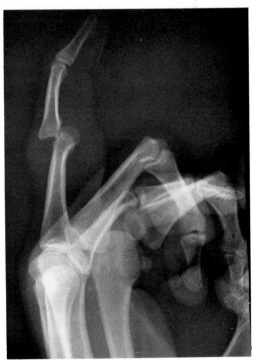

demonstrated. If the athlete heard or felt a snap or a pop and a hemarthrosis subsequently developed, the most likely diagnosis is an "isolated" tear of the anterior cruciate ligament. Failure to diagnose this lesion accurately may be attributed to uncertainty (among some physicians) as to whether such an injury can occur, the inability of the anterior drawer test to demonstrate a pure anterior cruciate ligament deficiency, and unfamiliarity with other clinical, arthrographic, and arthroscopic methods of confirming the diagnosis.

It has been our experience that the anterior cruciate ligament has been torn in

FIG. 30-30. Lateral roentgenogram of the index finger of a 16-year-old football player who had "sprained" his finger 6 weeks earlier shows obvious dorsal dislocation of the proximal interphalangeal joint, which is secondary to instability caused by disruption of the volar plate. McCue has called this lesion "coach's finger."

Drawer Sign. Classically, the orthopaedist has been taught that a clinical diagnosis of anterior cruciate instability is contingent upon demonstration of a positive anterior drawer sign. That is, anterior translation of the tibia in its relationship with the femur when the knee is flexed to 90° and anterior stress is applied. The origin of this maneuver is obscure, but for many its validity has remained unquestioned. However, the unreliability of the drawer sign has been noted by several authorities.

On the basis of my experience with more than 500 knees with anterior cruciate ligament disruption diagnosed at surgery, I agree with those who doubt the reliability of this diagnostic test. Analysis of the factors involved reveals four causes of false-negative results of the drawer test in instances of an isolated tear of the anterior cruciate ligament. First, in the face of acute injury, isolated anterior cruciate tears are often, but not always, accompanied by a tense hemarthrosis and reaction synovitis that precludes flexion of the knee to 90°. Second, protective spasm of the hamstring muscles secondary to joint pain can, in a well-muscled, well-conditioned athlete, generate considerable force. Simple vector analysis dictates that to effect translation of the tibia in the direction opposite such a force requires an effort on the part of the examiner that would tax the capabilities of most. Third, and perhaps most important, a consideration of the medial joint compartment with the knee flexed to 90° explains the cause for difficulty in effecting anterior translation of the tibia on attempting the drawer test (Fig. 30-31). The posterior surface of the medial femoral condyle is acutely convex. This convex femoral articulating surface lies in relationship with the concavity formed by the articulating surface of the medial tibial plateau and attached medial meniscus. The spatial relationship is almost like that of a ball-and-socket joint. From the practical standpoint, it is the posterior horn of the medial meniscus buttressed against the most posterior margin of the medial femoral condyle that precludes forward translation of the tibia. Fourth, my observations indicate that significant "anterior drawering" occurs only after peripheral separation of the posterior horn of the medial meniscus or disruption of the medial capsular or posterior oblique ligament.

Lachman's Test. Lachman has, for many years, taught a simple, reliable, and reproducible clinical test to demonstrate anterior cruciate ligament instability.*,[69] The examination is performed with the patient lying supine on the table with the involved extremity on the side of the examiner. With the patient's knee held between full extension and 15° of flexion, the femur is stabilized with one hand while firm pressure is applied to the posterior aspect of the proximal tibia in an attempt to translate it anteriorly (Fig. 30-32). A positive test, indicating disruption of the anterior cruciate ligament, is one in which there is palpable anterior translation of the tibia in relation to the femur, with a characteristic "mushy" endpoint. A corollary to interpreting the test is that if question remains in the examiner's mind as to whether the test is positive or negative, the ligament is torn.

The Lachman test for anterior cruciate instability obviates the problems inherent in the classic "drawer sign." First, the position of comfort of the acutely injured and distended knee joint is one of slight flexion, the position described for performing this test. Second, the force produced by hamstring spasm is negated by testing for anterior translation of the tibia with the knee extended. The physics of static friction resolves the force necessary to translate the tibia in a direction perpendicular to the opposing force of the hamstring muscles into simply that force necessary to overcome the friction of the two surfaces plus the weight of the leg. By extending the knee, the force of the hamstrings is negated, and that necessary to overcome the friction of articular surfaces is negligible. Third, with the knee extended, that area in contact with the tibial plateau and the attached medial meniscus is the slightly convex, weight-bearing surface of the femur (Fig. 30-33). The relatively flat configuration of this surface does not obstruct forward motion of the tibia, as previously described, when the joint is flexed to 90°.

---

* Lachman, J.: Personal communication.

FIG. 30-31. This diagram shows the relationship of the medial femoral condyle, medial meniscus (*MM*), and tibia in the sagittal plane with the knee flexed to 90°, the position in which the classic drawer test is elicited. The medial meniscus, being attached to the tibia and abutting against the acutely convex configuration of the medial femoral condyle, has a "doorstop" effect; it prevents anterior translation and precludes a "positive drawer sign." Disruption of the medial capsular ligament or posterior peripheral separation of the medial meniscus, however, will permit a positive drawer sign when the anterior cruciate ligament is torn.

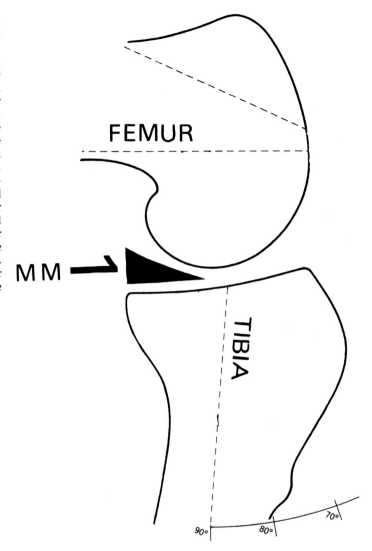

If the pitfalls of conservative management of injury to the knee are to be avoided, quite obviously, both an accurate diagnosis and an understanding of the effect of the particular deficiency on the joint are essential. Therefore, management of complications resulting from conservative treatment of the acutely injured knee first requires a diagnostic workup that, in addition to complete history, physical, and routine radiographic examination, should also include both arthrographic and arthroscopic examination of the joint. It is my opinion that with the modalities that we have at our disposal, diagnostic accuracy for the lesions occurring in the knee joint in the athlete should approach 100%. Furthermore, the orthopaedic surgeon who cares for these problems would find it to his best advantage to have facilities for reliable arthrography and to be proficient in the use of the arthroscope.

Popliteal artery thrombosis is a recognized complication of knee dislocation. If the artery is stretched to a point at which the inelastic intima is torn, with reduction of the dislocation the intima will roll up, like a window shade, and will subsequently act as a mechanical obstruction to the flow of blood (thus the term *intimal roll-up*).

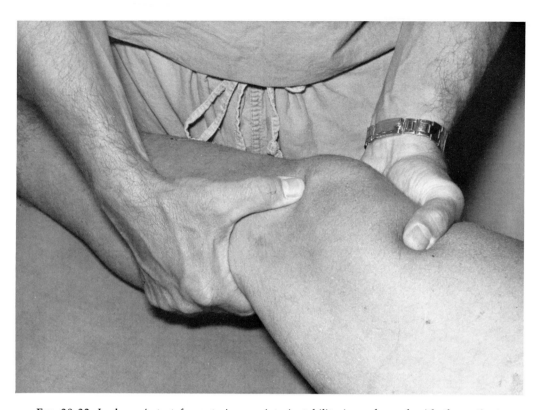

FIG. 30-32. Lachman's test for anterior cruciate instability is performed with the patient lying supine on the examining table, with the involved extremity to the side of the examiner. With the involved extremity in slight external rotation and the knee held between full extension and 15° of flexion, the femur is stabilized with one hand, and firm pressure is applied to the posterior aspect of the proximal tibia, lifting it forward in an attempt to translate it anteriorly. The position of the examiner's hands is important in performing the test properly. One hand should firmly stabilize the femur while the other grips the proximal tibia in such a way that the thumb lies on the anterior medial joint margin. When an anteriorly directed lifting force is applied by the palm and forefingers, anterior translation of the tibia with respect to the femur can be palpated with the thumb. Anterior translation of the tibia associated with a soft and mushy endpoint indicates a positive test.

Thrombosis ensues, and if the problem is not recognized, the limb is jeopardized. Green and Allen reported 51 cases of dislocated knees with popliteal artery injury.[29] Of 19 extremities with popliteal artery injury treated conservatively, 16 required amputation, while three survived. Of 21 patients who underwent arterial repair within 8 hours of the injury, 18 regained normal circulation to the leg, and only three patients required amputation. Another 11 patients had popliteal artery repair performed 8 hours or more following dislocation, and all 11 came to amputation.

The necessity of early diagnosis and arterial repair performed within 6 to 8 hours after injury is established if the limb is to survive. In view of the fact that a knee may dislocate and reduce while the patient is transported from the site of injury, the possibility of popliteal artery injury must be considered in all patients who have sustained significant trauma to the joint. Inordinate pain, paralysis, or diminution of pulses demands immediate evaluation and, if indicated, arterial surgery. An immediate arteriogram of the femoral popliteal system should be performed (Fig. 30-34); if positive,

FIG. 30-33. With the knee extended, the relationship of the femur, medial meniscus (*MM*), and tibia is significantly changed. The comparatively flat weight-bearing surface of the femur does not obstruct forward motion of the meniscus and tibia when anterior stress is applied. Thus, when there is an isolated tear of the anterior cruciate ligament, anterior stress of tibia with the knee extended will clinically demonstrate cruciate instability.

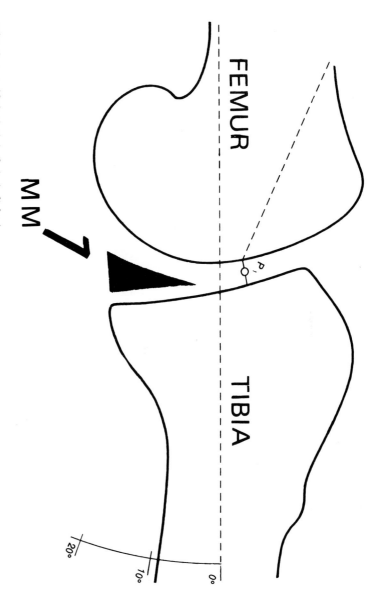

arterial surgery should ensue promptly. There is no place for expectant evaluation or treatment of this potentially catastrophic injury.

Complications of Operative Management of Knee Injuries. The most common postoperative complications seen in the knee are persistent effusion and synovitis. Causes of postsurgical effusion may be divided into four general groups: (1) persistent unresolved derangement, (2) inappropriate rehabilitation, (3) infection, and (4) joint surface erosion and/or degenerative changes.

Persistent Unresolved Derangement. The most common persistent postoperative knee effusion occurs after meniscectomy when there is associated anterior cruciate ligament insufficiency. Whereas the knee with an isolated meniscus tear will be free of effusion and synovitis within several weeks of surgery, the knee with an associated torn anterior cruciate ligament can have a persistent effusion for months following surgery. Provided that there is no other cause for the effusion and that the other supporting ligamentous structures are intact,

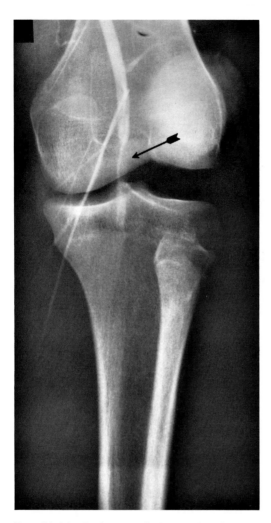

FIG. 30-34. Occlusion of the popliteal artery (*arrow*), resulting from dislocation of the knee with intimal roll-up and subsequent thrombosis formation, is demonstrated by femoral arteriography. Early arteriography is mandatory in significantly traumatized knees in which there is any question of the status of the arterial tree.

this problem is best managed by repeated aspirations to keep the joint decompressed, application of a compressive wrap, and patience; eventually the joint will dry up. It has been our experience that intra-articular corticosteroid injection and oral administration of anti-inflammatory drugs are of little benefit in resolving this postoperative problem.

Misguided surgery that has not resolved the basic mechanical abnormality will result in effusion, progressive atrophy of the thigh musculature, and persistence of preoperative symptoms. The person who has one or both menisci removed when, in fact, the primary problem is recurrent subluxation of the patella, is an excellent example of this situation; single meniscectomy when both menisci are deranged is another. Obviously, the solution to this problem is to establish an accurate diagnosis based on the principles mentioned above and to rectify the problem with more-precise surgery.

Inappropriate rehabilitation following surgery to the knee joint may well result in effusion and synovitis. That is, too little or too much exercise can present a problem. Also, stressing a knee with limited motion, either with weight bearing or with a premature isotonic exercise program, will precipitate a reactive synovitis. Rehabilitation of the joint following surgery is every bit as important in the management of the patient as is the surgery itself. Therefore, it remains the responsibility of the surgeon to ensure that the rehabilitation program is supervised by a physical therapist or athletic trainer experienced and knowledgeable in rehabilitating the postoperative knee.

Postoperative infection of the knee joint may be caused by organisms that are either highly virulent or less so. Determination of the nature of the organism is made on both the basis of the results of cultures and the clinical appearance of the patient. Management of the patient with a postoperative knee infection requires excellent judgment on the part of the surgeon. To return the patient to the operating room and open the knee infected with a low-virulence organism may well bring on more problems than it solves; failure to perform adequate drainage of an infection caused by a highly virulent organism may terminate in disaster.

A low-virulence postsurgical pyarthrosis of the knee is characterized by a boggy synovitis, relatively small effusion, low-grade fever, and minimal pain on joint motion. Unless the problem is recognized, the indolent synovitis may persist for weeks with associated marked quadriceps atrophy that only emphasizes the swollen appearance of the knee joint. Organisms responsible for this type of infection are *Staphylococcus epidermidis* and the streptococci.

When the diagnosis is entertained, the patient should be hospitalized and the synovial fluid cultured. Early definitive treatment should consist of immobilization in Buck's traction with the knee held in a position of comfort, aspiration and saline lavage of the joint twice daily until clear, and administration of 8 million to 10 million units of aqueous crystalline procaine penicillin by continuous intravenous drip.

It has been our experience that *S. epidermidis*, the organism responsible for indolent postoperative synovitis in the majority of instances, is most effectively treated by penicillin rather than by the other synthetic antistaphylococcal agents. If indicated, appropriate changes in antibiotic therapy can be made, pending results of the cultures and sensitivity studies. Usually, however, *S. epidermidis* infections are well on their way to resolving within 24 to 48 hours. When the patient has been afebrile for 48 hours, the white count has returned to normal, and the synovial fluid is sterile on culture, 8 mg of short-acting dexamethasone is injected intra-articularly. A marked improvement will be noted over the next 24 hours, and at that time a long-acting repository form of the corticosteroid is injected. With subsidence of the synovitis, the knee is then gradually mobilized to effect a return of motion, and the patient is then advanced to an isometric and isotonic exercise program, as indicated by the clinical situation. Oral antibiotic therapy is continued for a minimum of 2 weeks or until the sedimentation rate returns to normal.

Postoperative pyarthrosis with sepsis due to the more virulent organisms such as *Staphylococcus aureus* presents an entirely different situation. The distinguishing feature of the clinical picture is a septic febrile course associated with production of large quantities of purulent synovial fluid. The knee is warm, swollen, and markedly painful on motion. Deciding whether the situation warrants closed-tube or open drainage requires experienced clinical judgment. A sterile synovitis fitting the aforementioned clinical picture has been observed to follow surgery. Therefore, unless there is unequivocal evidence of bacterial sepsis, the patient should be hospitalized, placed in traction, and given intravenous antibiotics effective against penicillin-resistant *S. aureus*. Frequent joint aspirations should be performed to keep the synovial cavity decompressed. If there is no improvement within the next 24 to 48 hours and if cultures confirm a diagnosis of *S. aureus* pyarthrosis, the patient should be taken to the operating room for adequate drainage.

Complications in the Lower Leg

The anterior tibial compartment syndrome has been reported to occur as an acute entity following strenuous exercise of the lower extremities.[11,16,33,41,51,56] Pain in the muscles of the anterior compartment is the predominant symptom. Following strenuous exercise, discomfort begins as a dull ache and increases to a severe pain. It is not relieved by rest, and any motion, active or passive, exacerbates the discomfort. Weakness or paralysis of anterior compartment muscles, usually involving the anterior tibial muscle or the extensor hallucis longus, substantiates the diagnosis. Although the differential diagnosis may include stress fracture, thrombophlebitis, cellulitis, and shin splints, weakness or muscle paralysis is the differentiating factor.

Emergency fasciotomy of the anterior compartment is indicated once the diagnosis of anterior tibial compartment syndrome is made. Leach and co-workers report complete recovery if surgical release of the fascia is performed within 6 hours of the onset of symptoms.[41] If surgery is delayed, irreversible muscle necrosis and subsequent fibrosis may occur. The etiology of this syndrome is obscure.[23,27] Decreased arterial inflow has not been demonstrated to be the initial problem, so peripheral pulses may well be palpable in an acute episode.

Intermittent claudication[39] in athletes, described by Snook as ischemic myositis, is a symptom complex characterized by crampy pain in the involved muscles during exercise.[64] The discomfort is relieved by rest and returns with activity. There is no swelling, diminution of peripheral pulses, pallor, or paralysis. Pain (the predominant symptom) increases until the athlete is forced to discontinue his activity. Fasciotomy affords complete relief of symptoms and prevents the potentially catastrophic consequences of muscle necrosis.

Should muscle necrosis and subsequent fibrosis occur as a result of either acute anterior compartment syndrome or intermittent claudication, debridement of the fibrosed muscles may be indicated. Needless to say, termination of either process in frank muscle necrosis portends disaster for the athlete.

Achilles Tendon Rupture. Problems related to ruptures of the Achilles tendon are primarily the result of delay in diagnosis or rerupture due to inadequate length of immobilization. The unsuspecting examiner may fail to appreciate the lesion because the posterior tibial and peroneal tendons can perform active plantar flexion of the foot even in the presence of a complete Achilles tendon rupture. The diagnosis may be made with certainty, however, if a patient cannot stand on tiptoe and has a positive Thompson test and a palpable defect in the substance of the tendon. Also, rerupture is not uncommon in patients who underwent surgical reapproximation but were not kept immobilized long enough to ensure healing.

In managing a patient with a late diagnosis or rerupture of the Achilles tendon, institution of several basic principles will ensure success. Specifically, end-to-end apposition must be ensured by surgical intervention and fixation, and rigid immobilization of the part must be maintained for 10 weeks. My preferred method for dealing with this problem is to expose the proximal and distal segments of the tendon, freshen the ends of the tendinous stumps (back to normal-looking tendon), pass Bunnell sutures in each segment, and then approximate the ends by flexing the knee and plantar flexing the foot. The patient is then placed in a toe-to-groin cast for 6 weeks. At the end of 6 weeks, the cast is removed and a toe-to-below-knee cast is applied for an additional 6 weeks. We have not found it necessary to devise fascial flaps to effect contact.[1,12,15]

Complications in the Ankle

Incomplete Rehabilitation. The most common complication that beleaguers the athlete is the incompletely rehabilitated ankle. After healing of a moderate to severe sprain or fracture, there is always marked limitation of joint motion; specifically, the patient is unable to move the joint successfully through an effective range of dorsiflexion. The joint is put at a disadvantage during the mid-stance-through-toe-off stage of the gait cycle. As a result, with a return to vigorous activity the contracted posterior capsule is exposed to repeated microstraining, with a subsequent reactive synovitis, pain, and sensation of weakness. Such a patient complains of "weak ankles," which he believes to be due to residual ligamentous laxity resulting from the initial injury. Careful examination demonstrates a stable ankle, effusion, and limitation of dorsiflexion when compared with the normal contralateral joint. The characteristic physical finding is decreased dorsiflexion. This may be detected by having the patient lean forward while standing and flexing both knees and ankles, keeping the heels on the floor. Limitation of motion will be visible, or the patient will describe a distinct feeling of stiffness in the involved joint.

Treatment, therefore, should be directed toward restoring full motion. Since a reactive synovitis associated with effusion can limit dorsiflexion, as can capsular contractures, resolution of the problem must be directed toward both conditions. Once it has been established that the joint is roentgenographically negative and all ligaments are stable, it should be aspirated. Not infrequently, as much as 3 ml to 4 ml of clear or blood-tinged synovial fluid can be removed. Aspiration in itself, by decompressing the joint, will increase the motion. It is my practice also to instill 1 ml of dexamethasone to counteract the reactive synovitis. Most important, however, is the initiation of a clearly explained and closely supervised program of active assisted dorsiflexion exercises. When full motion is effected, unless some other complicating condition exists, the patient's complaints will abate.

Joint Instability. There are four basic instabilities that can occur at the ankle joint. Deficiency in the anterior talofibular ligament will produce a positive anterior drawer test. Insufficiencies of both the anterior talofibular ligament and the calcaneofibular ligament will result in varus instability, as demonstrated by the talar tilt sign. Diastasis of the mortise with instability in the coronal plane is due to disruption of the anterior tibiofibular ligament associated with lesions of the interosseous ligament or the bony structures. Abduction instability due to isolated deltoid ligament deficiency is most unusual; usually, this is a combination of deltoid ligament instability associated with malunion of a fibular fracture or anterior fibulotalar–interosseous membrane laxity. Such a lesion is quite rare and usually results from an eversion fracture-dislocation of the ankle joint.

The vast majority of ankle joint instabilities may be effectively managed by appropriate adhesive strapping of the joint. Garrick and Regva have demonstrated, in a study involving 2400 intramural basketball players, that prophylactic strapping of the previously injured ankle joint significantly reduces the incidence of re-injury.[26] In my experience, it is the rare patient who requires surgical reconstruction of an unstable ankle.

There are no effective surgical reconstructive procedures for deltoid ligament insufficiency or for tibiofibular–interosseous ligament insufficiency. For patients with a positive talar tilt sign and significant disability (indicating chronic disruption of both the anterior fibulotalar and fibulocalcaneal ligaments), a modified Watson-Jones procedure may be considered (Fig. 30-35).

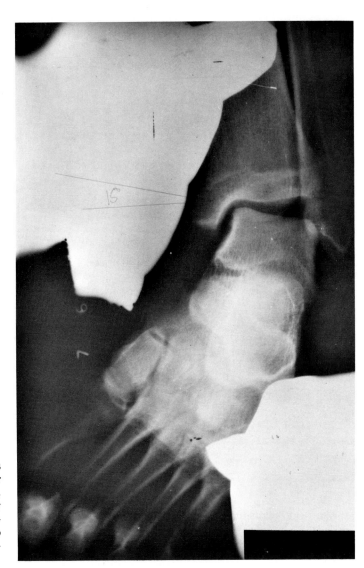

FIG. 30-35. Tibiotalar stress film demonstrates a 15° talar tilt. On the basis of this study, a diagnosis of lateral instability was rendered, and reconstructive surgery was proposed to the patient, who had complained of recurrent sprains.

However, it must be emphasized that what appears on roentgenograms to be "positive talar tilt" may represent physiologic laxity, and the films should be compared with views of the uninvolved contralateral joint (Fig. 30-36).

Anterolateral joint stability can be effected by a relatively simple modification of the Watson-Jones procedure. The peroneus brevis tendon and distal fibula are exposed through a curvilinear incision, following the course of the distal tendon. The tendon is transected 6.25 cm superior to the tip of the malleolus. The proximal segment is then sutured into the peroneus longus tendon. The distal segment of the brevis is then bisected just proximal to its point of insertion into the base of the fifth metatar-

sal. A $\frac{1}{4}$-inch hole is then drilled in the sagittal plane, through the distal tip of the fibula. The anterior segment of the sectioned tendon is then placed from anterior to posterior, and the posterior segment is placed from posterior to anterior through the hole. The distal ends are pulled taut and tied on themselves. With the foot placed in eversion and 10° of dorsiflexion, a cast is applied, which the patient wears for 8 weeks. At the end of the 8-week period, an intensive range-of-motion exercise program is initiated.

Osteophytes and Fracture Fragments in the Joint Space. The third form of complication following ankle sprain or fracture is secondary to osteophytes and fragments that have not united. The reactive hyper-

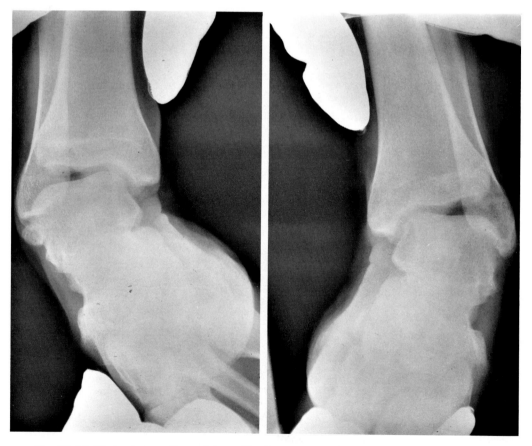

FIG. 30-36. Bilateral stress films of the ankle demonstrate symmetrical laxity in this patient. Further examination did demonstrate limitation of dorsiflexion of the involved side. It has been my experience that most complaints after an injury are due not to laxity but rather to incomplete rehabilitation and limitation of joint motion.

trophic spurring that is produced can be placed into two groups: mediolateral osteophytes and anteroposterior osteophytes. Although mediolateral osteophytes may produce clinical deformity and frightening-looking roentgenograms, they are seldom, if ever, a source of problems or disability.

Anteroposterior osteophytes, on the other hand, may be a source of considerable problems. Those that arise on the anterior neck of the tibia may, in fact, present a mechanical block to dorsiflexion and cause problems by limiting this motion (Fig. 30-37). When this does occur, surgical excision of the osteophytes may be indicated.

An ununited osteochondral fracture of the dome of the talus may be responsible for pain and effusion in a previously injured ankle joint. The lesion usually involves the lateral margin of the dome of the talus, and the diagnosis is made by a good-quality roentgenogram taken in the anteroposterior projection (Fig. 30-38). If complaints persist following adequate rehabilitation of the joint, surgical extirpation of the fragment may be indicated. A small anterolateral

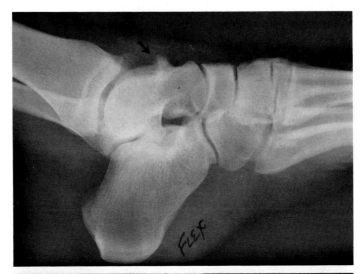

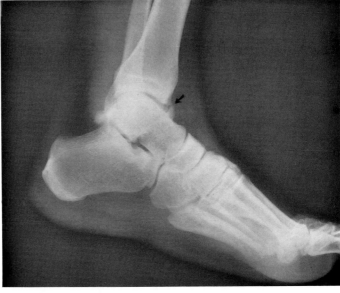

FIG. 30-37. Anterior tibiotalar osteophyte formation resulted from repeated microtrauma in this former collegiate oarsman. The lesions (*arrows*) created a mechanical block to dorsiflexion that caused the patient pain and "instability" when he participated in vigorous activities. Surgical removal of the lesions resulted in a significant increase in dorsiflexion and resolution of the patient's complaints.

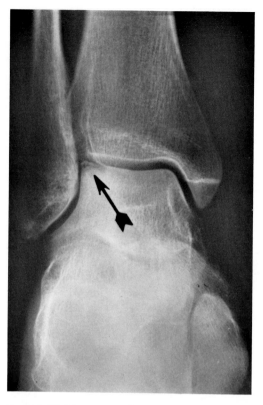

FIG. 30-38. Nonunion of an osteochondral fracture of the lateral dome of the talus (*arrow*) caused the patient pain and recurrent effusion with activity. Surgical removal of the fragment is indicated.

of this problem requires roentgenograms of good definition to pinpoint the location of the loose bodies and a well-planned surgical incision that does not disrupt supporting ligamentous structures.

Complications in the Foot

Ever since Robert Jones sustained a fracture through the tuberosity at the base of his fifth metatarsal while dancing, this lesion has been referred to as a Jones fracture. These lesions are frequently encountered and uniformly heal with conservative treatment. Dameron has pointed out, however, that fractures occurring in the 1.5-cm segment of the shaft just distal to the flare of the tuberosity can prove very difficult to manage.[20] A report on 20 fractures through the proximal part of the shaft of the fifth metatarsal indicated that five required bone grafting to effect union. My own experience with this lesion has been similar.[68] The lesion can present with one of four distinct courses. First, the fracture may go on to satisfactory healing with either plaster im-

incision into the joint, with the foot placed in maximum plantar flexion, will afford adequate exposure to retrieve the fragment.

Fibrous union of malleolar tip fractures is not uncommon (Fig. 30-39). In the nonathlete, these lesions rarely, if ever, present problems. However, persons involved in vigorous activity may experience disabling pain at the fracture site. If the joint is stable and has a full range of motion but there is a clearly defined lesion on roentgenograms and disabling pain, surgical removal of the fragment may be indicated. However, the surgeon must be certain that removal does not produce instability by removing bony support to the mortise, and care must be taken to avoid disrupting the supporting ligamentous structures.

Loose bodies in the ankle joint that cause locking, decreased motion, and recurrent effusion should be removed. Management

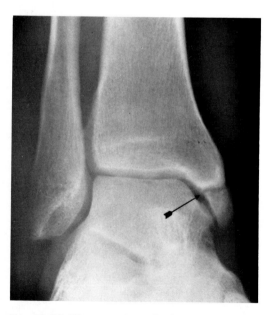

FIG. 30-39. Fibrous union of a fracture of the tip of the medial malleolus (*arrow*) causes pain with vigorous activity. If technically feasible, a satisfactory result can be effected by removing the fragment. Another option is internal fixation of the fragment with cancellous bone grafting for osteosynthesis.

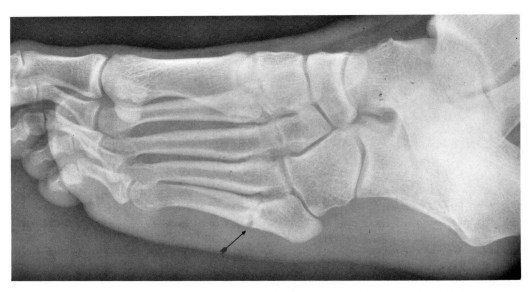

FIG. 30-40. Roentgenogram demonstrates refracture (*arrow*) through a healed fracture involving the fifth metatarsal distal to the tuberosity. Note the formation of sclerotic bone across the medullary canal. Effective management requires removal of sclerotic bone to effect medullary continuity, inlay bone grafting, and 6 weeks' plaster immobilization.

mobilization or simple rest and protection. Second, a patient who was not treated may present several months after the injury with a delayed union and a hypertrophic callus about the lesion. Third, following what appears to be satisfactory healing, the bone may refracture through the original site, which is characterized by dense, sclerotic bone (Fig. 30-40). A fourth eventuality is established nonunion, which may follow whether or not the injury was treated (Fig. 30-41).

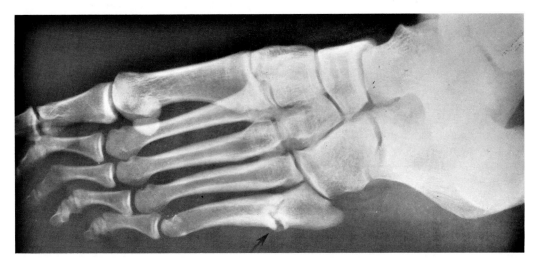

FIG. 30-41. Roentgenogram demonstrates an established nonunion of a fracture of the fifth metatarsal distal to the tuberosity (*arrow*). Widening and sclerosis of the fracture line are noted, as well as sclerosis of the medullary cavity. To effect healing, this lesion must be treated surgically with removal of sclerotic bone from the medullary canal, inlay bone grafting, and cast immobilization for 6 weeks.

Confronted with a fracture involving the proximal shaft of the fifth metatarsal distal to the tuberosity, the orthopaedic surgeon must be aware of the typical unpredictability of the course of this fracture. When seen initially, the lesion should be treated in a non-weight-bearing cast for 6 weeks. Should the lesion go on to delayed nonunion with characteristic sclerosis about the fracture site, or should refracture occur, an inlaid bone graft is indicated. The lesion is approached through a dorsolateral curvilinear incision that avoids the plantar skin and exposes the lateral aspect of the proximal shaft. A 1.5-cm square panel of cortical bone centered over the site of the fracture is removed. The medullary canal is characteristically obliterated by dense, sclerotic, poorly organized bone. It is important that this sclerotic bone be removed from the medullary canal, with either a drill or a small curette. A comparable plug of bone is then removed from the proximal tibia through a second incision and placed into the window. The graft should be truly inlaid without protruding, so that it will remain in place and will not create an elevated irregularity that would interfere with shoe fitting. A non-weight-bearing cast is then applied for 6 to 8 weeks, until healing is effected.

Peripheral Nerve Lesions

Injuries to the axillary, suprascapular, long thoracic, and common peroneal nerves are uncommon in athletes. The mechanism of injury can be either a direct blow or a stretch. After blunt trauma the prognosis is good; traction injuries, however, generally do not recover. It is important to recognize the nature of these problems if one is to initiate appropriate therapy and to apprise the patient of his problem accurately and intelligently.

Axillary nerve stretch injuries result from hyperabduction, glenohumeral subluxation, or dislocation. Although deltoid weakness occurs immediately, in a well-muscled athlete the correct diagnosis may not be made, unless he is carefully examined, until deltoid atrophy becomes evident weeks later. If permanent deltoid paralysis persists, the patient's athletic activities will have to be modified. An intensive isotonic exercise program for shoulder girdle musculature should be instituted to compensate for the deltoid weakness. Surgical exploration of the nerve is not indicated.

Suprascapular nerve paresis is generally due to a direct-blow injury. Paralysis of the infraspinatus muscle results in marked weakness of external humeral rotation and discernible muscle atrophy on careful examination. This lesion should not be mistaken for a rotator cuff tear. A course of "watchful neglect" is indicated, since complete recovery can always be expected.

Injury to the long thoracic nerve produces immediate winging of the scapula. Although it may take up to 12 to 18 months, recovery will be complete. No treatment—other than reassuring the patient—is indicated.[30]

Traction injuries to the common peroneal nerve can occur in association with disruption to the posterior and lateral structures of the knee, as seen in the lateral compartment syndrome. Surgical repair of the stretched nerve is not feasible, and the prognosis is poor. Because of footdrop, bracing is necessary. The polyurethane in-shoe orthosis proves quite satisfactory. Also to be considered at a later date is transfer of the posterior tibial tendon through the interosseous space to the midfoot.

Complications in the Cervical Spine

The vertebral bodies, soft tissue supporting structures, and cervical nerve roots are frequently injured. The majority of these problems are minor; however, some may be tragic. Although football has received a great deal of attention recently for its high incidence of related cervical spine injuries, water sports, wrestling, and gymnastics produce a significant number of such problems.

Injuries to the cervical area can be classified into five groups, on the basis of severity: mild, moderate, severe, very severe, and catastrophic. Stable cervical sprains, strains, and the pinch–stretch neuropraxias of the cervical roots, the so-called burners, can be considered mild. All patients recover, with or without treatment. In managing this type of injury the physician is well advised to protect the athlete who has less than full, pain-free range of motion by forbidding participation in contact sports.

Among the moderate cervical injuries are occult fractures and the effects of repeated microtrauma: early degenerative changes or intervertebral disc space narrowing. Presumably, repeated impact exerted on the cervical spine will produce specific roentgenographic findings, yet in most instances there are no associated clinical signs or symptoms. Albright and associates reported a study involving 75 University of Iowa freshmen football recruits who had cervical spine roentgenograms (after having played in high school but before college).[5] Of that group, 32% had one or more of the following: occult fracture of the posterior elements, vertebral body compression fracture, intervertebral disc space narrowing, or other degenerative changes. Only 13% admitted to a history of neck symptoms.

Management of the athlete with an injury in the moderate group is not concerned so much with treatment *per se* as with guidelines for exclusion from participation. In general, a person with roentgenographic evidence of instability or painful limitation of motion should not be permitted to participate in contact or high-velocity sports. If the spine is stable and there is full, pain-free motion (Fig. 30-42), participation may be permitted at the discretion of a young athlete's parents or of the adult athlete after he has been fully informed of the potential for further degenerative changes and associated problems.

Severe cervical injuries are those in which there is an unstable fracture, subluxation, or dislocation without neurologic involvement. The goal in the management of such a patient is to effect and maintain a stable reduction, preferably by closed methods. If the athlete is to return to vigorous physical activity, the spine must be stable. In instances of subluxation or dislocation without fracture, this may not occur without spine fusion (Fig. 30-43). Also, in the athlete who desires to return to contact activity, unstable cervical fractures are best treated by early fusion (Fig. 30-44).

Very severe cervical injuries are fractures or dislocations with disabling residual neurologic involvement. Catastrophic injuries are those that produce permanent quadriplegia. Management of the complications associated with these injuries is beyond the scope of this chapter.

Spondylolysis is a stress fracture involving the pars interarticularis. It is a common problem, the incidence in the general population being estimated at 5%. However, it appears that the incidence is considerably higher among female gymnasts, pole-vaulters, and weightlifters. Spondylolysis can be divided into two types: preroentgenographic, in which there is no roentgenographic evidence of the defect, and the more commonly recognized spondylolysis with roentgenographic findings. Preroentgenographic spondylolysis presents with a history of onset of low back pain, usually without preceding trauma. There is no radiation of pain into the lower extremities, and the patient identifies the painful area as the superior aspect of the sacroiliac joint, on one or both sides. There is decreased lumbar motion, with loss of the normal lordosis and absence of extension. In addition, the patient manifests significant hamstring spasm. A youngster with well-localized low back pain associated with limited extension and hamstring spasm should be considered to have spondylolysis, despite lack of roentgenographic findings. Initiating conservative management at this point and excluding the patient from athletic activity may produce healing of the lesion.

Roentgenographic findings in spondylolysis are a lytic and/or sclerotic lesion involving the pars interarticularis on one or both sides of a lumbar vertebra. The lesion usually involves L5. Treatment is directed toward keeping the patient at rest until the symptoms subside. In instances of persistence or frequent recurrence, it is recommended that conservative treatment be maintained for 6 to 12 months. Micheli and colleagues recommend use of a modified Boston brace.[53] Surgical intervention is indicated when symptoms persist despite a 6- to 12-month period of conservative management. My experience is that it is the extremely rare person with a spondylolysis who requires spine fusion. When indicated, however, a transverse process fusion, as described by Wiltse and associates, is mandatory.[77]

Spondylolisthesis is a progression of spondylolysis in which there is anterior translation of the superior vertebra in relation to the inferior one. Again, many youngsters with grade 1 or 2 spondylolisthesis participate in all forms of vigorous and contact sports. The nature of the dis-

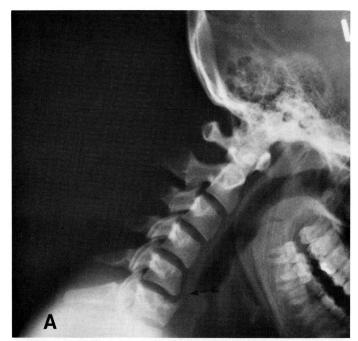

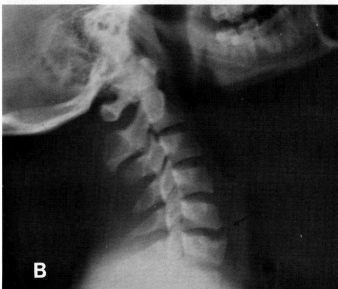

FIG. 30-42. Flexion (*A*) and extension (*B*) views demonstrate a stable cervical spine despite an anterior compression fracture of C6 (*arrows*). The patient had played 3 years of college football since sustaining the injury. He had a full, pain-free range of cervical spine motion and was neurologically intact, and he was permitted to continue his football career.

order is one of slowly progressive slip. There is no basis for the misconception, shared by many physicians, that participating in contact activities with a spondylolisthesis will result in acute encroachment on the spinal cord.

Management of spondylolisthesis is conservative and includes limitation of activity, bracing,[53] and use of a bedboard. An indication for surgery is slipping of one grade while under conservative management, or persistent disability despite a 6- to 12-month conservative program. Evaluation prior to fusion should include a complete neurologic workup as well as a myelogram. For patients who have no neurologic involvement and a negative myelogram, the fusion of choice is a transverse process fusion. Removal of the posterior element necessarily involves disruption of the posterior supporting soft tissue structures, which may contribute to further slipping.

FIG. 30-43. Flexion (*A*) and extension (*B*) views demonstrate an unstable cervical spine at C3–4 (*arrows*) despite 3 months' immobilization following injury.

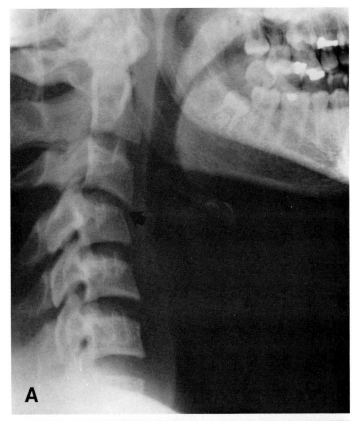

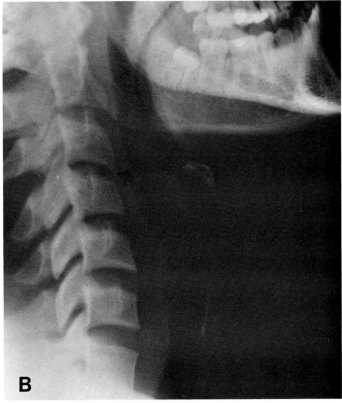

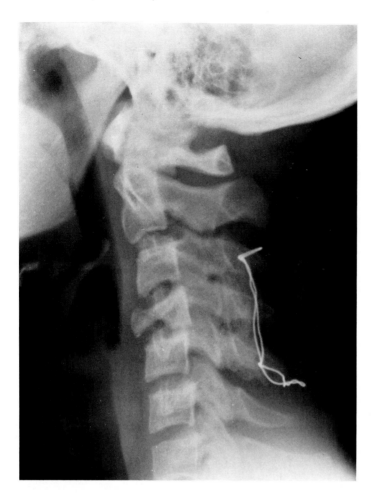

FIG. 30-44. Stability of the cervical spine was effected by early fusion. The patient returned to tackle football with no problem.

COMPLICATIONS OF ATHLETIC INJURIES IN OLDER ADULTS

For the athlete, the onset of middle age occurs somewhere between 30 and 35 years, when the components of the musculoskeletal system undergo a variety of attritional changes. Ligaments lose tensile strength, degenerative changes occur in the joints, bone mass decreases, and muscle mass diminishes, with subsequent decrease in strength. Common problems seen in this age group include intervertebral disc degeneration of the cervical and lumbar spine, musculotendinous rupture of the biceps and the gastrocnemius–soleus mechanism, degenerative capsulitis of the glenohumeral joint, and degenerative lesions of the menisci. With the exception of intractable degenerative disc disease associated with findings of neurologic impairment and

complete rupture of the Achilles tendon, as a general rule of thumb it is strongly recommended that these problems of middle life be treated conservatively. Specifically, the involved part is rested during periods of acute symptoms, and the patient is then placed on a very carefully supervised rehabilitation program after the symptoms subside.

Tennis Elbow

Tennis elbow, primarily an affliction of middle age, can best be attributed to repeated microstrain of the origin of the forearm extensor musculature in the area of the extensor aponeurosis. More specifically, Nirschl has identified the definitive pathology as involving the extensor carpi radialis brevis and describes the problem as a "microtear" of the tendon unit, which goes on to multiple repeated tears, with healing impaired by a granulation response.*

Tennis elbow may be due to improper form, improper equipment, or inadequate forearm extensor musculature. Tennis players who strike the ball on their backhand shot without proper use of body weight and shoulder girdle muscles may overload the forearm musculature and place excessive stress at the origin of the extensor mass. Obviously, the solution to this problem lies not with the physician but with the coach.

The racquet may contribute to tennis elbow if the grip is too large or too small or if the racquet is too rigid, too heavy, or strung too tightly. As a general rule, the racquet that will transmit the least strain on the extensor musculature is one with the largest comfortable grip, lighter in weight and more flexible, with a moderate string tension of 58 to 60 pounds. It may be metal, wood, or some other material.

Conservative Treatment. The single most important etiologic factor is weak extensor musculature. Especially in middle-aged tennis players, there is inadequate forearm muscle mass to absorb the impact created when the ball is struck. Therefore, the key to treating tennis elbow is to counteract the inflammatory response with appropriate physical modalities and drugs and to strengthen the forearm muscle mass with a well-supervised isotonic exercise program.

With regard to any inflammatory reaction, aspirin and phenylbutazone (Butazolidin) taken orally or a cortisone derivative injected into the painful site may achieve temporary relief of symptoms. Also, application of ice, ultrasound, and electric galvanic stimulation have a limited role. Most important is the institution of a muscle-strengthening exercise program. The patient should be instructed to do extensor curls using a 3- to 5-pound dumbbell. Three sets of 20 repetitions performed four times a day over a period of 3 to 4 months will increase muscle strength and alleviate symptoms. The patient must understand that this program must be carried out faithfully over a 3- to 4-month period before relief of symptoms will occur.

Operative Treatment. In 1% to 2% of patients treated for tennis elbow, surgery may be considered. Although a number of procedures have been described, I agree with Nirschl that a release of the extensor mass from the extensor aponeurosis, which includes the extensor brevis origin, is the procedure of choice.* At the same time, the joint should be explored and any hypertrophic synovium excised. Postoperative care includes immobilization in plaster for 3 weeks followed by an intensive range-of-motion and isotonic exercise program. In selected patients the results of surgery have been gratifying.

REFERENCES

1. Abraham, E., and Pankovich, A.M.: Neglected rupture of the Achilles tendon. J. Bone Joint Surg., 47A:253, 1975.
2. Adams, J.E.: Injury to the throwing arm: A study of traumatic changes in the elbow joint of boy baseball players. Calif. Med., 102:127, 1965.
3. ———: Little League shoulder—osteochondrosis of the proximal humeral epiphysis in boy baseball pitchers. Calif. Med., 105:22, 1966.
4. Aergerter, E., and Kirkpatrick, J.S.: Osteogenesis imperfecta. In Aergerter, E.E., and Kirkpatrick, J.A., Jr. (eds.): Orthopaedic Diseases. 3rd ed., p. 153. Philadelphia, W.B. Saunders, 1968.
5. Albright, J.P., Moses, J.M., Feldick, H.G. et al.: Nonfatal cervical spine injuries in interscholastic football. J.A.M.A., 235:1243, 1976.
6. Allman, F.: Course on Athletic Injuries of the Upper Extremities. Presented to the Committee on Sports Medicine, The American Academy of Orthopaedic Surgeons, Eugene, Oregon, 1974.
7. Allman, F.L., Jr.: Fractures and ligamentous injuries of the clavicle and its articulations. J. Bone Joint Surg., 49A:774, 1967.
8. Balasubramaniam, P., and Prathap, K.: The effect of injection of hydrocortisone into rabbit calcaneal tendons. J. Bone Joint Surg., 54B:729, 1972.
9. Bedi, S.S., and Ellis, W.: Spontaneous rupture of calcaneal tendon in rheumatoid arthritis after local steroid injection. Ann. Rheum. Dis., 29:494, 1970.
10. Bergfeld, J.A.: The fate of the acromioclavicular joint following first and second degree sprains. Orthop. Trans., 1:24, 1977.
11. Blandy, J.P., and Fuller, R.: March gangrene. J. Bone Joint Surg., 39B:693, 1975.
12. Bosworth, D.M.: Repair of defects in the tendo achilles. J. Bone Joint Surg., 38A:111, 1956.
13. Brogdon, B.G., and Crow, N.E.: Little Leaguer's elbow. Am. J. Roentgenol. Rad. Ther. Nucl. Med., 83:671, 1960.
14. Brown, R. et al.: Osteochondritis of the capitellum. J. Sports Med. Phys. Fitness, 2:27, 1974.
15. Bugy, E.I., Jr., and Boyd, B.M.: Repair of neglected rupture or laceration of the Achilles tendon. Clin. Orthop., 56:73, 1968.

* Nirschl, R.: Personal communication.

16. Carter, A.B., Richards, R.L., and Zachary, R.B.: The anterior tibial band syndrome. Lancet, 2:928, 1949.
17. Collins, H.R., and Wilde, A.H.: Shoulder instability in athletes. Orthop. Clin. North Am., 4:759, 1973.
18. Cowan, M.A., and Alexander, S.: Simultaneous bilateral rupture of Achilles tendons due to triamcinolone. Br. Med. J., 1:1658, 1961.
19. Cox, J.S.: Fate of the acromioclavicular joint in athletic injuries. Am. J. Sports Med., 9:50, 1981.
20. Dameron, T.B.: Fractures and anatomical variations of the proximal portion of the fifth metatarsal. J. Bone Joint Surg., 57A:788, 1975.
21. Devas, M.B.: Stress fractures in athletes. J. Sports Med. Phys. Fitness, 1:49, 1973.
22. Dotter, W.E.: Little Leaguer's shoulder—a fracture of the proximal epiphyseal cartilage of the humerus due to baseball pitching. Guthrie Clin. Bull., 23:68, 1953.
23. Edwards, E.A.: The anatomic basis for ischaemia localized to certain muscles of the lower leg. Surg. Gynecol. Obstet., 87:94, 1953.
24. Ellman, H.: Osteochondrosis of the radial head. Scientific exhibit presented at the Annual Meeting of The American Academy Orthopaedic Surgeons, Washington, 1972.
25. Elton, R.C.: Stress reaction of bone in Army trainees. J.A.M.A., 204:314, 1968.
26. Garrick, J., and Regva, R.: Role of external support in the prevention of ankle sprains. Med. Sci. Sports, 5:200, 1973.
27. Getzen, L., and Carr, J. III: Etiology of anterior compartment syndrome. Surg. Gynecol. Obstet., 125:347, 1967.
28. Gilmer, W.S., and Anderson, L.D.: Reactions of the somatic tissue which may progress to bone formation. South. Med. J., 52:1432, 1959.
29. Green, N.E., and Allen, B.L.: Vascular injuries associated with dislocation of the knee. J. Bone Joint Surg., 59A:236, 1977.
30. Gregg, J.R., Labosky, D., Harty, M. et al.: Serratus anterior paralysis in the young athlete. J. Bone Joint Surg., 61A:825, 1979.
31. Helfet, A.J.: Coracoid transplantation for recurring dislocations of the shoulder. J. Bone Joint Surg., 40B:198, 1958.
32. Holdsworth, F.: Fractures, dislocations, and fracture-dislocations of the spine. J. Bone Joint Surg., 52A:1534, 1970.
33. Horn, C.E.: Acute ischemia of the anterior tibial muscle and the long extensor muscles of the toes. J. Bone Joint Surg., 27:615, 1945.
34. Hughes, J.R.: Ischaemic necrosis of the anterior tibial muscles due to fatigue. J. Bone Joint Surg., 30B:581, 1948.
35. Hughston, J.C.: Myositis ossificans traumatica. South. Med. J., 55:1167, 1962.
36. Ismail, A.M., Balakrishnan, R., and Rajakumar, M.K.: Rupture of patellar ligament after steroid infiltration. J. Bone Joint Surg., 51B:503, 1969.
37. Jackson, D.W., and Feagin, J.A.: Quadriceps contusion in young athletes: Relation of severity of injury to treatment and prognosis. J. Bone Joint Surg., 55A:95, 1975.
38. Kennedy, J.C., and Willis, R.B.: The effects of local steroid injections on tendons: A biomechanical and microscopic correlative study. Am. J. Sports Med., 4:11, 1976.
39. Kennelly, B.M., and Blumberg, L.: Bilateral anterior tibial claudication. J.A.M.A., 203:487, 1968.
40. King, J.W., Brelsford, H.J., and Tullos, H.S.: Analysis of the pitching arm. Clin. Orthop., 67:116, 1969.
41. Leach, R.E., Zohn, D.A., and Stryker, W.S.: Anterior tibial compartment syndrome. Arch. Surg., 28:187, 1964.
42. Leavitt, D.G., and Woodward, H.W.: March fracture: A statistical study of forty-seven patients. J. Bone Joint Surg., 26:733, 1944.
43. Lee, H.B.: Avulsion and rupture of the tendo calcaneus after injection of hydrocortisone. Br. Med. J., 2:395, 1957.
44. Leveton, A.L.: March (fatigue) fractures of the long bones of the lower extremity and pelvis. Am. J. Surg., 71:222, 1946.
45. Lipscomb, A.B.: Baseball pitching injuries in growing athletes. J. Sports Med., 3:25, 1975.
46. Lipscomb, A.B., Thomas, E.D., and Johnston, K.J.: Treatment of myositis ossificans traumatica in athletes. Am. J. Sports Med., 4:111, 1976.
47. Lombardo, S.J., Kerlan, R.K., Jobe, F.W. et al.: The modified Bristow procedure for recurrent dislocations of the shoulder. J. Bone Joint Surg., 58A:256, 1976.
48. McBryde, A.M.: Stress fractures in athletes. J. Sports Med., 3:212, 1975.
49. McCue, F.D., Andrews, J.R., Michael, H., and Gieck, J.H.: The Coach's finger. J. Sports Med., 2:270, 1974.
50. Mann, T.P.: Fatigue fracture of the tibia: Three cases at a naval training establishment. Lancet, 2:8, 1945.
51. Mavor, G.E.: The anterior tibial syndrome. J. Bone Joint Surg., 38B:513, 1956.
52. May, V.R., Jr.: A modified Bristow operation for anterior recurrent dislocations of the shoulder. J. Bone Joint Surg., 52A:1010, 1970.
53. Micheli, L.J., Hall, J.E., and Miller, M.E.: Use of modified Boston brace for back injuries in athletes. Am. J. Sports Med., 8:351, 1980.
54. Mital, M.A., Matza, R.A., and Cohen, J.: The so-called unresolved Osgood-Schlatter lesion. J. Bone Joint Surg., 62A:732, 1980.
55. Moore, J.R.: Osteotomy–osteoclasis, a method for correcting long bone deformities. J. Bone Joint Surg., 29:119, 1947.
56. Mozes, M., Yochanan, R., and Jahr, J.: Anterior tibial syndrome. J. Bone Joint Surg., 44A:730, 1962.
57. Nickerson, S.H.: March fracture of insufficiency fracture. Am. J. Surg., 62:154, 1943.
58. Norman, A., and Dorfman, H.D.: Juxtacortical circumscribed myositis ossificans: Evolution and radiographic features. Radiology, 96:301, 1970.
59. Salter, R.B., and Harris, W.R.: Injuries involving the epiphyseal plate. J. Bone Joint Surg., 45A:587, 1963.
60. Savage, R.: Popliteal artery injury associated with knee dislocation: Improved outlook? Am. Surg., 46:627, 1980.

61. Siffert, R.S.: The growth plate and its affections. J. Bone Joint Surg., 48A:546, 1966.
62. Slocum, D.P.: Overuse syndromes of the lower leg and foot in athletes. Instr. Course Lect., 17:359, 1960.
63. ———: Classification of elbow injuries from baseball pitching. Tex. Med., 64:48, 1968.
64. Snook, G.A.: Intermittent claudication in athletes. J. Sports Med., 3:71, 1975.
65. Thompson, R.C., Jr., Morres, J.N., Jr., and Jane, J.A.: Current concepts in management of cervical spine fractures and dislocations. J. Sports Med., 3:159, 1975.
66. Thorndike, A., Jr.: Myositis ossificans traumatica. J. Bone Joint Surg., 22:315, 1940.
67. Tirnon, M.C., Anzel, S.H., and Waugh, T.R.: Surgical management of osteochondritis dissecans of the capitellum. Am. J. Sports Med., 4:121, 1976.
68. Torg, J.S., Balduini, F.C., Zelko, R.R. et al.: Fractures of the base of the fifth metatarsal distal to the tuberosity: Classification and guidelines for nonsurgical and surgical management. J. Bone Joint Surg., 66A:209, 1984.
69. Torg, J.S., Conrad, W., and Kalen, V.: Clinical diagnosis of anterior cruciate ligament instability in the athlete. Am. J. Sports Med., 4:84, 1976.
70. Torg, J.S., and Moyer, R.A.: Nonunion of a stress fracture through the olecranon epiphyseal plate observed in an adolescent baseball pitcher. J. Bone Joint Surg., 59A:264, 1977.
71. Torg, J.S., Pollack, H., and Sweterlitsch, P.: The effect of competitive pitching on the shoulders and elbows of preadolescent baseball players. Pediatrics, 49:267, 1972.
72. Torg, J.S., Truex, R.C., Jr., Marshall, J. et al.: Spinal injury at the level of the third and fourth cervical vertebrae from football. J. Bone Joint Surg., 59A:1015, 1977.
73. Tullos, H.S., and King, J.W.: Lesions of the pitching arm in adolescents. J.A.M.A., 220:264, 1972.
74. Unverferth, L.J., and Olix, M.L.: The effects of local steroid injections on tendon. J. Sports Med., 1:31, 1973.
75. Weaver, J.K., and Dunn, H.K.: Treatment of acromioclavicular injuries, especially complete acromioclavicular separation. J. Bone Joint Surg., 54A:1187, 1972.
76. Welling, R.E., Kakkasseril, J., and Cranley, J.J.: Complete dislocation of the knee with popliteal vascular injury. J. Trauma, 21:450, 1981.
77. Wiltse, L.L., Widell, E.H., Jr., and Jackson, D.W.: Fatigue fracture: Basic lesion in isthmic spondylolisthesis. J. Bone Joint Surg., 57A:17, 1975.
78. Zaccalini, P.S., and Urist, M.R.: Traumatic periosteal proliferation in rabbits. J. Trauma, 4:344, 1964.

Part Three

COMPLICATIONS OF ARTHROPLASTY AND TOTAL JOINT REPLACEMENT

31 Complications of Arthroplasty and Total Joint Replacement in the Shoulder

BRIAN A. ROPER AND MELVIN POST

This chapter is actually premature, insofar as there is little in the literature on the subject of total shoulder replacement, and therefore, of necessity, little is known of the complications. Orthopaedic surgeons have largely been concentrating their attention on arthroplasty in the major weight-bearing joints.

It is only comparatively recently that surgeons have started working on total shoulder replacement. The reason for this is that the numbers of suitable candidates is likely to be small. Patients with involvement of the shoulder with rheumatoid arthritis usually have severe involvement of other joints, and therefore the demands that they put on their shoulders are small. These patients are usually functioning around waist level with limited rotation. It is only when they need to comb their hair or wash their faces that the limitation of movement interferes, and they usually manage to alter their lifestyle to circumvent this limitation. It is only when they have severe pain that they are sufficiently concerned to inquire about surgery. With osteoarthrosis of the shoulder, pain does not seem to be a marked feature; in most cases it is limitation of movement that is predominant. Again, people seem to accept substantial limitation of movement before complaining. The other reason that shoulder arthroplasty has been slow to take off is that arthrodesis is a reasonably satisfactory procedure. A successful shoulder fusion permits the patient to raise the hand to the mouth, grasp objects in front, and forcefully push and pull if the scapula is held stable on its chest wall by strong muscles.

Shoulder arthrodesis is recommended (1) for low-grade infection of the shoulder, such as tuberculosis, with the expectation that the disease progression will cease and a stable, painless shoulder joint will result; and (2) for specific paralytic conditions such as a flail shoulder resulting from poliomyelitis, irreversible brachial plexus damage, or other disorders causing paralysis of the muscles associated with severe loss of shoulder function. Previously, shoulder arthrodesis was performed for failed treatment of massive rotator cuff tears and degenerative conditions caused by trauma. It is still occasionally performed for intractable, painful arthritis of the glenohumeral joint from any cause, especially when the patient has had multiple failed operations.

In 1942 the Barr Committee[1] recommended that the optimal position for arthrodesis of the shoulder was 50° of abduction of the arm as measured from the vertebral border of the scapula, 15° to 25° of forward flexion, and 25° to 30° of external rotation. On the other hand, Rowe[21] recommended an abduction angle of 20° measured from the side of the body, 30° of forward flexion, and 40° of internal rotation. He stated that poor results were obtained with excessive abduction and forward flexion of the arm and concluded that lifting and elevation of the hand to the face were achieved more efficiently when there was minimal humeral abduction.

Recently, it has been realized that rotation is probably more important than the degree of abduction or flexion. It is this fact that is encouraging more orthopaedists to experiment with arthroplasty of the shoulder.

REGIONAL CONSIDERATIONS

The main advantage to operating on the shoulder, compared with, for example, the hip joint, is that the shoulder joint is relatively superficial. Therefore, there are fewer tissue planes to cross, with less potential for accumulation of hematomas. It has the advantage over the knee joint of not being *too* superficial. The healing of the skin after knee joint replacement is a considerable source of concern. The tremendous vascularity around the shoulder joint should make infection less likely. This certainly does seem to be the case in most operations on the shoulder. However, the surgeon should not be complacent and should make every effort to use meticulous surgical technique to minimize infection and achieve optimal results. Unlike the hip or the knee, there is little or no room for error about the shoulder girdle, and once a mistake is made it is most difficult to rectify. Operations on the shoulder do not seem to be deviled by the problems of deep venous thrombosis, as is the case with the hip joint.

DISLOCATION: DESIGN CONSIDERATIONS

The shoulder is the pivotal point of the upper extremity. The shoulder girdle comprises the glenohumeral, acromioclavicular, and sternoclavicular joints and the "scapulothoracic articulation." These joints are completely dependent on their ligaments, tendons, and muscles so that they can interact in a harmonious manner. If a prosthetic replacement is considered, the surgeon should strive to use a procedure that creates the least stress on the bony parts of the shoulder joint and is durable. In any event, no artificial replacement can ensure against eventual failure. This is especially true of a constrained prosthesis because the forces are transmitted directly to the bone, while an unconstrained replacement depends on the integrity of its surrounding soft tissues.

There are three types of prosthetic total shoulder prostheses in vogue: the unconstrained, the semiconstrained, and the constrained. The unconstrained device does not fix a fulcrum, but it provides the least amount of force that is exerted on the contiguous parts of the shoulder. A semiconstrained replacement is basically the same as an unconstrained type, but because of the configuration of the cuplike device,

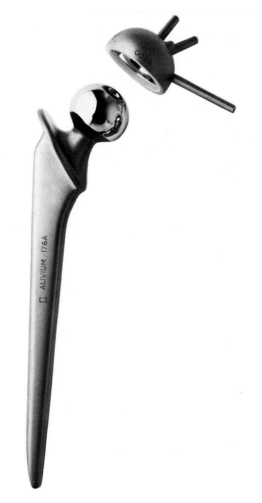

FIG. 31-1. The Stanmore prosthesis (courtesy of A. W. F. Lettin, M.D.).

as is employed by Lettin and associates[11,12] (Fig. 31-1), it acts as a concentric ball-and-socket joint and creates a semifulcrum that permits a semblance of stability of the prosthetic humeral head. Hemiarthroplastic and resurface cup devices behave like unconstrained replacements. A constrained-type prosthesis has a fixed fulcrum and causes the greatest force on the bony parts of the shoulder region. This last design may include a large or small spherical metal head. The large head has less chance of dislocating than does the small head. In the Imperial College London Hospital (ICLH) series in which an unconstrained large head (Fig. 31-2) was used, dislocation was not a feature. The metal head may be

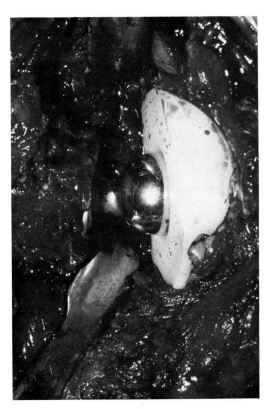

FIG. 31-2. The ICLH prosthesis, Mark I. The cup is cemented to the glenoid and acromion. The Mark II cup is shallower, and the head is totally unconstrained.

inserted in a reverse anatomical fashion, as employed by Bayley and Kessel (Fig. 31-3).[2] In the type employed by Post and colleagues[16–18] (the Michael Reese total shoulder [MRTS]), a small metal head is deliberately used so that controlled dislocation is achieved when a predetermined torque and the motion limits of the prosthetic device are exceeded. This design allows the metal head to snap apart from its prosthetic metal glenoid, thereby protecting the scapula from fracture through the suprascapular notch, the weakest portion of the scapula. Laboratory tests and clinical experience have shown that the scapula is best protected from fracture with controlled dislocation of the humeral head. No case is known in which this portion of the scapula has fractured with the use of a MRTS. When a traumatic dislocation occurs, revision surgery is relatively easy. But it follows

that each complication usually leads to additional operative procedures.

Whenever possible, an unconstrained replacement is always preferred over a constrained prosthesis. It is fortunate that unconstrained devices can be used in the vast majority of cases that require a total shoulder replacement. For an unconstrained joint to work, the rotator cuff mechanism must be functional. The greatest failure rate with unconstrained prosthesis is caused by a severely damaged rotator cuff. The rotator cuff must be capable of being closed effectively about the prosthesis. If a massive unrepairable rotator cuff tear is present, an unconstrained device such as the Neer prosthesis will not be functionally effective and can lead to dislocation (Fig. 31-4). In this case the constrained-type prosthesis is more desirable.

Post and co-workers[18] showed that when the deltoid and short rotator muscles of the rotator cuff are normal, the compression forces always exceed the shear of the humeral head on its glenoid. When the deltoid is normal and the short rotator muscles are ineffective, shear is always greater than the compression force of the humeral head on its glenoid during active elevation of approximately 30°. In pathologic states the deltoid is also usually weakened, and the situation is even worse. Thus, anything that destroys the function of the rotator cuff is more likely to give a poor result with an unconstrained replacement. Most rotator cuff tears can be repaired, with the exception of the most advanced cuff arthropathy and a significant number of massive tears. Pain relief is excellent with an unconstrained replacement, even with a poor or torn rotator cuff that can be repaired. Still, restoration of function is poor and the failure rate highest when there is severe cuff disease. In this case the surgeon must decide which prosthetic device to use. Use of a constrained replacement is the operation of last resort but sometimes must be used. It is no longer a matter of *which* is best, but *what device is required to achieve an optimal result.* The surgeon should keep in mind both long-term and short-term goals.

In general a constrained joint should permit lateral rotation, abduction, and a stable 360° arc of movement to allow the

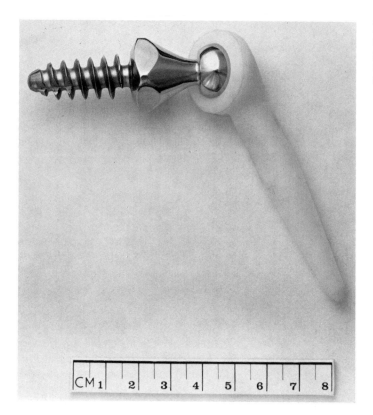

FIG. 31-3. The Kessel shoulder replacement, Mark II, with the glenoid and humeral components assembled. The ball screws into the glenoid.

prime movers to act on the joint where there is a nonfunctioning rotator cuff mechanism. Each patient should have four anatomical prerequisites to be considered a possible recipient of a constrained prosthesis: (1) an intact glenoid and scapular neck, (2) strong serratus anterior and trapezius muscles to stabilize the scapula, (3) either no soft tissue contracture or a contracture that can be effectively released, and (4) a strong deltoid muscle that allows active elevation of the arm. A weak or absent deltoid does not preclude the use of a constrained prosthesis if only passive—not active—overhead motion is acceptable to the patient. In many patients with shoulder disease the deltoid muscle is nonfunctional. If the glenohumeral joint is severely damaged and function of the rotator cuff is absent, a constrained prosthesis is intended to provide a fixed fulcrum independent of the stabilizing muscles to allow an adequate, stable range of lateral rotation, abduction, and forward flexion.

REASONS FOR DISLOCATION

The shoulder, unlike the hip, is relatively superficial and relies largely on a thin layer of superficial muscles for its stability. Certainly after replacement, the great mobility of the glenohumeral joint relates primarily to its large proximal humerus and shallow glenoid for the unconstrained replacement. Thus, unconstrained prostheses are highly dependent on a functional rotator cuff—or at least a capsule than can be repaired—if dislocation is to be avoided. The most common causes of subluxation and dislocation of an unconstrained prosthesis from its glenoid articular surface are (1) poor version of the prosthesis, (2) a deficient glenoid, in which the bone is lost, and (3) a severely destroyed rotator cuff (see Figs. 31-4 and 31-5). In the first instance this complication can be obviated by achieving a proper degree of version of the humeral component. The deficient anterior glenoid can be bone grafted and can then provide adequate

FIG. 31-4. This elderly woman had had multiple previous operations for a massive tear of the right rotator cuff. A Neer unconstrained total shoulder replacement was subsequently performed and promptly dislocated anteriorly because the soft tissues were not adequate to stabilize the prosthetic replacement. The patient has little pain but poor function.

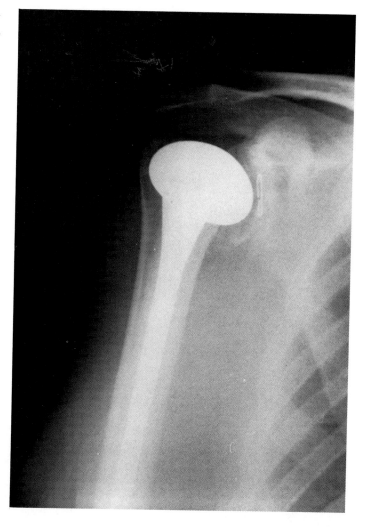

stability for the humeral component in most cases. With an irreparably destroyed rotator cuff, it may not be possible to cover the prosthesis with a functional capsule (Fig. 31-6). Clayton and colleagues[5] have attempted to prevent this complication by using a subacromial polyethylene spacer. Fortunately, even most large capsule tears can be repaired when an unconstrained prosthesis is used. When cuff tears cannot be repaired, the surgeon should consider the use of a constrained device, notwithstanding the increased number of complications associated with these prostheses. However, when an unconstrained plastic glenoid liner is used, it is not usually pos-sible to revise these cases later with a fixed-fulcrum device.

As mentioned previously, in the MRTS prosthesis, which employs a fixed fulcrum, controlled dislocation is designed to occur when a specific torque is exceeded. If an incorrect version of the glenoid component, an incorrect degree of retroversion of the humeral component, or incomplete locking of the metal ring on its metal glenoid is permitted, dislocation and eventual pullout of the metal glenoid from the bone is very likely to occur (Fig. 31-7). In these cases, revision surgery is needed to replace the old polyethylene component and to lock the metal ring securely on its metal glenoid.

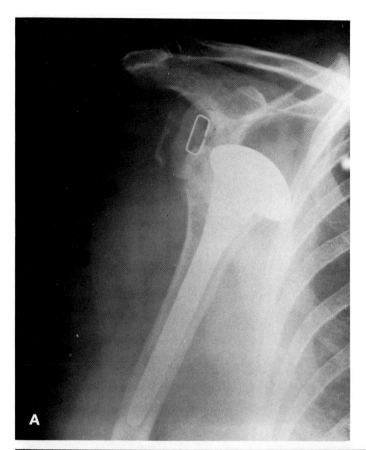

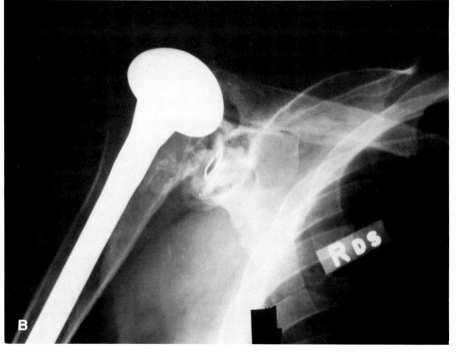

FIG. 31-5. (*A* and *B*) This man had been treated with multiple reconstructions of the rotator cuff. He developed severe pain and marked superior subluxation of the humeral head. The undersurface of the acromion became eroded by the humeral head, and shoulder pain increased. A Neer total shoulder replacement was performed, and the humeral metal head subluxated superiorly. The prosthetic replacement was unstable, and pain was intolerable.

FIG. 31-6. This elderly woman had undergone multiple operations for a traumatic fracture-dislocation of the right shoulder that resulted in a resection arthroplasty. The rotator cuff had been destroyed and apparently resected. A Neer hemiarthroplasty was inserted, with the false expectation that this would create stability and relieve pain. The result was poor.

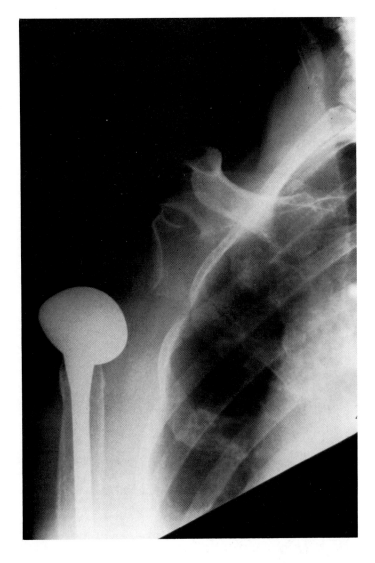

A poorly retroverted humeral component must be removed along with its cement from the intramedullary canal and the correct degree of retroversion (25°) achieved for the MRTS. An improperly positioned metal glenoid component cannot be corrected and will ordinarily have to be removed if recurring dislocation persists.[16]

Neer,[14] in his series of hemireplacements, stated that transitory subluxation was common but disappeared after the muscles regained tone. This is not always the case. Should the inferior subluxation persist for a lengthy period, neurapraxia or neurotmesis of the axillary nerve should be suspected.

Interestingly, Reeves[18,19] uses a tightly constrained joint in which a ball is restrained in a socket greater than a hemisphere by a polyethylene collar. Reeves reported no dislocations in his series. Lettin and associates[12] reported three dislocations in three patients within a few days of operation in their series of 36 surviving patients. In two the dislocation was reduced by manipulation under general anesthesia, and there were no further problems. The third patient underwent an open reduction of a fracture-dislocation of the shoulder, followed by a replacement of the head of the humerus with a Neer prosthesis. The shoulder muscles were grossly atrophic, the shoulder

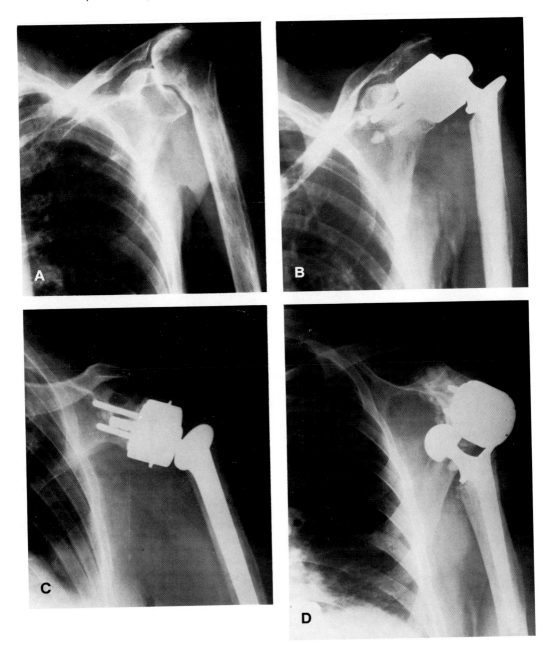

FIG. 31-7. (A) This elderly woman had a severely destroyed rotator cuff and demonstrated marked erosion of the superior half of the glenoid articular surface. Note the erosion of the medial proximal humeral shaft and the undersurface of the acromion. An MRTS replacement was performed at another institution. Unfortunately, the metal glenoid cup was inserted incorrectly after the articular surface was "smoothed" in such a manner as to permit the metal glenoid cup to be positioned in a tilt-up position rather than the required tilt-down position. If a constrained prosthesis was to have been inserted, the superior glenoid should have been bone grafted and the metal cup then inserted to permit the proper version of the glenoid cup. (B) The result was poor and showed a painless dislocation of the metal head from its glenoid. This view shows an obvious tilt-up position of the metal glenoid. The prosthesis behaved as it was designed to do and dislocated without causing fracture of the medial glenoid vault.

(Continued)

continued to dislocate, and removal of the prosthesis was required. In the series of Post and associates,[17] using constrained prostheses, 12 traumatic dislocations occurred in a group of 96 series I and II total shoulder replacements. Three of five patients had several recurring episodes that were due to alcoholism. In these cases the dislocations proved the merit of the prosthetic design by preventing a pullout of the metal glenoid from the vault or scapular fracture. Surgical revision with insertion of new plastic components was performed in each instance, since the metal humeral head cannot be forced back into the polyethylene cup. Other dislocations that had been operated on at other institutions and reported to one of the authors (MP) were related to incorrect humeral or metal glenoid version.

The question of constraint and dislocation is, of course, intimately concerned with postoperative management. With a constrained replacement, immediate full, active mobilization can be started. With an unconstrained prosthesis the likelihood is that postoperative immobilization may have to be slightly longer or even greatly prolonged for some patients and may be associated with a reduced total range of movement owing to adhesions or capsular contraction. When inadequate external rotation is achieved with a constrained replacement, dislocation is more likely to occur, especially if the prosthesis is forced beyond its motion limits. Therefore, under no circumstances should a constrained replacement be forced or "stretched" during rehabilitation exercises.

SPECIFIC COMPLICATIONS

Early Complications

Infection. In a series of 43 patients, Neer records one case of infection in a prosthetic replacement of the humeral head for a fracture.[14] This was promptly controlled by removal of the prosthesis. In a series of 54 patients having had total shoulder replacements, Reeves did not encounter any early infection.[19,20] Lettin reported one deep infection in a series of 35 patients who had total shoulder replacements.[11] This required removal of the prosthesis. Cofield reported two infections in a series of 104 total shoulder replacements (1.9%), including six revisions done before 1975.[6] Both required removal of the prosthesis, creating a resectional arthroplasty. Post and colleagues[17] reported two infections in a series of 96 constrained total shoulder replacements. Both required removal and created a resectional arthroplasty.

If care is taken with surgery, particularly with respect to hemostasis and the use of suction drainage, it would appear that infection is unlikely to be a problem. If methylmethacrylate is used, incorporation of antibiotic into the cement may reduce the incidence of infection, according to Bucholz and Engelbrecht[4] and Elson and McGechie.[8]

Loosening. Lettin and co-workers[12] reported loosening of the prosthesis in ten shoulders in 36 surviving patients. Eight occurred with rheumatoid arthritis and two with arthritis caused by trauma. One patient was sensitive to cobalt, a factor that may have contributed to the loosening. Seven of the ten required removal of the device and had excision arthroplasties. They were surprisingly stable, with an average range of active motion that was no worse before replacement was attempted. Beddow and Elloy[3] have used a semiconstrained prosthesis to prevent the superior subluxation that is common to unconstrained prostheses and have had four cases loosen in a total of 19 patients. One of the four cases followed a scapular fracture after a fall. In

FIG. 31-7. (*Continued*) (C) Another elderly woman had severe arthritis and rotator cuff arthropathy that had been operated on elsewhere. The metal glenoid cup was incorrectly inserted upside down, causing a tilt-up position of the cup. This caused excessive impingement of the medial humeral metal neck on the inferior aspect of the plastic glenoid rim of the metal cup. Torque was excessive. (D) When the arm was brought to the side, the metal head dislocated from its cup without fracture of the medial vault.

reports by Post and colleagues[16-18] and in recent follow-up evaluations, seven loose glenoids occurred in a series of 96 constrained total shoulder replacements. Five were due to severe trauma, one was related to infection and had to be removed, and one was related to a metastatic carcinoma of the lung to the scapular vault. More recently, in two patients receiving series I arthroplasties whose operations were performed from 1973 to 1975, and in five patients receiving series II arthroplasties whose operations were performed after January 1976, the glenoid screws broke owing to metal fatigue.[16-18] In each instance the glenoid components loosened, requiring removal in two patients thus far. The screws always broke at the midportion with the glenoid vault after prolonged use. These older screws were made by casting. The newer screws that are now used are made by a cold-rolling process and have much greater strength. Whenever a constrained prosthesis is employed, loosening is of great concern on both the humeral and glenoid sides of a component. The forces that can weaken the bond of the metal glenoid to

its glenoid are certainly transmitted to the humerus, which can cause a similar weakening of the prosthesis in the shaft. Loosening has not been a problem with unconstrained prostheses, except for the humeral prosthesis when it has been inadequately press-fitted.

The diagnosis of loosening is just as difficult to determine in the shoulder as it is in the hip joint. Pain on active and passive movements is the clinical sign. The sedimentation rate is unreliable. Plain films showing halos around the tips of stems and screws (Fig. 31-8) are suggestive but not conclusive. Arthrography has been tried by Murray and Rodrigo in the hip joint and found to be difficult to interpret.[13] It appears that a layer of dye can penetrate between the fibrous tissue lying between bone and cement without indicating true loosening. Evidence is accumulating that radioactive technetium scanning showing increased radioactivity may well be a very valuable means of detecting loosening. The problem of metal sensitivity remains a big, as yet unanswered, question.[9]

It would appear that when loosening

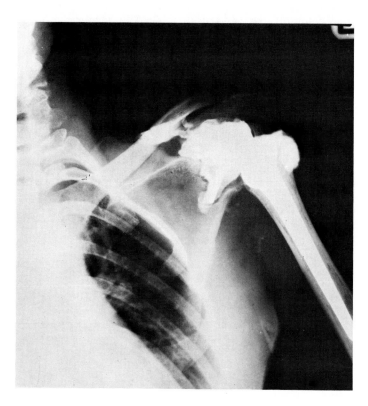

FIG. 31-8. A loose Stanmore prosthesis, showing a lucency around the cement in the glenoid.

occurs, it may well be possible, as in the hip, to replace the device. Should this be technically impossible, total removal seems to give a very acceptable, pain-free range of movement. The greatest density of trabeculae in the spongelike structure of the glenoid vault is located beneath the subchondral bone of the glenoid. That is the part that provides the greatest support for the glenoid component. It is therefore essential that the subchondral plate and its underlying trabeculae be preserved, since the trabeculae not only act as shock absorbers but also serve to disperse cement homogeneously in the bone. If the cortical cover of the cancellous vault is weakened by severe osteoporosis, destruction by tumor tissue, or surgical excavation, the strength of the bone and the resulting bond of the prosthetic metal component will be poor, and the attachment will certainly doom a constrained prosthesis to eventual failure (Fig. 31-9).[16-18]

Vessel Damage.   Particularly in fracture-dislocation of the humeral head and in rheumatoid arthritis with gross joint destruction, the axillary vessels may be placed in jeopardy at the time of surgery, especially if there is severe chronic dislocation. Lettin[11] had three cases in which the vein was damaged, leading to edema that subsequently resolved. Otherwise, this is not usually a problem.

Nerve Damage.   Cofield[6] reported two instances in which the axillary nerve was injured. In one case it was lacerated and repaired but did not recover, and later the patient required a trapezius transfer to the proximal humerus. During mobilization of the rotator cuff (supraspinatus) the suprascapular nerve may also be injured, and care should be taken during such a procedure when attempting to cover an unconstrained prosthetic device. In chronically and anteriorly dislocated humeral heads the brachial plexus can sustain injury during the dissection of the capsule from the surrounding structures.

Immediate Complications of Anesthesia.   One of us (MP) had one patient awaken with an ipsilateral hemiparesis following general anesthesia. Beyond this, we are unaware of complications related to anesthesia in total shoulder replacement.

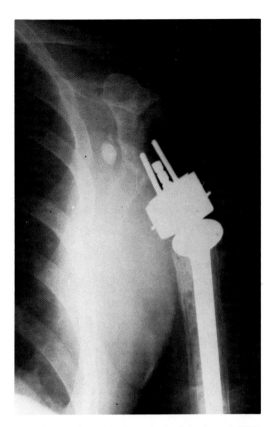

FIG. 31-9. This elderly man had had an MRTS replacement performed several years before. He developed carcinoma of the lung that metastasized to the glenoid vault and destroyed the bone, causing the prosthesis to simply drop from its previous space. The shoulder was relatively painless, and the patient went downhill owing to his tumor.

Mechanical Failure.   The greatest incidence of mechanical failure occurs with constrained prostheses. Post and colleagues[16-18] have had ten bent or broken prosthetic necks in series I prostheses used before 1975, in which 4-mm-diameter stainless steel humeral necks with a yield strength of 824 lb were used. In series II prostheses, used after January 1976, there have not been any bent or broken humeral necks. The series II device is made of Vitallium, has an 8-mm neck, and has a yield strength of 4970 lb. However, as previously described, glenoid screws that were made by casting methods have broken. Moreover, an analysis of these cases shows that these patients were active.

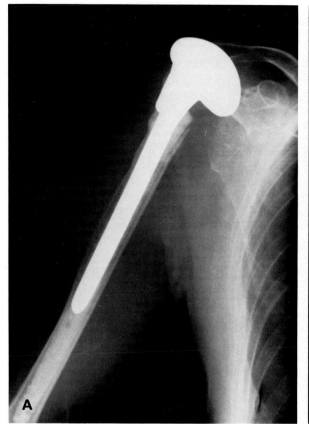

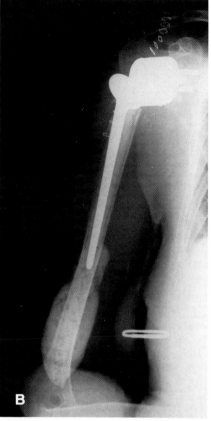

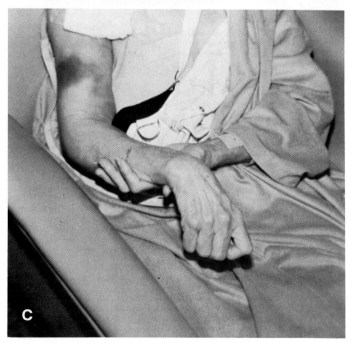

FIG. 31-10. (A) This elderly woman had sustained a fracture-dislocation and had undergone multiple operations elsewhere. A Neer prosthesis had been incorrectly inserted and was not seated deeply enough. In addition, the rotator cuff was nonexistent, and the patient had an unstable shoulder that was painful. (B) The shoulder was revised, and an MRTS prosthesis was inserted. Note the severe osteoporosis and thinning of the humeral cortices. During removal of the cement from the intramedullary canal, one cortex was inadvertently perforated; when methylmethacrylate was injected under pressure, it extruded into the surrounding tissues.

(Continued)

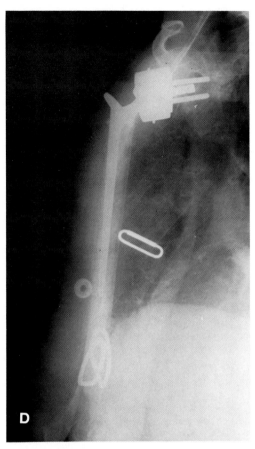

D

FIG. 31-10. (*Continued*) (C) At the close of surgery, the patient could extend the wrist, and an immobilizer was applied. Within 24 hours the patient demonstrated wristdrop. A discoloration about the lower arm coincided with the use of a strap that held the arm to the side of the body in the immediate postoperative phase. This apparently caused compression of the radial nerve against the cement. (D) Several days later, the patient underwent an exploration of the radial nerve. The nerve had indeed been compressed against a 1-inch segment of extruded cement. The cement was removed without difficulty and the nerve freed. At 3½ months the patient still had wristdrop, providing some suspicion that in addition to the compression of the nerve, the nerve tissue had somehow received a thermal injury from the hardening methylmethacrylate. There was full recovery at 8 months.

Late Complications

Infection. The occurrence of infection some years after the insertion of a prosthesis is well known in the hip joint. The nature of the process, however, remains a mystery.

Is the infection introduced at the time of surgery, or do the prosthesis and cement act as a focus for a subsequent introduction of bacteria? So far, the answer to this crucial question remains unknown.

It is strongly recommended that patients with joint replacements receive antibiotic coverage for several days if dental work is performed, especially work on the gums. Lettin and associates[12] reported one patient who developed an infection 15 months after operation as a result of staphylococcal infection that spread in the bloodstream. The bacteria was the same type as that from a pyogenic arthritis in the opposite shoulder. Continuous irrigation with antibiotics initially controlled the infection, but it eventually required removal of the prosthesis, resulting in a resection arthroplasty.

Reeves,[19,20] in his series, had a case of deep infection 4 years after the insertion of a total shoulder replacement for severe osteoarthritis. The entire prosthesis had to be removed. Interestingly, the range of motion in this patient was absolutely full and was the best range in all directions in the entire series! The best results from a Girdlestone excision arthroplasty are from those cases in which a total replacement has been excised because of loosening or infection.

MISCELLANEOUS CONSIDERATIONS

Most total shoulder replacements that are now performed, whether of the unconstrained or of the constrained variety, can be performed by a longitudinal 16-cm incision over the deltopectoral groove. If the anterior deltoid is detached from its origin and inadequately reattached to the bone at its origin at the close of surgery, this muscle may be severely weakened or may later detach. It is often possible to perform an arthroplasty of the shoulder without detaching the deltoid, provided that the arm is kept abducted to relax the muscle. The early results of this technique seem much better, in terms of recovery of function, than with those in which the muscle was detached. Leaving an intact deltoid, combined with use of a continuous passive motion machine in two cases following introduction of an ICLH unconstrained prosthesis, has resulted in an almost full range of active motion. Many patients come to surgery having had a radical acromionectomy that certainly destroys the fulcrum for the deltoid. Those cases previously operated on usually show severe fibrosis in the anterior, and occasionally in the lateral, deltoid, especially if branches of the axillary nerve have been injured.

Revision operations of total shoulder replacements in which bone cement has been employed can be most difficult and can cause unique complications even under the best of circumstances (Fig. 31-10).

Occasionally, the subscapularis must be lengthened and freed from adhesions to allow adequate external rotation of the shoulder with unconstrained replacements. Impingement at the anterior acromion, coracoacromial ligament, or acromioclavicular joint requires an anterior acromioplasty and occasionally a resection of the lateral clavicle distal to the coracoclavicular ligaments to free the rotator cuff.[15]

Prominent Greater Tuberosity

When the head of the prosthesis is positioned below the level of the greater tuberosity, an unconstrained arthroplasty procedure will give less than optimal results owing to impingement of the tuberosity at the acromion. This can be corrected by removing the protruding bone from the humerus or raising the humeral component above the level of the tuberosity. The acromion should not be shortened.

REFERENCES

 1. Barr, J.S., Freiberg, J.A., Colonna, P.C., and Pemberton, P.A.: A survey of end results on stabilization of the paralytic shoulder. J. Bone Joint Surg., 24:699, 1942.
 2. Bayley, J.I.L., and Kessel, L.: The Kessel total shoulder replacement. In Bayley, J.I.L., and Kessel, L. (eds.): Shoulder Surgery, pp. 160–164. Berlin, Springer-Verlag, 1982.
 3. Beddow, F.H., and Elloy, M.A.: Clinical experience with the Liverpool shoulder replacement. In Bayley, J.I.L., and Kessel, L. (eds.): Shoulder Surgery, pp. 164–167. Berlin, Springer-Verlag, 1982.
 4. Bucholz, H.W., and Engelbrecht, H.: Über die Depotwirkung einiger Antibiotica bei Vermischung mit dem Kunstharz Palacos. Chirurg, 41:511, 1970.
 5. Clayton, M.L., Ferlic, D.C., and Jeffers, P.D.: Prosthetic arthroplasties of the shoulders. Clin. Orthop., 164:184, 1982.
 6. Cofield, R.H.: Total joint arthroplasty. The shoulder. Mayo Clin. Proc., 54:500, 1979.
 7. Crenshaw, A.H.: Arthrodesis. In Campbell's Operative Orthopaedics, p. 1185. St. Louis, C.V. Mosby, 1971.
 8. Elson, R.A., and McGechie, D.B.: Antibiotics and acrylic bone cement. J. Bone Joint Surg., 58B:134, 1976.
 9. Evans, E.M., Freeman, M.A.R., Miller, A.J., and Vernon-Roberts, B.: Metal sensitivity as a cause of bone necrosis and loosening of the prosthesis in total joint replacement. J. Bone Joint Surg., 56B:626, 1974.
10. Kessel, L.: Personal communication.
11. Lettin, A.W.F.: Personal communication, 1976.
12. Lettin, A.W.F., Copeland, S.A., and Scales, J.T.: The Stanmore total shoulder replacement. J. Bone Joint Surg., 64B:47, 1982.
13. Murray, W.R., and Rodrigo, J.I.: Arthrography for the assessment of pain after total hip replacement. J. Bone Joint Surg., 57A:1060, 1975.
14. Neer, C.S. II: Displaced proximal humeral fracture. II. Treatment. J. Bone Joint Surg., 52A:1090, 1970.
15. Neer, C.S. II, and Kirby, R.M.: Revision of humeral head and total shoulder arthroplasties. Clin. Orthop., 170:189, 1982.
16. Post, M., Haskell, S.S., and Jablon, M.: Total shoulder replacement with a constrained prosthesis. J. Bone Joint Surg., 62A:327, 1980.
17. Post, M., and Jablon, M.: Constrained total shoulder arthroplasty: Long-term follow-up observations. Clin. Orthop., 173:109, 1983.
18. Post, M., Jablon, M., Miller, H., and Singh, M.: Constrained total shoulder joint replacement: A critical review. Clin. Orthop., 144:135, 1979.
19. Reeves, B.W.: A total shoulder endoprosthesis. Eng. Med., 1:64, 1972.
20. Reeves, B.W.: Proceedings Treiziene Congres International Chirurgie Orthopedique et de Traumatologie. Brussels, Imprimerie des Sciences, 1975.
21. Rowe, C.R.: Re-evaluation of the position of the arm in arthrodesis of the shoulder in an adult. J. Bone Joint Surg., 56A:919, 1974.

32 Complications of Arthroplasty of the Elbow

ROGER DEE

GENERAL CONSIDERATIONS

Soft Tissue Problems

Delayed wound healing can follow any incision, particularly on the extensor surface of the elbow. In the case of a prosthetic replacement, wound breakdown can have disastrous consequences. The risk can be minimized by placing the incision intelligently and handling tissue gently, avoiding undermining large flaps and paying particular attention to patients who have often been on corticosteroid therapy, in whom the skin may be wafer thin. Posterior incisions should be curved to avoid the point of the olecranon, and on occasion, separate medial and lateral incisions may be a wiser choice for some of the nonprosthetic arthroplasties, provided that the intervening skin bridge is sufficiently wide. The skin sutures or clips may safely be left *in situ* for a minimum of 3 weeks and even longer in patients with post-steroid changes.

Despite these precautions, there may be sloughing of portions of the skin at the edges, owing to ischemia. Under these circumstances it is necessary to immobilize the arm in plaster. The wound may be adequately dressed and any necessary skin grafting performed through an appropriate window in the plaster. The graft will not take over the extensor surface if the elbow is immobilized in a simple sling and allowed to move.

Hematoma formation is common following the extensive dissection involved in many of these procedures. It can be avoided by meticulous hemostasis after removal of the tourniquet. In addition, it is essential to use two suction drains, one down to the articular surface and one in the subcutaneous area. These drains can be withdrawn proximally through any supporting dressing or plaster. If a hematoma develops, it will inevitably lead to a delay in wound healing. The wound may break down as late as 1 month from primary surgery, so as soon as hematoma is detected, it should be evacuated under appropriate surgical conditions.

Circulatory Problems

Direct damage to major blood vessels has not been described following arthroplasty but poses a theoretical risk. Should it occur, appropriate repair at the time of surgery is indicated.

Postoperative circulatory embarrassment may be caused by an overtight compression dressing or cast and can usually be remedied by splitting the dressing down to the skin. I have relieved the compression of a hematoma postoperatively, but I have not had to perform radical fasciotomies for compartment syndrome after this operation. Once again, it is a possibility, and one should be aware of this as a possible complication.

Extending the elbow following arthroplasty can cause circulatory problems if the arm has been fixed in a flexed position for many years, and under these circumstances, flexing the elbow may be all that is necessary to restore adequate blood flow. The usual methods may be used to monitor compartmental pressures, together with the acceptable clinical criteria of watching for limitation of extension of the fingers, a severe degree of pain, diminished capillary blood flow, or absent radial pulse. One should be ready to take instant action, since delay can very rapidly result in loss of forearm muscle function.

Neurologic Problems

Because the ulnar nerve is most at risk in the operative field, it is wise to identify and protect it at all times during the surgery.

993

In the region of the sublimis tubercle of the ulna, it is directly applied to bone and may be very firmly bound and difficult to define. The usual care must be exercised at the end of the operation by relocating the ulnar nerve, if necessary. This is particularly important in the case of prosthetic arthroplasty, a proper muscle bed being essential. The nerve that is transplanted to a subcutaneous position often continues to give symptoms postoperatively for an indefinite period, and this is particularly true if it is adjacent to metal.

Wristdrop that was not apparent immediately after surgery can develop a few hours later when an elbow long flexed has been immobilized in extension after a mobilizing operation. The radial nerve recovers quickly—within an hour or so—after the elbow is placed in a more appropriate position of 90° of flexion. Although the nerve could be damaged directly by excessive stripping of soft tissues proximally as far as the spiral groove, I am unaware that this complication has ever occurred; if so, it has not been reported. Similarly, one might expect occasional thermal damage from the excesive use of cement in the medullary cavity of the lower half of the humeral shaft during revision in which the cortex is thinned or perforated, but I know of no accounts of this.

The posterior interosseous nerve, in contrast to the radial nerve, is at direct risk during these procedures, where it passes around the neck of the radius, for example, from the injudicious or inexpert use of Homan-type retractors. Great care is necessary particularly when removing a radial ulnar synostosis, and overenthusiastic resection of the radial head should be avoided.

COMPLICATIONS OF NONPROSTHETIC ARTHROPLASTY

In the literature, if we exclude simple excision of the radial head and arthrolysis, three principal groups of arthroplasties may be distinguished. There are minor variations in each of the three categories in the exact amount of bone removed, the surgical approach made to the joint, and the postoperative care. Each of the three groups,

however, has fundamental differences in operative technique that differentiate them from one another. Each group also relies on a distinctive process of repair. Failure to appreciate this can lead to an inappropriate choice of operation.

Subcapsular, Subperiosteal Excision of the Elbow Joint

In subcapsular, subperiosteal excision of the elbow joint the humerus is sectioned at or above the level of the epicondyles, and part of the olecranon and radial head is also removed to give a bone gap of some 3 cm with the elbow extended. The dissection is performed subperiosteally, and there is some immediate postoperative stability created by the preservation of the ligaments that are in continuity with the periosteal flap. The operation depends for its success on the regenerative properties of the periosteum. Thus it was first described by Ollier[26] for use in young patients with ankylosis following tuberculosis and has later been used with success by Kirkaldy-Willis[18] in a similar age group and again in patients with stiff elbows following tuberculosis or trauma. For this type of patient, Kirkaldy-Willis described just over half of his results as being either good or excellent, but he stressed the importance of a meticulous postoperative regime. This regime is similar to the one used by Ollier and involves progressive mobilization of the new joint with some form of hinged splint that maintains lateral stability. He emphasizes the importance of increasing physiotherapy after the first 3 weeks and points out that muscle strength must be built up over a period of at least 3 months. He also notes that if the gap excised is too large, the result is a flail joint; if the gap is too small, reankylosis occurs. According to Kirkaldy-Willis,* the results are not satisfactory in rheumatoid arthritis.

Hurri and associates[15] also described results of the use of this technique in the rheumatoid elbow and noted that although it gave good pain relief in 81% of 53 cases, poor primary motion was achieved in 10

---

* Kirkaldy-Willis, W.H.: Personal communication.

FIG. 32-1. The result of excision arthroplasty for rheumatoid arthritis. There is a fulcrum as flexion approaches 90°.

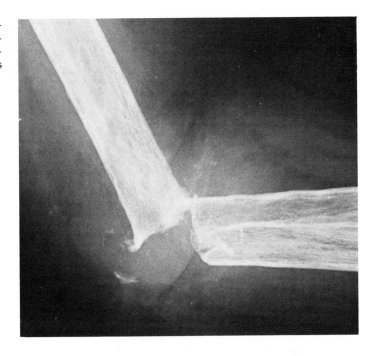

cases, which required correction by reoperation, and ankylosis occurred in one case. In addition, paresthesia in the region of the ulnar nerve was present in 17%, and resorption of bone at the region of the olecranon fossa was present in 26%. In patients with rheumatoid arthritis, stability and strength were found to be better when a modified Hass arthroplasty was used (see below).

Excision of the Elbow Joint

Simple excision of the olecranon and distal humerus together with their periosteal covering was condemned by Ollier for leading to "absence of articulation."[26] The development of gross instability is the most common complication of this procedure, as reported by Dee (Figs. 32-1 and 32-2).[6,8,9]

The technique of Hass gives the best results if care is taken to preserve the collateral ligaments of the joint and to refashion the bone ends to form a "functional ginglymus."[14] There is, therefore, not a large gap between the bone ends, and a stable fulcrum is preserved. Hass used a fat-flap interposed between the bone ends. Even so, 20% of his cases gave poor results

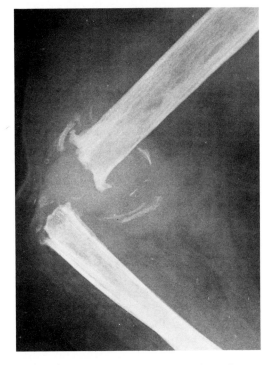

FIG. 32-2. The dramatic moment when, as flexion exceeds 90°, the stability of the fulcrum is lost. Severe pain was experienced at this moment, and the patient had immediate loss of grip.

owing to recurrent ankylosis. Once again, the margin for error is small. Hass used skin traction to avoid contact between the bone ends because of the fear of reankylosis, but Unander-Scharin and Karlholm[37] reported two postoperative flail elbows in patients with rheumatoid arthritis when they used a modification of the Hass technique. They point out that the operation is unsuccessful in the painful but mobile joint, indicating that in patients with rheumatoid arthritis the operation is best performed for ankylosis.

Hurri and colleagues[15] report that elbow joints after this operation are posturally "quite unstable" at rest but only "fairly stable" with tightened muscles. Vainio reports that resorption of bone at the region of the olecranon fossa is present in 46% after this procedure, but the complication can be diminished by filling the olecranon fossa with bone chips beneath an interposed skin graft. Without some form of interposition the operation is unsatisfactory in patients with rheumatoid arthritis.*

Anatomical Arthroplasty

When the elbow joint in question has relatively normal bone architecture and the ligaments are preserved, it is possible to excise a fine sliver of bone from each articular surface and refashion a stable articulation in a long-standing case of ankylosis. This operation, first described by Defontaine,[11] can also be used together with soft tissue interposition to relieve pain and improve stability in a rheumatoid joint.

A procedure has been developed by Scudder,[31] Campbell,[3] and MacAusland[22] using fascial interposition. Their results confirmed that a range of motion of 90° or so in a useful arc may be expected but that the joint remains a little loose collaterally. Any error of judgment that results in removal of too much bone will produce an elbow that is unstable and may dislocate. Dee[8,9] has described bone erosion leading to late subluxation or even dislocation following this sort of procedure. The author has also pointed out the ease with which reankylosis can occur in patients who have rheumatoid arthritis.

MacAusland[22] stressed the importance of building some stability into the arthroplasty by fashioning a crest longitudinally in the floor of the trochlear notch of the ulna and notching the distal end of the humerus. It is interesting that all authors agree that the best results are achieved when the operation is performed for posttraumatic stiffening and that the penalty for too little excision of bone is reankylosis.

Knight and VanZandt[19] observed medial subluxation in five of their 45 cases and lateral subluxation in eight. They reiterate the contraindications stressed by Campbell (tuberculosis, extensive scar tissue, extreme muscle atrophy) and state that patients who need to use the arm for heavy physical labor should not have this procedure because strength and stability will not be adequate postoperatively. To prevent subluxation due to progressive bone erosion after surgery, they recommend that more bone be taken from the olecranon and the radius than from the humerus. As bone erosion proceeds, if it involves the humerus, it will certainly wear away the condyle, which may fracture and become detached. With the dissolution of the condyle (Figs. 32-3 and 32-4), subluxation occurs, and instability develops. Knight and VanZandt[19] recommend excision of the head of the radius, which they regard as a potent factor in causing erosion of the lateral epicondyle. They also feel that subluxation is more likely if an attempt is made to fashion a carrying angle.

Froimsen and co-workers,[13] in 1976, reiterated the value of skin interposed between the bone ends, and my personal experience with this operation has indicated that it is excellent as an adjunct to anatomical arthroplasty following trauma that leaves the architecture of the joint relatively intact. The problem in rheumatoid arthritis, however, is getting a successful piece of dermis from these patients, who often have poor skin. When it is possible, it is an excellent conservative procedure.

COMPLICATIONS OF PROSTHETIC ARTHROPLASTY

Because consistently high-grade results cannot be achieved with nonprosthetic arthroplasty in patients with rheumatoid ar-

---

* Vainio, K.: Personal communication, 1975.

FIG. 32-3. The early result of this anatomical arthroplasty seems good 6 months from surgery. Note the central notch in the distal humerus. No material was interposed.

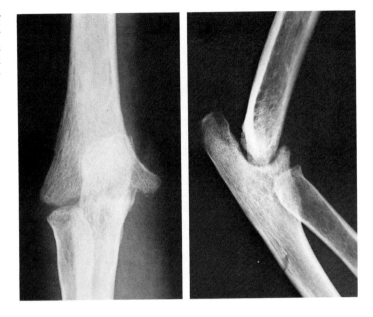

thritis or with flail elbows, the search continues for a prosthetic replacement. A strong motivation is the increasing number of younger patients with flail arms resulting from severe compound fractures following traffic accidents.

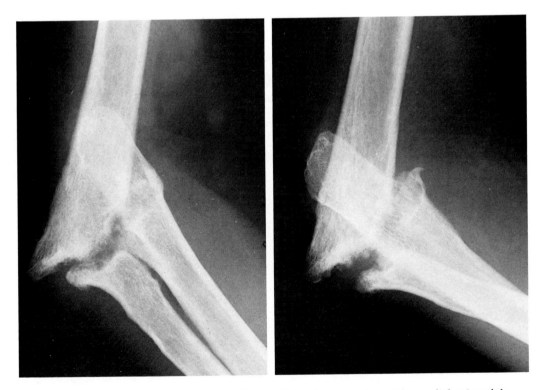

FIG. 32-4. The same patient shown in Figure 32-3 a few years later. The medial epicondyle has been completely eroded, and subluxation has occurred.

Replacement Hemiarthroplasty

No large series has been published, but for many years an occasional case has been reported in which the lower end of the humerus,[1,22,23,32,38] or, alternatively, the proximal end of the ulna,[17] has been replaced by a custom-made, anatomically shaped prosthesis usually made of metal but occasionally of acrylic, nylon, or Teflon. It seems that good pain relief in the short term is achieved, but the wear properties of the nonmetallic materials have led to rapid fragmentation and the development of sinuses. In the case of metal components, erosion of bone in contact with the metal can cause late complications.

I have used fresh frozen allografts to replace the deficient distal humerus on several occasions in younger patients in whom the only alternative would have been a large metal replacement.[10] Although these large allografts may fracture, the fractures do then seem to heal, and function is maintained despite the wear and erosion that take place at the bearing surface of the graft. This is a good, conservative alternative in the young patient who has lost 3 inches or so of distal humerus, and it has the advantage that no more of the patient's bone stock is damaged by methylmethacrylate insertion, since the allograft can be fixed in place by standard compression plating.

I do not recommend transplantation of the whole elbow joint, since my only two cases of this procedure, unlike humeral allografts alone, have been failures.

Hinge Arthroplasty

A custom-built chrome–cobalt hinge prosthesis was available in the 1950s (Fig. 32-5). Its insertion involved removal of the olecranon, so the hinge was relatively near the surface. Wound breakdown was a common complication.

In England both Shiers and McKee developed elbow hinges, but they were not originally designed for use with acrylic cement, and difficulty was often encountered in inserting their straight stems into the anatomical curves of the bones.

Dee[7] reported the results of arthroplasty using a prosthesis of his own design with suitable curved medullary stems and using acrylic cement. An early complication noted at this stage was avascular necrosis of the olecranon, which occurred from a combination of overenthusiastic stripping of sur-

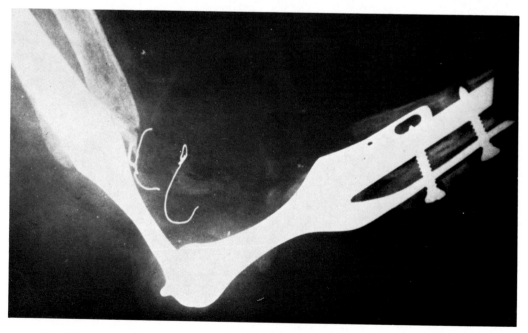

FIG. 32-5. An early type of elbow hinge. Note the loosening of the Vitallium screws.

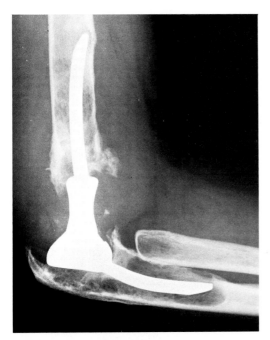

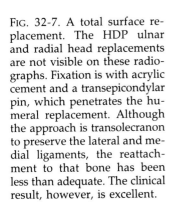

FIG. 32-6. The typical appearance of a loose prosthesis, in this case a Dee hinge 2 years after insertion. Both components are loose, and it is interesting that the patient was sensitive to cobalt. Note the characteristic cortical destruction.

an ominous note when he detailed his initial results of 20 elbow hinge replacements, principally using McKee's design and its modification but including six Dee elbows. He noted that 25% of his series were loose at 3 years. Dee's personal series in which his own design of a fully constrained hinge joint was used now confirms that loosening is a serious inherent defect of the fully constrained total hinge; 25% of his 40 elbow replacements reviewed at 5 years were loose. The loosening is a serious matter because there is considerable damage to the bone both proximally and distally as the loose acrylic plug abrades the inner cortex (Fig. 32-6). The rotatory forces generated by the action of pronation and supination are not dissipated at the articulation but are transmitted directly to the bond between the acrylic and the bone of the proximal segment. It is now apparent that the high rate of loosening is common to all fully constrained joint prostheses of this design. The problem is exacerbated when there is existing limitation of pronation and supination.

rounding soft tissues and packing an eroded olecranon with large quantities of cement. He described an operative technique to avoid this complication. Souter[33] sounded

Molds and Surface Replacements (Fig. 32-7)

The late Geoffrey Platt was using a chrome–cobalt mold interposed between the bone surfaces in the early 1960s in Aylsbury, England, but he did not report on his

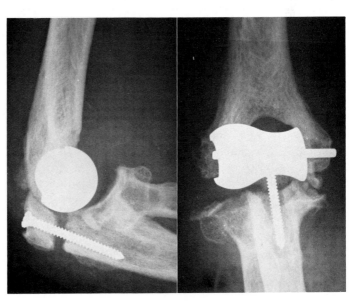

FIG. 32-7. A total surface replacement. The HDP ulnar and radial head replacements are not visible on these radiographs. Fixation is with acrylic cement and a transepicondylar pin, which penetrates the humeral replacement. Although the approach is transolecranon to preserve the lateral and medial ligaments, the reattachment to that bone has been less than adequate. The clinical result, however, is excellent.

results. Personal observation of six cases by one of the authors indicates that good movement was achieved but that there was a high incidence of ulnar nerve irritation.

Street and Stevens[34] described a surface replacement of the articular surface of the distal humerus in 10 cases. The operation is not suitable for patients with active rheumatoid arthritis or hemophilia or for the very young. There has been one subluxation due to improper placement of the prosthesis. Accurate placement of the prosthesis is essential for success, and a Kirschner wire is used as a guide placed so as to obtain the correct carrying angle. It is doubtful whether this prosthesis will be useful in patients with atrophic bone or rheumatoid arthritis, since avascularity, fracture, or erosion of the bone embraced by the prosthesis will lead to loosening.

"Semiconstrained" Prostheses (Fig. 32-8).   In the flail elbow with loss of bone, perhaps following a compound fracture or a failed hinge, one has the most difficult problem, because none of the soft tissue arthroplasties are really satisfactory. One needs the stability that can be given only by a linked replacement, and a surface replacement is not satisfactory. The use of a fully constrained hinge in these circumstances, however, will certainly lead to failure in a young, vigorous person with strong musculature developing rotation forces.

Swanson[35] first tackled this problem by using a flexible hinge of silicone rubber, but he noted that although it was possible to obtain an adequate result with this method in a sedentary patient, it is probably not indicated in a manual worker, for whom Swanson preferred arthrodesis.

Many semiconstrained designs have been in use for several years following the failure of the original constrained devices. They will remain in use, since they answer the clinical need to stabilize an elbow when there has been severe bone loss or ligament damage and when stabilization does not seem to be possible in any other way. The short-term results seem to indicate that allowing some varus–valgus motion and some rotation into these designs has resulted in an acceptable degree of loosening. This has been the experience with the revised Coonrad prosthesis,[4] the Dee semicon-

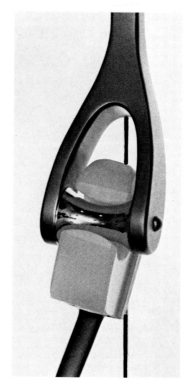

FIG. 32-8. A semiconstrained total elbow replacement with a snap fit (Dee). Note the built-in carrying angle and the amount of lateral movement possible at the prosthesis. It is still undergoing clinical trial.

strained design,[10] the triaxial prosthesis of Inglis,[16] and also the Schlein device.[29] Also in this category are the designs from the Mayo Clinic[24,25] and the Volz Arizona HSC[2] prosthesis. These devices allow some of the stresses in the articulation to be transmitted to the surrounding soft tissues and thus dissipated and not all transmitted to the cement mantle. The trade-off is often a more complicated design with some loss of strength compared with the massive hinges. Thus there have been component failures in most series.[2,16,24] The treatment of component failure and loosening is revision (see below).

A complication described in many of these series is fracture of the humeral shaft or humeral condyles during insertion.[2,16] Conservative treatment thereafter seems to be the treatment of choice, 6 weeks of immobilization usually being sufficient to stabilize the intraoperative fracture. Careful surgery, together with good preoperative radiographic evaluation and careful implant selection and sizing, should prevent this complication.

REVISION

The revision operation is difficult and requires patience and delicacy. A cement-removal tool, such as a "cement eater" set or a Midas instrument, is necessary. Use of a fiberoptic headlight and combined Water-Pik/suction device is also advisable. To minimize the risk of perforation of the cortex, I advise formal exposure of at least 6 inches of visible cortex of both ulna and humeral shaft so that the direction of the tool can be accurately lined up.[10] Primary orientation is of course given by the view down the inside of the shaft between passes with a power instrument.

The salvage procedure of choice varies with circumstance. Certainly the worst thing to do is to insert a long-stem version of the device that has already failed (*e.g.*, a constrained hinge) or to try to recement the loosened component. When the bone erosion of the cortex was not severe, I have successfully revised with a semiconstrained stemmed device and obtained durable results in a dozen cases. This is now my standard procedure in such circumstances.

When the bone stock is very severely damaged, an alternative is to insert cortical cancellous bone graft into the cleared portion of the medullary cavity and to insert another prosthesis a year later. The architecture of the bone is reasonably restored in this time.[10] This two-stage procedure may be particularly helpful when porous-coated stems are available in revision prostheses.

UNCONSTRAINED PROSTHESES AND THEIR COMPLICATIONS

When the architecture of the joint is well preserved and the ligaments are intact, it is possible to insert a surface-replacement prosthesis that is unlinked. The congruity of the new articulating surface, combined with appropriate soft tissue balancing and the integrity of the major ligaments, is responsible for providing postoperative stability. Severe rheumatoid arthritis (grades III and IV) is the usual indication.

Kudo and co-workers[20] have described 24 cases, all of them in patients with rheumatoid arthritis and a 46-month average follow-up, and had only one case of loosening and one case of instability. Reports of three series in which Ewald's capitello-condylar design was used have been published, all cases with rheumatoid arthritis.[4,12,27] Good or satisfactory results were reported in more than 80% of the cases (with an average follow-up of 35 to 42 months and a total of 127 cases).

Loosening does not seem to be a problem in these unconstrained designs, but these authors report cases of instability as 5.7%,[12] 13.3%,[4] and 14.3%,[27] with average residual flexion contractures of 31°, 35°, and 33°, respectively.

Instability following these types of procedures usually occurs because the anterior oblique portion of the medial collateral ligament (MCL) is violated at surgery or damaged preoperatively and not repaired. Its important stabilizing role has been well documented.[30]

Use of the lateral Kocher approach is stressed by several authors as critical in avoiding damage to the MCL during insertion of these prostheses.[12,27] This is particularly important because the lateral radiocapitellar side of the radial head is often removed and not replaced. When replaced, it is doubtful whether the replacement radiocapitellar arthroplasty is as efficient as the original congruent fit of the natural joint in functioning as a secondary stabilizer.

Although some slack in the MCL may be taken by having different thicknesses of prostheses and different angles of valgus on the humeral component available, as in the Ewald design, it is not surprising that occasionally a clinical case of instability is manifest. In my experience, if the joint is unstable at the end of surgery, it may not stabilize even with 6 weeks of postoperative immobilization in a cast, and it is as good to evaluate the situation carefully before leaving the operating room and to try to obtain a more stable solution.

Reconstruction of the MCL may be performed at surgery with the methods described in the literature.[36] Alternatively, it may be necessary to insert a semiconstrained prosthesis. The occasional case of instability will not be completely eliminated as a complication until we have the ability to balance the soft tissues and jig the elbow in extension and flexion at the correct degree of carrying angle. Such sophisticated prosthetic designs, together with more appropriate instruments, will also take care of the residual flexion contractures seen in one in three of these operated cases.

INFECTION

Infection rates differ widely among the various series of semiconstrained arthroplasties. Morrey and colleagues[25] reported 8.8% in 80 cases in which Mayo and Coonrad designs were used, whereas Brumfield and associates,[2] in the same year, reported only one case of superficial infection in 30 arthroplasties in which the Mayo and the AHSC designs were used.

Schlein[29] reported 1% infection in 400 cases in which his prosthesis was inserted by various surgeons, and Inglis and Pellicci[16] reported 3.2% of cases infected of 31 replacements with Pritchard-Walker or triaxial prostheses. The three principle series in which the capitellocondylar unconstrained joint was used have an average infection rate of 8% in 127 cases, whereas by contrast Kudo and co-workers reported no cases of infection in their 24 unconstrained prosthetic replacements.[20]

My own experience does not lead me to believe that total replacement of the elbow is particularly more at risk of infection than is total joint replacement of the knee joint. These procedures are often lengthy and tedious, and they are often performed on patients who are particularly prone to infection (patients with severe rheumatoid arthritis). Nevertheless, when associated with the injection of large quantities of methylmethacrylate into the long bones of the arm, this high infection rate continues to be disturbing.

A voluminous literature exists on the treatment of infection following total joint replacement, and the same general principles apply in the elbow. Early diagnosis is essential, and organisms may be obtained

by aspiration or blood culture. If caught early, it is worth one attempt at vigorous irrigation and open debridement without removing a tight joint. Following this, immobilization of the joint in a cast plus appropriate intravenous medication for 6 weeks with careful monitoring of blood antibody levels for proper efficacy is required. When the infection is more established and there is obvious spread around the cement mantel, nothing less than total removal of the device together with *all* of the cement will suffice.

Morrey and Bryan state that if significant function is lost, the elbow remains painful, and there is no evidence of sepsis at 1 year, "reimplantation may be considered in certain instances, although it is generally not recommended."[24]

REFERENCES

1. Barr, J.S., and Eaton, R.G.: Elbow reconstruction with a new prosthesis to replace the distal end of the humerus. J. Bone Joint Surg., 47A:1408, 1965.
2. Brumfield, R.H., Jr., Volz, R.G., and Green, J.F.: Total Elbow Arthroplasty, a review of 30 cases employing the Mayo and the A.H.S.C. prosthesis. Clin. Orthop., 158:137, 1981.
3. Campbell, W.C.: Mobilization of joints with bony ankylosis. J.A.M.A., 83:976, 1924.
4. Coonrad, R.W.: Coonrad total elbow replacement. Presented at the Annual Meeting of the American Orthopaedic Association, June 27, 1978.
5. Davis, R.F., Weiland, A., Hungerford, D.S. et al.: Nonconstrained total elbow arthroplasty. Clin. Orthop., 171:156, 1982.
6. Dee, R.: Elbow arthroplasty. Proc. R. Soc. Med., 62:1031, 1969.
7. Dee, R.: Total replacement arthroplasty of the elbow for rheumatoid arthritis. J. Bone Joint Surg., 54B:88, 1972.
8. Dee, R.: Total replacement of the elbow joint. Mod. Trends Orthop., 6:250, 1972.
9. Dee, R.: Total replacement of the elbow joint. Orthop. Clin. North Am., 4:415, 1973.
10. Dee, R.: Reconstructive surgery following total elbow endoprosthesis. Clin. Orthop., 170:196, 1982.
11. Defontaine, L.: Osteotomie trochleiforme. Rev. Chir., 7:716, 1887.
12. Ewald, F.C., Scheinberg, R.D., Poss, R. et al.: Capitellocondylar total elbow arthroplasty. J. Bone Joint Surg., 62A:1259, 1980.
13. Froimsen, A.J., Silva, J.E., and Richey, D.G.: Cutis arthroplasty of the elbow joint. J. Bone Joint Surg., 58A:863, 1976.
14. Hass, J.: Functional arthroplasty. J. Bone Joint Surg., 26:297, 1944.
15. Hurri, L., Pulkki, T., and Vainio, K.: Arthroplasty of the elbow in rheumatoid arthritis. Acta Chir. Scand., 127:459, 1964.

16. Inglis, A.E., and Pellicci, P.M.: Total elbow replacement. J. Bone Joint Surg., 62A:1252, 1980.
17. Johnson, E.W., Jr., and Schlein, A.P.: Vitallium prosthesis for the olecranon and proximal part of the ulna. J. Bone Joint Surg., 52A:721, 1970.
18. Kirkaldy-Willis, W.H.: Excision of the elbow joint. Lancet, 1:53, 1948.
19. Knight, R.A., and VanZandt, I.L.: Arthroplasty of the elbow: An end result study. J. Bone Joint Surg., 34A:610, 1952.
20. Kudo, H., Iwano, K., and Watanabe, S.: Total replacement of the rheumatoid elbow with a hingeless prosthesis. J. Bone Joint Surg., 62A:277, 1980.
21. MacAusland, W.R.: Arthroplasty of the elbow. N. Engl. J. Med., 236:97, 1947.
22. MacAusland, W.R.: Replacement of the lower end of the humerus with a prosthesis: A report of four cases. West. J. Surg. Gynecol. Obstet., 62:557, 1954.
23. Mellen, R.H., and Phalen, G.S.: Arthroplasty of the elbow by replacement of the distal portion of the humerus with an acrylic prosthesis. J. Bone Joint Surg., 29:348, 1947.
24. Morrey, B.F., and Bryan, R.S.: Complications of total elbow arthroplasty. Clin. Orthop., 170:204, 1982.
25. Morrey, B.F., Bryan, R.S., Dobyns, J.H., and Linscheid, K.L.: Total elbow arthroplasty. J. Bone Joint Surg., 63A:1050, 1981.
26. Ollier, L.: Traite des Resections et des Operations Conservatrices qu'on peut Praetiquer sur le Systeme Osseaux. Paris, G. Masson, 1885.
27. Rosenberg, G.M., and Turner, R.H.: Nonconstrained total elbow replacement. Clin. Orthop., 1984.
28. Rosenfeld, S.R., and Anzel, S.H.: Evaluation of the Pritchard total elbow arthroplasty. Orthopaedics, 5(6):713, 1982.
29. Schlein, A.R.: Semiconstrained total elbow arthroplasty. Clin. Orthop., 121:222, 1976.
30. Schwab, G.H., Bennett, J.B., Woods, G.W., and Tullos, H.S.: Biomechanics of elbow instability: The role of the medial collateral ligament. Clin. Orthop., 146:42, 1980.
31. Scudder, C.: Arthroplasty for complete ankylosis of the elbow. Ann. Surg., 48:711, 1908.
32. Silva, J.F.: Arthroplasty of the elbow. Singapore Med. J., 8:222, 1967.
33. Souter, W.A.: Arthroplasty of the elbow. Orthop. Clin. North Am., 4:395, 1973.
34. Street, D.M., and Stevens, P.S.: A humeral replacement prosthesis for the elbow. J. Bone Joint Surg., 56A:1147, 1974.
35. Swanson, A.B.: Flexible Implant Resection Arthroplasty in the Hand and Extremities. St. Louis, C.V. Mosby, 1973.
36. Tullos, H.S., Schwab, G., Bennett, J.B., and Woods, G.W.: Factors influencing elbow instability. Instr. Course Lect., 32:185, 1983.
37. Unander-Scharin, L., and Karlholm, S.: Experience of arthroplasty of the elbow. Acta Orthop. Scand., 36:54, 1965.
38. Venable, C.S.: An elbow and an elbow prosthesis: Case of complete loss of the lower third of the humerus. Am. J. Surg., 83:271, 1952.

33 Complications of Arthroplasty and Joint Replacement at the Wrist

ALFRED B. SWANSON, JAMES H. HERNDON,
AND GENEVIEVE DEGROOT SWANSON

The wrist is the key joint for proper function of the hand.[11] Wrist movements can place the hand in any plane in space with respect to the forearm and allow the hand to assume optimal position for the performance of functional adaptations; these are greatly facilitated by wrist motion, especially flexion, even if it is limited. This is particularly true if the fingers are partially disabled. A few degrees of wrist movement increases the reach of the fingers in space by 5 cm to 6 cm, greatly improving their functional potential. Writing is difficult for patients who have a wrist fusion if the function of the fingers is also inadequate. Personal hygiene can be a problem for patients with fused wrists, especially if fixed in extension. A great many of the functional adaptations require flexion of the wrist and rotation of the forearm. The loss of these actions can result in severe disability, even more so if the fingers, elbow, or shoulder is also disabled.

A stable wrist is necessary for proper transmission of muscle forces from the forearm to the digits. However, a mobile wrist is most important in moving objects toward the body, as in activities of daily living. Disabilities of the wrist are a common result of fractures or dislocations of the carpal bones and of the distal end of the radius or ulna, and they may also follow the destructive changes of rheumatoid arthritis or osteoarthritis. The goal of reconstructive procedures of the wrist would be an ideal compromise between stability and mobility.

A brief discussion of the anatomy and physiology of the wrist will help in understanding the pathomechanics of deformities and the indications, goals, and pitfalls of the reconstructive procedures most commonly used. A critical review of past and current reconstructive procedures is presented, since they apply to the radiocarpal and distal radioulnar joints and to individual carpal bones.

ANATOMY OF THE WRIST

The wrist is a multiple-link system between the forearm and the hand. It is composed of interrelated articulations between the distal radius, the distal ulna, the proximal and distal carpal rows, and the metacarpal bases. These articulations can be classified as (1) the radiocarpal joint, between the distal radius and the proximal carpal row, (2) the distal radioulnar joint, between the distal radius and the ulna, and (3) the midcarpal joint, between the proximal and distal carpal rows.

The proximal carpal row includes the scaphoid (navicular), lunate, and triquetral bones. The scaphoid and lunate articulate with facets on the radius. These bones are united by short interosseous ligaments (Figs. 33-1 and 33-2). The distal carpal row includes the trapezium, trapezoid, capitate, and hamate. These bones are also linked by short interosseous ligaments. The ulnar and radial collateral ligaments help provide lateral support of the wrist. The dorsal and especially the palmar radiocarpal ligaments are extremely important in maintaining support of the carpal area. The fibers of the palmar radiocarpal ligament extend distally and obliquely from the radius, the triangular fibrocartilage complex, and the radial styloid process. Short, deep ligamen-

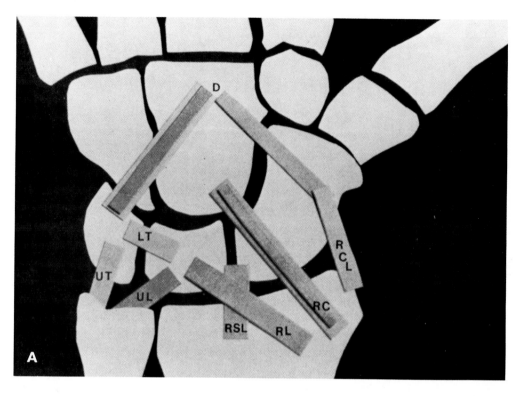

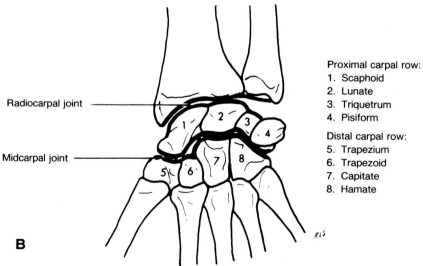

FIG. 33-1. (*A*) Schematic representation of the carpal ligaments. *D*, deltoid; *RCL*, radial collateral; *RC*, radiocapitate; *RL*, radiolunate; *RSL*, deep radioscaphoid-lunate; *UL*, ulnolunate; *UT*, ulnotriquetral (volar attachment of the ulnocarpal meniscus); *LT*, lunotriquetral. (*B*) Diagram of the radiocarpal and midcarpal joints and the relationship of the carpal bones. (*A*, Taleisnik, J.: Post-traumatic carpal instability. Clin. Orthop., 149:73, 1980)

tous bands connect the trapezium and trapezoid to the scaphoid, and the hamate to the triquetrum. The dorsal ligamentous structures are not as dense as the volar ones. Taleisnik has classified these ligaments into two groups: extrinsic and intrinsic.[90,91]

Classification of Wrist Joint Ligaments

Extrinsic
 Proximal (radiocarpal)
  Radial collateral
  Volar radiocarpal
   Superficial
   Deep
    Radioscaphoid-capitate
    Radiolunate
    Radioscaphoid-lunate
  Ulnocarpal complex
   Meniscus (radiotriquetral)
   Triangular fibrocartilate
   Ulnolunate ligament
   Ulnar collateral ligament
  Dorsal radiocarpal
 Distal (carpometacarpal)
Intrinsic
 Short
  Volar
  Dorsal
  Interosseous
 Intermediate
  Lunotriquetral
  Scapholunate
  Scaphotrapezial
 Long
  Volar intercarpal (V deltoid)
  Dorsal intercarpal

(Modified from Taleisnik, J.: The ligaments of the wrist. J. Hand Surg., 1[2]:111, 1976)

The integrity of these ligaments must be maintained in carpal bone surgery.[74,76]

The anatomy of the triangular fibrocartilage complex of the wrist has recently been clarified by Palmer and Werner.[59] It is a homogeneous structure composed of, but not dissectible into, an articular disc, the meniscus homologue, the dorsal and volar radioulnar ligaments, the ulnar collateral ligament, and the sheath of the extensor carpi ulnaris (Fig. 33-3).

MOTIONS AT THE WRIST

Movements at the wrist include flexion, extension, adduction-ulnar deviation, and abduction-radial deviation and are combined with pronation and supination of the forearm. The wrist motions are complex and are integrated between the various joints and the individual carpal bones. Rotation of the scaphoid is necessary for full

radial deviation because of the radial styloid process. Kinematics of the normal wrist are complicated, and only recently, with the use of sophisticated techniques, have they been clarified. The center of wrist motion in both the anteroposterior and lateral planes is located at the head of the capitate, and not in the body or the neck of the capitate.[48] The wrist behaves similar to a universal joint, with motion possible in all planes, including 6° to 9° of rotation.

Flexion, extension, and radial and ulnar deviation at the wrist occur in both the radiocarpal and midcarpal joints.[36,37] Rotation of the forearm is most important for adapting the wrist joint to movements of the hand and requires integrity of the distal radioulnar joint. Circumduction movement of the wrist is formed by a combination of flexion and extension and ulnar and radial deviation. This motion traces a conical configuration in space that is irregular, because the participating movements are not symmetrical in their range. Motions added by forearm rotation compensate for this asymmetry and allow the axis of the hand to lie anywhere within a cone with an angle of aperture of approximately 170°.

Flexion and extension of the wrist are maximal when there is no lateral deviation. The average extension is from 60° to 80°, and the palmar flexion is from 70° to 90°; abduction or radial deviation is greatest when the hand is in 0° of extension and has a range of approximately 15°; adduction or ulnar deviation is usually two to three times greater and may reach 45°.

Ulnar and radial deviation of the wrist occur mainly at the radiocarpal joint. However, because a bony crest separates the distal radial surface in two cavities and a strong interosseous ligament unites the scaphoid and lunate bones, approximately 20% of radial deviation movements also rise at the midcarpal joint, mainly around the head of the capitate. Not only do the intercarpal ligaments restrict motion, but impingement of the distal row at each end of the proximal row limits motion as well.[54]

During wrist extension, approximately two thirds of movement is located principally at the radiocarpal joint and one third at the midcarpal joint (Fig. 33-4). In flexion, approximately 60% of excursion occurs at

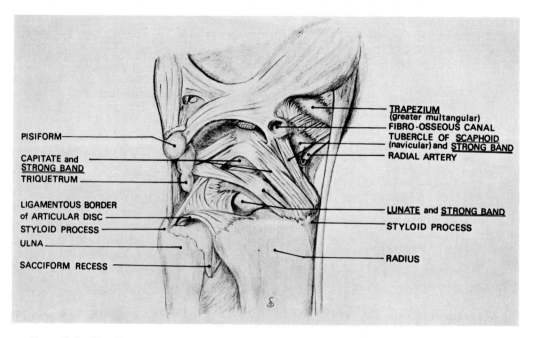

FIG. 33-2. The ligamentous structures on the palmar aspect of the carpus. The very important strong bands are noted. Note also the prominences of the lunate, scaphoid, and trapezium. When these bones are surgically removed, weak areas are produced between the strong bands. These areas may allow palmar dislocation of an implant. This can be prevented by leaving a thin layer of bone attached to the ligaments or by bringing the adjacent bands together with sutures or a strip of tendon material.

the midcarpal level and the rest at the radiocarpal level.[87] As noted, the scaphoid bone bridges the midcarpal joint. However, from a functional point of view, the midcarpal joint continues distally between the trapezium, the trapezoid, and adjacent surfaces of the first and second metacarpals; the thumb, trapezium, and scaphoid act as a unit that plays only a small part in midcarpal movements. Motion around the scaphoid takes place in all three body planes: vertically at its proximal pole, horizontally at the distal pole, and coronally at the scaphoid-capitate articulation.

Integrated movements of the radiocarpal and midcarpal joints are made possible by important displacements of the carpal bones. The shape of the proximal carpal row changes in various hand positions, and the shape of the distal carpal row becomes modified accordingly. Link systems are present in the hand, as they are in the digits. Proper balance of this link system depends on the shape of bones and the integrity and tension of their ligaments. Palmer and colleagues have recently shown that the functional range of wrist motion appears to be between 10° of palmar flexion and 35° of dorsiflexion, 10° of radial deviation, and 15° of ulnar deviation.[60]

THE RADIOCARPAL JOINT

PATHOMECHANICS OF RHEUMATOID DEFORMITIES

Rheumatoid arthritis is a common cause of severe impairment of the wrist. It may affect the soft tissues and joints of the wrist, including the radiocarpal, intercarpal, and radioulnar joints, singly or in combination. The destructive synovitis of the rheumatoid disease at the wrist causes loosening of the ligaments and erosive changes of bone, disturbing the multiple-link system of the wrist. In some cases spontaneous fusion of

FIG. 33-3. The components of the triangular fibrocartilage complex: *MH*, meniscus homologue; *AD*, articular disc; *UCL*, ulnar collateral ligament; *RUL*, dorsal and volar radioulnar ligaments. The extensor carpi ulnaris sheath (another component of the complex) is not shown. Other structures shown are the metacarpal bones (2, 3, 4, and 5), the carpal bones (*S*, scaphoid; *L*, lunate; *TQ*, triquetrum; *H*, hamate; *C*, capitate; *TZ*, trapezoid; *TP*, trapezium), and the radius (*R*) and ulna (*U*). (Palmer, A.K., and Werner, F.W.: The triangular fibrocartilage complex of the wrist—anatomy and function. J. Hand Surg., 6:153, 1981)

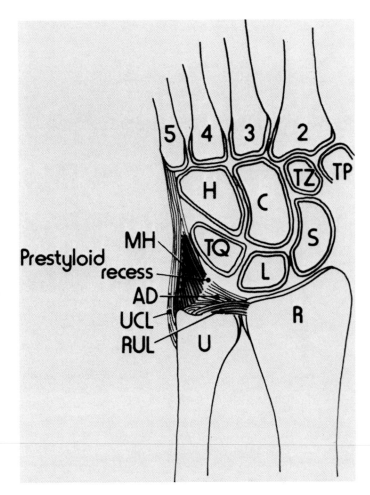

the wrist may occur before subluxation. In severe cases a complete dislocation of the wrist can also be present. Loosening of the ligaments of the radial aspect of the joint is common and allows an ulnar displacement of the proximal row, resulting secondarily in radial deviation of the hand. The associated subluxation of the distal radioulnar joint causes a loss of stability on the ulnar aspect of the wrist. Loosening of the palmar radiocarpal ligament allows a collapse in the long axis, followed by buckling of the radiocarpal linked system. However, a palmar subluxation of the proximal row on the radius is more common.

Rheumatoid insults to the radiocarpal joint are common and especially disabling when associated digit deformities are present. The resulting deformities may be summarized as follows: fusion and/or fibrosis and associated stiffness; ulnar shift of the carpus on the radius, which may or may not result in radial deviation of the hand; palmar subluxation of the carpus on the ulna with associated absorptive changes in the proximal carpal row; occasional radial and palmar dislocation of the hand off the radius; and associated ruptures of extensor tendons. These deformities are usually associated with marked instability and serious loss of hand function.[84]

SURGICAL PROCEDURES

The more common procedures used in attempts to control pain, correct wrist alignment, and provide stability or mobility to the wrist have included osteotomy of the

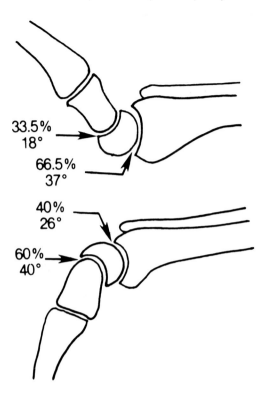

33.5%
18°

66.5%
37°

40%
26°

60%
40°

FIG. 33-4. Approximately two thirds of the arc of carpal extension (*top*) occurs at the proximal carpal radial articulation, while most (60%) carpal flexion (*bottom*) arises at the midcarpal joint. (Volz, R.G., Lieb, M., and Benjamin, J.: Biomechanics of the wrist. Clin. Orthop., 149:112, 1980)

radius, arthrodesis or pseudoarthrodesis of the wrist joint, dorsal wrist stabilization, proximal row carpectomy, palmar shelf arthroplasty, and implant arthroplasty.

Osteotomy of the Radius

When a small degree of pain-free wrist movement is present but in a nonfunctional plane, an osteotomy of the radius is indicated to relocate the available motion into a more functional plane.

Arthrodesis

The majority of hand adaptations are associated with forearm supination and wrist flexion. The critical importance of even a few degrees of wrist motion, especially flexion, has already been discussed. For these reasons, we have avoided per-

forming surgical arthrodesis of the wrist in patients with rheumatoid arthritis. In the past, the wrist has been fused only in cases of marked instability, in which adequate rotation of the forearm and finger function were present to compensate for the loss of motion at the wrist. Fusion of the wrist is occasionally indicated in certain cases of wrist disability in patients who do heavy manual work.[46,78,85]

When all motion at the wrist is lost following arthrodesis, the angle of fusion is an important consideration for preservation of maximal hand function. The so-called functional position of the wrist corresponds to the position of maximal efficiency of the flexor muscles. It usually is described as slight extension of the wrist, to approximately 30°, and slight ulnar deviation, to 15°. It is in this position of the wrist that the hand is best adapted for the handling of most objects. Early reports suggested fusing the wrist in 20° to 30° of extension and from neutral to 20° of ulnar deviation.[66] Leibolt noted that any ulnar deviation tended to weaken the first three radial digits.[46] Pahle and Raunio reported that of 20 wrists disabled by rheumatoid arthritis and fused in greater than 5° of radial deviation, 17 developed ulnar deviation of the fingers. Of 18 wrists fused in greater than 5° of ulnar deviation, 14 developed a radial deviation of the fingers. The authors also noted that only six of 31 wrists fused in a neutral position developed any radial or ulnar deviation of the fingers.[58] In our center, we have also observed that the wrist should be fused in approximately 15° of extension and in neutral radial-ulnar deviation. In the rare case in which bilateral wrist fusion would be indicated, the dominant side should be fused in 0° to 15° of extension for power use, and the nondominant hand should be fused in slight palmar flexion (up to 10°, as suggested by Dupont and Vainio) for facilitating personal hygiene care and other activities of daily living.[22] We do not recommend bilateral wrist fusions or any type of wrist arthrodesis in a paralytic extremity. We avoid wrist fusion in patients with rheumatoid arthritis.

The pitfalls of wrist arthrodesis must be carefully avoided. The common approach for wrist fusion is between the fourth and fifth extensor compartments. An *en bloc* mobilization and dorsal radial retraction of the entire contents of the fourth compartment, including the tendons, must be carried out to avoid intracompartmental scarring, which could result in restriction of gliding of the finger extensor tendons; this could also occur if the patient fails to mobilize the digits postoperatively. Smith-Petersen advocated an ulnar exposure of the wrist to avoid this complication and used the excised distal ulna as a bone graft.[67] This dissection is more difficult and requires excision of the distal ulna, even in cases in which the distal ulnar-carpal joint is adequate. A dorsolateral approach, such as that described by Haddad and Riordan, is preferred.[30] The wrist joint is exposed between the third and fourth compartments. The dorsal sensory branch of the radial nerve and the dorsal branch of the radial artery must be identified and preserved during this dissection.

The fusion can include the proximal carpal row only, or both carpal rows, or it can extend to include the carpometacarpal joints; however, great care must be taken not to incorporate the basal joint of the thumb in the fusion procedure (Fig. 33-5). Campbell and Keokarn described two cases of limited prehension following inclusion of the basal joint of the thumb in arthrodesis of the wrist.[12] Whenever possible, the carpometacarpal joint should be preserved for motion and shock absorption, as recommended by Dupont and Vainio.[22]

Nonunion following arthrodesis of the wrist joint is an uncommon complication that has been reported by The Hospital for Special Surgery to have occurred in only one of 18 wrists reviewed.[71] This complication occurs more frequently in patients with tuberculosis. Haddad and Riordan reported one case of nonunion in a patient who removed his cast prematurely.[80] Clendenin and Green, however, reported a 20% incidence of pseudarthrosis with wrist fusion and a 7% fracture rate in healed fusions.[13] Millender and Nalebuff and Mannerfelt and Malsten have reported good success in fusions of rheumatoid wrists with the use of an intramedullary Steinmann pin inserted retrograde through the third metacarpal and into the radius.[51,56] Based on our experience, we prefer using as a bone-formation inducer a corticocan-

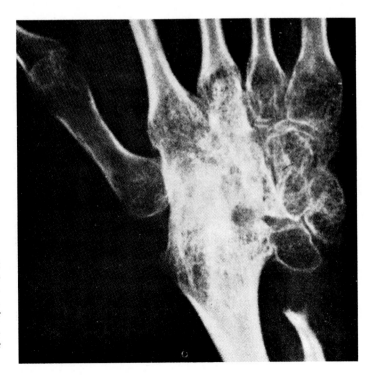

FIG. 33-5. A fusion of the wrist in which the basal joint of the thumb has been partially included in the fusion mass, interfering with the mobility of this important joint. (Carroll, R.E., and Dick, H.M.: J. Bone Joint Surg., 53A:1365, 1971)

cellous bone graft, with or without intramedullary fixation, to provide good stability.

Petrie has described 12 cases of compression arthrodesis in which he used an AO plate and screws to maintain the bone graft, with no occurrence of nonunion.[62] Kay has reported a similar procedure for radiocarpal and intercarpal arthrodesis in six patients.[39] Heiple and associates have described a method of "instant fusion" that employs a titanium implant fixed in position with methylmethacrylate.[32] Other complications that have been reported with arthrodesis are skin necrosis, superficial radial nerve palsy, median nerve palsy, infection, and iliac donor site pain.[13]

Pseudarthrodesis

Fair results have been obtained after a pseudarthrodesis procedure for wrist stabilization. In this method the same surgical technique used for wrist arthrodesis is carried out, except that the postoperative immobilization period is deliberately curtailed in an effort to obtain fibrous union instead of bony union and so to retain some wrist motion. A heavy Kirschner wire is introduced retrograde through the third metacarpal into the radius and removed after approximately 4 to 6 weeks. Guarded movements of the wrist in the desired arc are then allowed. The results of this method, however, have been unpredictable because of the difficulty in evaluating the appropriate degree of healing.

Dorsal Wrist Stabilization

A dorsal wrist stabilization procedure in which the radiocarpal ligament and the extensor retinaculum are used following synovectomy and resection of the distal ulna was reported by Straub and Ranawat to be a useful substitute for arthrodesis.[71] However, of the 37 reported cases, 16 developed a spontaneous fusion, and 16 had an arc of motion of less than 30°; 16 of these patients had no improvement in their activities of daily living, and six had recurrent pain. In a more recent follow-up, range of motion decreased in virtually all patients.[43]

Proximal Carpal Row Resection

Resection of the proximal carpal row has also been used as a method of treatment in certain severely impaired wrists with destruction of the proximal carpal row and/or subluxation of the radiocarpal joint.[53] This method was described by Stamm in 1944 and consisted of excision of the scaphoid, lunate, triquetrum, and radial styloid process.[70] This procedure was popular following World War II; however, the results were not reliable and resulted in restricted wrist motion.[68] Cave has stated that this procedure was "to be deplored."[35] Crabbe and Jorgensen each reported a large series of proximal carpal row resections and found that, in most cases, grasp strength was weakened, especially in the dominant hand.[16,35] Jorgensen's best results were obtained in patients operated on shortly after they were injured. Crabbe noted that the results were worse in patients who presented with degenerative changes. Even though there was often a decrease in pain following surgery, most patients had persistent pain, especially after strenuous use. All patients had a decrease of wrist motion, ranging from 40% to 87% of the preoperative arc. Inglis and Jones have reported a series of 12 cases of proximal row carpectomy in which they state that the results obtained were satisfactory.[34] However, we feel that arthrodesis or implant arthroplasty should be preferred in most cases.

Palmar-Shelf Arthroplasty

Other procedures, such as palmar-shelf arthroplasty, have been performed in an attempt to retain some movement in wrists severely involved with rheumatoid arthritis. In this technique the carpus is brought dorsally over a prepared shelf of the anterior cortex of the radius. This method is designed to prevent palmar dislocation of the carpus. However, we have found its outcome to be unreliable. Albright and Chase have reported that in some patients there was continued erosion of the carpus and radius, with a collapse deformity of the wrist and a tendency to radial or ulnar deviation (Fig. 33-6).[4] Clayton has also reported that one of his two patients who had palmar-shelf arthroplasty developed severe ulnar deviation requiring prolonged splinting.[4] It appears that soft tissue reconstruction alone is not sufficient to prevent further deformity in a wrist that is subjected to heavy use and that sufficient stability with adequate

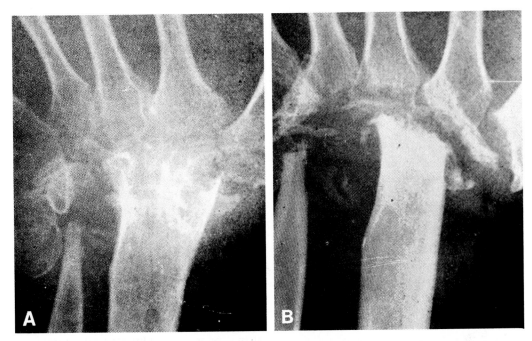

FIG. 33-6. (*A*) Preoperative roentgenogram of a wrist with severe destruction secondary to rheumatoid arthritis. (*B*) The same patient 3 years after palmar-shelf arthroplasty. Continued erosion has occurred in the remaining carpal bones, the metacarpals, and the distal radius. (Albright, J.A., and Chase, R.A.: Palmar-shelf arthroplasty of the wrist in rheumatoid arthritis: Report of nine cases. J. Bone Joint Surg., 52A:896, 1970)

mobility can be provided only by an implant arthroplasty.

Implant Procedures

There has been a rapidly growing interest in implant procedures of the wrist joint. One of the earliest wrist prostheses was reported by Gold in 1965. He described the use of an acrylic prosthesis for the distal portion of the radius following resection of a recurrent giant cell tumor.[28] However, the implant fractured after 2 years and was replaced with a Vitallium prosthesis; this procedure was complicated by gangrene, and a below-elbow amputation was carried out.

Flexible Implant Resection Arthroplasty. A reconstructive procedure that would provide a disabled wrist with reasonable stability and strength but enough mobility to assist in hand adaptations would be ideal. Such a result can be achieved with an implant resection arthroplasty. In the light of our experience, gained with the development of the silicone rubber finger-joint implant, the concept of a flexible-hinge intramedullary stemmed implant was applied to the wrist joint.[72,86] In 1967 we developed a silicone elastomer hinged implant for the radiocarpal joint. Several different implant designs were tested.[76,85] The implant is a one-piece, intramedullary, stemmed, flexible hinge fabricated of High-Performance Silicone Elastomer* and is available in five anatomical sizes. The core of the implant contains a Dacron reinforcement, to provide axial stability and resistance to torque. The implant is well tolerated by the bone and soft tissues and has a high flexural durability (more than 200 million flexion repetitions to 90° without evidence of material failure).[83,87,88] The proximal stem of the implant fits into the intramedullary canal of the radius, and the distal stem passes through the capitate bone into the intramedullary stem of the third metacarpal. This implant has been designed as an adjunct to resection arthroplasty of the wrist, to maintain the joint space and alignment

---

* Dow Corning Corporation, Midland, MI.

while supporting the capsuloligamentous structures around the implant. It allows reconstruction and balancing of the musculotendinous system and early postoperative mobilization. The degree of pain relief, mobility, and stability obtained with this method has been most encouraging. It would appear that a properly done flexible implant resection arthroplasty of the radiocarpal joint, including proper capsuloligamentous reconstruction and balancing of the muscle power to obtain adequate active movements in all planes, is superior to arthrodesis, pseudarthrodesis, and other simple resection arthroplasty procedures for the arthritic wrist.[85]

The use of flexible materials as an adjunct to resection arthroplasty provides a new and different approach to joint reconstruction; it allows us to take an easier and safer alternative in helping nature build her own new joint system through resection arthroplasty.[50,76]

The concept of flexible implant resection arthroplasty could be expressed simply as follows: bone resection + implant + encapsulation = new joint.[70,73,78] In realizing the goal of a simplified and dependable joint reconstruction, we chose the route of improving the well-established concept of resection arthroplasty. We reasoned that by minimizing the demands on synthetic materials and simulating the biomechanics of the human joint system, it is much more likely that the improved resection arthroplasty will be long lived and free of disastrous complications. The concept of flexible implant resection arthroplasty has as one of its greatest advantages the fact that after a time, if the implant fails, the option of a functional resection arthroplasty still remains. If a fusion procedure is contemplated, it can easily be accomplished with an iliac bone graft.

Indications.   The flexible-hinge wrist implant resection arthroplasty is indicated in cases of instability of the wrist due to subluxation or dislocation of the radiocarpal joint, severe deviation of the wrist causing musculotendinous imbalance of the digits, stiffness or fusion of the wrist in a nonfunctional position, and stiffness of a wrist when movement is required for hand function.[66,68,73] These disabilities are most com-

monly the result of rheumatoid arthritis but may also be secondary to degenerative or posttraumatic arthritis. Reconstruction of the wrist should be performed before surgery of the finger joints unless there are extensor tendon ruptures.

Surgical Technique (Fig. 33-7).   A straight longitudinal incision is made over the dorsal wrist, preserving the superficial sensory nerves. The extensor retinaculum is incised to prepare a radially based flap between the first and second dorsal compartments. A narrow proximal flap is prepared for later resuture over the extensor tendons to prevent bow-stringing.

Another retinacular ligament flap can be prepared to relocate the extensor carpi ulnaris tendon in associated implant reconstructions of the ulnar head. The necessary synovectomy of the extensor compartments is performed, care being taken to remove only the synovium. The capsuloligamentous structures are carefully preserved for later resuturing. A distally based flap is formed, and the ligamentous structures are stripped from the dorsum of the radius.

Usually, parts of the scaphoid and lunate are partially destroyed and may be dislocated and fused to the anterior surface of the distal radius. Resection of the remaining lunate bone is done carefully with a rongeur. Part of the distal scaphoid, capitate, and triquetrum can be retained in some cases. The anatomy of the flexor compartment should be kept in mind to avoid injury to the underlying tendons and neurovascular structures. The end of the radius is squared off to fit against the distal carpal row. The distal row of carpal bones should be left intact because of their importance in maintaining the stability of the metacarpal bases. The radiocarpal subluxation should be completely reduced. The intramedullary canal of the radius is prepared to receive the proximal stem of the implant. If there has been marked radiocarpal dislocation with subsequent soft tissue contracture, it is preferable to shorten the distal radius rather than to remove more of the carpal bones. The distal stem of the implant fits through the capitate bone into the intramedullary canal of the third metacarpal. The intramedullary canal of the third metacarpal is prepared by carefully passing a wire or very thin broach through the capitate bone and the base of the metacarpal and into its canal. The final reaming procedure is carried out with an air drill.

A research project to develop a bone liner (grommet) has been carried out from 1976 to date, using a variety of materials to protect the silicone flexible-hinge implants for finger and wrist joints from cutting by sharp, thin bone edges, as seen in some cases.[81] The results of this work have shown that unfixed metal or bovine pericardium is accepted by the host tissues and can successfully protect the implant from cutting by sharp bone ends.

The distal ulna is trimmed back to approximately 1 cm from the distal end of the radius and capped with an ulnar head implant. The hand is then centralized over the radius. The proximal stem of the implant is inserted first into the intramedullary canal of the radius, and the distal stem is then introduced through the capitate into the intramedullary canal of the third metacarpal. If an implant resection arthroplasty of the metacarpophlangeal joints is contemplated, the end of the distal stem may be shortened so that both implant stems can fit into the third metacarpal. Enough bone should have been resected so that extension of the wrist is possible on passive manipulation. Usually 1 cm to 1.5 cm of separation between the bone ends is adequate. To obtain good results, it is essential that the implant be properly seated and the bone ends smoothly prepared.

Repairs of both the palmar and dorsal capsuloligamentous structures around the implant are critical to obtain an adequate result. The palmar ligaments are reefed proximally and/or distally, according to where they are loose. The proximal palmar reefing is done by passing 2-0 Dacron sutures through two small drill holes made in the palmar distal edge of the cut end of the radius. The distal palmar reefing is done by passing a 2-0 Dacron suture through a small drill hole made in the cut end of the capitate bone (see Fig. 33-7, *E* and *F*).

The dorsal capsuloligamentous structures are firmly sutured over the implant. Sutures are passed through small drill holes in the dorsal cortex of the radius to ensure good capsular fixation. The repair should be tested so that approximately 30° of extension and flexion and 10° of ulnar and radial deviation are possible on passive manipulation. The distally based ligamentous flap is brought back to the radius and sutured to the bone with 2-0 Dacron sutures. More than 30° of postoperative extension or flexion may increase the potential for implant failure and does not improve wrist function significantly. In patients with significant bone loss or loose ligaments who may have excessive extension or radial or ulnar deviation after implant arthroplasty, it may be necessary to add sutures to the palmar, radial, and ulnar cortex of the radius to tighten the capsule in these areas. Adequate ligamentous repair is very important in achieving proper function and durability with this type of arthroplasty. The previously prepared distal extensor retinacular flap is brought down over the wrist joint under the extensor tendon and sutured in place to provide further capsular support. The pull of the extensor tendons of the wrist is then evaluated; they should be shortened or transferred as required to obtain wrist extension without lateral deviation. The extensor tendons of the digits are repaired as necessary. The proximal retinacular flap is then sutured in place over the extensor tendons to prevent bowstringing. The reconstruction of the distal radioulnar joint is completed by using a retinacular flap from the sixth dorsal compartment to relocate the extensor carpi ulnaris tendon. The wound is closed, and a small drain is inserted subcutaneously. A voluminous conforming dressing is applied, including a plaster splint to maintain the wrist in a neutral position.

The extremity is elevated for 3 to 5 days. A short arm cast with the wrist in neutral position is then applied and fitted with outriggers to hold rubber band slings to keep the fingers in extension if the tendons have been repaired. This is worn for approximately 2 to 4 weeks. We desire a good ratio of mobility and stability; a joint that is too loose may be unstable. We attempt to obtain 50% to 60% of the normal flexion-extension movements as the ideal goal. The patient is started on an exercise program following cast removal to obtain active flex-

(Text continues on page 1018.)

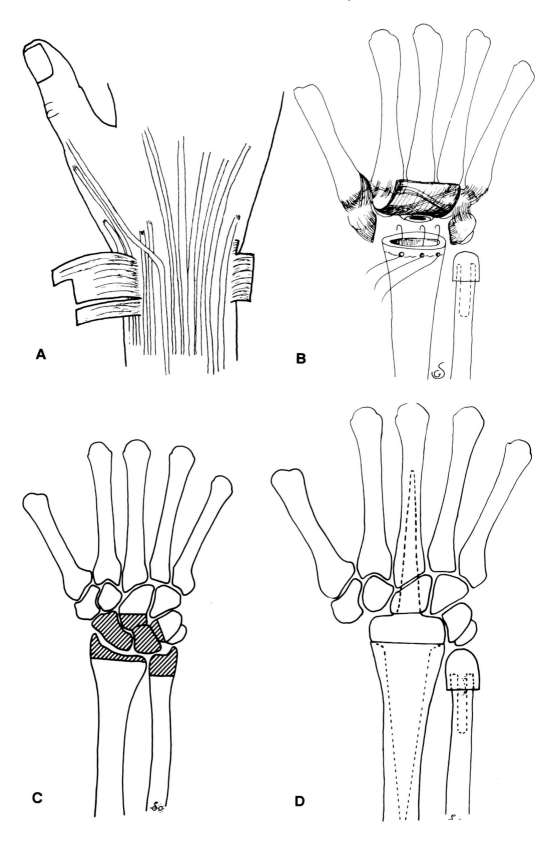

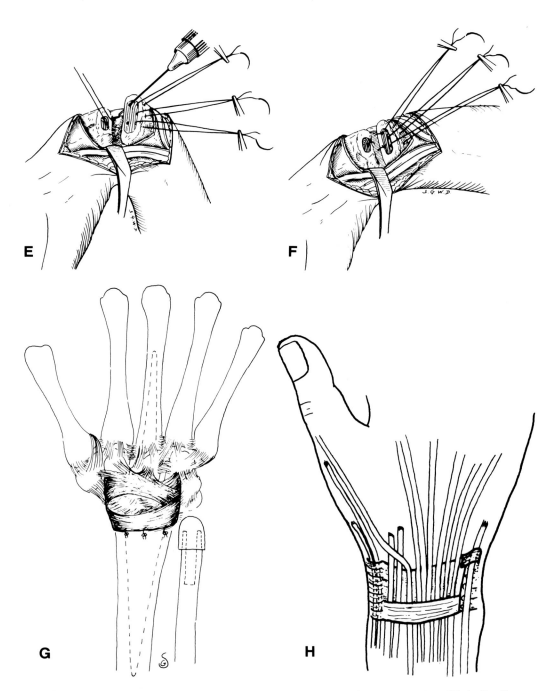

Fig. 33-7. (A) The preferred technique of extensor retinaculum preparation. (B) A distally based radiocarpal flap is prepared by elevating the dorsal capsuloligamentous structures from the underlying radius and carpus. (C) The usual area of resection of the distal radius, ulna, and carpus used in wrist implant resection arthroplasty. (D) The flexible wrist implant and ulnar head implant are in place. (E and F) The palmar ligaments are reefed proximally and/or distally, according to where they are loose, and 2-0 Dacron sutures are passed through small drill holes in the distal palmar edge of the radius and/or through the cut end of the capitate. (G) The radiocarpal capsuloligamentous flap is firmly sutured over the wrist implant with 3-0 Dacron sutures passed through small drill holes made in the dorsal distal edge of the resected radius. An inverted-knot technique is used. (H) The distal retinacular flap is placed under the extensor tendons. The proximal flap is placed over the tendons to prevent bow-stringing. The small flap used to relocated the extensor carpi ulnaris is illustrated.

ion and extension. If there is a tendency for tightness, some active and passive stretching exercises are prescribed.

Results. Flexible implant arthroplasty was performed in 181 wrists in 139 patients (42 bilateral cases) in our clinic from January 1970 through April 1983 (Fig. 33-8). Most patients were women, and most had rheumatoid arthritis. A follow-up ranging from 6 months to 10 years (average 4 years) was available for 170 wrists. After surgery, there was complete pain relief in 90% of the wrists, 7% had mild pain, and 3% had moderate pain after prolonged activity. The average postoperative flexion (34°) and extension (26°) provided a 60° range of motion in a more functional arc of movement. The motion obtained within 6 to 12 months after surgery was noted to be maintained in most patients throughout their follow-up.

The power of grip is related to a number of factors, including the condition of the proximal and distal joints, musculotendi-

nous status, and pain. There were no statistically significant differences between the preoperative and postoperative grip strengths, except in those patients with rheumatoid arthritis who presented less than 5 pounds of grip preoperatively; this group showed a significant improvement postoperatively. The complications and revision procedures in this group of patients were reviewed. There were no postoperative infections. A delay in wound healing requiring no secondary procedure was noted in three wrists (two with rheumatoid and one with psoriatic arthritis). The importance of proper tissue handling in surgery and avoidance of pressure on the dorsal wrist through tight or improperly padded dressings or braces must be emphasized in this group of patients, who are largely corticosteroid dependent and present poor tissues. For this same reason, surgical knots placed in the superficial layers must be inverted.

Revision procedures were carried out on 25 wrists in 23 patients, nine for fractured

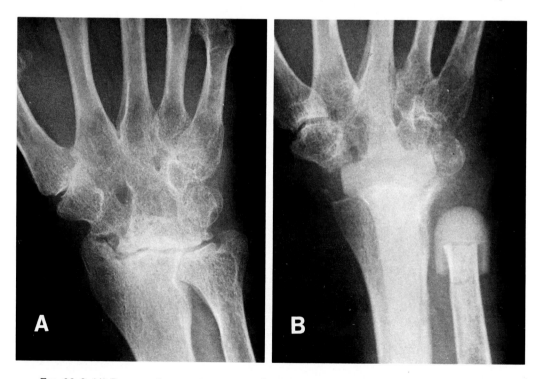

FIG. 33-8. (*A*) Preoperative roentgenogram shows a wrist severely destroyed by rheumatoid arthritis. (*B*) Postoperative roentgenogram demonstrates an excellent result with the flexible silicone wrist implant.

implants, four for tendon imbalance, five for tendon imbalance and recurrent synovitis, and seven for retrieval studies at the time of other surgery on the same extremity. In 22 of these cases the implant was removed and replaced, including the insertion of metal grommets in three of these cases (Fig. 33-9). A wrist fusion was carried out in these wrists, two with a fractured implant and one with a severe tendon imbalance. One of these fusions was later reconverted to a successful radiocarpal implant arthroplasty. A 16% fracture rate was noted for the implants made of silicone elastomer No. 372, and a 4% fracture rate was noted in the high-performance silicone elastomer implants. In two of these patients no revision procedure was carried out because of lack of clinical symptoms. Restricting wrist motion to no more than 30° of flexion and extension and 10° of ulnar and radial deviation through proper capsuloligamentous reconstruction and musculotendinous balance is critical. It is equally important to reduce wrist subluxation properly, to obtain proper soft tissue balance, and to correct proximal and distal deformities that could compromise the balance at the wrist. The bone preparation must be meticulous to obtain smooth bone edges against the implant midsection. Bone liners (grommets) have been used in 35 wrists to date to protect the implant midsection in cases in which the bones are sharp and thin; a favorable bone remodeling at the bone–implant interface and no evidence of implant fracture where the grommets have been used have been observed to date (Fig. 33-10). Radiologic survey has shown the formation of thin bone plates around the intramedullary stems of the implants, with smooth remodeling about the midsection in the great majority of cases. Bone overgrowth across the implant midsection was seen in one wrist of a patient with scleroderma. In two patients with an aggressive, recurrent synovitis of the hand and wrist, some bone absorption was present around the implant.

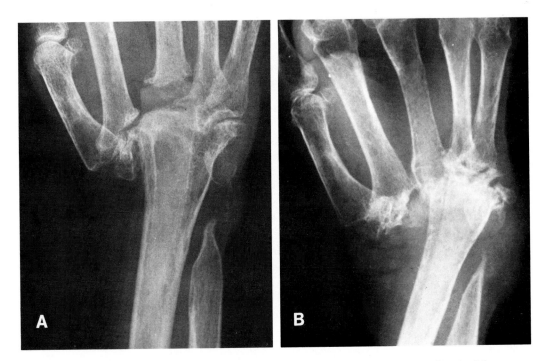

FIG. 33-9. (*A*) A silicone rubber wrist implant was placed in a carpus that had been severely destroyed by rheumatoid arthritis. (*B*) The implant broke at the junction of the stem and waist, allowing radial drift of the hand. The implant was later replaced with the newer high-performance rubber implant.

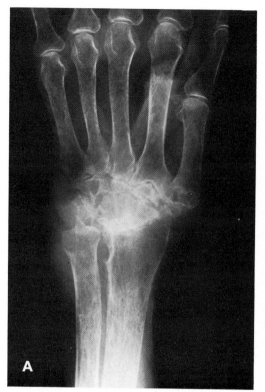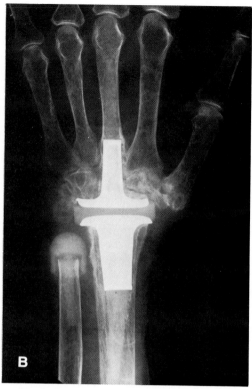

FIG. 33-10. (*A*) Preoperative roentgenogram of the wrist of a 77-year-old woman shows severe changes secondary to rheumatoid arthritis. (*B*) Postoperative roentgenogram shows a silicone flexible-hinge radiocarpal implant protected proximally and distally by a metal grommet. The distal radioulnar joint was reconstructed with an ulnar head implant. Note the favorable bone production around the intramedullary portion of the grommets.

The distal stem of the implant was not properly fitted in the third metacarpal and protruded through its side wall in two cases; no clinically or radiologically significant consequences resulted from this technical error. It is our opinion that this method has a place in the reconstruction and rehabilitation of the upper extremity in patients with rheumatoid arthritis.

Other Radiocarpal Joint Implants. It appears that three different concepts for wrist joint arthroplasty have emerged: resection arthroplasty, flexible implant resection arthroplasty, and total joint replacement. Many implants for the wrist joint are now appearing in the market. These are mainly made of rigid materials, employ rigid fixation to the bone with methylmethacrylate, and are based on the concept of total joint replacement. They include the

Mayo Clinic implant, the Volz implant, the Loda implant, the Meuli implant, the GSB implant, and others (Figs. 33-11 and 33-12).[33]

Total joint replacement is a method in which the function of the joint is completely substituted by a mechanical model. This approach has certain attractive possibilities from an engineering standpoint. The concept of total joint replacement with rigid materials has found success in the weight-bearing knee and hip joints. A problem remains, however, with the total dependency on insubstantial synthetic materials at the interface or boundary between the artificial material and the human tissues. This boundary must always exist, and as a result, any implanted device is only as successful as its biochemical and biologic tolerance by the human host tissues. These

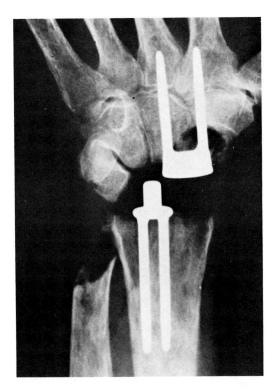

FIG. 33-11. Dislocation of a Meuli implant is a complication that may occur in the early post-operative period.

methods as applied to the smaller joints of the hand and the wrist have met with mixed success and limited acceptance. However, the goal of prosthetic replacement is excellent, since restoration of early motion with stability has obvious advantages over simple resection arthroplasty or fusion procedures. We should be cautious in the evaluation of these implants for use in patients until there has been time for critical evaluation.

Initial early reports on the Meuli total wrist prosthesis demonstrated good relief of pain (92% of patients), with an average of 59° of flexion-extension and 25° of radioulnar deviation. An initial rate of re-operation of 35% has been reduced by improved technique.[8] No long-term results reporting loosening or implant failure have been published. This device, like the Volz total wrist prosthesis, was designed with the center of rotation to radial, and ulnar deviation of the hand often occurred. This

has been corrected in the Volz prosthesis by replacing the two distal stems with a single stem that inserts into the third metacarpal. No loosening has occurred in Volz's first 100 cases, and he is now designing a prosthesis for use without bone cement.[94] Results have improved, with less ulnar deviation of the hand. In 100 patients followed a year or more, 48% had excellent results, 38% good, and 8% fair, and 6% of the procedures were failures.

In these cemented prostheses, infection and loosening remains a serious complication.[44] Two deep infections in the Mayo Clinic series required removal of the pros-

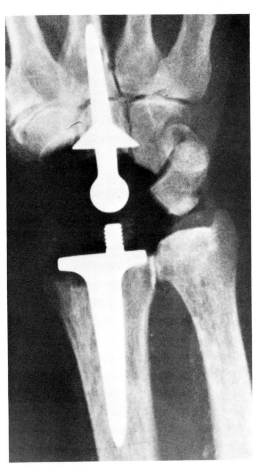

FIG. 33-12. The Loda implant is a type of total wrist unit that requires methylmethacrylate for fixation. It is an important design, because the center of axis of rotation is offset from the long axis of the radius (*i.e.*, at the head of the capitate). It requires considerable bone resection.

thesis. Loosening occurred in five patients in the metacarpal. In Volz's series, 18% had a motor imbalance that was subsequently corrected, 5% had inadequate range of motion, 5% had delayed wound healing, 4% experienced dislocations, 2% became infected, and 17% had loosening.[94]

THE DISTAL RADIOULNAR JOINT

PATHOMECHANICS OF DEFORMITIES

The function of the distal radioulnar joint may be compromised in certain posttraumatic situations, such as following a Colles' fracture, or it may be secondary to a proximal displacement of the radial shaft, such as seen after simple resection of the radial head. However, dysfunction of this joint occurs most frequently from the destructive synovitis of rheumatoid arthritis, which sets off a chain of disabilities that impair the normal function of the wrist and hand. Bäckdahl has described this problem in his comprehensive essay "The Caput Ulnae Syndrome in Rheumatoid Arthritis."[5] Approximately one third of our patients with rheumatoid arthritis undergoing hand surgery had associated distal radioulnar joint disability, which is characterized clinically by dorsal prominence and instability of the ulnar head, with increasing weakness of the wrist, pain and crepitation on movement, especially rotation, and a decrease of rotation and dorsiflexion. There may be increased flexion of the fourth and fifth metacarpals owing to the loss of the normal action of the extensor carpi ulnaris, which is displaced palmarly, and ruptures of the extensor tendons of the little, ring, and long fingers, which must be differentiated from the above.

Dysfunction of the extensor carpi ulnaris in this syndrome is an important and frequently ignored problem that can lead to further imbalances in the complex musculoskeletal disabilities of the rheumatoid hand. Normally, the extensor carpi ulnaris acts in dorsiflexion and ulnar abduction of the wrist and helps stabilize the wrist during abduction and extension of the thumb and when the hand is opened for grasp. It also contracts during palmar flexion of the wrist, whereas the other extensors relax. The extensor carpi ulnaris crosses the dorsal surface of the distal ulna to assist in stabilization of the wrist and maintain the integrity of the distal radioulnar joint. It helps stabilize the fifth metacarpal through its insertion, and its dysfunction allows greater flexion of the fourth and fifth metacarpals, with secondary deformity and impaired finger function.

As the destructive synovial hypertrophy increases, the ligamentous support of the distal ulna formed mainly by the triangular fibrocartilage and its ligaments, the ulnar collateral ligament, and the surrounding capsule undergoes attritional changes: the ulnar head now can dislocate dorsally to the line of least resistance. The sixth dorsal compartment is stretched by the synovial hypertrophy, and the extensor carpi ulnaris is subluxated ulnarly and palmarly. Roentgenographic examination may show early subluxation and erosive changes of the ulnar head and the ulnar notch of the radius. The ulnar head loses its smooth, rounded contour and becomes sharp and irregular. The ulnar styloid may become prominent or may disappear, or severe absorption of the distal ulna may occur. Extensor tendons may rupture over the jagged distal ulnar or secondary to attritional changes from severe invasive synovitis.

SURGICAL PROCEDURES

Resection Arthroplasty

Resection of the ulnar head for disabilities of the distal radioulnar joint was popularized by Darrach in 1912.[18] This procedure has been used for posttraumatic conditions, congenital defects, and, more recently, disabilities secondary to rheumatoid arthritis.[17,25,41,49,65] Removal of less than 2 cm to 3 cm of the distal ulna does not usually result in instability, because the interosseous membrane and the pronator quadratus can stabilize the remnant distal ulna. In rheumatoid arthritis, however, instability of the distal ulna is more common because of the destruction of the ligamentous support by synovitis.

Problems reported after simple resection of the ulnar head include excessive resection of bone, causing wrist weakness and instability, dorsal instability of the ulna, and progression of carpal shift in the ulnar direction (Fig. 33-13). Loss of the action of

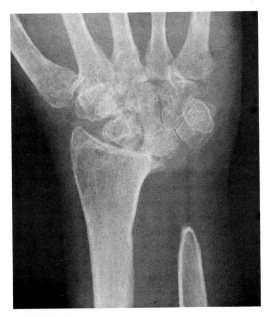

FIG. 33-13. Roentgenogram of a patient with rheumatoid arthritis who has had a Darrach procedure in which an excessive amount of bone was removed from the distal ulna, allowing for ulnar shift of the carpus.

as an adjunct to ulnar head resection arthroplasty.[65,66] This implant is now fabricated of High-Performance Silicone Elastomer and is available in eight sizes with a pretied polyester suture (Fig. 33-14). We have demonstrated that this procedure has definite advantages in preserving the anatomical relationship and physiology of the distal radioulnar joint. Less bone has to be removed because the implant allows smooth articulation of the distal ulna with the radius. The physiological length of the ulna is maintained to help prevent ulnar carpal shift and provide greater wrist stability. A smooth articular surface for the radius and carpus is provided to allow freer movements of the distal radioulnar and carpoulnar joints, and a smoother surface is provided for the overlying extensor tendons. Reconstruction of ligaments is made possible to maintain the distal ulna in position without creating bony impingement, and the important extensor carpi ulnaris tendon can be rerouted over the dorsum of the ulna. Bone overgrowth is decreased and the appearance of the wrist improved.

the extensor carpi ulnaris, rupture of extensor tendons over the cut end of the bone, symptomatic bone overgrowth at the resected end of the ulna, and loss of cosmesis due to narrowing of the wrist have also been reported. Colwill, in an attempt to prevent dorsal subluxation of the distal ulna, has designed a distally based volar flap of capsule that is sutured to the dorsal cut surface of the distal ulna.*

Lauenstein Procedure.   The Lauenstein procedure is an attempt to accomplish what a Darrach procedure does while avoiding the weakness, instability, and flattening on the dorsoulnar side of the wrist that may result after a Darrach procedure. It is a fusion of the distal ulna to the radius and resection of a portion of the ulna proximal to this fusion to allow for pronation and supination.

Ulnar Head Implant Resection Arthroplasty

In 1968 we developed a silicone rubber intramedullary stemmed implant to be used

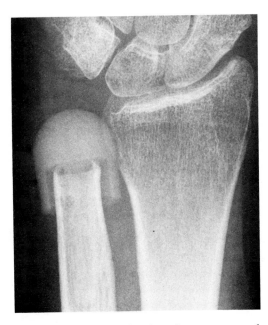

FIG. 33-14. This ulnar head implant was sutured in place. High-performance rubber is now used, with preservation of the distal periosteum. The skirt of the implant fits over the distal ulna with its intact periosteum. The skirt must not be too tight over the amputated bone end.

---

* Colwill, J.C.: Personal communication.

Indications. The ulnar head implant replacement arthroplasty may be considered for disabilities of the distal radioulnar joint in rheumatoid, degenerative, or posttraumatic dysfunctions. Specific indications include pain and weakness of the wrist not improved by conservative treatment, instability of the ulnar head with radiologic evidence of dorsal subluxation, and erosive changes. This procedure can also be used for the symptomatic sequelae of a failed Darrach procedure or of a failed flexible hinge arthroplasty.

Surgical Technique (Fig. 33-15). A longitudinal incision of 6 cm to 8 cm, centered over the ulnar head, is used to expose the extensor retinaculum of the sixth dorsal compartment. The dorsal cutaneous branch of the ulnar nerve must be identified and carefully preserved. The extensor retinaculum of the sixth dorsal compartment is incised in such a fashion as to preserve a narrow radially based flap and a broad ulnarly based flap. If a synovectomy of the dorsal compartments is indicated, it must be carried out at the same time. The extensor carpi ulnaris tendon, which is usually in palmar subluxation off the ulnar head, is retracted. After adequate exposure, retractors are placed under the neck of the ulnar head to protect the underlying structures, and the bone is sectioned at the neck. The periosteum is not stripped off the distal ulna, but muscular attachments on the anterior surface of the ulna are released over the distal 2 cm. The ulnar head and attached synovial sac are removed *en bloc*, and a complete synovectomy of the joint is performed. Bone irregularities that may be present at the end and undersurface of the ulna are smoothed so that the bone presents a cylindrical shape to fit the contour of the implant.

The intramedullary canal is prepared to receive the stem of the implant. An implant of appropriate size is selected; the stem of

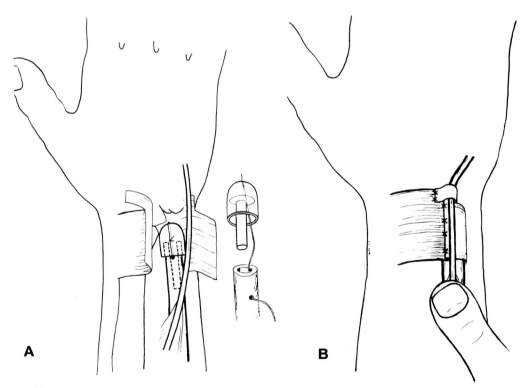

A   **B**

Fig. 33-15. (*A*) The extensor retinaculum of the sixth dorsal compartment is incised in such a fashion as to preserve a narrow, radially based distal flap and a wide, ulnarly based proximal flap. The preferred method for securing the ulnar head implant to the distal bone end is shown. (*B*) Closure of the retinacular flaps, including the check ligament for the extensor carpi ulnaris.

the implant must fit snugly in the intramedullary canal, and the cuff must fit loosely over the bone end. The implant should be secured to the end of the ulna to prevent the slight tendency for the implant to extrude from the intramedullary canal in the early postoperative course. The ends of the nonabsorbable polyester retention cord are passed through two small drill holes made in the distal ulna and securely tied together once the implant is well seated over the bone end. Passing of the nonabsorbable polyester retention cord through the end of the bone is facilitated by the use of a looped wire. Occasionally, digital extensors are ruptured as a result of the ulnar head irregularities or synovitis and must be repaired. Prior to implant insertion, sutures are placed through the interosseous ligament close to the radioulnar border to secure the preserved capsule over the ulnar head implant. Sutures may be placed through small drill holes in the radius if the local tissues are inadequate.

The retinaculum of the sixth dorsal compartment is used as a check ligament to hold the dorsally subluxated ulna in a reduced position. While an assistant maintains the palmar reduction of the ulna, retinacular flaps are sutured as follows: the broad proximal ulnarly based flap is placed under the extensor carpi ulnaris tendon and sutured over the ulna into the remaining ligaments of the distal radioulnar joint, the soft tissues of the radius, and the retinaculum of the fifth dorsal compartment with five to six 3-0 Dacron sutures. It is important to release the extensor carpi ulnaris tendon proximally and distally to allow free excursion. The narrow, radially based distal retinacular flap is looped under and around the extensor carpi ulnaris tendon and sutured to itself; it acts as a pulley to maintain this tendon over the dorsum of the ulnar head.

A small drain is inserted into the wound, and a voluminous conforming dressing is applied, including a plaster palmar splint; this is worn for 4 to 5 days. On the third postoperative day the drain is removed and, if there is no swelling, a short arm cast or splint is applied to protect the wrist from excessive activity for 3 to 6 weeks.

Results. A meticulous evaluation of all of our patients was carried out both before and after surgery and included clinical and radiologic studies to analyze the possibility of improving the surgical technique and the implant design. A study of our first 22 cases showed a significant amount of absorptive change in the distal 1 cm of the resected ulna in two of these cases and a distal migration of the implant in five cases (Fig. 33-16). These findings were essentially roentgenographic and were of no clinical consequence to the patients. The absorptive problems were considered to have been caused by an excessively tight fit of the cuff. The design of the implant was modified slightly in 1969 to increase the space between the cuff and the stem and to decrease the thickness of the wall of the cuff. With this modification, an improved fit of the implant could be obtained, and the rim of the cortical bone covered by the cuff was no longer submitted to excessive pressure. The slight tendency for the implant to

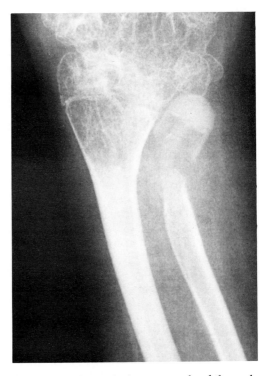

Fig. 33-16. This wrist is an example of the early technique of ulnar head replacement arthroplasty. The implant has migrated distally and ulnad. Moderate bone resorption is present. These complications have been prevented with the newer techniques.

extrude from the intramedullary canal in the early postoperative course was explained by the fact that there is no contiguous articulation to support the distal end of the implant and help maintain its position in the early stages of healing of the capsuloligamentous structures. This problem can be corrected by fixing the implant to the distal end of the ulna. The implant is now available with a pretied polyester cord around the base of its stem and is fabricated of High-Performance Silicone Elastomer.

Patients showed relief of pain and crepitation; they were satisfied with their functional and cosmetic result and reported a greater ability to use the hand, including those operated on earlier who presented some of the problems discussed above. It was noted that the improvement in the appearance of the wrist was greater following implant arthroplasty than after simple resection of the ulnar head, because the width of the wrist was maintained. No cases of carpal shift were noted. Improvement in the strength of grip was reported by the patients and measured clinically, but the gain in strength that could be attributed to the ulnar head replacement is difficult to evaluate because most of these patients had other reconstructive procedures of the fingers and thumb in the same extremity. Improvement in the range of pronation, supination, and wrist extension was noted after surgery. A recent report on 11 years' experience with 400 ulnar head implant arthroplasties has shown that, provided that the proper surgical indications and techniques are followed, satisfactory results can be obtained in the greater majority of cases.[80] Patients with disability of the distal radioulnar joint requiring an ulnar head resection would benefit from a reconstructive procedure of the joint by implant resection arthroplasty.

CARPAL SCAPHOID AND LUNATE

PATHOMECHANICS OF DEFORMITIES

The proximal carpal row represents a link between the region of the forearm and the distal carpal row and the hand. If the midcarpal joint becomes unstable, the lunate rotates dorsally and the capitate becomes hyperflexed. The resultant shortening of the long axis of the carpus causes rotation of the scaphoid, which is usually seen only in normal radial deviation. Instability of the midcarpal joint may follow a hyperextension injury of the wrist in which the volar carpal ligaments are partially ruptured and the joint capsule between the capitate, scaphoid, and lunate bones is damaged. In extreme cases of instability the scaphoid dislocates spontaneously and shifts horizontally so that its distal articular surface points straight forward. Carpal instability is most vulnerable in dorsiflexion and ulnar deviation. Collapse deformity of the wrist can also occur after dislocations of the lunate or loosening of ligaments of the wrist by an arthritic process.

Aseptic necrosis and arthritis of the carpal bones, either primary or secondary to trauma, continue to be common causes of disability of the wrist joint.[42,64,73] Conservative treatment for Preiser's and Kienböck's aseptic necrosis of the scaphoid and lunate bones has produced unpredictable results. Some cases go to permanent bone absorption and deformity, followed later by intercarpal and radiocarpal arthritis. Fractures, fracture-dislocations, and dislocations of these bones are also complicated by aseptic necrosis and arthritic changes, no matter how carefully treated. The resultant stiffness of the wrist joint, pain on activity, and weakness of grip noted by these patients are severe handicaps to normal function. These lesions frequently occur in young, active people whose requirements for function are great. Because work and sport activities are usually disturbed, these conditions have important economic and personal significance.

SURGICAL PROCEDURES

Reports on the surgical treatment of these conditions have included local resection, proximal row carpectomy, bone grafting, intercarpal fusion, wrist fusion, radial styloidectomy, radial shortening, ulnar lengthening, soft tissue interposition arthroplasty, and implant arthroplasty.

Resection Arthroplasty

Local resection procedures embody a basic principle of surgery: the removal of irreversibly damaged parts. However, they have frequently been complicated by migration of adjacent carpal bones into the space left by the resection, wrist weakness, and instability. These problems have been discussed in the literature as sequelae of excision of the lunate for Kienböck's disease and excision of the scaphoid for ununited fractures.[19,20,23,24,26,97]

There have been few and isolated reports of good results following excision of the lunate; however, the follow-up period evaluated in these cases was relatively short. Stähl reported migration of adjacent carpal bones in the space left by excision of the lunate and increasing osteoarthritis of the wrist.[69] Dornan compared the results of treatment of Kienböck's disease in patients treated with prolonged immobilization in a cast to those for patients treated by excision of the lunate: both groups were relieved of pain but presented marked weakness of the wrist, and fewer than 70% of these patients were able to return to work.[21] Tajima published similar findings, and, in his quest for a more effective treatment, he has been curetting the necrotic area of the lunate and bone-grafting the cavity.[89]

Böhler reported that he had never seen a normal wrist after excision of the scaphoid.[10] On the other hand, Keon-Cohen reported acceptable results after complete excision of the scaphoid but poor results after excision of only the proximal avascular fragment.[40] The Pennsylvania Orthopaedic Society, in their evaluation of treatment of nonunion of the scaphoid, reported unsatisfactory results in patients who attempted to return to heavy work (66% following total excision of the scaphoid and 27% in those treated by partial excision).[20] Patients doing only light work appeared to do better. Edelstein condemned partial or complete excision of the scaphoid after evaluating 60 patients who underwent such treatment.[24]

The problems resulting from proximal row carpectomy have already been discussed and also apply if this procedure is used for treatment of disabilities of individual carpal bones.

In the past, nonunion of the scaphoid has been treated by radial styloidectomy, with or without bone grafting of the scaphoid.[9,14,52,93] Most reported series are small, and the results are unpredictable. Mazet and Hohl compared a group of patients treated by radial styloidectomy alone with those treated by radial styloidectomy and bone grafting of the scaphoid; of the 11 wrists treated in the first fashion, six were failures, three had fair results, and only two had good results.[52] We feel that styloidectomy of the radius is not recommended, not only because of the unreliability of the results, but because it removes an important support for the scaphoid implant, should this arthroplasty be desired.

Intercarpal Fusion

There has been an increased interest in intercarpal fusion as a method of treatment for disabilities of the scaphoid and lunate. Peterson and colleagues reviewed eight cases of intercarpal fusion performed at the Mayo Clinic over a period of 20 years; fusion of the scaphoid to the trapezium to the trapezoid was performed, and a failure of fusion of the scaphoid occurred in two wrists, leading to the conclusion that arthrodesis of a single carpal bone to another in the proximal carpal row is unwise.[61] A follow-up study of a series of 27 cases of intercarpal fusion reported by Graner and associates showed the results to be unsatisfactory: there was a decreased range of motion in all wrists operated on, development of radiocarpal fusion in four wrists, persistent pain in two cases, and decreased grip strength in one case.[29]

Cooney recently reported on a longer follow-up of 38 patients at the Mayo Clinic.[15] The types of fusion were radius–proximal row, scapholunate, scaphoid–lunate–triquetrum, scaphoid–lunate–capitate–triquetrum–lunate, lunate–triquetrum, and scaphoid–trapezoid–trapezium. Most patients had no change in their grip strength, 15 patients had 50% of normal wrist motion, and the rest had 30% or less of normal wrist motion. Eleven of 41 wrists required additional surgery for nonunion to extend the fusion or insert a silicone rubber lunate implant.

A more popular limited wrist arthrodesis, the scaphoid–trapezium–trapezoid, or triscaphoid, arthrodesis, has been reported to be successful for scapholunate dissociation, rotary subluxation, of the scaphoid, or arthritis of these joints (Fig. 33-17). Watson and Hempton reported two initial nonunions, but none since they began using

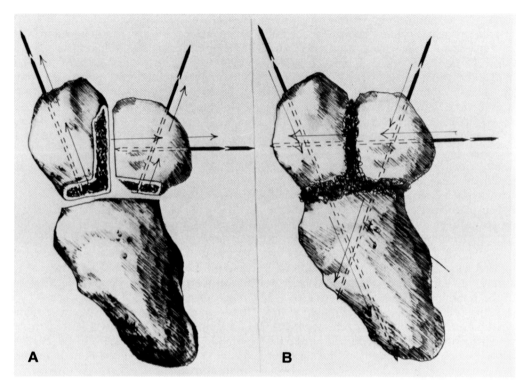

FIG. 33-17. (*A*) Articular surfaces are removed, and three pins have been "preset" in a retrograde fashion. (*B*) Cancellous bone grafts have been packed between the bones, the external shape of the triscaphoid unit is maintained, and the pins are driven across the arthrodesis sites. (Watson, H.K., and Hempton, R.F.: Limited wrist arthrodesis. I. The triscaphoid joint. J. Hand Surg., 5:320, 1980)

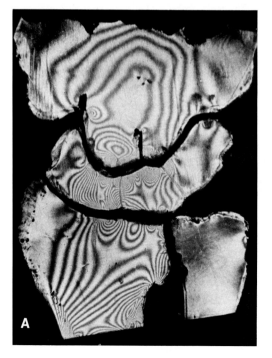

autogenous bone grafts from the distal radius.[96] The authors have had three cases of shoulder–hand syndrome, which resolved with treatment and achieved 80% of flexion-extension and 66% of radial and ulnar deviation of the wrist.

Kashiwagi and associates did a very interesting evaluation of 70 patients with Kienböck's disease.[38] They noted a higher incidence of disease (46%) in heavy manual workers and, with the use of tomograms,

FIG. 33-18. Photoelastic studies demonstrate areas of maximum stress on the lunate with the wrist in different positions. (*A*) Anteroposterior view of wrist in neutral position. (*B*) Anteroposterior view of the wrist in maximum ulnar deviation. Note the increase in stress lines in the lunate. (*C*) Sagittal section of the wrist in neutral position. (*D*) Sagittal section of the wrist in maximum dorsiflexion. Note the increase in stress lines in the lunate. (Courtesy of D. Kashiwagi, M.D., and A. Fujiwara, M.D.)

FIG. 33-18. *(Continued)*

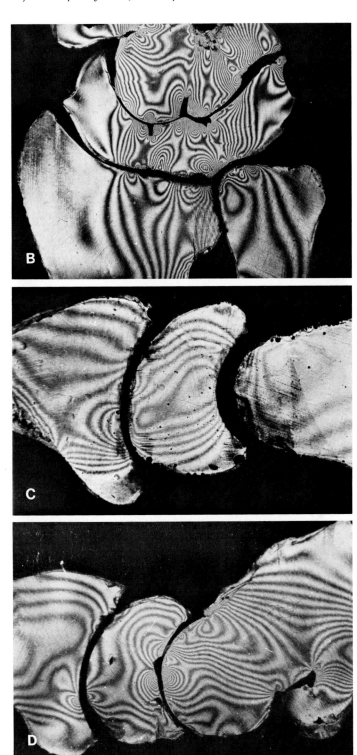

demonstrated previously undiagnosed fractures of the lunate in 75% of the patients; biomechanical and photoelastic studies of the lunate in various wrist positions demonstrated the locations of areas of increased stress, allowing them to postulate that trauma may be an important etiologic mechanism of this poorly understood entity (Fig. 33-18). In this series, three wrists were treated by curettage and bone grafting of the lunate, 29 by intercarpal fusion, 21 by excision of the lunate, and 17 by silicone implant resection arthroplasty. Intercarpal fusion brought improvement of grip strength in all cases; however, there was persistent pain on activity in five patients and pseudarthrosis in three patients. Some improvement in wrist motion was noted in those wrists in which the lunate fused to the triquetrum; however, motion was restricted in those wrists in which the lunate was fused to the triquetrum, hamate, and capitate. Patients treated by excision of the lunate presented improved wrist motion and relief of pain; however, migration of the carpal bones occurred in three of the 21 patients. All 17 patients who underwent silicone implant resection arthroplasty of the lunate showed a gain of 35° of wrist motion, no residual pain, and an increased grip strength; the implant migrated in one case (Fig. 33-19).

The ideal treatment would be a method that would relieve pain but maintain stability, power, and mobility of the wrist joint. We find that although intercarpal bone fusions may retain some wrist motion, they have not been satisfactory. Arthrodesis of the wrist joint may relieve pain, as has already been discussed; however, the resultant impairment from loss of mobility should limit this procedure to strict surgical indications. We prefer silicone implant resection arthroplasty for treatment of disabilities of individual carpal bones. Arthrodesis or flexible implant resection arthroplasty of the wrist may be indicated in certain cases of severe instability or generalized arthritic involvement.

Interpositional Arthroplasty

A method of interpositional arthroplasty in which local fatty tissues are used for treatment of Kienböck's disease has been studied by Therkelsen and Andersen, who reported poor results in 12 of their 19 operated cases.[92] Nahigian and co-workers reported the use of a dorsal flap arthroplasty to prevent carpal bone migration after excision of the lunate in long-standing cases of Kienböck's disease.[57] The flap was fashioned from the dorsal capsule of the wrist. The authors reported the results to be satisfactory after 28 months' follow-up. However, more long-term results are necessary to establish the effectiveness of this method in the treatment of Kienböck's disease.

Rigid Implant Arthroplasty

Metallic and acrylic implants have been used to replace the scaphoid and lunate.[2,3,6,27,45,47,55,63,97] Barber and Goodfellow evaluated the long-term follow-up of acrylic lunate prostheses in 14 operated wrists; slight pain persisted in ten patients, and the prosthesis maintained the carpal architecture in most cases, but subluxation and collapse did occur (Figs. 33-20 and 33-21).[6]

The Fett metal ball for replacement of the scaphoid has been reported to give acceptable results, but there is little documentation of long-term follow-up of wrist strength, mobility, pain relief, and use of the hand.[55] Bone resorption seems to be a common problem, subluxation of this rigid implant occurs, and the use of a circular implant to replace a bone as complicated as the scaphoid does not seem physiological (Fig. 33-22).

Acrylic prostheses for replacement of the scaphoid have not been reported to be successful. Agerholm and Lee used scaphoid acrylic implants made from molds fashioned after anatomical specimens in cadavers in 16 patients.[2] The implants were removed in two cases, one for anterior dislocation and one for fracture of the implant that occurred 5 years after surgery. Loss of wrist motion and power were found to be common, only four of these wrists were pain free, and collapse of the carpus occurred in one patient. Agner described the use of acrylic implants in seven wrists; five implants were removed because of increasing pain and stiffness, and radiocarpal arthrodesis was indicated.[3]

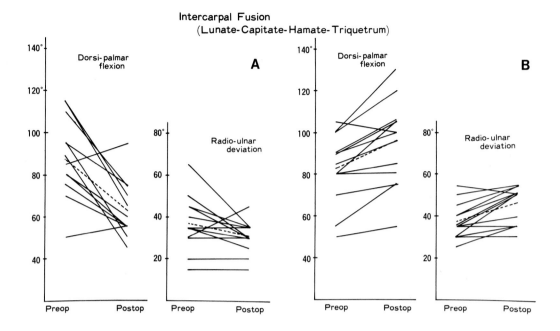

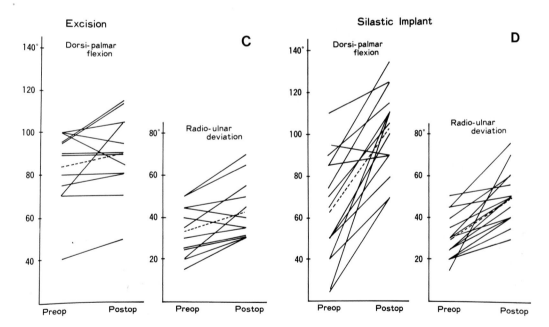

FIG. 33-19. Comparison of preoperative and postoperative range of motion in patients treated for Kienböck's disease by (*A*) intercarpal arthrodesis, (*B*) limited intercarpal arthrodesis, (*C*) excision of the lunate, and (*D*) silicone rubber implant arthroplasty. (Courtesy of D. Kashiwagi, M.D., and A. Fujiwara, M.D.)

The basic concept of the use of metallic and acrylic implants appears sound; however, this method has been unsatisfactory because of problems relating to progression of the arthritic process, migration of the implant, poor anatomical sizing, breakdown

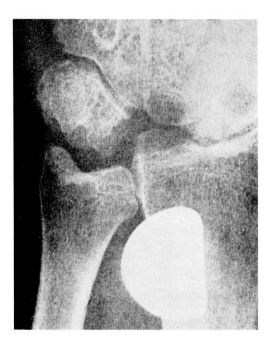

FIG. 33-20. Carpal collapse occurred after dislocation of a Vitallium lunate prosthesis. (Barber, H.M. and Goodfellow, J.W.: Acrylic lunate prosthesis. J. Bone Joint Surg., 56B:706, 1974)

of the material, and absorption of bone due to the hardness of the material.

Flexible (Silicone) Implant Resection Arthroplasty

In 1967, Swanson designed and developed intramedullary stemmed silicone rubber implants for the replacement of the carpal scaphoid and lunate bones.[74] These implants act as an articulating spacer to maintain the relationship of the adjacent carpal bones after excision of the scaphoid or lunate while preserving the mobility and stability of the wrist. These implants are

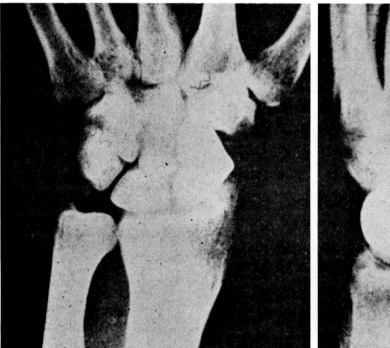
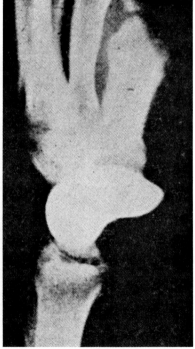

FIG. 33-21. Roentgenograms show subluxation and malrotation of a metal replacement prosthesis for the scaphoid. (Waugh, R.L., and Reuling, L.: United fractures of the carpal scaphoid: Preliminary report of the use of Vitallium as replacements after excision. Am. J. Surg., 67:184, 1945)

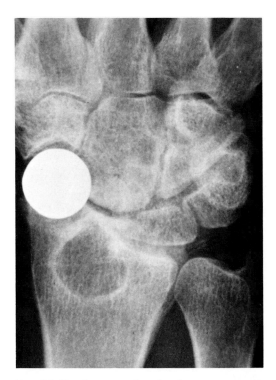

FIG. 33-22. An example of a long-term result after insertion of a Fett ball for a damaged scaphoid. Note the erosion of the implant into the trapezoid, capitate, and distal radius. Some collapse of the carpus has also developed, with the hamate now articulating with the distal radius.

made of silicone elastomer, which is well tolerated by the bone and soft tissues.

Anatomical shaping and sizing were studied by means of cadaver bones and x-ray films of a variety of hands. These implants have essentially the same shape as their anatomical counterparts, the concavities being more pronounced, however, to provide greater stability. These implants have a stabilizing stem that fits into an adjacent carpal bone to facilitate their localization and early postoperative stability. The stem of the scaphoid fits into the trapezium and the stem of the lunate into the triquetrum; these bones were selected for fixation points because there is the least intercarpal motion between these bones and the replaced one.

Spacer implants, especially for a single carpal bone, require good anatomical fitting and firm support on all sides by the adjacent bones, as well as tight capsuloligamentous structures around the implant. The implants act similar to a ball bearing, which must be surrounded by its housing to function. Adequate capsuloligamentous support and continuity around these implants is essential for early and late stability and must be obtained at surgery. If there is a collapse deformity at the wrist, as may follow a hyperextension injury, with associated damage to the carpal ligaments and the scaphoid and lunate bones, instability will continue unless the ligamentous structures are repaired. When carpal stability is good and a firm capsuloligamentous system can be reconstructed, good long-term results can be obtained. This method has been used successfully in our clinic for 15 years.

Scaphoid Implant Arthroplasty. In-dications. Flexible implant resection arthroplasty of the scaphoid is indicated for acute fractures of the scaphoid, either grossly displaced or comminuted, for pseudarthroses, especially with a small proximal fragment, for Preiser's disease, for avascular necrosis, and for failures from previous surgery.

If complete relief of symptoms is to be expected, the procedure should be used only in cases in which the arthritic involvement is localized to the scaphoid articulations and in which there is adequate support of and the implant and carpal stability (Fig. 33-23). If the radial styloid has been removed, there is no provision for lateral stability of the implant. Some surgeons have attempted to get around this problem by reconstructing a ligamentous structure on the radial aspect of the radius. In cases of old fracture-dislocation of the wrist with injury to the scaphoid and associated disruption of ligaments, especially the radiocarpal ligament, satisfactory results will probably not be achieved unless the carpal relationships and the ligamentous integrity have been reestablished. In cases in which there is severe diminution in the size of the scaphoid through long-standing disease, there may be inadequate room for placing an implant. Based on a review of our first 100 cases of scaphoid implant arthroplasty, we have developed a classification of var-

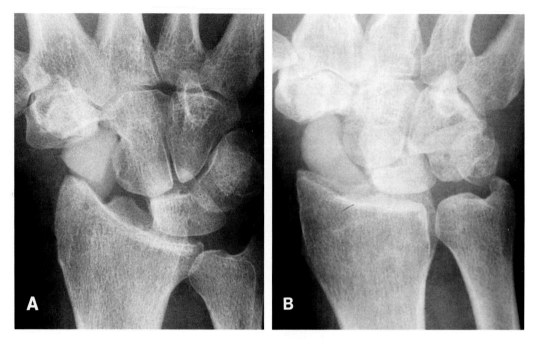

FIG. 33-23. (*A*) Malrotation and anterior subluxation of a silicone rubber implant after replacement arthroplasty of the scaphoid may be compared with (*B*) a properly seated and stable silicone rubber scaphoid implant.

ious possible treatments according to the presenting scaphoid pathology (Table 33-1).

Surgical Technique (Fig. 33-24). A 7-cm to 10-cm dorsoradial longitudinal incision is made across the radiocarpal joint midway between the tip of the styloid and Lister's tubercle. Dissection is carried to the retinaculum, with the longitudinal veins and the branches of the superficial radial nerve spared. The extensor pollicis longus tendon is identified and its retinaculum incised to release the tendon and retract it radially. The extensor retinaculum is dissected from the third compartment radially, as a flap, to expose the second compartment. The extensor carpi radialis longus and brevis tendons are dissected from the surrounding tissues and each other to their insertions. The transverse metacarpal vessels are protected. The extensor tendons can be retracted radially, ulnarly, or apart from each other to expose the dorsoradial capsule of the wrist joint. The dorsal capsule of the wrist is incised in a T fashion, with the tip of the longitudinal incision directed toward the trapezoid and the horizontal arm of the

incision placed over the distal radius at the insertion of the dorsal capsule. Dissection of the dorsal capsule is done with the wrist flexed. It is elevated by sharp dissection close to the bone to preserve adequate tissues for later reattachment. By retracting the wrist extensor tendons radially, the scapholunate junction and the capitate can be identified. By retracting the extensor tendons ulnarly, the distal portion of the scaphoid can be identified, and its articulations with the trapezoid and trapezium, as well as with the radius, can be shown. If necessary, intraoperative radiographs are obtained to identify the carpal bones. This is usually not necessary with this rather wide anatomical dissection.

The scaphoid is removed piecemeal with a sharp rongeur, with great care taken to avoid injury to the underlying palmar ligaments and both dorsal and palmar scapholunate ligaments. It is usually wise to leave flakes of bone in the area of the palmar ligament to avoid injury to these important structures. This is particularly true at the distal pole. If the distal pole is completely

Table 33-1. Classification of Scaphoid Pathology and Its Treatment

STAGE	PATHOLOGY	TREATMENT(S)
I	Acute scaphoid fracture Acute scaphoid fracture-dislocation	Immobilization Open or closed reduction
II	Nonunion of scaphoid	Bone grafting Treatment with a bone stimulator
III	Avascular necrosis of a fragment with 0–5% carpal height collapse Minimal lunate dorsiflexion (RL angle* 0–10°)	Partial scaphoid implant replacement Scaphoid implant replacement
IV	Comminuted or grossly displaced fracture Avascular necrosis with degenerative arthritic changes in the scaphoid Subluxation of the scaphoid with degenerative arthritic changes Nonunion of the scaphoid with cystic changes and 5–10% carpal height collapse Minimal to moderate lunate dorsiflexion (RL angle* 10–39°) Mild degenerative arthritic changes of contiguous bones	Scaphoid implant replacement
V	Stage IV pathology of the scaphoid with Carpal height collapse greater than 10% Moderate to severe lunate dorsiflexion (RL angle* > 30°) Mild to moderate degenerative changes of contiguous bones	Scaphoid implant replacement with or without intercarpal fusion Scapholunate implant replacement Proximal row carpectomy
VI	Stage IV pathology of the scaphoid or previous surgery with Carpal height collapse > 15% Severe lunate dorsiflexion (RL angle* > 30°) Severe intercarpal and radiocarpal degenerative arthritic changes	Radiocarpal implant arthroplasty Wrist arthrodesis Ulnar impingement treatment as needed

* Radiolunate angle

removed, a hole will be left in the palmar supporting structures, through which the implant could protrude. To avoid this problem we usually leave a thin wafer of bone just distal to the radiocapitate ligament and up to the trapezium.

The condition of the contiguous bones should be evaluated for the presence of arthritic or cystic changes, surface irregularities, cartilage loss, and instability patterns. Traction and compression on the hand across the wrist joint help evaluate instability patterns, particularly the position of the lunate to the capitate and radius. The presence and severity of dorsiflexion instability (DISI) or palmar flexion instability (VISI) patterns can be noted and related to the space available for the implant. A decision can be made to do an intercarpal fusion in association with the scaphoid implant replacement, depending on the severity of the degenerative arthritic changes

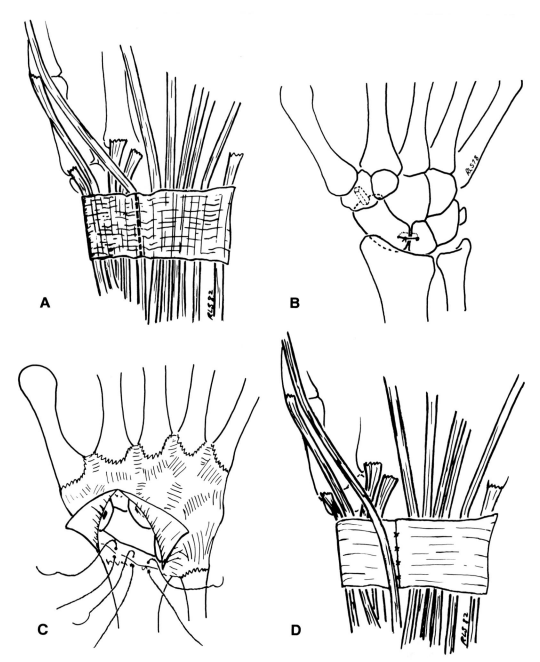

FIG. 33-24. (A) The extensor retinaculum is incised over the extensor pollicis longus, which is retracted radially. The extensor digitorum communis tendons are retracted ulnarward. The extensor carpi radialis longus and brevis tendons can be retracted ulnarly, radially, or from each other as needed. (B) The scaphoid implant is fixed to the lunate by passing a 2-0 nylon suture on an FS needle through a small hole made in the lunate. The implant stem fits in the trapezium, or between the trapezium and trapezoid. (C) The wrist capsule is securely sutured by passing 3-0 Dacron sutures through three small drill holes in the distal radius. The closure is completed with small Dacron and Dexon sutures with the knots inverted so that there will be no adherence to the overlying extensor tendons. (D) The extensor retinaculum is closed over the extensor tendons, except for the extensor pollicis longus, which is left free in the subcutaneous tissues.

and the instability pattern noted. An iliac bone graft is usually preferred, but resected bone, if healthy, could also be used. We usually fuse only the capitate–lunate area using an inlay graft, with either buried Kirschner wires or staples for immobilization. The posterior sensory branch of the interosseous nerve is identified in its course between the distal radius and ulna. Approximately 10 mm of nerve is resected to provide a sensory denervation of part of the carpal area. Care is taken to avoid injury to the associated small arteries and veins.

The correct implant size is determined by trial fitting with the sizing set. Sizing should start with the smallest implant to allow better visualization around it and to determine the proper spatial relationship of the implant to the contiguous bones. An implant size that fits easily into the space is selected from the seven available sizes. Scaphoid implants are made for either the right or the left hand. It is very important that the implants not be too large. With the smallest implant fitted into the space, it is possible to see where the stem of the implant should be directed. This may vary according to the carpal anatomy of the individual patient. The stem hole is usually fashioned in the trapezium, but the stem may also be inserted between the trapezium and the trapezoid or in the trapezoid. The hole is started with a small broach, curette, or drill to accept the implant stem and is gradually enlarged, by impacting the bone rather than removing it, to accept the implant stem comfortably. The hole should be directed at such an angle that the implant will be anatomically oriented; this is usually in the long axis of the trapezium. Repeated insertion of the sizers helps one to evaluate the final implant orientation, which is so important to the results. When a satisfactory fit has been otained, with the implant in position the wrist joint is moved passively in all directions to verify the stability of the implant in all ranges of motion. Shortening of the end of the stem is permissible, although reshaping of the implant body should be avoided whenever possible.

The scaphoid implant is fixed to the lunate at the scapholunate junction with a loop-suture technique. A hole is made in the lunate bone with a 0.045-inch Kirschner wire as the wrist is markedly flexed; the hole is started at the dorsal portion of the bone and angled palmar and radiad to exit approximately two thirds down on its scaphoid facet. A 2-0 nylon suture swaged on a FS needle has been used. The needle is straightened and is first passed from dorsal to palmar through the hole in the lunate. The needle is then curved back to a semicircle and passed through the upper third of the scaphoid implant at its lunate facet to exit dorsally, taking at least a 5-mm to 7-mm bite through the implant. The suture is then pulled through the lunate and the scaphoid implant. The implant is placed in position with the stem appropriately located and the sutures pulled tight and securely tied with multiple surgical knots. This should provide excellent positioning and immobilization of the implant. Prior to implant insertion, the palmar ligaments and capsule should have been observed and if necessary, adequately tightened with sutures.

The dorsal capsule, which has been preserved during the dissection, is securely sutured with three 2-0 or 3-0 Dacron sutures with the knots inverted; three 1-mm drill holes placed in the distal radius help secure the capsular repair. The dorsocarpal ligament is further sutured with small Dacron sutures and absorbable Dexon sutures, with the knots inverted so that a smooth surface is restored for the overlying tendon compartments. The tendon compartments are brought back over the area of the dorsocarpal ligament, and the retinaculum is resutured to enclose the extensors of the wrist and fingers. The extensor pollicis longus tendon is usually left outside the retinacular repair in the subcutaneous tissue, and one must make sure that there is no constriction of its muscle. The retinaculum is carefully closed, as are the subcutaneous layers. Multiple small drains are inserted subcutaneously, or a small suction apparatus can be used. The skin is closed with interrupted sutures. A secure conforming dressing, including longitudinally oriented Dacron batting strips and an anterior and posterior splint, is applied. We prefer to use a nonelastic conforming wrapping material, such as Kling.

Postoperative Care. The extremity is kept elevated for 3 to 5 days, and shoulder movements and finger wiggling are encouraged. A long-arm thumb spica cast is applied for 4 weeks, and a short-arm thumb spica cast is then used for an additional 4 weeks. If a plaster cast is applied at the end of the operative procedure, the cast should be bivalved. The skin sutures can be removed at 3 weeks through a cast window, and the cast can be adjusted as necessary, or changed. Rehabilitation of the hand and forearm is started at 8 weeks and consists of isometric gripping exercises to develop the extrinsic and intrinsic muscles. Full use of the wrist is usually resumed at the end of 12 weeks. Intraoperative or postoperative roentgenograms should be made to evaluate the position of the implant. Serial roentgenograms should be made in the long-term postoperative course to evaluate the maintenance of the position of the implant and the condition of the wrist bones.

Results. A Field Clinic survey of scaphoid implant resection arthroplasty included a total of 321 wrists operated on in various centers around the world. The procedure was performed for nonunion of the scaphoid in 163 wrists, for dislocation of the scaphoid in 11 wrists, for failed bone grafting in 48 wrists, for avascular necrosis in 71 wrists, for radioscaphoid arthritis in 49 wrists, and for panscaphoid arthritis in 13 wrists. Relief of pain was noted in 271 wrists; there was no change in the preoperative pain in 25 wrists and an increase of pain in five. There were five fractured implant stems (1.5%), rotation of the implant with the stem in position occurred in 47 wrists (14.7%), and subluxation of the implant with the stem out of the trapezium was reported in 12 wrists (3.7%). Secondary surgery was required in 3.7% of the reported cases; this included implant replacement in six wrists, proximal row carpectomy in two wrists, and wrist fusion in four wrists.

Postoperative pain may be due to injury of a superficial sensory branch of the radial nerve, subluxation of the implant, or a continued arthritic process. The surgical indications and techniques of this procedure must be followed meticulously. Fracture of the implant stem can be caused by inadequate alignment of the implant, poor bone preparation, or injury to the implant during surgery. This problem should be decreased with the advent of the High-Performance Silicone Elastomer. Rotation and subluxation of the implant are mainly due to failure to secure the capsuloligamentous continuity properly around the implant and to insertion of an implant of improper size.

Lunate Implant Arthroplasty. Indications. The lunate implant resection arthroplasty is indicated for avascular necrosis (Kienböck's disease), long-standing dislocation, localized arthritic changes, and resistance to conservative treatment. The contraindications to the procedure are similar to those stated for the scaphoid implant arthroplasty.

From a recent review of our first 69 cases of lunate implant arthroplasty, we have developed a classification of severity of lunate pathology based on lunate status, carpal height collapse, angular alterations of the relationships among the carpal bones, and arthritic involvement of contiguous carpal bones (Table 33-2).

Surgical Technique (Fig. 33-25). A 7-cm to 10-cm dorsal longitudinal incision is used in cases of Kienböck's disease. When the lunate is dislocated, a palmar approach is suggested. The superficial sensory branches of either the radial or ulnar nerve must be respected. The extensor pollicis longus is dissected and retracted radially. Dissection is carried down to the fourth extensor compartment of the extensor digitorum communis tendons. These are dissected with their synovial cover and retracted ulnad to expose the dorsocarpal ligament. With the wrist flexed, the dorsocarpal ligament is incised in a T shape, with its vertical extension placed over the lunate in the direction of the capitate and third metacarpal, and its horizontal extension at the insertion of the capsule over the distal radius. The capsule is dissected close to bone to preserve enough material for later reattachment. Positive identification of the lunate is essential. The scaphoid and lunate, at their junction, may appear to be one bone; after incising the interosseous scapholunate lig-

Table 33-2. Classification of Avascular Necrosis of the Lunate and Its Treatment

STAGE	PATHOLOGY	TREATMENT(S)
I	Sclerosis of the lunate with Minimal symptoms Normal carpal bone relationships	Splinting and rest Revascularization Lengthening or shortening of the ulna and radius

II	Sclerosis of the lunate with cystic
	    changes and
	Clinical symptoms
	Normal carpal bone relationships
		Lunate implant replacement
		Lengthening or shortening of the ulna
		    and radius

III	Sclerosis, cysts, and fragmentation of the lunate with Scaphoid–radius angle of 40–60° 0–5% carpal height collapse Minimal carpal translation	Lunate implant replacement

IV	Sclerosis, cysts, and fragmentation of
	    the lunate with
	Scaphoid-radius angle < 70°
	5–10% carpal height collapse
	Moderate carpal translation
		Lunate implant replacement with
		    scaphoid stabilization by soft tissue
		    reconstruction
		Intercarpal fusion if there are early
		    changes in contiguous bones

V	Sclerosis, cysts, and fragmentation of
	    the lunate with
	Scaphoid–radius angle > 70°
	Carpal height collapse > 10%
	Severe carpal translation
	Cystic changes in contiguous bones
		Lunate implant replacement and
		    intercarpal fusion
		Scapholunate implant replacement
		Wrist arthrodesis
		Ulnar impingement treatment as
		    needed

VI	Sclerosis, cysts, and fragmentation of
	    the lunate with
	Scaphoid–radius angle > 70°
	Carpal height collapse > 15%
	Severe carpal translation
	Cystic changes in contiguous bones
	Significant intercarpal and
	    radiocarpal degenerative arthritic
	    changes
		Radiocarpal implant arthroplasty
		Wrist arthrodesis
		Ulnar impingement treatment as
		    needed

ament, identification of the two bones is easy. Radiographs are taken, if necessary, for proper identification of the carpal bones.

The lunate is removed *en bloc* or piecemeal with great care to avoid injury to the palmar radiocarpal and ulnocarpal ligaments. A very thin layer of bone may be left with the ligaments to avoid injuring them. The integrity of the anterior capsuloligamentous structures in the depths of the wound must be verified. Frequently, there is ligament inadequacy immediately under the lunate because the two strong bands of the palmar radiocarpal and ulno-

carpal ligaments are attached on each side of the lunate and are separated by bone removal. The ligament structures are brought together with 3-0 Dacron sutures to ensure a firm palmar capsular support. Repair of the defect in this area may occasionally require a tendon graft or a slip of the flexor carpi ulnaris or radialis.

The associated bones should be evaluated for the presence of arthritic changes, loss of cartilage, surface irregularities, cystic changes, and collapse patterns. It is our feeling that in the presence of moderate to severe collapse patterns, intercarpal fusions

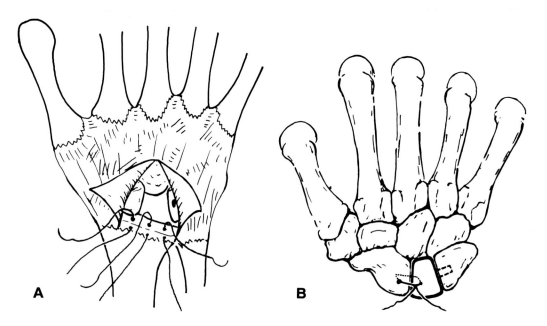

FIG. 33-25. (*A*) The wrist capsule is securely sutured by passing 3-0 Dacron sutures through three small drill holes in the distal radius. The closure is completed with small Dacron and Dexon sutures with the knots inverted so that there will be no adherence to the overlying extensor tendons. (*B*) Lunate implant in position with the stem in the triquetrum. Temporary fixation is accomplished with a 2-0 nylon suture on an FS needle passed through the implant and the scaphoid.

are indicated. If the radioscaphoid angle is greater than 70°, the vertical rotation of the scaphoid can be corrected by fusion of the scaphoid to the capitate with an inlay iliac bone graft. The corrected position may be maintained with buried Kirschner wires or small staples.

The posterior sensory branch of the interosseous nerve is identified in its course between the distal radius and ulna. Approximately 1 cm of nerve is resected to provide a sensory denervation of part of the carpal area. A size implant that will comfortably fit into the space left by the excision of the lunate is selected from the five available sizes. The implant should not be too large. Sizing should start with the smallest sizer to allow appreciation of the spatial relationships of the implant to the contiguous bones. The deep concavity of the lunate implant seats over the head of the capitate. A small awl, curette, or drill is used to make a hole in the triquetrum to accept the stem of the implant. The hole may then be enlarged with a small, curved

hemostat. This hole should not be larger than the implant stem. The bone should be impacted rather than removed. There should be minimal trauma to the triquetrum during this procedure. The direction of the hole should be such that the stem placement will orient the implant in an accurate anatomic relationship to the contiguous bones. Repeated insertion of the sizers will help evaluate the final implant orientation and the direction of the hole in the triquetrum. Shortening of the end of the stem of the implant is permissible, but reshaping of the implant should be avoided.

A loop-suture technique is used to fix the lunate implant to the scaphoid at the scapholunate junction. A hole is made with a 0.045-inch Kirschner wire from the dorsum of the scaphoid to exit palmarward approximately two thirds of the way on its lunate facet. The hole is very carefully placed with the wrist in marked flexion. A 2-0 nylon suture swaged on an FS needle is used for fixation. The needle is straightened and is first passed through the hole in the scaphoid from dorsal to palmar. The needle is then curved back to its semicircular shape and passed through the lunate implant, taking a 5-mm to 7-mm bite through the scaphoid facet of the implant approximately one third of the way from its dorsal surface. The suture is securely tied with multiple surgical knots. Tightening the suture pulls the implant down snugly against the scaphoid.

The dorsal capsular flap, which is preserved during the dissection, is tightly sutured with 3-0 Dacron sutures with the knots inverted. Three small drill holes are made in the distal radius to place sutures that will help secure the capsular closure. A strip of extensor retinaculum can be used to reinforce the dorsal carpal ligaments. The tendon compartments are brought back into position so that there will be no adherence to the underlying structures.

The stability of the capsular repair should be verified by passive movement of the wrist in all directions. An excessively tight repair could prevent an adequate range of motion of the wrist. At least 30° of flexion should be obtainable. The overlying extensor tendons are placed back in anatomic position with the retinaculum sutured over them. However, the extensor pollicis longus is left free in the subcutaneous tissue, and it is important that its muscle belly not be constricted by the retinaculum. The subcutaneous tissues are closed with absorbable sutures and the skin with interrupted sutures. Multiple small drains are inserted subcutaneously. A secure, voluminous conforming dressing that includes anterior and posterior plaster splints is made of Dacron batting and a conforming Kling bandage wrap. The extremity is elevated for 3 to 5 days, and the patient is instructed in movement of the shoulder and some finger wiggling. A short- or long-arm thumb spica cast is applied, depending on the stability of the carpal bones. If a cast has been applied at surgery, it should be bivalved.

When the implant arthroplasty is done for patients with palmar dislocation of the lunate, a palmar incision is used; the lunate is usually displaced into the carpal canal and is easily exposed. The capsuloligamentous structures should be carefully dissected from the lunate so that they are preserved

for later repair. The implant procedure is then carried out as described. A meticulous repair of the anterior radiocarpal ligaments must be performed to achieve good stability of the implant. A free graft of the palmaris longus can be used to stablize the carpus volarly and to reinforce the radiocarpal ligaments. The graft can be threaded through drill holes in the radius, scaphoid, and capitate and back across the lunate implant to the radius. This method is especially useful in cases of carpal bone instability, as may be seen with lunate dislocations. The transverse carpal ligament is left unsutured to decompress the carpal canal. Frequently, in long-standing dislocations a smaller implant is required because of the decreased space. If there is intercarpal instability associated with the dislocation, the possibility of subluxation of the implant in the postoperative period may be present. If severe instability of the carpus is present, or if it is impossible to reconstruct the ligaments, simple resection of the lunate without using the implant is indicated.

Postoperative Care. Skin sutures are removed at 2 to 3 weeks through a window in the cast or by changing the cast. The cast is worn for 6 to 8 weeks and may be tightened or changed during this time. The rehabilitation program includes isometric gripping exercises for development of the extrinsic and intrinsic muscles of the hand and forearm. Full use of the wrist is usually resumed at 12 weeks unless an intercarpal fusion was done; this requires a longer immobilization. Intraoperative and postoperative roentgenograms can be made to evaluate the position of the implant. Long-term postoperative serial roentgenograms should be made to evaluate the maintenance of the position of the implant and the condition of the wrist bones.

Results. A Field Clinic survey of 225 cases of lunate implant arthroplasty operated by surgeons in various centers around the world showed that the implant was used for Kienböck's disease in 184 wrists and for trauma in 41 wrists. Symptoms were reported to have been present for more than 2 years in 57 cases, for less than 2 years in 100 cases, and for less than 1 year in 74 cases. There was excellent relief of pain in 162 wrists; the pain was decreased in 48 wrists and remained unchanged in 15 wrists. Complications reported included fracture of one implant and subluxation of 27 operated wrists (11%). Of these subluxations, 14 were asymptomatic, 13 were painful, and seven were associated with median nerve compression (Figs. 33-26 and 33-27).

Scapholunate Implant Arthroplasty.
Indications. Use of a silicone scapholunate implant may be considered when both the carpal scaphoid and lunate are involved upon diagnosis of the following clinical conditions: (1) acute fractures of both lunate and scaphoid, or when one bone is fractured and the other inadequate (comminuted or grossly displaced), (2) avascular necrosis, (3) pseudarthrosis, (4) localized osteoarthritic changes, (5) long-standing dislocation, and (6) failed previous surgery.

Wrist reconstruction with the scapholunate implant should not be used in cases that have extensive arthritic involvement not localized to the scaphoid and lunate articulations. Any situation in which loss of support for the implant or instability of the carpus would be present is a contraindication to the use of this implant. If the radial styloid has been removed, there is no provision for lateral stability of the implant. In cases of old fracture-dislocations of the wrist with injury to the scaphoid or lunate and associated disruption of the ligaments, especially the radial carpal ligaments, satisfactory results are unlikely unless the carpal relationships and the ligamentous integrity have been reestablished. In cases in which there is severe diminution in the size of the scaphoid or lunate through long-standing disease, there may be inadequate space to accept the implant.

Surgical Technique (Fig. 33-28). A longitudinal incision 8 cm to 13 cm long is made, starting from the base of the second metacarpal and directed proximally along the central axis of the dorsal radius. Dissection is carefully carried down through the subcutaneous tissues, avoiding injury to the skin, longitudinal veins, and branches of the superficial radial and ulnar nerves. This provides exposure to the extensor retinaculum, which is longitudinally incised between the third and fourth compartments (extensor pollicis longus, extensor digitorum communis, and extensor indicis proprius). The digital extensors of the fourth compartment are mobilized *en bloc* with the extensor retinaculum and are reflected ulnad

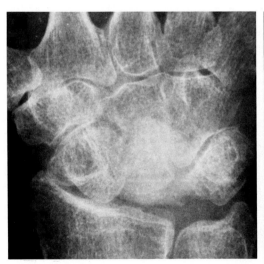 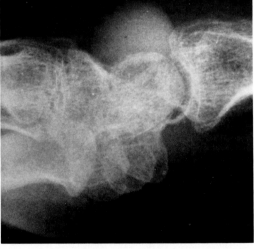

FIG. 33-26. In this unusual case, the lunate implant dislocated dorsally. A secure reconstruction of the dorsal capsule is necessary, with reattachment of the capsule to the radius by sutures placed through drill holes in the bone, to prevent dorsal migration of the implant. If the capsule is not sufficient, a strip of the extensor retinaculum or tendon may be used to reconstruct the capsule.

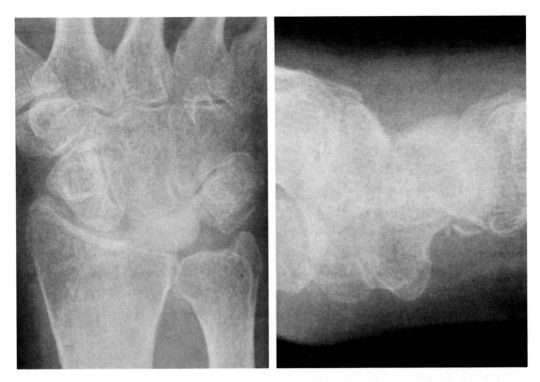

FIG. 33-27. Roentgenograms show a properly seated silicone rubber implant for replacement of a diseased lunate.

to expose the dorsal carpal ligament. The extensor pollicis longus is released and retracted radially. The extensor retinaculum is reflected from the extensor carpi radialis longus and brevis tendons. The wrist radial extensors and the extensor pollicis longus can be retracted radially or ulnarly to facilitate exposure; these tendons are then retracted radially, and the dorsal carpal ligament is incised in a T fashion. The dissection is carried out close to the bones to retain as much tissue as possible. Elevation of the dorsal carpal ligament exposes the radial styloid, scaphoid, lunate, triquetrum, capitate, trapezoid, and trapezium. Careful identification of the carpal bones is essential, and an intraoperative radiograph may be useful. The diseased carpal scaphoid and lunate are identified, along with their articulations with the adjacent carpal bones, and are removed piecemeal with a rongeur, with care taken not to injure the underlying structures. Small flakes of bone are left on the underlying capsule to preserve the integrity of the palmar capsuloligamentous

support for the implant. The palmar ligaments are inspected through the dorsal incision, and if loose, they can be tightened by suturing them to the distal palmar edge of the radius with 2-0 Dacron sutures on a PR-4 needle passed through 0.5-mm to 1-mm drill holes. Any bone spur or irregularities are smoothened with the round burr. The correct size of the implant is determined by trial fitting with the sizing set. An implant size that fits comfortably into the space left by the excision of the scaphoid and lunate is selected from the four available sizes. The implant should not be too large; sizing should start with the smallest sizer to allow appreciation of the spatial relationships of the implant to contiguous bones. Adequate fit of the implant is verified by passively moving the wrist in all directions. The implant must be stabilized in position with sutures to the trapezium, triquetrum, and distal radius. Small drill holes (0.5 mm to 1 mm) are made in these bones, and a 2-0 nylon suture on an FS needle is passed through the drill holes in the tra-

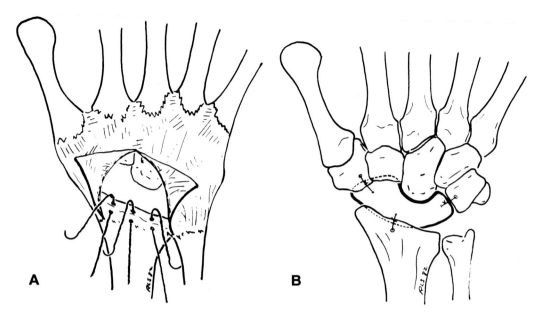

FIG. 33-28. (*A*) Repair of the dorsal carpal ligaments. Prior to implant insertion, three to four small drill holes are made in the dorsal distal edge of the radius, and 2-0 Dacron sutures on a PR-4 needle or 3-0 Dacron sutures on a PR-2 needle are passed. After repair on the palmar capsule, if necessary, and implant fixation, these are tied with inverted knots as the wrist is held in neutral position. (*B*) Method of implant fixation. Sutures of 2-0 nylon on a PS-3 needle are passed through small drill holes (0.5–1 mm) made in the trapezium and triquetrum; a 0 Dexon suture on a T-5 needle is used for fixation through a small drill hole in the distal radius; 7-mm bites are taken through implant.

pezium and triquetrum. A 7-mm bite is taken through the implant. A 0 Dexon suture on a T5 needle is used to stabilize the implant to the distal radius. The sutures are passed prior to implant insertion and are firmly tied, with the knots inverted as the assistant maintains the wrist in a neutral position. Prior to inserting the implant, a series of three to four small drill holes are made in the dorsal distal edge of the radius to secure the dorsal wrist capsule with 2-0 Dacron sutures on a PR-4 needle or 3-0 Dacron sutures on a PR-2 needle. Multiple 6-0 Dexon sutures with inverted knots, complete with sutures of the dorsal wrist capsule, provide a smooth gliding surface for the overlying extensor tendons. The extensor retinaculum is sutured back over the extensor tendons with a 4-0 Dexon suture, except for the extensor pollicis longus, which is left subcutaneous. The subcutaneous tissues are reapproximated with inverted 5-0 Dexon sutures and the skin with 5-0 interrupted nylon sutures. Several small drains are inserted subcutaneously,

and a voluminous conforming dressing is applied, including palmar and dorsal plaster splints to secure the wrist in a neutral position.

Postoperative Care. The extremity is kept elevated with a special arm sling. Finger and shoulder movements are encouraged. After 3 to 5 days the dressing is changed and the drains removed. The extremity is then placed in a long-arm thumb spica cast for 4 weeks and then in a short-arm thumb spica cast for 4 more weeks. In the postoperative rehabilitation program the patient is instructed to carry out strengthening exercises for the hand and forearm. Protective hand activities are prescribed 3 months following surgery. Activities are then progressively increased as tolerated (Fig. 33-29).

Discussion of the Results of Carpal Scaphoid and Lunate Implant Resection Arthroplasty

We have studied the movement of the carpal bones with roentgenograms and cinefluoroscopy in the normal wrist, the

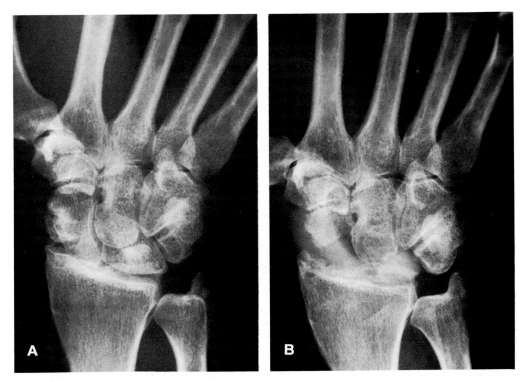

FIG. 33-29. (*A*) Preoperative and (*B*) postoperative roentgenograms show the results of a silicone scapholunate implant arthroplasty. Note on the postoperative film the presence of remnant bone at the distal scaphoid palmar surface. This flake of bone is left at surgery to maintain the stability of the palmar ligaments to help prevent vertical rotation of the implant.

injured wrist, and the wrist with silicone implants of the carpal bones. The implant spacer seems to move as did the bone it has replaced. Normal wrist ranges of motion are never completely recovered because of the tightening of the wrist ligaments, which does not lessen after carpal bone replacement. The slightly decreased range of wrist motion actually increases the stability, which we consider a desirable feature. Complete freedom from pain, adequate range of motion, good stability, and ability to perform normal work, including heavy labor or sports, have been achieved in most of our patients operated on with this method. It is our opinion that replacement of the scaphoid and lunate should be done early, as soon as the disease process of the affected bone is considered irreversible. The arthritic process, which has a tendency to spread to associated joints, may then be avoided. We have been using this method since 1967; the implant appears to be well

tolerated both biologically and mechanically. If the indications for their use are properly understood and followed, excellent clinical results can be expected.

We believe that these space-occupying implants minimize the displacement of the other carpal bones after excision of the lunate or scaphoid and that the maintenance of a normal carpal architecture is important in avoiding the development of osteoarthritis of the remaining joints. The follow-up of our cases suggested that when the operation is technically successful, degenerative changes do not occur despite prolonged and heavy use of the wrist. The presence of osteoarthritis of the wrist, other than around the affected bone, is not an absolute contraindication to implant replacement; however, some continued pain may be expected in the untreated joints. Cystic changes can occur when a silicone implant abrades with pressure against adjacent tissue if there is a break in the cortical bone. A subcortical cyst can be aggravated by foreign-body particles of silicone, as it can be with any synthetic material. Implants should not be too large to avoid concentrated load bearing on adjacent bone. If, on long-term follow-up, disabling degenerative changes in other areas of the wrist are noted, a proximal carpal row resection or wrist fusion can still be done. The carpal implant procedures are relatively simple, entail a short postoperative course, and provide a potential of wrist motion with adequate stability, mobility, and freedom from pain.

REFERENCES

1. Agerholm, J.C., and Goodfellow, J.W.: Avascular necrosis of the lunate bone treated by excision and prosthetic replacement. J. Bone Joint Surg., 45B:110, 1963.
2. Agerholm, M.C., and Lee, M.L.: The acrylic scaphoid prosthesis in the treatment of united carpal scaphoid fracture. Acta Orthop. Scand., 37:67, 1966.
3. Agner, O.: Treatment of nonunited navicular fractures by total excision of the bone and the insertion of acrylic prosthesis. Acta Orthop. Scand., 33:235, 1963.
4. Albright, J.A., and Chase, R.A.: Palmar-shelf arthroplasty of the wrist in rheumatoid arthritis: Report of nine cases. J. Bone Joint Surg., 52A:896, 1970.
5. Bäckdahl, N.: The caput ulnae syndrome in rheumatoid arthritis. Acta Rheum. Scand., 5[Suppl.]:1, 1963.
6. Barber, H.M., and Goodfellow, J.W.: Acrylic lunate prosthesis. J. Bone Joint Surg., 56B:706, 1974.
7. Barnard, L., and Stubbins, S.: Styloidectomy of the radius in the surgical treatment of nonunion of the carpal navicular. J. Bone Joint Surg., 30A:98, 1948.
8. Beckenbaugh, R.D., and Linscheid, R.L.: Total wrist arthroplasty: A preliminary report. J. Hand Surg., 2:337, 1977.
9. Bedeschi, P., and Luppino, T.: Sostituzione prostesica contemporanae dello scafoide e del semilunare, in endoprotesi articolari del polso e della mano. Capitolo, 3:31, 1974.
10. Böhler, L.: The Treatment of Fracture, 47th ed. Baltimore, William Wood, 1935.
11. Boyes, J.H.: Bunnell's Surgery of the Hand, 5th ed. Philadelphia, J.B. Lippincott, 1970.
12. Campbell, C.J., and Keokarn, T.: Total and subtotal arthrodesis of the wrist. J. Bone Joint Surg., 46A:1520, 1964.
13. Clendenin, M.B., and Green, D.P.: Arthrodesis of the wrist—complications and their management. J. Hand Surg., 6:253, 1981.
14. Cobey, M.C., and White, R.K.: An operation for nonunion of fractures of the carpal navicular. J. Bone Joint Surg., 45A:1321, 1963.
15. Cooney, W.P.: Intercarpal fusion. Presented at the 39th Annual Meeting of the American Society for Surgery of the Hand, Atlanta, February 1984.
16. Crabbe, W.A.: Excision of the proximal row of the carpus. J. Bone Joint Surg., 46B:708, 1964.
17. Cracchiolo, A., and Marmor, L.: Resection of the distal ulna in rheumatoid arthritis. Arthritis Rheum., 12:415, 1969.
18. Darrach, W.: Anterior dislocation of the head of the ulna. Ann. Surg., 56:802, 1912.
19. Davidson, A.J., and Howitz, M.T.: An evaluation of excision in the treatment of ununited fractures of the carpal scaphoid bone. Ann. Surg., 108:291, 1938.
20. Donaldson, W.F. et al.: Evaluation of treatment of nonunion of the carpal navicular. J. Bone Joint Surg., 44A:169, 1962.
21. Dornan A.: The results of treatment in Kienböck's disease. J. Bone Joint Surg., 31B:518, 1949.
22. Dupont, M., and Vainio, K.: Arthrodesis of the wrist in rheumatoid arthritis. Ann. Chir. Gynaecol. Fenn., 57:513, 1968.
23. Dwyer, F.C.: Excision of the carpal scaphoid for ununited fractures. J. Bone Joint Surg., 31B:572, 1949.
24. Edelstein, J.M.: Treatment of ununited fractures of the carpal navicular. J. Bone Joint Surg., 21:902, 1939.
25. Flatt, A.E.: The Care of the Rheumatoid Hand, 3rd ed. St. Louis, C.V. Mosby, 1974.
26. Gillespie, H.S.: Excision of the carpal lunate bone in Kienböck's disease. J. Bone Joint Surg., 43B:245, 1961.
27. Girzadas, D.V.: Limitation of the use of metallic prosthesis in the rheumatoid hand. Clin. Orthop., 67:169, 1969.
28. Gold, A.M.: Use of a prosthesis for the distal portion of the radius following resection of a recurrent giant cell tumor. J. Bone Joint Surg., 47A:216, 1965.
29. Graner, O., Lopes, E.I., Carvalho, B.C., and Atlas, S.: Arthrodesis of the carpal bones in the treatment of Kienböck's disease: Painful ununited fractures of the navicular and lunate bones with avascular necrosis and old fracture dislocations of carpal bones. J. Bone Joint Surg., 48A:767, 1966.
30. Haddad, R.J., and Riordan, D.C.: Arthrodesis of the wrist. J. Bone Joint Surg., 49A:950, 1967.
31. Harris, W.H., Jones, W.N., and Aufranc, O.E.: Problem Cases From Fracture Grand Rounds at Massachusetts General Hospital, p. 291. St. Louis, C.V. Mosby, 1965.
32. Heiple, K.G., Burstein, A.H., and Gradisar, I.: Instant wrist fusion—a preliminary report. Presented at the 29th Annual Meeting of The American Society for Surgery of the Hand, Dallas, January 1974.
33. Herndon, J.H., and Hubbard, L.F.: Total joint replacement in the upper extremity. Surg. Clin. North Am., 63:715, 1983.
34. Inglis, A.E., and Jones, E.C.: Proximal row carpectomy for disease of the proximal row. J. Bone Joint Surg., 57A:726, 1975.
35. Jorgesen, E.C.: Proximal row carpectomy: An end-result study of 22 cases. J. Bone Joint Surg., 51A:1104, 1969.

36. Kaplan, E.B.: Functional and Surgical Anatomy of the Hand, 2nd ed. Philadelphia, J.B. Lippincott, 1965.
37. Kapandji, I.A.: The Physiology of the Joints, 2nd ed. London, E. & S. Livingstone, 1970.
38. Kashiwagi, D. et al.: An experimental and clinical study of lunatomalacia.
39. Kay, G.D.: A method of radiocarpal and intercarpal arthrodesis. J. Bone Joint Surg., 57B:531, 1975.
40. Keon-Cohen, B.: To speke of phisik and of surgerye. J. Bone Joint Surg., 52B:597, 1970.
41. Kessler, I., and Hecht, O.: Present application of the Darrach procedure. Clin. Orthop., 72:254, 1970.
42. Kienböck, R.: Über traumatische Malazie des Mondbiens und ihre Folgezustände. Fortschr. Geb. Roentgenstr., 16:77, 1910–1911.
43. Kulick, R.G., DeFiore, J.C., Straub, L.R., and Ranawat, C.S.: Long term results of dorsal stabilization in the rheumatoid wrist. J. Hand Surg., 6:272, 1981.
44. Lamberta, F.J., Ferlick, D.C., and Clayton, M.D.: Volz total wrist arthroplasty in rheumatoid arthritis: A preliminary report. J. Hand Surg., 5:245, 1980.
45. Legge, R.F.: Vitallium prosthesis in the treatment of fracture of the carpal navicular. West. J. Surg., 58:468, 1951.
46. Liebolt, F.L.: Surgical fusion of the wrist joint. Surg. Gynecol. Obstet., 66:1008, 1938.
47. Lippman, E.M., and McDermott, L.J.: Vitallium replacement of lunate in Kienböck's disease. Milit. Surgeon, 105:482, 1949.
48. Littler, J.W.: Principles of reconstructive surgery of the hand. In Converse, J.M. (ed.): Reconstructive Plastic Surgery. Philadelphia, W.B. Saunders, 1964.
49. Lugnegard, H.: Resection of the head of the ulna in posttraumatic dysfunction of the distal radioulnar joint. Scand. J. Plast. Reconstr. Surg., 3:65, 1969.
50. Madden, J.W., and Peacock, E.E., Jr.: Studies on the biology of collagen during wound healing: Dynamic metabolism of scar collagen and remodeling of dermal wounds. Ann. Surg., 174:511, 1971.
51. Mannerfelt, L., and Malmsten, M.: Arthrodesis of the wrist in rheumatoid arthritis. Scand. J. Plast. Reconstr. Surg., 5:124, 1971.
52. Mazet, R., Jr., and Hohl, M.: Radial styloidectomy and styloidectomy plus bone graft in the treatment of old ununited carpal scaphoid fractures. Ann. Surg., 152:296, 1960.
53. McLaughlin, H.L., and Baab, O.D.: Carpectomy. Surg. Clin. North Am., 31:451, 1951.
54. McMurthy, R.Y., and Youm, Y.: Wrist motion: A new approach. Presented at the 30th Annual Meeting of The American Society for Surgery of the Hand, San Francisco, February 1975.
55. Metcalfe, J.W.: Vitallium sphere prosthesis for nonunion of the navicular bone. J. Int. Coll. Surg., 22:459, 1954.
56. Millender, L.H., and Nalebuff, E.A.: Arthrodesis of the rheumatoid wrist: An evaluation of sixty patients and a description of a different surgical technique. J. Bone Joint Surg., 55A:1026, 1973.
57. Nahigian, S.H., Li, C.S., Richey, D.G., and Shaw, D.T.: The dorsal flap arthroplasty in the treatment of Kienböck's disease. J. Bone Joint Surg., 52A:245, 1970.
58. Pahle, J.A., and Raunio, P.: The influence of wrist position on finger deviation in the rheumatoid hand. J. Bone Joint Surg., 51B:664, 1969.
59. Palmer, A.K., and Werner, F.W.: The triangular fibrocartilage complex of the wrist—anatomy and function. J. Hand Surg., 6:153, 1981.
60. Palmer, A.K., Werner, F.W., and Glisson, R.: Normal wrist motion. Presented at the 39th Annual Meeting of the American Society for Surgery of the Hand, Atlanta, February 1984.
61. Peterson, H.A. et al.: Intercarpal arthrodesis. Arch. Surg., 95:127, 1967.
62. Petrie, D.P.: Compression arthrodesis of the wrist. J. Bone Joint Surg., 57B:531, 1975.
63. Picaud, A.: Treatment of pseudoarthrosis of the scaphoid with acrylic prosthesis. Mem. Acad. Chir., 79:200, 1953.
64. Preiser, G.: Über eine typische posttraumatische und zur spontanfraktur führende Ostitis des Naviculare carpi. Fortschr. Geb. Roentgenstr., 15:189, 1910.
65. Ranawat, C.S., DeFiore, J., and Straub, L.R.: Madelung's deformity: An end-result study of surgical treatment. J. Bone Joint Surg., 57A:772, 1975.
66. Robinson, R.F., and Kayfetz, D.O.: Arthrodesis of the wrist. J. Bone Joint Surg., 34A:64, 1952.
67. Smith-Petersen, M.N.: A new approach to the wrist joint. J. Bone Joint Surg., 22:122, 1940.
68. Stack, J.K.: End results of excision of the carpal bones. Arch. Surg., 57:245, 1948.
69. Stähl, F.: On lunatomalacia (Kienböck's disease). Acta Chir. Scand., 95[Suppl. 26], 1947.
70. Stamm, T.T.: Excision of the proximal row of the carpus. Proc. R. Soc. Med., 38:74, 1944.
71. Straub, L.R., and Ranawat, C.S.: The wrist in rheumatoid arthritis. J. Bone Joint Surg., 51A:1, 1969.
72. Swanson, A.B.: A flexible implant for replacement of arthritic and destroyed joints in the hand. New York Univ. Inter-Clin. Info. Bull., 5:1, 1966.
73. ———: Finger joint replacement by silicone rubber implants and the concept of implant fixation by encapsulation. Ann. Rheum. Dis., 28[Suppl.]:47, 1969.
74. ———: Silicone rubber implants for the replacement of the carpal scaphoid and lunate bones. Orthop. Clin. North Am., 1:299, 1970.
75. ———: Flexible implant arthroplasty for arthritic disabilities in the radiocarpal joint. Orthop. Clin. North Am., 4:383, 1973.
76. ———: Flexible Implant Arthroplasty in the Hand and Extremities. St. Louis, C.V. Mosby, 1973.
77. ———: Implant arthroplasty for disabilities of the distal radioulnar joint. Orthop. Clin. North Am., 4:373, 1973.
78. ———: Flexible implant arthroplasty in the hand. Clin. Plast. Surg., 3:141, 1976.
79. ———: Reconstructive surgery in the arthritic hand and foot. Ciba Found. Symp. 31(6):1979.
80. Swanson, A.B.: Flexible implant arthroplasty of the distal radioulnar joint—long term results. Presented at the 36th Annual Meeting of the American Society for Surgery of the Hand, Las Vegas, February 1981.

81. ———: A grommet bone liner for flexible implant arthroplasty. Bull. Prosth. Res. Rehab. Eng. Res. Devel., BPR10-35, 1:108, 1981.

82. ———: Implant arthroplasty in the hand and upper extremity and its future. Surg. Clin. North Am., 61:369, 1981.

83. ———: Bone remodeling phenomena in flexible (silicone) implant arthroplasty in the hand: Long term study. Kappa Delta Award Lecture, presented at the 49th Annual Meeting of the American Academy of Orthopaedic Surgeons, New Orleans, January 21–26, 1982. Orthop. Rev., 11:129, 1982.

84. Swanson, A.B., and deGroot Swanson, G.: Pathogenesis and pathomechanics of rheumatoid deformities in the hand and wrist. Orthop. Clin. North Am., 4:1039, 1973.

85. ———: Flexible implant arthroplasty of the radiocarpal joint: Surgical technique and long-term results. In Inglis, A. (ed.): The American Academy of Orthopaedic Surgeons Symposium on Total Joint Replacement of the Upper Extremity, pp. 301–306. St. Louis, C.V. Mosby, 1982.

86. ———: Joint replacement in the rheumatoid metacarpophalangeal joint. In Inglis, A. (ed.): The American Academy of Orthopaedic Surgeons Symposium on Total Joint Replacement of the Upper Extremity, pp. 217–237. St. Louis, C.V. Mosby, 1982.

87. Swanson, A.B. et al.: Durability of silicone implants—an in vivo study. Orthop. Clin. North Am., 4:1097, 1973.

88. Swanson, A.B., deGroot Swanson, G., and Frisch, E.E.: Flexible (silicone) implant arthroplasty in the small joints of the extremities: Concepts, physical and biological considerations, experimental and clinical results. In Rubin, L.R., (ed.): Biomaterials in Reconstructive Surgery, pp. 595–623. St. Louis, C.V. Mosby, 1983.

89. Tajima, T.: An investigation of the treatment of Kienböck's disease. J. Bone Joint Surg., 48A:1649, 1966.

90. Taleisnik, J.: The ligaments of the wrist. J. Hand Surg., 1:10, 1976.

91. Taleisnik, J.: Post-traumatic carpal instability. CORR, 149:73, 1980.

92. Therkelsen, F., and Andersen, K.: Lunatomalacia. Acta Chir. Scand., 07:503, 1949.

93. Verdan, C., and Narakas, A.: Fractures and pseudoarthrosis of the scaphoid. Surg. Clin. North Am., 48:1083, 1968.

94. Volz, R.G.: The development of a total wrist arthroplasty. CORR, 116:209, 1976.

95. Volz, R.G., Lieb, M., and Benjamin, J.: Biomechanics of the wrist. CORR, 149:112, 1980.

96. Watson, H.K., and Hempton, R.F.: Limited wrist arthrodesis. I. The triscaphoid joint. J. Hand Surg., 5:320, 1980.

97. Waugh, R.L., and Reuling, L.: United fractures of the carpal scaphoid: Preliminary report on the use of Vitallium replicas as replacements after excision. Am. J. Surg., 67:184, 1945.

34 Complications of Implant Surgery in the Hand

JOHN P. ADAMS AND ROBERT J. NEVIASER

Arthroplasty of the hand is essentially joint resection, with or without interposing materials.[1,3–10,14–22,25] In the past two and one half decades, various linked and unlinked interposition materials have been used with varying effectiveness. These have included metal, fascia, silicone rubber, metal–polyethylene combinations, and polypropylene–steel–silicone combinations.

Along with the variations in arthroplasty techniques, an assortment of tendon transfers have been reported by numerous surgeons. The complications of some techniques will not be discussed, either because they have largely been abandoned or because they are so new that adequate follow-up of sufficient numbers is not available. This discussion will be limited to complications of resection arthroplasty without the use of a spacer and to those with interposition material that has silicone rubber as its principal ingredient.

The joints that will be discussed are the interphalangeal joints of the fingers and thumb, the metacarpophalangeal joints of the fingers and thumb, and the metacarpotrapezial joint of the thumb. Resection and resection with an interposition material have been carried out in each of these joints. Some of the complications, such as infection, are applicable to all joints and will be discussed in a general manner, while certain complications are relatively limited to specific joints and will be discussed as problems of individual joints.

INFECTION

The hazard of infection is present in all implant surgery; the reported incidence is less than 1%.[13] When it occurs, treatment requires drainage of the joint, administration of appropriate antibiotics, and, usually, removal of the implant, although in mild cases healing will occur with the implant in place. Chronic drainage of an infected joint requires implant removal. The removal of the implant usually allows speedy healing of the joint, which can then be treated as a resection arthroplasty. The anticipated end result of an infected arthroplasty is healing of the joint but with a somewhat decreased range of motion; most of these joints are stable and pain free. Additional arthroplasty procedures should not be attempted until a long time has elapsed during which clinical evidence of infection is absent. This period should probably not be less than 6 months to 1 year.

Spontaneous fusion after infection is rare. If this is anticipated, the joint should be stabilized in a position of optimal function with respect to other joints of the same digit. Fusion is more likely to occur in the interphalangeal joints than in the metacarpophalangeal joints. Prompt treatment of suspected infection gives the best prospect for a functional end result and usually prevents major bone involvement. The prophylactic use of antibiotics, though recommended by some, has no reported basis for general acceptance, except in previously infected joints that are being reoperated on, or perhaps in high-risk patients with other potential sources of infection.

DISLOCATION OF THE IMPLANT

Dislocation of the implant at the metacarpophalangeal joint occurs infrequently in both the proximal phalanx and the metacarpal.[2,6,11] It may be due to improper placement, overdrilling of the anterior cortex with subsequent erosion and displacement, or fracture of the anterior cortex during reaming of the medullary canal. It may also be due to use of an implant that is too small or one not properly seated.

The treatment for a dislocation is replacement with an implant of the proper size and correction of any deformity that may contribute to dislocation (*e.g.,* severe ulnar drift). In case of loss of bone stock, removal of the implant and conversion to a resection arthroplasty are required.

In chronic subluxation of the metacarpophalangeal joints there is usually erosion of the dorsal portion of the proximal phalanx, which may include up to half of its articular surface. It is necessary to estimate the extent of this erosion before any bone resection is carried out; otherwise, injudicious bone resection may lead to a joint so loose that implant stability is difficult or impossible to obtain. After dislocation has occurred and a second procedure is necessary, it should be approached as being a more difficult procedure than the initial one. The medullary canals must be reopened to adequate size and depth, a synovectomy should be done if there has been a recurrence of synovial hypertrophy, the volar ligaments again must be released to allow slight passive hyperextension of the joint with the implant in place, the radial collateral ligament must be reassessed and its function ensured, and the extensor mechanism should be well centered over the joint and should remain there through passive flexion.

The implant should be as large as the bony resection and the medullary canals will accept; a too-small canal may lead to stem extrusion. The implant should not be trimmed or the stem shortened. Suture anchorage of the Dacron-covered implant has been advocated. After insertion of the implant and closure of the dorsal capsule, the finger must be retested for intrinsic tightness; if this is present, the involved muscle(s) should be released by tenotomy, first on the ulnar side and including radial intrinsics if necessary. The second arthroplasty for dislocation usually requires additional capsular surgery directed toward increased stability with (ultimately) reduced range of motion. Postsurgical care should include the details applied to establishing the desired arc of motion.

Dislocations of interphalangeal joint implants are extremely rare. These could occur for the same reasons as those listed above;

in selected cases, management might also include interphalangeal arthrodesis.

The dislocation of the proximal interphalangeal implant may have been due to instability of the implant, which in turn is frequently due to the small circumference of the intramedullary canal of the middle phalanx. Redrilling of the medullary canals (preferably with mechanically powered high-speed drills) and selection of a larger implant may be essential. The resection of collateral ligaments usually does not lead to medial-lateral instability with implant dislocation. However, a subluxation of the middle slip of the extensor tendon will, and a recentering of this with repair of the oblique retinacular ligaments is often necessary. In cases in which there is intrinsic contracture, it must be relieved so that the resting posture of the finger assumes a slightly "intrinsic-minus" position.

FRACTURE OF THE IMPLANT

Implant fracture was mentioned often in the early use of implants.[24] It has decreased with improved surgical technique and will probably decrease further with the recent introduction of a stronger, more tear resistant silicone rubber. The experiences reported here are related to the materials in use prior to 1975. In 1974 the Mayo Clinic group reported an incidence of breakage of 25.4% with the Swanson design and 38.2% with the Niebauer type.[2]

The technical causes of failure are injury to the implant in handling, improper trimming of the joint margins (which may erode the implant and lead to fracture), and fatigue fracture due to chronic implant failure (Fig. 34-1).

The treatment for a fractured implant, whether in the interphalangeal or metacarpophalangeal joint, is careful replacement if there are symptoms that warrant additional surgery. The stress placed on the index metacarpophalangeal and proximal interphalangeal joints with pinch makes these joints more prone to implant failure.

It should be emphasized that many implant fractures are found only on roentgenographic examination and present minimal symptoms. When symptoms do occur and surgical reexploration is carried out, careful

FIG. 34-1. (*A*) This fracture of
an implant in an index proximal interphalangal joint occurred approximately 2 years
after insertion. (*B*) Fracture of
an index metacarpophalangeal
joint implant.

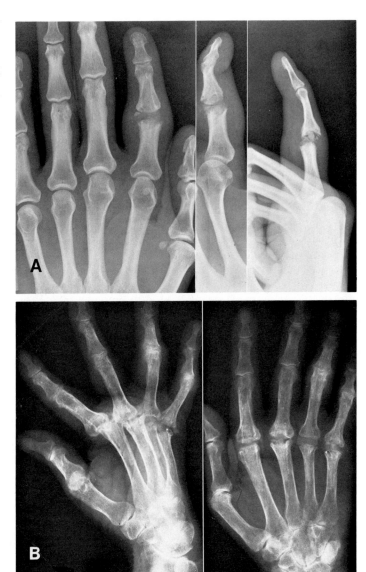

attention to soft and bony tissues is mandatory to correct any conditions that may
have contributed to the failure.

Early fracture, within a few weeks or
months of surgery, is usually due to a faulty
implant, although the fault is less likely to
be in its manufacture than in some accidental and unrecognized damage in handling
at the time of surgery. In such cases, when
other aspects of the surgery have been
properly performed, reinsertion (after redrilling or curettage of the medullary canals
and removal of any bony spurs) of an

implant of proper size may be all that is
necessary.

In late fracture of implants, factors other
than material failure must be considered.
As mentioned, early implant fracture in the
index finger may lead one to recommend
arthrodesis of the metacarpophalangeal joint
when there is adequate interphalangeal joint
function, or, conversely, fusion of the proximal interphalangeal joint when there is
stability and a suitable range of motion in
the metacarpophalangeal joint. Also, in the
index finger a reinforcement of the abduc-

tion position of the pinch mechanism by tendon transfer to reinforce the first dorsal interosseus muscles may be considered.

The role of the thumb in producing the stress leading to implant failure must also be determined, since an unstable thumb will produce a variety of stresses on the index finger. A thumb metacarpophalangeal joint fixed in flexion will place maximum stress just distal to the proximal interphalangeal joint, whereas a metacarpophalangeal joint fixed in hyperextension will force the index to seek the thumb, usually with the interphalangeal joints in maximum flexion and the metacarpophalangeal joint extended and rotated. Therefore, correction of a thumb deformity may be essential for maintenance of index finger joint correction.

In fractures of ulnar implants the implants for the long and ring fingers should be replaced if there is adequate bone stock and the soft tissues are still present in a condition that will allow their reconstruction. In the little finger, fusion or resection to produce a stable joint may be the treatment of choice.

Implant fracture in the proximal interphalangeal joint may be treated by simple replacement when there is adequate bone stock and the tendons and soft tissues are of adequate quality to permit a movable joint.[23] If there is a question of stability or motion, arthrodesis is most often the treatment of choice. Arthrodesis is difficult and may require bone grafting with a graft in the shape of an intramedullary peg. Immobilization with crossed Kirschner wires usually provides the stability required until fusion occurs.

STIFFNESS

Normal joint motion never returns after resection or implant surgery, and the average return after implant surgery is not much greater than that after resection alone. The major advantage of implant surgery lies in providing greater stability and earlier motion.

The complication of stiffness may occur in both flexion and extension, the latter being less functionally disabling than the former.

Management of severe stiffness may require a repeat of the surgical procedure. Stiffness early in the postoperative period can be recognized and addressed. In the metacarpophalangeal joint the optimal range of motion is related to interphalangeal joint motion. If interphalangeal joint motion aproaches normal, then stability, rather than mobility, will be the goal. Therefore, the surgeon should decide where he wants the useful arc of motion to fall, and by placing due emphasis on flexion and extension splinting, the desired range can be achieved in most instances. This attention to range of motion must begin early, usually as soon as the bulky supportive postoperative dressings have been removed at 5 to 7 days. A splinting program combined with active exercises must be continued through the first 6 to 8 weeks of the postoperative period and sometimes longer.

Proximal interphalangeal joint stiffness is more difficult to manage. If maximal flexion is functionally desirable, some loss of extension (up to 30°) may be a necessary compromise. As in the metacarpophalangeal joint, the details of splinting and exercise must be carefully taught to the patient and must be enforced early and continuously through the period of connective-tissue remodeling. If a fixed, stiff joint results, a secondary operative procedure will probably be necessary. Stiffness is more likely to occur in osteoarthritis than in rheumatoid arthritis, and anticipation of this should alert the surgeon to modify both his operative technique and his postoperative management.

RECURRENT DEFORMITY

There is a recurrence of ulnar deviation in approximately half of the operated cases with implant surgery, and the incidence is higher in resection arthroplasty. Recurrent deformity is time related, so in assessing postoperative results one should differentiate between 2- and 5-year follow-ups. The causes of recurrent deformity are many and include inadequate surgery at the outset—soft tissue release or synovectomy, improper placement of an implant of improper size, extensor tendon and extensor hood reconstruction, and inadequate intrinsic muscle release—and inadequate or improper postoperative care. In a progressive disease such as rheumatoid arthritis there may be further destruction of supportive soft tissues with resultant recurrence of the deformity.

The role of the radial wrist extensors is still being debated, but it may be important in the treatment of certain patients with recurrent deformity.

If the deformity is severe, a second procedure may be necessary. Reoperation usually leads to a decreased range of motion but can restore some of the function lost because of recurrent deformity.

Recurrent ulnar drift will occur in the majority of metacarpophalangeal joint arthroplasties that exhibit a reasonable range of motion and have had a follow-up of more than 2 years (Fig. 34-2). Mild deformity requires no treatment. Early severe deformity is usually caused by inadequate soft tissue correction or fracture or dislocation of the implant. When there is severe recurrence, the cause must be determined and corrected in the manner described earlier. Fusion of the metacarpophalangeal joints, particularly in the ring and little fingers, should be considered if there is a functional range of interphalangeal joint flexion.

Recurrent angular deformity in the proximal interphalangeal joints is common, particularly in nonrheumatoid joints. Mild deformity should be tolerated; the more severe degree of deformity, if symptomatic, is probably best handled by arthrodesis.

Patients should be told preoperatively that some recurrence of ulnar deviation is likely to occur but that in most instances it will not equal the preoperative degree and will infrequently require reoperation.

Recurrent deformity in flexion may accompany ulnar deviation; if it is severe and abrupt in onset, it usually signals implant fracture. If it occurs early, it is usually related to inadequate bone resection, volar capsular release, or both. Although extension splinting may sometimes help, it will not overcome this deformity. In the proximal interphalangeal joint, angular deformity may be reduced, but it usually recurs in

spite of meticulous attention to soft tissue reconstruction of both joint and tendons.

In instances in which secondary procedures are deemed necessary to correct recurrent deformity, a careful preoperative analysis of the likely cause of the deformity is essential so that those forces contributing to the deformity—whether active or passive—can be corrected.

THE METACARPOPHALANGEAL JOINT OF THE THUMB

Only one series of metacarpophalangeal joint implant arthroplasties has been reported. In selected cases and with careful capsule and tendon repair, a painless, stable joint can be achieved. The complication rate to date has been low. Painful arthroplasties can be converted to arthrodeses in those thumbs that have adequate interphalangeal and carpometacarpal joint function. Fractured or displaced implants may require replacement. Infected implants require the same management as infected implants elsewhere.

THE METACARPOTRAPEZIAL JOINT

Arthroplasty of the metacarpotrapezial joint has been practiced successfully for many years.[12,26]

Resection Arthroplasty

Resection arthroplasty, in which the joint is debrided and the trapezium excised, has as its usual complications mild discomfort and modest motion. Properly carried out and with proper attention to the other thumb joints, this procedure has rather uniformly successful results.

Subluxation may occur, however, when collapse or hyperextension deformity of the metacarpophalangeal joint occurs and goes unrecognized or untreated. When such a deformity exists, it may lead to failure of the carpometacarpal arthroplasty; once recognized as such a contributing factor, it should be corrected.

Implant Arthroplasty

Implant arthroplasties fall into two categories. In the first there is minimal joint

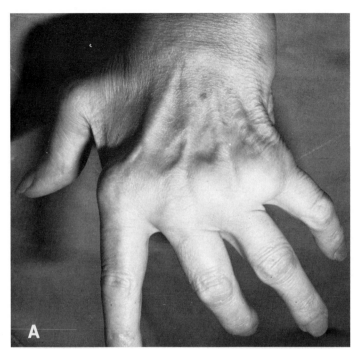

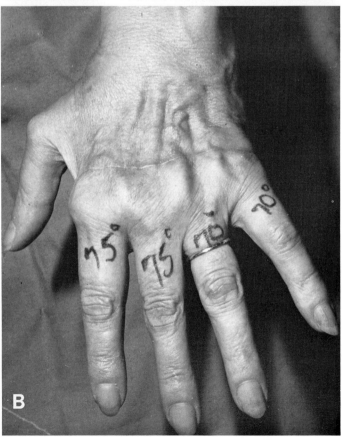

FIG. 34-2. (*A*) Preoperative view indicates the degree of extension and illustrates ulnar deviation. (*B*) Appearance at follow-up 2 years later, showing extension: the numbers on the fingers indicate ranges of flexion. (*C*) Appearance at follow-up at 5 years shows some loss of extension and slight recurrence of ulnar drift.

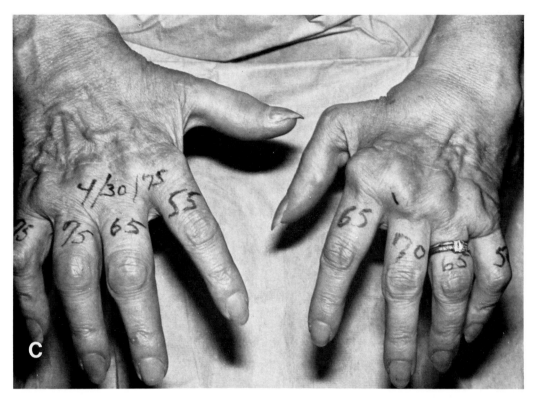

FIG. 34-2. (*Continued*)

resection and insertion of a thin layer of silicone, with or without a stem. In the second there is removal of the entire trapezium and insertion of a trapezium replacement with a stem.

In the first category the problem of subluxation is a factor if careful capsular and tendon reconstruction is not carried out. The presence of a hyperextension deformity of the metacarpophalangeal joint and an adduction-flexion deformity of the first metacarpal will contribute to subluxation and deformity. These must be corrected.

The most common complication of complete trapezial replacement is subluxation or dislocation (Fig. 34-3). In certain cases, chronic subluxation may lead to fracture of the stem of the implant. Once subluxation occurs, it will probably not be correctable by nonsurgical means. Minor degrees of subluxation and instability are usually asymptomatic and will be tolerated by the patient.

The technique of total implant surgery has been modified to ensure greater implant stability. If the implant is not stable at the completion of surgery, postoperative immobilization is unlikely to produce stability. This type of arthroplasty must be immobilized longer than others, and internal fixation with Kirschner wires in addition to casting may be indicated.

The role of the hyperextended metacarpophalangeal joint and the adducted flexed first metacarpal must again be emphasized as contributing to recurrent subluxation of the total trapezial replacement. Infected implants require adequate local treatment. In severe cases the implant should be removed, thereby converting the arthroplasty to a resection arthroplasty.

CONCLUSIONS

Arthroplasty of the hand has been broadened somewhat with the introduction

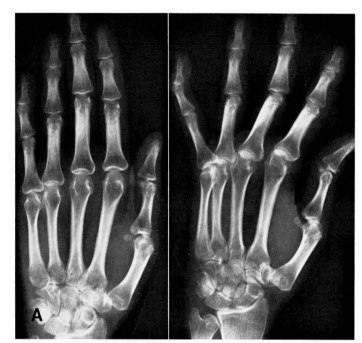

FIG. 34-3. (*A*) Preoperative roentgenogram shows dislocation of the metacarpotrapezial joint. (*B*) Early postoperative view shows the implant in place. (*C*) The implant dislocated approximately 8 weeks after immobilization was removed. (*D*) Complete dislocation of the implant occurred in spite of ligamentous reconstruction, tendon transplant, Kirschner wire fixation, and cast fixation for 6 weeks.

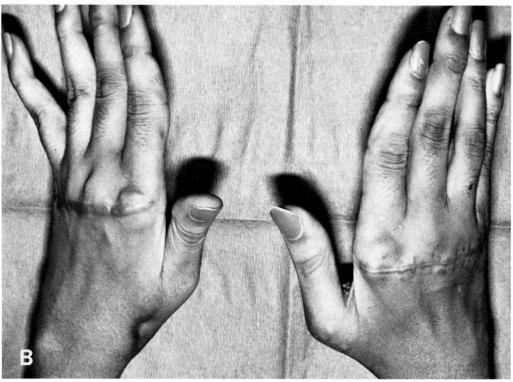

of newer interposition materials. Surgeons who have not had experience with the early types of resection arthroplasties in all of the joints in which interposition materials may now be used are not as likely to be familiar with the meticulous techniques that

FIG. 34-3. (*Continued*)

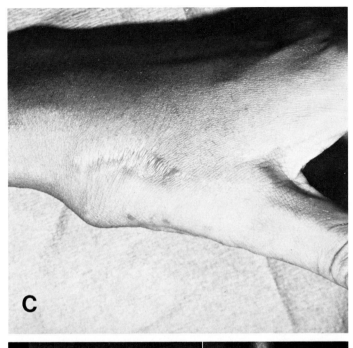

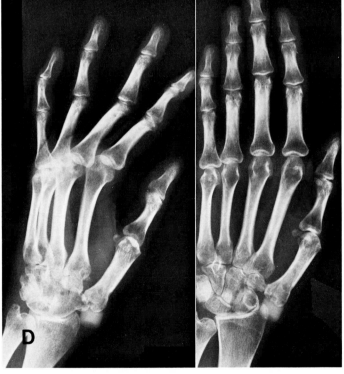

were required to achieve success in the pre-implant days. Insertion of implants is simple. A successful surgical result is difficult, however, and requires meticulous surgical technique built around a thorough understanding of the pathophysiology and pathologic anatomy of the deformity to be corrected. If such care is given to the deformed joint, the complications can be kept at a predictably low level and, when recognized, can be treated with minimal compromise of the end result.

REFERENCES

1. Aptekar, R.G. et al.: Metacarpophalangeal joint surgery in rheumatoid arthritis: Long-term results. Clin. Orthop., 83:123, 1972.
2. Beckenbaugh, R.D., Linscheid, R.L., Dobyns, J.H., and Bryan, R.S.: Review and analysis of 532 Silastic MP implants. J. Bone Joint Surg., 57A:724, 1975.
3. Bolton, N.: Arthroplasty of the metacarpophalangeal joints. Hand, 3:131, 1971.
4. Burton, R.I.: Implant arthroplasty in the hand: An introduction. Orthop. Clin. North Am., 4:313, 1973.
5. Flatt, A.E.: The Care of the Rheumatoid Hand, 2nd ed. St. Louis, C.V. Mosby, 1968.
6. ———: Studies in finger joint replacement: A review of the present position. Arch. Surg., 107: 437, 1973.
7. Goldner, J.L. et al.: The clinical experience with silicone–dacron metacarpophalangeal and interphalangeal joint prostheses. J. Biomed. Mater. Res., 7:137, 1973.
8. Griffiths, R.W., and Nicolle, F.V.: Three years' experience of metacarpophalangeal joint replacement in the rheumatoid hand. Hand, 7:275, 1975.
9. Gschwend, N.: Comparison of results obtained by excisional arthroplasty and silicone rubber prostheses. Ann. Rheum. Dis., 28[Suppl.]:104, 1969.
10. Harrison, S.H.: The proximal interphalangeal joint in rheumatoid arthritis. Hand, 3:125, 1971.
11. Heuston, J.T. et al.: The role of the intrinsic muscles in the production of metacarpophalangeal

subluxation in the rheumatoid hand. Plast. Reconstr. Surg., 52:342, 1973.
12. Kessler, I.J.: Silicone arthroplasty of the trapezio-metacarpal joint. J. Bone Joint Surg., 55B:285, 1973.
13. Millender, L.H., Nalebuff, E.A., Hawkins, R.B., and Ennis, R.: Infection after silicone prosthetic arthroplasty in the hand. J. Bone Joint Surg., 57A: 825, 1975.
14. Millender, L.H. et al.: Metacarpophalangeal joint arthroplasty utilizing the silicone rubber prosthesis. Orthop. Clin. North Am., 4:349, 1973.
15. Nalebuff, E.A.: Present status of rheumatoid hand surgery. Am. J. Surg., 122:304, 1971.
16. Page, D. et al.: A study of the wear resistance of a prosthesis for the metacarpophalangeal joint of the thumb. Clin. Orthop., 100:301, 1974.
17. Swanson, A.B.: Finger joint replacement by silicone rubber implants and the concept of implant fixation by encapsulation. Ann. Rheum. Dis., 28[Suppl.]: 47, 1969.
18. ———: Arthroplasty in traumatic arthritis of the joints of the hand. Orthop. Clin. North Am., 1: 285, 1970.
19. ———: Disabling arthritis at the base of the thumb: Treatment by resection of the trapezium and flexible (silicone) implant arthroplasty. J. Bone Joint Surg., 54A:456, 1972.
20. ———: Flexible implant arthroplasty for arthritic finger joints: Rationale, technique, and results of treatment. J. Bone Joint Surg., 54A:435, 1972.
21. ———: Flexible implant resection arthroplasty. Hand, 4:119, 1972.
22. ———: Flexible Implant Resection Arthroplasty in the Hand and Extremities. St. Louis, C.V. Mosby, 1973.
23. ———: Implant resection arthroplasty of the proximal interphalangeal joint. Orthop. Clin. North Am., 4:1007, 1973.
24. Urbaniak, J.R.: Prosthetic arthroplasty of the hand. Clin. Orthop., 104:9, 1974.
25. Vaughn-Jackson, O.J.: Excisional arthroplasty. Ann. Rheum. Dis., 38[Suppl.]:43, 1969.
26. Wilson, J.N.: Arthroplasty of the trapezio-metacarpal joint. Plast. Reconstr. Surg., 49:143, 1972.

35 Complications of Arthroplasty and Total Joint Replacement in the Hip

ARNOLD D. SCHELLER, RODERICK H. TURNER,
AND J. DRENNAN LOWELL

HISTORICAL OBSERVATIONS

In Philadelphia in 1825, John Rhea Barton created an artificial hip joint in the intertrochanteric area of a 21-year-old sailor who had developed ankylosis of the hip in a poor functional position secondary to injury.[4,135] In describing the procedure "to a large medical class and many respectable physicians assembled," he made the following comment: "I wish it to be distinctly understood that a submission to my contemplated plans had not been urged upon my patient by any false or delusory promises; but that an explanation of his existing condition, and of the means proposed to be attempted for his relief, was fully made to him, in language adapted to his right comprehension of the matter." He then went on to describe the technique of his operation and its requirements for success. At the conclusion of his remarks, he made another comment on the indications for surgery that is as sage today as it was at the time it was made: ". . . where the deformity or inconvenience is such as will induce the patient to endure the pain and incur the risks of an operation."

Barton was describing the first arthroplasty to have been done in the United States. The arthroplasty antedated anesthesia, antiseptic and aseptic surgery, antibiotics, blood replacement, and many other important adjuncts to surgery that we take for granted. Yet the conclusions he drew and the advice he gave to his patient are no different from the approach each of us should be taking as we plan surgical relief of distress in our own patients today.

Total hip arthroplasty has met with such success that few, if any, of us would elect to return to earlier methods of management of the painful hip. Ring, McKee, Charnley, Aufranc, and others who have followed the path they created have reported success rates in total joint reconstruction well in excess of 90%, and this rate of success continues to inch up, based on the continued contributions of these pioneers and their followers.[30,31,34,56,100,116,122,139,163] There is, however, a debit side to the ledger, and it is with this that we propose to deal in this chapter. Complications may be minor and inconsequential or catastrophic and life threatening; immediate or delayed; local and related to the operated hip, at some distance from the operative site, or general and of concern to the patient's well-being as a whole, or of such nature as might occur with any procedure of comparative magnitude.

A review of the current literature on total hip arthroplasty reveals a few specific complications to have been reported by almost all authors: death, infection, dislocation, subluxation, trochanteric problems, metaplastic ossification, phlebitis, embolism, wear, loosening, and stem failure. The reported incidence of each varies; ranges are listed in Table 35-1.

Some of the complications are related to the general medical condition of the patients with whom we deal, others to the technical aspects of the surgery, and others to the devices and materials available. Some are within our control, and others are not.

In looking at these problems in detail, it would be good to consider first the patient

Table 35-1. Reported Incidence of Complications Following Hip Arthroplasty

COMPLICATION	INCIDENCE RANGE
Death	0–2%
Dislocation	0–5%
Subluxation	0–3%
Trochatneric problems	0–3%
Myositis ossificans	3–67%
Phlebitis	10–60%
Pulmonary embolism	0–5%
Loosening	1–67%
Stem failure	0–1%
Infection	0.3–11%
Wear (≤1.5 mm in 10 yr)	86%

population that presents for total hip arthroplasty, for, in a review of the first 131 patients presenting at the Peter Bent Brigham Hospital for total hip arthroplasty and seen by Koide and co-workers,[97] only 20% were considered to be otherwise normal, healthy persons. Eighty percent had either mild or severe systemic disease that limited their activities but was not totally incapacitating. The most common problems were cardiovascular and pulmonary; 40% were hypertensive, 33% showed various ECG abnormalities, and 16% showed old coronary artery disease or ECG changes. Others had congestive heart failure or valvular disease under treatment or had chronic obstructive pulmonary disease diagnosed by x-ray or pulmonary function testing. Half of the patients were over the age of 60, and 87% were over the age of 50 years.

It is essential that patients hospitalized for total hip arthroplasty be given a thorough medical workup in advance of their surgery, if we are to avoid postoperative cardiac or pulmonary problems. It is our practice to admit patients to the hospital 2 days in advance of surgery and have them seen by an internist who is in the hospital regularly, so that he can be familiar with their overall condition and make appropriate recommendations in advance of the procedure. Every effort is made to obtain outside medical information about these patients in advance of their admission and to have this

available for the examining internist. Only by doing so can we hope to return them to their regular practitioners in as good a state as we originally found them.

The complications arising in association with total hip arthroplasty may conveniently be divided into three general categories: intraoperative, postoperative, and late. At the beginning of each section of this chapter, under each of the general headings, are listed those specific problems that have been reported in the orthopaedic literature, have occurred in the cumulative experience of the Brigham and Women's Hospital and at the New England Baptist Hospital, or have been brought to our attention from outside our institutions.

INTRAOPERATIVE COMPLICATIONS

Cardiovascular Complications

Adverse cardiovascular effects associated with the use of bone cement have been reported by many authors, and a transient drop in blood pressure at the time of insertion of the acetabular or femoral component (particularly the latter) is a common experience. This is usually benign and shows prompt, spontaneous reversal. More dramatic—and sometimes catastrophic and not reversible—is cardiac arrest.

A number of studies have been undertaken to determine the mechanism of these effects, with varying conclusions. Ellis and Mulvein concluded that these effects were entirely due to the monomeric methylmethacrylate, based on a series of studies with anesthetized dogs.[58] Breed, on the other hand, blamed the effects on the mechanical embolization of fat and marrow elements as the cause of both hypotension and death, based on studies done on anesthetized rabbits.[12] It is of interest that he could produce the same lowering of blood pressure by forceful injection of methylmethacrylate or bone wax with finger pressure into the femoral canal of these animals, and he was able to demonstrate both fat and marrow embolized to the lungs in postmortem specimens. In this same series of experiments, he noted that as little as 5 ml of saline solution injected rapidly into the femoral canal of a rabbit could completely clear the canal of fat and marrow elements and produce instant death. Once again, the marrow elements were identified in the lungs postmortem.

Tronzo and colleagues looked at the problem in human subjects undergoing total joint replacement and measured the elevation of intramedullary pressure when methylmethacrylate and the femoral component were inserted in total hip arthroplasty.[171] From baseline pressures measured through drill holes in the supracondylar area of the femur, elevations to a level of 300 torr were noted during packing and insertion. These pressures are on the same order of magnitude as those found by Breed in his laboratory experiments.[12] It was Tronzo's conclusion that venting distal to the area of cement insertion was desirable, but it was found that plastic vent tubes inserted from above did not produce satisfactory pressure reduction. Others feel that the problem is a more complex one and include the possible roles of hypovolemia reflex vasodilatory reaction to the heat produced in the curing of the cement, chemical interaction between methylmethacrylate and the anesthetic used, the use of beta-adrenergic blocking agents, and inadequate oxygenation.[97] Until there is better understanding of the causative mechanisms, there seems to be general agreement that prior to insertion of cement, there should be adequate volume replacement, the patient should be well oxygenated, and (because the fall in blood pressure is rapid) there should be close observation of vital signs during and immediately after the cementing.

Markolf and Amstutz and Harris advocate plugging the femoral canal just distal to the tip of the stem of the femoral component before inserting the cement, as an effective means of increasing pressure and improving fixation of the component.[81,109] This appears to have the added benefit of eliminating the pressure below the plug normally seen at the time of femoral cementing. This should also ameliorate the potential problems of fat and marrow embolization.

Biomechanical Complications

As an element in planning the surgical steps to be carried out in the performance of total hip arthroplasty, consideration must be given to the altered biomechanics of the joint occasioned by the presenting problem and its correction. It is the consideration of these factors that makes the proper total hip procedure a reconstruction rather than a replacement. If a normal person stands on one leg and with the pelvis in equilibrium, the abductor muscles must balance the weight of the body about a center of motion within the hip joint. The lever arms through which these forces act are in a ratio of 1:2 in a normal person, and the load across the joint will be the sum of these two forces (Fig. 35-1). A common finding in degenerative hip disease is medial buildup of bone in the base of the acetabulum, resulting in lateral translation of femoral head and lengthening of the lever arm through which the body weight acts. At the same time, progressive external rotation contracture may reduce the length of the lever arm for the abductors so that the ratio of the length of the lever arm may increase to as much as 3:1 or 4:1, as noted by Charnley (Fig. 35-2).[26] Restoration of more nearly normal joint forces must include medialization of the acetabulum, as advocated by Charnley, Greenwald and Nelson, and Denham; and Charnley and Greenwald and Nelson recommend lateralization of the trochanter as well.[26,49,78] Improvement of the ratio of the lever arm reduces joint force, reduces the power that must be developed by the abductors to walk with a normal gait, and should reduce component wear.

If the acetabulum should be medialized to improve the abductor force, at the same time it should not be medialized too much. Excessive medialization may follow reconstruction in patients whose initial problem is rheumatoid arthritis, ankylosing spondylitis, old congenital dislocation of the hip, or old central fracture-dislocation. As noted by Welch and Charnley, excessive reaming of the medial wall or perforation of the medial wall in the patient with rheumatoid arthritis may predispose, ultimately, to central migration and central dislocation of the acetabular component.[179] This has been observed by MacNab in a patient with rheumatoid disease (Fig. 35-3). Similar admonitions for caution have been written by Harris in relation to the location of the socket in patients being treated for painful

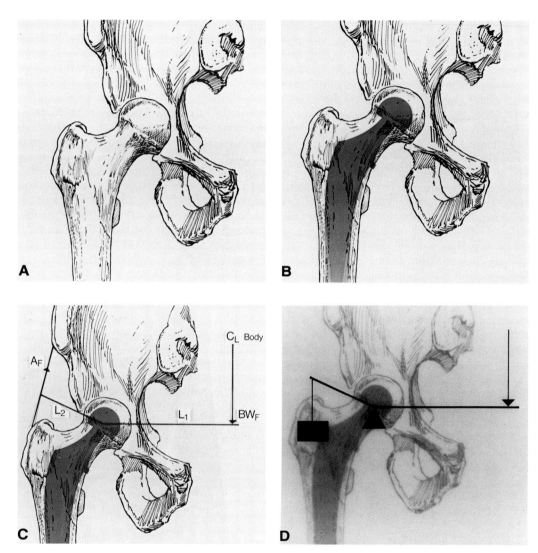

FIG. 35-1. (*A* through *D*) When a normal person stands on one leg with the pelvis in equilibrium, the abductor muscles must balance the weight of the body about a center of motion with the hip joint. The lever arms through which these forces act are in a ratio of 1:2 in a normal person, and the load across the joint is the sum of these two forces.

residuals of congenital dysplasia or dislocation of the hip.[83] Coventry reported medial dislocation of an acetabular component following a fall on the trochanter in a young patient who had had a total hip arthroplasty for a painful hip following central fracture-dislocation.[40] In this instance, no medial bony wall was present a year and a half after injury, and there was inadequate medial support for the cement to withstand the shock of injury. If the

apex of the weight-bearing dome of the acetabulum should be medial to the lateral lip to avoid lateral displacement of the acetabular component, it would also be lateral to any medial lip formed as a result of injury or disease; this medial lip, for practical purposes, can be considered to be at the juncture of the iliopectineal and ilioischial lines on the normal anteroposterior roentgenogram of the pelvis.[94] If the upward and medial thrust of the apex of

FIG. 35-2. Degenerative arthritis of the hip is frequently associated with medial buildup of bone in the depths of the acetabulum, lateral and proximal translation of the femoral head, and fixed external rotation of the proximal femur. These changes lengthen the lever arm through which the center of gravity acts on the femoral head and reduce the lever arm of the abductors. As a result, joint forces are greatly increased if the patient attempts to walk without limping. Proper reconstruction in total hip arthroplasty requires correction of each component deformity if more nearly normal mechanics are to be restored and forces across the joint favorably reduced. (Charnley, J.: Total hip replacement by low-friction arthroplasty. Clin. Orthop., 72: 7, 1970)

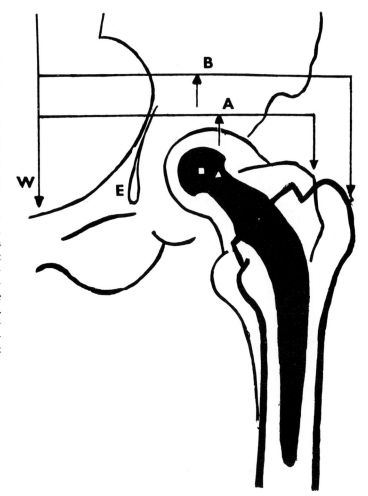

the acetabulum toward the ischium is through the sciatic notch and not through bone, medial migration of the components is more likely.

Penetration of the Medial Acetabular Wall

Deliberate penetration of the medial wall to obtain adequate coverage for the acetabular component should be avoided whenever possible. When working stock is deficient, the bony coverage for the head can be increased by using the resected head of the femur as a lateral lip graft. This can be bisected and shaped to fit the side of the ilium and held in place with bicortical bone screws (Fig. 35-4).

Penetration of the medial wall of the acetabulum, the pubic ramus, or the ischium

is not uncommon. Such penetration may be of minor consequence, the end result being only a small mass of cement seen outside of its usual location on a postoperative roentgenogram, or it may be instantly catastrophic, producing massive hemorrhage with injury to the internal iliac artery or vein, or both, as reported by Mallory.[107] Hemorrhage will be rapid, and immediate abdominal exploration and ligation of the bleeding vessel or vessels are mandatory for the survival of the patient (Fig. 35-5). Lesser holes in the medial pelvic wall may lead to interference with normal muscle function, if the herniation of cement that follows intrudes on normal gliding mechanisms, or, as Lowell and Davies reported, there may be late occurrence of a bladder fistula and joint sepsis, ultimately necessi-

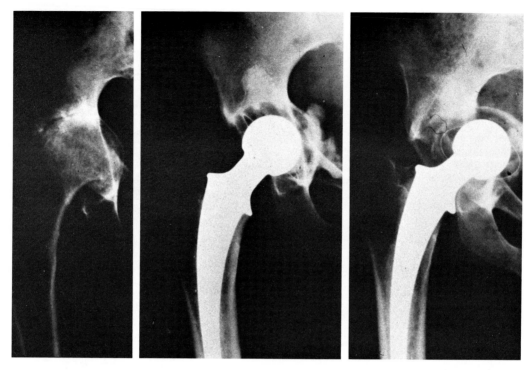

FIG. 35-3. Excessive medial translation of the acetabulum in this patient contributed to further spontaneous medial migration of the acetabular component and ultimate central dislocation. The apex of the weight-bearing dome of the acetabulum should be well supported by the bony roof of the acetabulum so that upward forces are directed toward the sacroiliac joint and not toward the sciatic notch. (Courtesy of Ian MacNab, M.D.)

tating removal of the total hip components (Fig. 35-6).[106]

If one visualizes a coronal section of the pelvis through the dome of the acetabulum, it is evident when the acetabulum is in its normal location that the bone in the region of the dome is thick, but medially the inner wall is thin, and the margin for error is limited (Fig. 35-7).[104] When the acetabulum is reamed to the depths of the old acetabular notch in preparation for insertion of the acetabular component, the biomechanics of hip function are improved, but the distance between the depths of the acetabulum and the interior of the true pelvis becomes small indeed. The internal iliac vessels lie just above and medial to this wall, in a groove between the iliac muscle and the internal obturator, and are not protected from a penetrating reamer by a layer of muscle.[107] Recognition of these anatomical relationships is particularly important in reconstruction of the hip in a patient who already

has medial translation of the acetabulum secondary to disease, injury, previous mold arthroplasty, or medial migration of the femoral prosthesis.

Identification of the medial surface of the pubic ramus may be easy or difficult. If one elects to make one of the anchoring holes for cement in the pubic ramus, the location for the beginning of this hole may be identified in most patients by a blush in the cancellous bone just anterior to the acetabular notch. Cautious curettage of this area usually leads the curette down the proper path in the direction of the pubic ramus. Problems arise, however, when the total hip arthroplasty is a revision procedure and the anatomical landmarks are altered. In such instances, it may be good to dissect around the anterior lip of the acetabulum and up, underneath the iliopsoas, so that the pubic ramus may be visualized directly and palpated. Scarring in the region of previous surgery may make this difficult.

Palpation of the ischium below and behind the posterior lip of the acetabulum—in planning the posterior-inferior anchoring hole—is rarely a problem.

Malposition of the Acetabular Component

The ideal position of the acetabular component varies with the device chosen. Ideally, the Charnley acetabular component is placed in 45° valgus, 0° to 5° anteversion, and 0° retroversion. The Charnley-Muller, Aufranc-Turner, and other 30-mm- and 32-mm-diameter components are designed for placement in 30° valgus but may be placed in up to 45° valgus and anteverted 5° to 15°. The Charnley acetabular component should be placed precisely as recommended by its designer, for modest variations may lead to instability, subluxation, or dislocation. The new Charnley socket design, with a long posterior wall, may help eliminate some of the problems of posterior instability, particularly when there have been minor degrees of variation from the planned positioning.

The larger-sized Charnley-Muller and Aufranc-Turner acetabular components seem to be more forgiving of minor or modest variations in socket placement, but no matter what device is chosen, retroversion in any degree is unacceptable if posterior instability is to be avoided (Fig. 35-8).[24] When this position is found at surgery, the component should be changed. At least 30° anteversion appears to be acceptable, but if the socket is placed in further anteversion and there is anterior instability when the hip is extended and rotated laterally, again, the socket should be changed.

Changing the socket should not be difficult, and the surgeon has two options (Fig. 35-9). If the pelvic wall is of normal thickness, the curved gouge of the Smith-Petersen type can be passed along the prosthesis–cement interface beginning at several locations along the periphery of the socket and working toward the apex; following this, the socket can gradually be pried loose from the ilium. We caution the surgeon in using this technique to remove acetabular components. Not infrequently, iatrogenic fracture of the osseous socket occurs. Acetabular fracture decreases the integrity of the final component fixation. We recommend that the surgeon cut the polyethylene component into pie-shaped sections with either an osteotomy or a Midas Rex cutting instrument. Each of these should be pried toward the center of the acetabulum until enough sections have been generated to allow the remaining portion to fall out. This technique is extremely useful in revision arthroplasty or in any situation in which the ilium is thin. The lugs of cement of the ilium, ischium, and pubis can usually be removed easily with a curette or small gouges. The acetabular component can then be cemented into the proper position after preparation of the acetabular bed.

Excessive varus angulation should be avoided (Fig. 35-10) to prevent impingement of the neck or trochanter against the lateral lip of the acetabular component, which limits abduction and causes impact loosening. Excessive valgus angulation (Fig. 35-11) leads to instability when the hip is adducted. In each situation, correction should be carried out.

If trochanteric osteotomy is not carried out and the approach is posterior, the error of positioning is often one of retroversion. If an anterior or anterolateral approach is used and a trochanteric osteotomy is not performed, the error of positioning is one of anteversion.

The surgeon should be particularly conscious of the hazards of malpositioning the acetabular components when dealing with old posterior fractures of the acetabulum with imperfect reduction of fracture fragments. When sufficient time has followed the injury to allow for remodeling of the fracture surfaces, the still posterior and medial translation of the posterior lip fragments may not be immediately evident. If this displaced lip is used as a guide for placement of the acetabular component, it will easily lead the surgeon to misplace the socket in retroversion (Fig. 35-12). In these cases, particularly, the stability of the hip should be tested in all positions before the wound is closed.

Malposition of the Femoral Component

Malposition of the femoral component is another cause of postoperative instability, as well as a source of variation from the

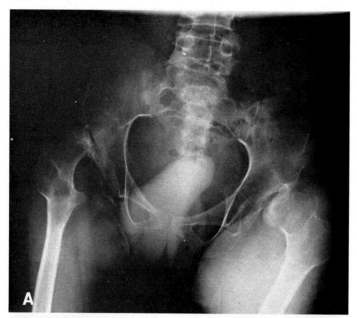

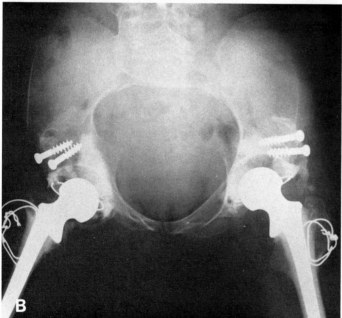

Fig. 35-4. Deficient stock on the iliac side of the joint secondary to an old congenital dislocation may make it difficult to obtain adequate coverage of the acetabular component. (*A*) The thickness of the acetabular dome may be increased by fixing a portion of the femoral head to this side of the ilium with screws or bolts (*B, C*). In this instance, fair but tenuous fixation was obtained with iliac fixation alone. The graft is expected to supply long-term support when it has healed and become revascularized. In the interim, the patient's hips are protected by crutch support.

expected arc of motion, particularly internal and external rotation. The Charnley component should be placed in neutral with regard to anteversion and retroversion; any significant variation from this may lead to instability. Components with larger heads, such as the Muller and the Aufranc-Turner, may be placed in neutral or preferably in 10° to 15° anteversion. Whether the tro-

chanter is removed as part of the surgical approach or not, if rotatory malposition is to be avoided, the position of the knee and the path of its flexion-extension arc must be carefully assessed at the time of femoral reaming and of placement of the components. The posterior approach without trochanteric osteotomy can lead to retroversion of the femoral component, and the anterior

FIG. 35-4. (*Continued*)

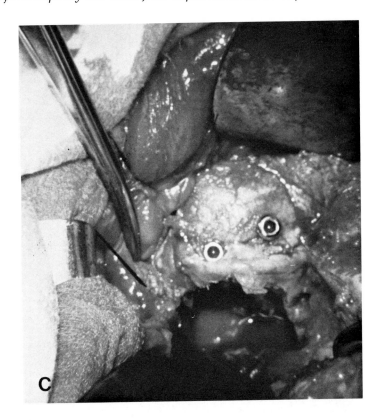

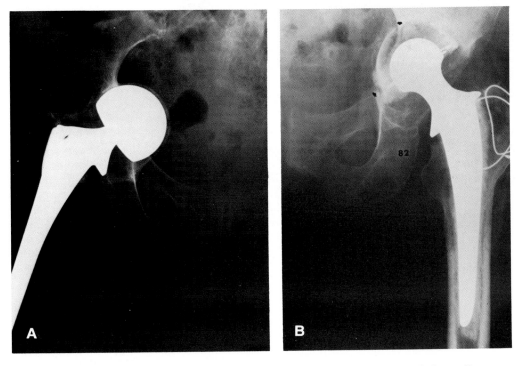

FIG. 35-5. (*A* and *B*) Varying degrees of penetration of the medial acetabular wall.

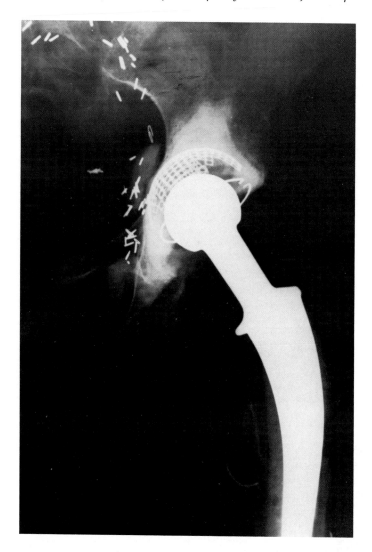

FIG. 35-6. Medial wall penetration that caused intrapelvic hemorrhage, necessitating retroperitoneal exposure for control of the bleeding.

and anterolateral approaches can lead to anteversion, just as occurs with positioning of the acetabular component. While the cement is hardening, it is particularly important that the assistant not allow the limb to rotate in such a manner that the femoral head is pressed against the acetabular margin and rotated out of planned position. A retroverted femoral head should be removed and replaced. Up to 30° anteversion may be tolerated, and the position may be stable, but it will affect the ultimate location of the arc of rotation. Careful testing on the table prior to wound closure should help determine the static stability of the hip.

Varus malposition of the femoral component is increasingly recognized as a threat to the durability of the reconstruction and may lead to component loosening with breakdown of the medial buttress of cement, stem failure, or both (Fig. 35-13). Measures should be taken to avoid malposition at the time of prosthesis placement, and it should be corrected when recognized.

Intraoperative Femoral Shaft Fracture

The incidence of intraoperative fractures ranges between 0.4% and 3%, depending on the report.[167] The cause of these fractures is related to the quality of the bone and

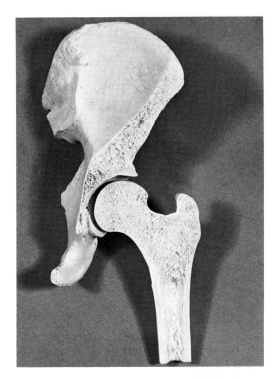

FIG. 35-7. The acetabular dome, as seen in this coronal section of the pelvis, is thick and strong if the acetabulum is in its normal location. Any degree of proximal displacement of the acetabulum secondary to disease or developmental anomaly leads to a rapid decrease in bony structure available for support of the acetabular component.

the handling of the femur during arthroplasty. Fractures were noted to occur at different stages of the operation. These stages are, in order of increasing frequency: (1) dislocation of the hip, (2) seating of the new femoral component, (3) reaming of the proximal femur, and (4) removal of the already-present methylmethacrylate. During removal of the methylmethacrylate, the femur appears to be at its highest risk for fracture. Johanssen and co-workers noted that 50% of the fractures in their series occurred during this stage of the operation.[91]

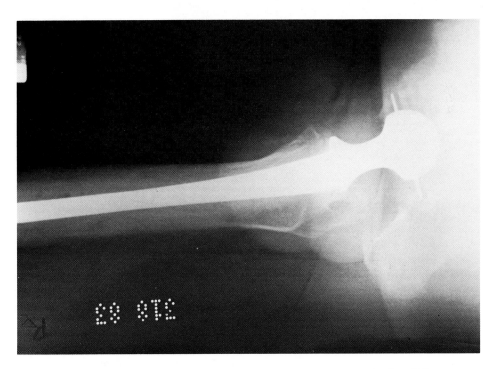

FIG. 35-8. Retroverted acetabular components increase posterior instability.

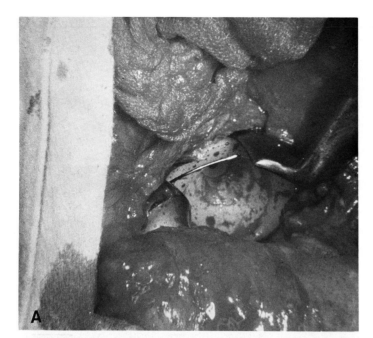

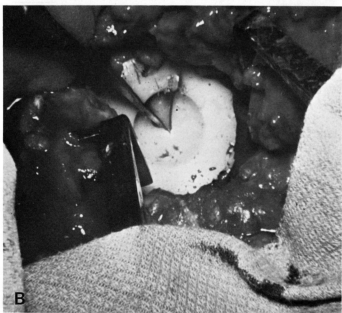

FIG. 35-9. (*A*) Socket removal presents a problem if the ilium is thin and working stock deficient. In most instances a Smith-Petersen acetabular gouge can be passed safely between the cement and bone in several locations, allowing the socket to be pried loose. (*B*) Where bone stock is limited, the acetabular component may easily be cut into pie-shaped pieces with an osteotome or power instruments; then each piece can be tipped forward in succession until the remaining portion is free.

The location of these fractures is primarily proximal, with the fracture usually at the tip of the femoral component. Scott and associates had 88% of their fractures in the proximal third,[155] whereas Johanssen and colleagues had 90% of their fractures in the proximal third; of these, 75% occurred at the tip of the prosthesis.[91]

Factors that put the patient at risk for intraoperative fracture are consistent in the two larger series. Previous surgery is the most common, followed by femoral bone defects (*i.e.*, cortical windows or defects from previous internal fixation), and osteoporosis was especially noted in patients with rheumatoid arthritis. All 22 patients

FIG. 35-10. Excessive varus angulation of the cup can cause trochanteric impingement.

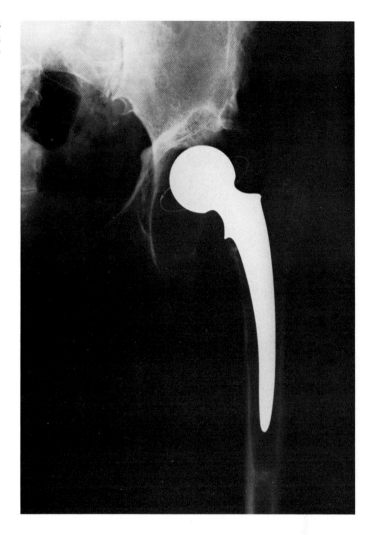

in the series of Johanssen and colleagues had undergone previous surgery (20 patients had previous total hip replacement).[91] In the series by Scott and colleagues, 75% of the 18 patients had had previous surgery.[155] In the series of Taylor and co-workers, 73% of the 11 patients had a failed total hip arthroplasty.[167]

In dealing with a normal-sized femur, splitting of the proximal portion at the time of preparation for insertion of the femoral component is unlikely. The situation is entirely different when the proximal femur is undersized, as in a congenitally dislocated hip. Whenever congenital anomalies are present in the proximal femur, appropriate measuring roentgenograms should be taken to ensure that the appropriate size prosthesis will be available at the time of surgery (Fig. 35-14). The line of planned resection must be marked on the measuring film so that the location of the transverse shaft diameters that determine the width of the prosthetic stem can be measured. A lateral film is also advisable to assess anterior curve in the area of concern. Templates for making these measurements are available from most prosthesis manufacturers, and if stems of appropriate size are not available, custom prostheses can be manufactured. Templates do not always give an accurate assessment of the dimensions of the lateral medullary canal. Fortunately, as noted by Dunn, the diameter of the medullary canal is always

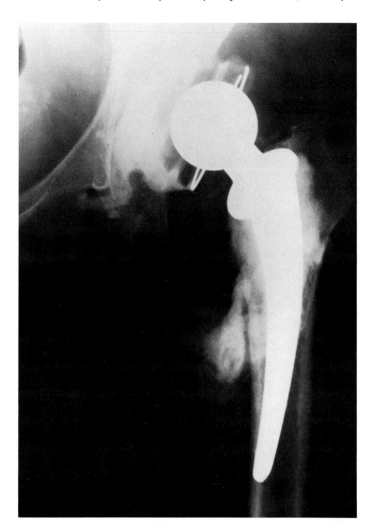

FIG. 35-11. Excessive valgus angulation increases instability with adduction.

less in the coronal plane than in the sagittal plane, so anteroposterior roentgenograms for purposes of measurement are reliable in determining internal shaft diameters, except when the diameter has been altered by previous surgery or fracture.[10]

The goal of treatment is recognition of the fracture, adequate internal fixation with fracture healing, and a functional hip arthroplasty. If the proximal shaft is split minimally, it may be reconstructed with circlage wires at the time of arthroplasty. Caution must be exercised to avoid extrusion of cement into the soft tissues, to remove any extravasating cement, and to bone-graft the defects. Methods of treatment for these proximal fractures have been multiple.

Various authors have detailed the results using traction, circlage wiring around a standard component, and the use of long-stem femoral components with and without additional internal fixation. The success of the modes is outlined in Table 35-2. Traction was used but once. The data suggest that the use of long-stem femoral components with or without circlage fixation and bone grafting is the method of choice. Although fracture healing will usually occur with the other methods outlined, the long-term incidence of component loosening is minimized with the use of long-stem femoral components and bone grafting. In the series by Scott and associates, there was a 33% failure rate secondary to loosening of the

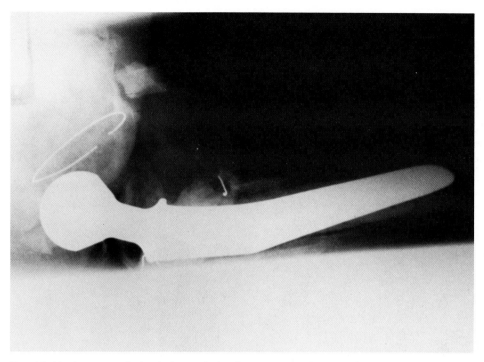

FIG. 35-12. A previously healed acetabular fracture with displaced acetabular margins can lead the surgeon to misplace the socket.

femoral component in the 12 proximal fractures when the long-stem components were not used. When a long-stem femoral component was used in four cases, there was healing in all four fractures and no evidence of loosening. Additional circlage fixation had been used in two of these four cases. Johanssen and co-workers found that if a long-stem femoral component was used with internal fixation, healing occurred uniformly with no evidence of loosening in most cases. In contrast, when they used a long-stem femoral component *without* additional internal fixation, only two of the five cases healed without loosening. Of the three remaining, two became symptomatic with loosening, and one had a nonunion.

Prevention is the key to success in these fractures. Proper preoperative planning, wide exposure, cautious cement removal, avoidance of cortical windows, and the use of biplane fluoroscopy to monitor cement removal aid in preventing intraoperative fractures of the femur. If intraoperative fracture occurs, the fracture should be

reduced anatomically and splinted with a longer-stem femoral component. After component insertion, the fracture site should be inspected, extravasated cement removed, and the fracture site autogenously bone-grafted.

Protrusion of the Stem of the Femoral Component

Protrusion of the stem of the femoral component—medially, laterally, posteriorly, or anteriorly—has been observed (Fig. 35-15). The most common type of stem protrusion is lateral protrusion. This frequently occurs during the conversion of a previous fracture of the proximal femur to a total hip replacement (Fig. 35-16). Instead of passing down the femoral shaft, the femoral component follows an old nail hole from the previous nailing. The abnormal varus orientation of the neck of the prosthesis that results should signify to the surgeon that this problem is present. While one is preparing the femoral shaft, particularly when there has been a previous nailing or

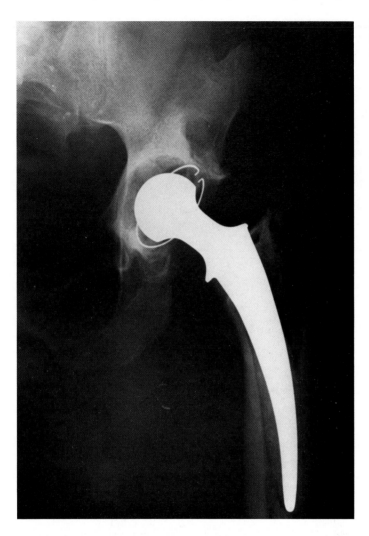

FIG. 35-13. Varus positioning increases the rate of femoral component loosening.

osteotomy, the tapered rasp designed by Charnley is useful because the rasp length readily determines whether the hole pre- pared for the seat of the femoral stem is truly within the axis of the femoral shaft or outside of it.

Table 35-2. Treatment Success of Intraoperative Fractures of the Proximal Third of the Femur

	SUCCESS RATE	
TREATMENT	SCOTT ET AL.	JOHANSSEN ET AL.
Traction	0/1(0%)	Not reported
Short-stem prosthesis insertion		
With fixation	4/7(64%)	2/6(33%)
Without fixation	3/4(75%)	Not reported
Long-stem prosthesis insertion		
With fixation	2/2(100%)	7/8(88%)
Without fixation	2/2(100%)	2/5(40%)

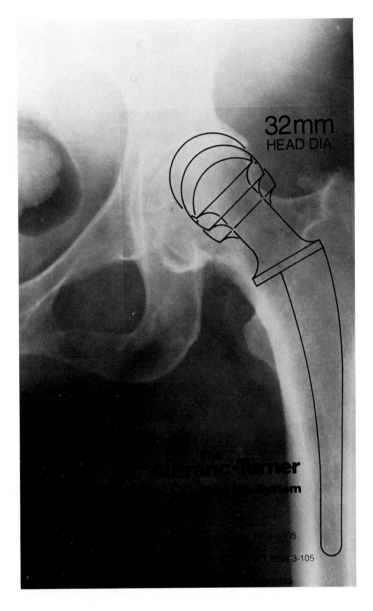

F<small>IG</small>. 35-14. Templates aid in predicting femoral component size and decreasing the incidence of fracture during stem insertion.

Medial stem protrusion usually occurs when the surgeon attempts to place a varus-stemmed prosthesis in valgus (see Fig. 35-15, *A*). Posterior stem protrusion occurs most frequently in patients with excessive femoral anteversion (CHD), or in whom the femoral neck osteotomy is excessively long (Fig. 35-15, *C*). Anterior stem protrusion occurs with the use of longer stem lengths or excessive anterior femoral bows (Fig. 35-15, *B*).

Proper preoperative roentgenographic planning and attention to surgical detail can decrease the incidence of stem protrusion. Correction of stem protrusion is a difficult and time-consuming operation that necessitates drilling-out all of the misplaced cement and repreparing the shaft. In cases of minimal stem protrusion we have utilized a high-speed, pneumatic, metal-cutting drill to shave down the protruded stem and bone-grafted the defect. When the protrusion is extensive, formal revision of the femoral component is necessary. Adequate exposure and lighting are crucial, and the use of special cement instruments, high-

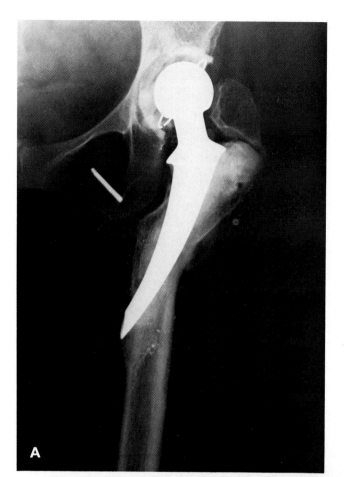

FIG. 35-15. Femoral stem protrusions: *A,* medial; *B,* anterior; *C,* posterior.

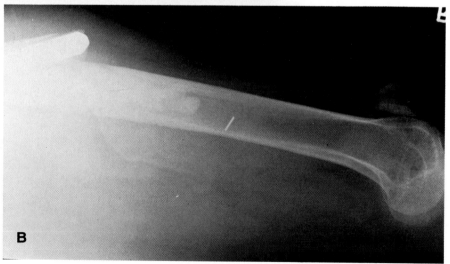

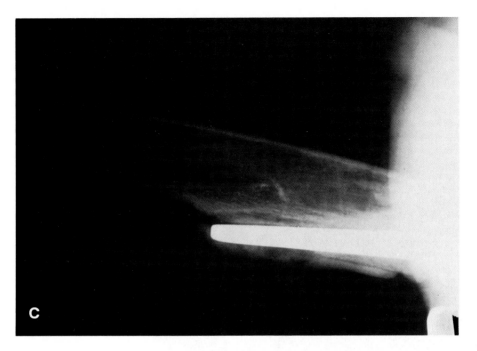

FIG. 35-15. (*Continued*)

speed pneumatic drills, and biplane fluoroscopy are necessary for safe removal of the cement (Fig. 35-17). It is important to bone-graft the femoral defect after insertion of the femoral component into the medullary canal to decrease the incidence of a permanent stress riser.[172] Other patients in whom location of the femoral shaft may be difficult are those with a restricted arc of motion secondary to a disease process and those who have had previous surgery. This may make visualization of the femoral shaft and the use of instruments for preparing the shaft difficult and awkward, and in such circumstances, trochanteric osteotomy can make visualization much simpler.

Cement Debris

Prior to wound closure, careful inspection for and debridement of all fragments of bone, cement, and devitalized tissue should be carried out. Retained cement fragments have been found within the joint and along the margins of the acetabulum and femur, and they can be a source of pain or (with frequent impact loading) can lead to fragmentation and foreign-body reaction or to component loosening (Fig. 35-18). Devitalized bone retained in soft tissue is a good

culture medium and nidus for infection. Hallel and colleagues reported on the extension of polymethylmethacrylate into the knee joint of a patient undergoing total hip arthroplasty for a failed Austin-Moore prosthesis.[80] The long stem of the Moore prosthesis had entered the knee and provided a channel for the cement to follow—an unusual complication but one that is preventable if one realizes the possibility of its occurrence.

Over-lengthening

Over-lengthening of the femur with total hip arthroplasty is a complication seldom reported but occasionally seen. Minor degrees should not produce a problem, but discrepancies of ½ inch or more are often noticed and are a source of patient complaints. It may result from the selection of prostheses with different-length necks in bilateral hip disease; it may occur, as noted by Dunn and Hess, in a reconstruction of a previously dislocated hip, when it was not possible to seat the femoral component low enough in the femoral shaft[53]; but most often it follows difficulty in assessment of the amount of neck to be resected at the time of femoral component placement. A

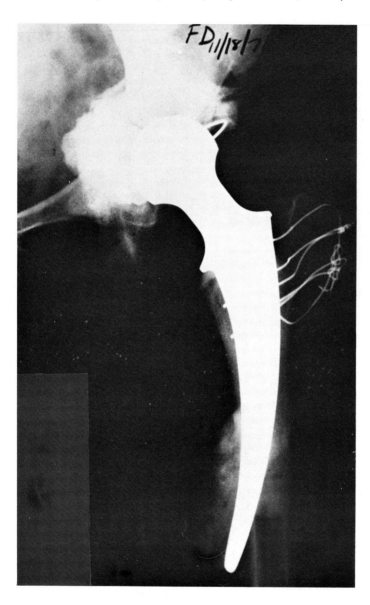

FIG. 35-16. Stem protrusion is difficult to avoid in patients who have rheumatoid arthritis and limited motion, a history of hip nailing, a stiff hip from previous surgery, or a prosthesis that is seated distally. When hip motion is limited, trochanteric osteotomy helps to facilitate identification of the medullary cavity of the shaft, but it is not a substitute for careful assessment of the preoperative films and the prosthesis to be employed.

judgment can be made prior to operation based on the use of templates and tracings on the patient's roentgenograms, but there seems to be no reliable method for checking these measurements during the course of the operative procedure. We have devised some simple jigs to improve our accuracy but find them to be reliable only within about ¼ inch (Fig. 35-19).[105]

Thermal Injury to Bone

The exothermic reaction of polymerizing cement continues to be a concern to ortho-

paedic surgeons and a source of much debate. In looking at this problem, Jeffries and colleagues noted that nonpermanent changes take place in tissue proteins subjected to temperatures of 45°C and that irreversible changes take place between 60°C and 65°C.[90] In spite of this observation, it was their conclusion that the mechanical and vascular injury occurring to bone at the time of acetabular and femoral preparation and the chemical insult to tissue from the monomer are the principal causes of bone cell death. The cement is not the

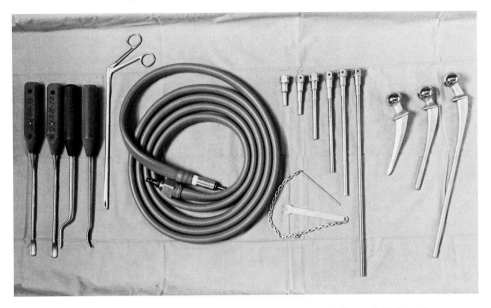

FIG. 35-17. Special cement instruments, high-speed pneumatic drills, and biplane fluoroscopy aid in safe cement removal.

source of damage. Others differ. DiPisa and associates reported the surface temperature on polymerizing polymethylmethacrylate to be 70.4°C and advocated precooling the high-density polyethylene socket with liquid nitrogen.[50] Their published study is based on laboratory experimentation, and they did not report trying this clinically. Whatever the ultimate outcome of this issue, it is fortunate that bone seems to take kindly to the presence of cement, that cement seems to produce little or no foreign-body reaction, and that whatever necrosis does occur is replaced by repair, as noted by Willerty and co-workers.[181] Ideally, in the future a filler or grouting agent will be developed that will produce the desired large area of surface contact between prosthesis and living tissue and no tissue necrosis.

POSTOPERATIVE COMPLICATIONS

Fat Embolism

Fat embolism at the time of femoral component insertion has been reported by a number of authors; Tronzo and associates found some 20 cases in the literature, 13 of which were fatal.[171] This appears to be a mechanical problem associated with increased intramedullary pressure occurring during cementing and component seating. More recently, Spenglar and co-workers have reported on a relatively typical case of fat embolism syndrome simulating that seen after fracture, which occurred some 14 hours after total hip arthroplasty in a 38-year-old woman who was otherwise well.[160] She had symptoms of tachypnea, hypoxemia, and cyanosis, with laboratory findings of a diminished PaO_2, thrombocytopenia, decreased perfusion on lung scan, and alveolar infiltrates on chest roentgenograms. Treated aggressively with nasal oxygen and intravenous corticosteroids, she survived. This represents an isolated report, but others may follow.

Hematoma

Excessive bleeding following total hip arthroplasty was reported in 1% of patients treated at the Mayo Clinic, and six of these 19 patients required reoperation.[41] We have seen it in our own institutions and have drained large hematomas and allowed smaller ones to resorb. Exploration was followed by infection in one patient, ultimately requiring a girdlestone resection. Preventive measures include careful inspection of the wound prior to closure with

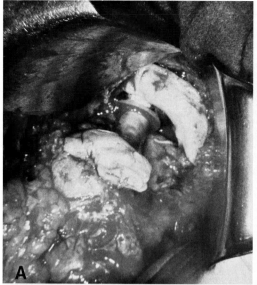

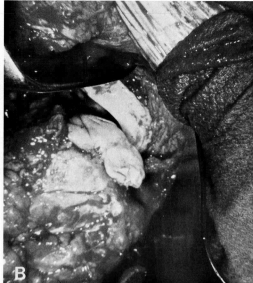

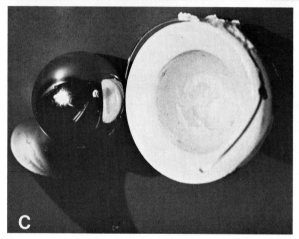

FIG. 35-18. Great care must be taken to avoid leaving adventitious fragments of cement in the wound. In this patient, cement was left on the margins of both the acetabular and femoral components (*A*). These masses came into contact with each other as the hip moved into external rotation. Continued impact loosened the femoral and acetabular components and seeded the synovium with particles of methylmethacrylate (*B*). In another patient, soft cement became entrapped in the acetabular component as the femoral component was placed. The hip never felt right after operation. An arthrogram was negative. Surgical exploration revealed the true nature of the problem (*C*).

correction of all persisting bleeding points, suction drainage for 48 hours after closure, and careful wrapping of the operated leg to include the buttock area with a wide elasticized bandage. This is kept in place for at least 48 to 72 hours. The bandage compresses dead space and helps close small venous bleeders that might otherwise ooze indefinitely. We have found that it produces softer wounds and greater comfort for the patient in the immediate postoperative period.

Recently, Ring and Oppenheim have reported on the arteriographic management of hemorrhage following pelvic trauma in major hip surgery.[131,137,138] With arteriography, bleeding points can be identified and, with almost uniform success, occluded either by embolization of autogenous clot with Gelfoam pellets or by insertion and inflation of a balloon catheter into the offending vessel or one of its tributaries.

Complications of Blood Replacement

Although major reconstructive surgery of the hip would be almost impossible if compatible blood were not available for transfusion, it is well recognized that blood transfusions are not without hazard. There is a 2.2% incidence of recognized hepatitis for each unit of blood given.[39] The safety of homologous transfusion is inversely proportional to the use of professional donors. The more frequent the use of professional donors, the more frequent the problem of hepatitis in the postoperative period. Although careful history taking and Australia antigen testing pick up 25% of the infectious blood, we are currently unable to identify all potentially infectious blood.

There are a number of ways around this problem, including the use of frozen blood, which is expensive ($50–$100 per unit), the use of packed cells and plasmanate, hypotensive anesthesia, acute isovolemic hemodilution, autotransfusion by prebleeding of the patient and storage of the blood in advance of surgery, and intraoperative autologous blood transfusion.[46,98,99,119,170] All of these should be encouraged and used where feasible.

Fortunately, the problem of ABO incompatibility is rare. If 100 ml of incompatible blood is given, the chances of survival are in the 90% range. If 500 ml is given, the chances of survival are in the 10% range.

Intraoperative autologous blood transfusion avoids many of the problems of homologous transfusion. This practice becomes cost-efficient when more than 2 units of blood are lost at surgery, since 62% to 65% of the shed red blood cells are salvaged. We have found this technique particularly useful in patients whose religious beliefs preclude the use of homologous transfusion, during difficult primary arthroplasty, and in most cases of revision arthroplasty.

Thromboembolic Disease

Thromboembolic disease with pulmonary embolism and potential death can be one of the most frightening complications of any surgery about the hip, including total hip arthroplasty. Its incidence and prevention have been eloquently described by Evarts, Harris, Salzman, and Hume.[64,84,85,88,148] There is variation in the published incidence of clinically recognized thromboembolic disease in this country and in Europe, and, consequently, there is great debate over the necessity and advisability

of using the preventive measures currently available, particularly since none are without some hazard. In patients managed without prophylactic anticoagulation, the incidence of fatal pulmonary embolism varies between 0% and 3.4%. In 106 patients given prophylactic warfarin or aspirin, Harris and colleagues recently reported an incidence of nonfatal pulmonary embolism of 0% to 1%.[84] The incidence of thrombophlebitis (based on clinical diagnostic criteria) was reduced from approximately 35% to 7% by prophylactic anticoagulation. The incidence of thrombi identified on venograms was reduced from an expected 56% to 33% by these measures.

It is our practice to use anticoagulant prophylaxis against thromboembolic disease and pulmonary embolism whenever it is not contraindicated by associated medical problems. In patients who have no history of prior thromboembolic disease, aspirin (600 mg twice daily, morning and evening) is given beginning the day after surgery. Where there is a history of thrombophlebitis or thromboembolic disease, warfarin is given in a dose of 10 mg to 15 mg intramuscularly the night after surgery, and then oral doses are begun at 48 hours and regulated in accordance with prothrombin times.[84] It is our preference to keep the prothrombin time of the patient one and one quarter to one and one half times the control value. Using this regime, we have experienced no fatal pulmonary emboli; there are occasional hematomas and occasional phlebitis, but none that was not manageable by simple measures. Based on current literature, at least three agents appear to be effective: warfarin, aspirin, and low-molecular-weight dextran.

When venous thrombosis is suspected postoperatively, physical signs are notoriously unreliable. Plethysmography is reliable if normal, but a phlebogram should be done if less-invasive diagnosis is not available or is not entirely normal. Ventilation/lung scans must be compared immediately with the chest x-ray if embolism is suspected. Pulmonary angiography is occasionally needed to resolve equivocal findings. Blood gas determinations do little to increase the accuracy of diagnosis and

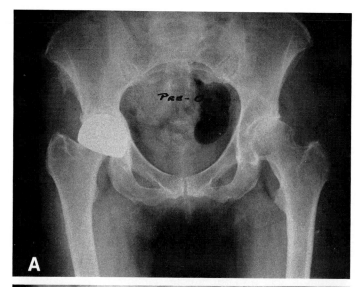

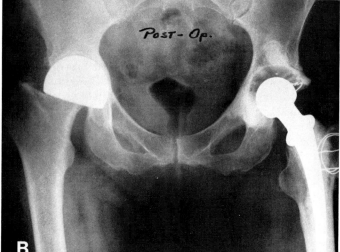

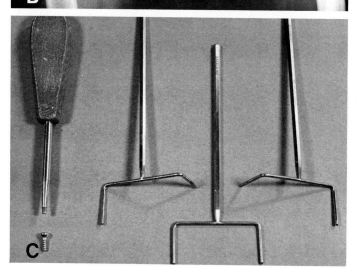

FIG. 35-19. Leg-length changes of moderate degree are a common postoperative finding. Increased length appears to be the most common direction of change. This patient's leg was lengthened ¼ inch by total hip arthroplasty; this created a discrepancy of ¾ inch compared to the opposite side, where an earlier mold arthroplasty had been done (*A* and *B*). A series of measuring devices used in conjunction with a socket–head compression screw were devised to reduce the occurrence of the problem (*C*). With the guide in place, a mark is made with the cutting cautery current on the fascia overlying the vastus lateralis or near the vastus lateralis tubercle at the base of the femoral neck; this provides a point of reference, permitting later comparison when the prosthesis is in place prior to removal of the femoral head (*D* and *E*). The screw is removed after final measurement. (Lowell, JD: Complications of total hip replacement. In The Hip: Proceedings of the Fourth Open Scientific Meeting of The Hip Society. St. Louis, C.V. Mosby, 1976)

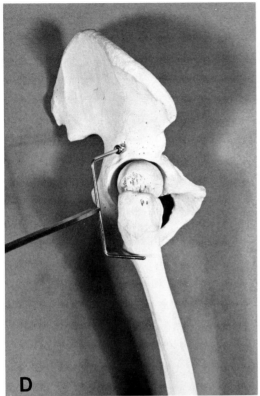
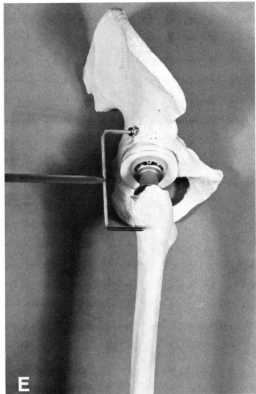

FIG. 35-19. (*Continued*)

should not be a reason to omit an appropriate lung scan. Management includes administration of heparin and warfarin, and in complicated cases venacaval interruption may become obligatory.

Cholecystitis

In a detailed discussion of general surgical complications following major hip surgery, Camer gives particular emphasis to the potentially lethal complication of acute cholecystitis.[20] Over the past 37 years, there have been multiple reports of acute cholecystitis following surgery remote from the biliary system.[76,77,87,96,152,166,169] Other series have indicated that severe trauma may be a causal factor in the development of acute cholecystitis and point out that the mortality rate is high if the disorder is not diagnosed properly.[143,184] We have seen more than 40 instances of acute cholecystitis at the New England Baptist Hospital in the past 16 years. In this period there were approximately 10,000 major joint (hip or knee) arthroplasties performed at this institution. Thirty-six cases of acute cholecystitis followed hip arthroplasty, and four cases followed knee arthroplasty. The overall incidence of acute cholecystitis after major joint replacement is approximately 1 per 250 cases. Camer reported on the first 25 cases, of whom 23 had had emergency surgery.[20] Although there was a wide age range, the incidence of cholecystitis was highest in women over the age of 60. There have been two deaths from gram-negative septicemia associated with gallbladder disease, so the incidence of mortality is approximately 1 per 5000 major arthroplasties.

Cholecystitis is most likely to occur shortly after the resumption of oral intake of food.[20] This may be related to the bile stasis and increased viscosity that occur when the patient is recumbent and not eating. Another possible causal factor is narcotic medication, which is known to increase the tone of the sphincter of Oddi.[20,38,77,152] Diagnosis can usually be suspected on clinical grounds, but more accurate definition of the problem is accomplished by ultrasound and by radionuclide hepatic imiondiacetic acid (HIDA) scanning.[20] Both of these tests are noninvasive and can be performed without disrupting the patient's postoperative hip convalescence. A final decision about cholecystitis must, however, be made on clinical grounds, since these noninvasive tests can occasionally be negative when the patient has acalculous cholecystitis. If surgery is prompt, the chances of gangrene, empyema, and perforation with subsequent biliary peritonitis are minimized. Surgery should be prompt and should be excisional, not simple drainage.[20]

Because of the seriousness of this disease, we recommend that patients who have a history of biliary symptoms have cholecystography and/or ultrasonography prior to elective orthopaedic surgery of any nature. In our series of 40 patients, the 38 patients who had excisional surgery survived, and none seeded the sepsis to their hips. In the two patients who died, the acalculous cholecystitis was diagnosed at autopsy, and the cause of death was gram-negative septicemia.

Neurologic Complications

Sciatic, femoral, and obturator neuropathies are well-documented complications of total hip replacement. In our experience they seem to follow release of a stiff hip resulting from a previously shortened extremity, or to wound hematoma. Most nerve injuries are transient, rarely lasting beyond a year. The reported incidence has been approximately 1%.[53,70] Comparison of preoperative and postoperative electromyographic studies, however, reveals a much higher incidence of subclinical nerve damage.[165,176] The majority of nerve injuries consist of neurapraxia due to retraction, limb position, or leg lengthening. Leg lengthening, especially that resulting from reconstruction of long-standing dislocation, may produce a much more severe and lasting neurapraxia. So also may direct surgical trauma, cement entrapment, and thermal injury cause more severe and lasting neurologic complications.[23,70] Hemorrhage

and the resulting hematoma, whether the result of surgery or anticoagulant medication, produce a neuropathy of more fleeting duration.[57,70,162]

We have seen three cases of permanent sciatic neuropathy in conjunction with recurrent dislocation of total hip replacements. We have also seen neuropathy when efforts to gain leg length are overly zealous. We would not agree with the report of Dunn and Hess indicating that it is safe to lengthen the leg as much as 9.4 cm.[53] Our rule of thumb is that it is dangerous to try to achieve leg lengthening in excess of 3 cm beyond the position that can be obtained on a "pull" radiograph. Although Dunn and Hess had only one case of sciatic palsy, this was a small series, and one case represents a 4.5% complication rate in their small group of 22 patients.[53,57]

Trochanteric Nonunion

Trochanteric osteotomy is strongly recommended by Charnley and by Eftekhar,[56] both to improve exposure at the time of hip reconstruction and to allow for lateral or distal transplantation to improve hip joint biomechanics postoperatively.[26,54] Others favor leaving the trochanter intact when possible and performing limited osteotomy for patients with a limited arc of motion and those undergoing revision surgery. Volz and Turner report trouble with trochanteric wiring in 4% to 80% of patients.[174] Parker and colleagues report problems in 17% of patients with trochanteric osteotomy treated at the Robert Breck Brigham Hospital (Fig. 35-20).[132] At that institution, two consecutive series of 100 patients each who had total hip arthroplasty were compared; one group was treated with trochanteric osteotomy, the other was not. The findings were as follows: those who did not have trochanteric osteotomy had shorter operating times (2 as compared to 3 hours), less intraoperative and postoperative blood loss (3 as compared to 4 units), fewer hematomas and infections, less ectopic bone formation, and more rapid rehabilitation. Sixteen of 100 patients thought to be candidates for leaving the trochanter intact at the time of surgery were not, and trochanteric osteotomy was necessary. The series of patients treated without

FIG. 35-20. Trochanteric non-union.

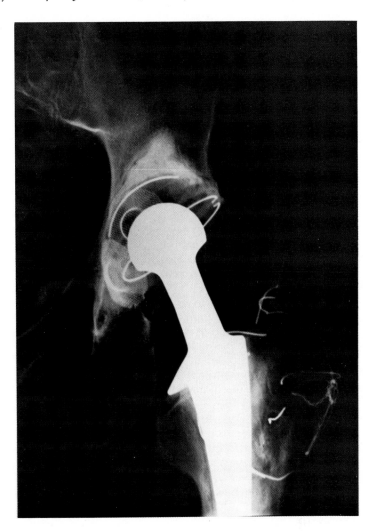

osteotomy included revisions of seven mold arthroplasties, two Austin-Moore arthroplasties, and two osteotomies.

Our own experience parallels that of the surgeons of Robert Breck Brigham Hospital, and whenever the range of motion is good and satisfactory visualization of the hip can be obtained without trochanteric osteotomy, we prefer to avoid this step and its postoperative problems of nonunion and trochanteric bursitis. Volz and Turner report that the use of a bolt to reattach the greater trochanter was followed by nonunion in only 1.3% of patients.[174]

English has reported on a trochanteric approach to the hip consisting of osteotomy of the greater trochanter located so as to keep the vastus lateralis and the abductor musculature intact and attached to the trochanter.[59] He reattached the trochanter with wire in his first series and with a bolt in his second series; the reported rates of nonunion were 4.3% and 2.5%, respectively. Bronsen has described a patient in whom a fragment of a broken trochanteric wire become interposed between the articular surfaces of the two components.[13] This issue, too, is not settled, leaving room for improvement in our methods of reattachment of the trochanter when osteotomy is necessary. Also needed are better identifying criteria for that group of patients for whom osteotomy of the trochanter is not necessary. It is interesting to note that when trochanteric osteotomy is not performed, the reported incidence of component malpositioning is slightly higher on both the femoral and acetabular sides, and, hence, particular attention should be paid to position if this structure is left intact.

LATE COMPLICATIONS

Infection

General Principles. Infection is the one local complication of the arthroplasty itself that can lead to total and irrevocable failure. Deep wound infection is reported in all series that are followed up for any length of time, and the incidences range from less than 1% to 11% when both primary and secondary procedures are included, to a high of 17% in revisions of previous total hip arthroplasties.[43,45,89,100,108,120,123,126,129,182,183] Because of the magnitude and gravity of the problem, wound sepsis has commanded much attention in the literature.

Burke assessed the level of bacterial wound contamination intraoperatively in a series of 50 "clean" laparotomies and found positive cultures in 100% of the procedures.[17] In 92%, coagulase-positive *Staphylococcus aureus* was found, and the average number of strains of staphylococci in each wound was 5.8. Fitzgerald and colleagues cultured 658 total hip arthroplasty wounds in the operating room and obtained positive cultures in 30%.[68] Twenty-five percent of patients undergoing primary hip surgery had positive cultures, as did 38% undergoing revision hip arthroplasty. Seven superficial and seven deep infections followed, an incidence of 1%. It is clear that bacterial contamination of operative wounds does occur during surgery, and there is an appreciable incidence of postoperative wound infection. Whether there is a direct connection between the two observations, however, is a matter of great debate. Sources of wound infection appear to be endogenous or exogenous, infections occurring through direct contamination or indirect contamination through fallout from organisms in the ambient air.

Prevention. Preventing infection has long been a challenge to surgeons, and many measures have been devised, including aseptic technique, careful and gentle handling of tissue, preoperative preparation of the patient, postoperative protection of the wound, and measures to decontaminate the environment in which the operative procedure is performed—traffic control, ultrafiltered air, helmet aspirator units, ultraviolet radiation. Sherr and Dodd have reported on the effectiveness of solutions of cephalothin, carbenicillin, polymyxin B, bacitracin, and neomycin used as antimicrobial irrigating solutions.[157] They showed also that povidone-iodine (Betadine), 25% by volume, is effective as an irrigating solution, but they have not used it clinically. Our practice at New England Baptist Hospital is to use a preparation of polymyxin B.

After detailed and repeated reviews of the literature on prophylactic antibiotics in hip surgery, we strongly endorse their routine use in all cases of reconstructive hip surgery, both primary and revision. The reader is referred to the writings of Boyd and colleagues,[11] Ericson and co-workers,[60] Burnett and co-workers,[18] Fogelberg and associates,[71] Lidwell and colleagues,[103] and Nelson and Schurmann[127] for clinical documentation of the effectiveness of prophylactic antibiotics. Recommendations on the duration of antibiotic therapy after surgery vary, but there seems to be no proven value in continuing antibiotic therapy beyond 48 hours following uncomplicated surgery.[134]

The cephalosporins have been very widely used for prophylaxis in total hip replacement since the introduction of cephalothin in 1964. Cefamandole nafate was introduced in 1978, as were several other second-generation cephalosporin antibiotics. Schurmann and colleagues pointed out that cefamandole has a much broader antimicrobial spectrum than does cephalothin, especially for gram-negative organisms.[151] These authors have also demonstrated that cefamandole is concentrated in bone and hematoma fluids at concentrations three times higher than cephalothin. They further conclude that antibiotic bone concentration occurs so rapidly that antibiotics need not be administered to the patient prior to entering the operating room in routine cases of total hip replacement. Our recommendation in the case of primary hip surgery in which there is no suspicion of sepsis is to initiate intravenous cefamandole, 1 g, at the time of intubation and to continue 1-g doses every 6 hours for 48 hours. If there has been previous surgery, or if there is any suspicion of sepsis, intravenous cefamandole is withheld until immediately after cultures are taken from joint fluid, hip capsule, and bone. As soon as these intraoperative cultures have been harvested, a 1-g intravenous bolus is given and repeated every 6 hours for 5 days. If sepsis seems likely or probable, the dosage is increased to 2 mg every 4 hours for 72 hours, then 1 g every 6 hours for an additional 2 days. By 5 days, the issue of sepsis should be clarified by information from the bacteriology laboratory as well as from the pathological analysis of the tissues. In revision cases in which the possibility of sepsis seems unlikely, prophylaxis is continued at a dosage of 1 g of cefamandole every 6 hours for 5 days to be certain that all cultures and subcultures are negative.

Preoperative Evaluation. For the successful treatment of sepsis there must be good cooperation among the orthopaedic surgeon, infectious-disease consultant, anesthesiologist, physical therapist, nursing team, microbacteriology laboratory, and orthopaedic radiologist. Complete medical evaluation should be undertaken prior to the surgical treatment of any hip that has potential sepsis. We strongly recommend that all patients who have had prior surgery have an aspiration of their hip to rule out the possibility of low-grade infection. Any intercurrent infection in the body, such as urinary tract infection, psoriatic skin, venous stasis ulcers, or other potential foci of infection, should be eliminated if possible. Stinchfield and associates,[164] Downes,[51] D'Ambrosia and colleagues,[44] Rubin and co-workers,[145] Eftekhar,[56] Turner and colleagues,[173] and others have reported metastatic seeding via the hematogenous route. The radiographic techniques useful in this evaluation of sepsis are described in detail by Wetzner and associates[180] and by Eftekhar.[56] Draining sinuses should be evaluated with a sinogram, and if the sinogram fails to show communication with the joint, a separate aspiration and arthrogram should be done through a clean portal.

Antibiotic Program. We continue to use a triple antibiotic protocol, as initially outlined by Fremont-Smith in 1974[73] and further refined by Turner and colleagues in 1982.[173] Table 35-3 shows the major groups of antibiotics used and their cellular mode of action. If a definitive organism has been identified by history and preoperative aspiration, antibiotic treatment is begun preoperatively. Our current practice is to initiate administration of at least two intravenous antibiotics appropriate for the individual organism based on sensitivity patterns. If no bacteria have been identified preoperatively, administration of the drugs in groups one, two, and three of Table 35-3 is initiated intravenously after the appropriate intra-

Table 35-3. Three Groups of Drugs Used in the Triple Antibiotic Protocol

ANTIBIOTIC GROUP	ANTIMICROBIAL AGENT(S)	SITE OF ACTION	AVERAGE DOSE (70-KG ADULT)	DURATION OF THERAPY
Group 1	Cefamandole Oxacillin Cephalothin	Interferes with cell wall "linkage"	2 g IV every 4–6 hours	21–28 days
Group 2	Clindamycin	Interferes at the 50S ribosomal subunit	600 mg IV every 6 hours	21–28 days orally; 2 mo. if appropriate
Group 3	Gentamicin Tobramycin Amikacin	Interferes at the 30S ribosomal subunit	80 mg IV every 8 hours; 300 mg IV every 8 hours (for amikacin)	10–14 days for gram-positive organisms; 21–28 days for gram-negative organisms

capsular cultures have been harvested at surgery. Adjustments in the drug selection are made depending on the results of intra-operative cultures and sensitivity patterns.

The standard protocol for staphylococcal infections (60% of all joint sepsis is staphylococcal) is to continue intravenous therapy for 3 to 4 weeks for the group one and two drugs and 2 weeks for the group three drugs. If one is treating a virulent gram-negative infection, the group three aminoglycoside drugs should be continued for 4 and even 6 weeks with extremely careful aminoglycoside monitoring, as has been outlined by Miley and colleagues.[117]

Monitoring of all patients on triple therapy should include the following: CBC with differential, SGOT, urinalysis, and creatinine studies, each done every 3 days. Audiovestibular monitoring is performed weekly to detect any possible aminoglycoside toxicity. Aminoglycoside levels are measured once every 5 days or as clinically indicated. Patients on aminoglycoside therapy for more than 14 days or patients with any history of renal disease should have serum creatinine levels carefully checked every day, 7 days a week. Upon completion of the intravenous therapy, the patient is put on a long-term oral treatment program for at least 1 year.

Clindamycin is a proven drug for the treatment of osteomyelitis and has good antistaphylococcal spectrum, so it is often chosen for long-term suppression when sensitivity testing permits. Cephalexin and ampicillin are other antibiotics often used for long-term oral suppression, depending on the sensitivity pattern of the principal organism cultured. Regrettably, there are few good antimicrobial agents for long-term oral suppression in the face of gram-negative sepsis. This is undoubtedly part of the reason that the clinical end results of single-stage conversion are poorest in the presence of gram-negative sepsis.

Surgical Approach. The surgical technique for either a one-stage conversion or a Girdlestone resection should include extensive debridement of all capsule, cement, sinus tracts, and prosthetic components. Only after such thorough debridement can one make a final decision on a single-stage conversion versus a Girdlestone resection.

The surgeon who is operating in the presence of known sepsis should be prepared to perform either a one-stage revision or a Girdlestone resection arthroplasty. Factors favoring single-stage revision, as advocated by Buchholz,[15,16] Salvati,[146] Turner,[173] and others[15,16,120,146,182] include the following:

Organisms that are sensitive to at least three, and preferably six, antibiotics
Gram-positive organisms
Absence of superinfection and multiple organisms
Healthy, well-vascularized tissues
Absence of draining sinuses
Radiographic evidence of healthy femoral cortical bone
Reasonably good bone, to support cement fixation, both in the acetabulum and in the femur

Of paramount importance is the assessment of soft tissue and bone quality. Factors indicating the potential success of a Girdlestone resection are as follows:

Virulent, resistant organisms
Gram-negative organisms
Two or more concomitant strains of organisms
Unhealthy and edematous soft tissues
Draining sinus(es)
Radiographic evidence of well-established osteomyelitis with bone erosion
Severe loss of bone substance

None of these indications is absolute, and judgment must be used, especially concerning the nature of the organism and the health of the soft tissues. An infected total hip replacement with radiolucent resorption lines and evidence of component subsidence is seen in Figure 35-21, *A*. A Girdlestone resection was done, and the postoperative appearance is seen in Figure 35-21, *B*.

Figure 35-22, *A*, shows an infected total hip prosthesis with radiolucent shadows and component subsidence. The tissues were healthy, and the offending organism was a coagulase-negative *Staphylococcus aureus*, so one-stage revision was performed to a long-stem Aufranc-Turner prosthesis (Fig. 35-22, *B*).

Results of One-Stage Revision Arthroplasty. Buchholz and colleagues have reported a 77% success rate in 583 patients after the first attempt at one-stage revision in the face of documented deep infection.[15,16] It is important to note that Buchholz does a single-stage conversion even in the presence of draining sinuses and virulent gram-negative organisms.[16] We have experienced too high a failure rate when these conditions prevail, and, consequently, we consider these to be among the important contraindications to single-stage total hip conversion. The clinical results of one-stage conversion at the New England Baptist Hospital have been published by Turner and associates,[173] and Miley and co-workers.[117] Eighty-six percent of 101 patients had no drainage, were free of pain, and ambulated with the support of a single crutch or less. These patients were considered to have good to excellent results. At the time of the report, there was a mean follow-up of 4 years. In the ensuing 2 years since this report, there were four revisions for nonseptic loosening in the patients who were graded good to excellent, so this figure must now be readjusted to 82%. To date, however, there have been no late infections beyond 4 postoperative years.

Conversion of Girdlestone Resection Arthroplasty to Total Hip Replacement (Reimplantation). Evaluation for reimplantation of a total hip replacement is not recommended until at least 12 months following a Girdlestone resection arthroplasty. When possible, we prefer to wait 24 months so that the patient achieves a mature end result of his Girdlestone resection and is both informed and realistic about the surgical alternatives for the future. Turner and colleagues[173] have recommended that the patient meet the following criteria:

An eager patient who is willing to undergo further major reconstructive hip surgery

A patient who has significant residual hip pain, despite the full-time use of a cane

A patient with healthy acetabular and femoral bone with stable radiographs and negative radionuclide bone scans (technetium and gallium) for 12 months

A patient with no wound drainage for at least 12 months

A patient whose sedimentation rate and white blood count are normal for at least 12 months

A patient with a negative hip aspiration and/or biopsy

A patient with realistic expectations about the end result of further surgery

Use of Antibiotic-Impregnated Cement. Buchholz has pioneered the use of antibiotic-impregnated cement for the prophylaxis and treatment of infection.[15,16] In the U.S., Food and Drug Administration regulations have not permitted the manufacture or marketing of antibiotic cement compounds, but the clinical practice of adding antibiotics to acrylic cement is widespread, although not uniform.[124]

If the operating surgeon elects to add an antibiotic to surgical cement such as polymethylmethacrylate, the antibiotic should ideally have all of the following properties:

A broad spectrum of coverage for gram-negative, gram-positive, and anaerobic organisms

No demonstrable evidence of patient sensitivity

No erosion of the physical properties of the cement by the addition of antibiotic powder

Ability to leech from the cement in sufficient quantity to saturate the wound hematoma

Thermostability at the polymerization temperature of the cement

In addition, the patient should not be sensitive to the cement used, and there should be no evidence of the emergence of a resistant bacterial strain.

There is sufficient information on the leeching of thermostable antibiotic from methacrylate cement to encourage consideration of this therapeutic combination in the prophylaxis and treatment of infections, especially in high-risk patients. There are 12 high-risk circumstances in which there has been documented evidence of an enhanced possibility of wound infection. In these 12 circumstances, we recommend the use of a fine crystalline-powdered antibiotic at the dosage level of at least 500 mg, but no more than 1000 mg, per 40 g of powdered cement. These circumstances are as follows:

Revision major joint surgery involving methacrylate

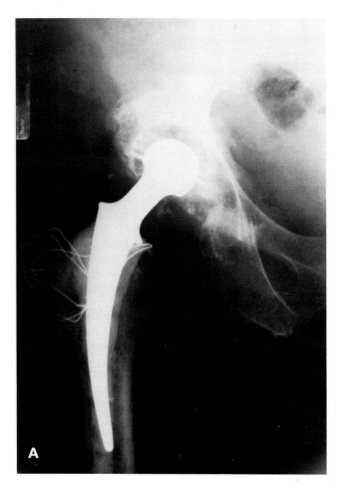

FIG. 35-21. (*A*) Total hip replacement with *Pseudomonas aeruginosa* infection. (*B*) Girdlestone resection following removal of all prosthetic components and cement.

Patient committed to long-term cortisone treatment

Rheumatoid arthritis or its variants (lupus, scleroderma, etc.)

Patient with an altered coagulation profile who is prone to develop postoperative wound hematoma

Traumatized soft tissues

Diabetes mellitus

Malignant tumors or leukemia

Immunosuppressive therapy (*i.e.,* renal transplant patients)

Poor general health (malnutrition, cirrhosis, etc.)

Recurrent foci of infection in the body (cystitis, dermatitis, pancreatitis, etc.)

Poor dental hygiene

Morbid obesity

In patients who are primarily at risk for staphylococcal infection, we use 1 g of ce-famandole. In patients who are primarily at risk for gram-negative infection, we use 600 mg of the aminoglycoside tobramycin per package of cement. In patients who are at risk for a methicillin-resistant staphylococcal infection, we use 1 g of tobramycin per package of cement.

Instability in the Total Hip Replacement

Dislocation or subluxation of the femoral component from the acetabulum is one of the more common complications of total hip arthroplasty.[24] Reported incidences range from 0.5%[54,61] to 5%.[141] Most of the larger and more recent published series have dislocation rates of 3% or less.[44,54,61,65,95,102,129,185] Several factors have been implicated as causes of dislocation.

There is a definite association between previous surgery and a higher incidence of

FIG. 35-21. (*Continued*)

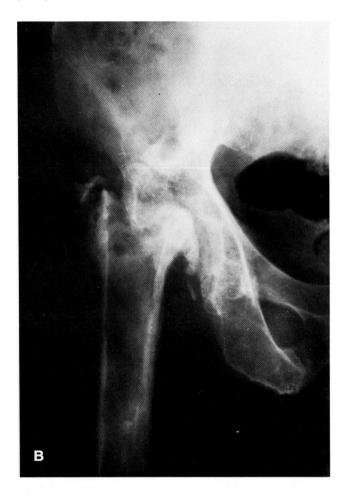

dislocation. In Fackler and Poss's series, only 1% of the hips not previously operated on dislocated.[65] In contrast, 5% of hips previously operated on dislocated, and 20.8% of those hips that had had a previous total hip arthroplasty dislocated. Up to 70% to 80% of the dislocated hips in the same series had had previous surgery.[65] These dislocations may be due to surgical damage to hip abductor muscles, the tension of which is necessary for hip stability.

Most authors agree that age and sex of the patient, as well as the primary pathologic process necessitating total hip replacement, have nothing to do with the rate of dislocation.[41,54,65,129,141] In a recent Mayo Clinic series, however, females had a higher rate of dislocation than did males.[185] The overall medical condition of the patient also has a bearing on the rate of dislocation.

Fackler and Poss note that the incidence of severe medical or neurologic problems (including alcoholism, uremic psychosis, senile dementia, cerebral palsy, and muscular dystrophy) was 14% in their control group, 22% in patients who underwent single dislocation, and 75% in those with recurrent dislocation.[65] This may be due to poor motor control of the involved limb or to lack of understanding and cooperation in avoiding positions of the limb that risk dislocation. Most authors feel that the surgical approach chosen is not a significant factor in influencing the rate of dislocation. Woo and Morrey, however, report a dislocation rate of 2.3% after an anterolateral approach and a 5.8% incidence after a posterior approach.[185] Woo and Morrey also showed that the incidence of dislocation is significantly greater in patients who develop

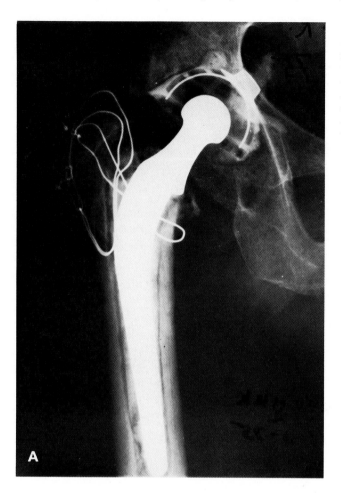

FIG. 35-22. (*A*) Preoperative x-ray of an infected Bechtol total hip replacement. Note the radiolucent lines at the bone–cement interface. (*B*) Postoperative x-ray shows a long-stem femoral component secured with radiolucent cement on the femoral side and radiopaque cement on the acetabular side of the joint.

a nonunion of the greater trochanter (17.6%) than in those who have trochanteric healing (2.8%).[185] The diameter of the head of the femoral prosthesis does not make a substantial difference in the clinical dislocation rate, even though laboratory studies have demonstrated more *in vitro* instability for the small, 22-mm head.[1,140,185]

Malpositioning of the prosthetic component has been implicated in dislocation.[95,140,141] The most serious error of positioning is retroversion of either the acetabular or femoral component. We believe that the correct position of the acetabulum should be less than 45° of abduction and 10° to 15° of anteversion. The femoral component should be placed in 5° to 10° of anteversion. Retroversion of either component must be strictly avoided. Proper soft tissue tension should be maintained by not placing the prosthetic acetabulum too ceph-

alad, not shortening the neck of the femur excessively, and, if a trochanteric osteotomy is done, transferring the trochanter both distally and laterally.[29,55]

Other possible causes of dislocation are remnants of methylmethacrylate or osteophytes around the rim of the acetabulum that allow the femoral neck to lever out.[41,54,129,133] The presence of methylmethacrylate, bone, or wire in the acetabulum[55,140] and the presence of too much fluid in the joint capsule[141] are additional possible causes of dislocation. Most dislocations occur less than 6 weeks postoperatively.[41,65,102,133,185] Therefore, proper education of the patient and staff in avoiding positions that predispose to dislocation, especially flexion, adduction, and internal rotation of the hip, is critical. Some attention must be paid to these details for the life of the patient, since up to 23% of all disloca-

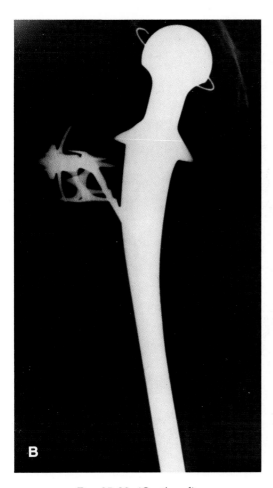

B

FIG. 35-22. (*Continued*)

tions in the series of Woo and Morrey occurred more than 1 year postoperatively.[185]

When a total hip replacement does dislocate, it can be successfully relocated without further surgery in the majority of the cases with the use of intravenous sedation, spinal anesthesia, or general anesthesia.[41,65,185] Between 18% and 31% of hips will, however, continue to redislocate.[61,65,185] These may then require further surgery, depending on the cause of the problem. Sellergren and Scheller have provided a logical clinical approach for dealing with a dislocated total hip replacement.[156] This may involve reattachment or advancement of the greater trochanter, removal of impinging osteophytes or pieces of methylmethacrylate, removal of foreign bodies from the acetabulum, plication of the cap-

sule, or revision of the components. If further surgery is not medically necessary, possible, or successful, bracing may sometimes be used to prevent further dislocation.[156]

Heterotopic Bone Formation

Heterotopic ossification of soft tissues is a common complication, although it does not usually cause pain or significantly decreased hip function (Fig. 35-23). The exact mechanism that triggers this untoward event is unknown, but it is apparent that in affected patients, pluripotential mesenchymal cells lay down an osteoid matrix in which there is calcium deposition with ultimate ossification.[93] In some patients, heterotopic ossification is seen only in a few isolated islands of bone visible on postoperative radiographs but in no way comprising hip motion or the ultimate functional result.[48] In others, large masses that ultimately coalesce and lead to complete joint ankylosis develop. Brooker and co-workers have classified ectopic ossification into four recognized categories:[14]

Class I: Islands within soft tissue
Class II: Spurs from the pelvis or femur leaving 1 cm or more distance between the pelvis or femur
Class III: Spurs from the pelvis or femur leaving less than 1 cm distance between the pelvis and femur
Class IV: Apparent bony ankylosis

The problem with heterotopic ossification remains incompletely resolved. However, three high-risk groups have been identified: (1) males who have not had previous hip surgery and who present with osteoarthritis and a limited range of hip motion; (2) males or females who have had previous hip surgery and developed heterotopic ossification during convalescence and for whom revision hip surgery is planned; (3) patients with ankylosing spondylitis in an active phase.[7]

The incidence of heterotopic ossification following total hip arthroplasty varies widely,[14,27,93,159] from a low of 2% to 4% reported by Riegler and Harris[136] to a high of 53% reported by Nollen and Slooff.[130]

Complete ankylosis following total hip arthroplasty reportedly occurs in 2% to 7% of patients.[27,42,93,130,136,159] Statistics on the

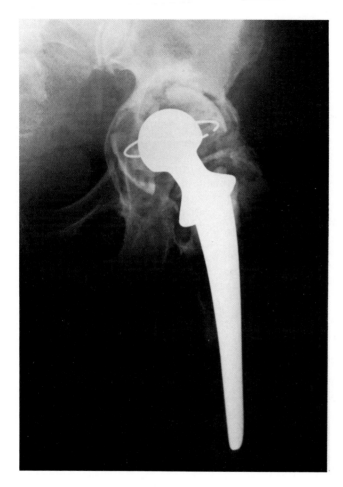

Fig. 35-23. Class IV heterotopic bone formation following total hip replacement.

frequency of occurrence of this complication, as they exist in the literature, deal almost exclusively with a random patient population presenting for total hip arthroplasty in major clinics. When high-risk patients are isolated from the general population (*e.g.*, males with osteoarthritis), the incidence of heterotopic ossification rises to 65%, with the condition being severe in one third of the cases.[114] There is, to date, no sizable series dealing with the limited issue of heterotopic ossification and its occurrence in patients undergoing revision surgery in whom heterotopic ossification was already present. It can be presumed to be at least as likely as in any of the recognized high-risk groups.

Several general preventive measures are currently considered useful in reducing the likelihood of heterotopic ossification and are practiced by the great majority of re-

constructive hip surgeons. These measures are as follows:

Use of a lateral or posterolateral surgical approach rather than an anterior approach

Avoidance of periosteal stripping if an anterior approach is indicated or preferred

Avoidance of detachment of the greater trochanter in most cases of primary hip surgery

Gentleness in handling of tissues

Cauterization and/or bone-waxing of raw bone surfaces

Careful institution of hemostasis and meticulous debridement of any devitalized tissues

Use of pulsating jet irrigation to remove fragments of bone and other particulate debris

Use of soft tissue compression with wound

suction drainage for 24 to 48 hours to reduce both dead space and the likelihood of hematoma formation

Prophylactic cortisone administration during convalescence does not seem to be useful. The usefulness of oral diazepam is debated, but the use of indomethacin during convalescence shows some promise.[142]

There are two therapeutic regimes with established effectiveness in reducing the incidence of heterotopic ossification in the patient convalescing from primary or revision total hip replacement arthroplasty: oral administration of diphosphonate (EHDP) and radiation therapy.[42,69,93] EHDP inhibits the growth of hydroxyapatite crystals *in vitro* and thus may be responsible for the prevention of pathologic calcification and, ultimately, heterotopic ossification *in vivo*.[93] There has been no evidence offered that EHDP inhibits the formation of osteoid matrix. EHDP should be administered orally at a dosage of 20 mg/kg beginning 2 to 4 weeks prior to surgery and continuing for 3 months after surgery. Local radiation of the operated area during early convalescence appears to have the potential to prevent mesenchymal cells from laying down osteoid matrix, which would ultimately calcify and ossify.[42,93] It is a regime that must be approached with caution, particularly in younger patients, since the long-term effects of radiation are not known. If radiation therapy is used, it should be started within the first week after surgery and should be given at a dosage level of 2000 rad in ten divided doses.

It appears that EHDP and localized radiation are treatments that are independently effective. Each addresses the biology of the problem at different phases of its development; it would thus appear that the suggestion of the Mayo Clinic group that EHDP therapy be considered a supplement to radiation therapy in particularly high-risk patients is worthy of serious consideration.

Cement Fracture

Isolated instances of cement fracture around the stem of the femoral head prosthesis have been reported by Weber and Charnley.[177] In a review of 6649 patients

operated on at Wrightington, 1.5% exhibited this finding, usually present by 6 months but asymptomatic in the majority. Often this was associated with some measure of pain in the thigh that was temporary and accompanied by slight subsidence of the prosthesis in 79 patients. Usually, the fracture occurred within 2 cm of the distal end of the prosthesis. None of the patients in this series went on to stem failure, and the finding is not felt to be an indication for revision. We have seen this finding in only one of our patients, and the patient has been asymptomatic in the 3 years since the fracture occurred (Fig. 35-24).

Loosening

Of the mechanical causes for late failure, loosening—whether septic or aseptic—appears to be on the increase (Fig. 35-25). Nolan and colleagues found femoral loosening in 0.3% of 3204 total hip arthroplasties done at the Mayo Clinic.[129] Salvati, in a late review of 100 cases operated on between 1968 and 1970, reported a 4% incidence of sterile loosening in patients followed more than 5 years.[147] Dandy and Theodorou, reviewing 1042 total hip replacements done by the McKee-Farrar technique, found that 6.6% of the patients had a loose prosthesis (3.5% cups, 2.2% stems, 0.9% cups and stems).[45]

Marmor found loosening in 6% of 160 patients and noted that the average age of the patients was 51.8 years, none being older than 62. Their average weight was 199 pounds, with a range from 174 to 225, and six patients were more than 6 feet tall.[112] In Marmor's series, then, relative youth, excessive weight, and above-average height were major contributing factors. Analyzing the first 20 failures of total hip arthroplasty at the Hospital for Special Surgery, Charvosky and associates noted that 12 failed secondary to infection and eight secondary to loosening, again attesting to the seriousness and frequency of this complication.[33] Coventry and colleagues, in a series of 2012 arthroplasties from the Mayo Clinic, reported acetabular loosening in two cases and femoral loosening in 4.2% of 333 hips followed for more than 2 years (Fig. 35-26).[41] Charnley found that 24% of patients had radiographic or clinical evi-

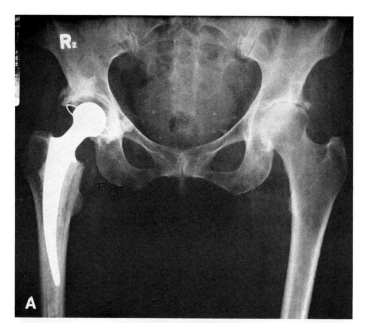

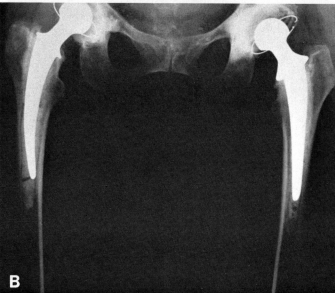

FIG. 35-24. Cement fracture without clinical evidence of loosening is not an indication for prosthetic revision. This patient had been knocked to the ground by her dog. Minimal transient hip pain followed. The prosthesis settled ⅛ inch, but 4 years later it remains asymptomatic (*A*). (*B*) Immediate postoperative roentgenogram 4 years after right total hip arthroplasty. (Lowell, J.D.: Complications of total hip replacement. In The Hip: Proceedings of the Fourth Open Scientific Meeting of The Hip Society. St. Louis, C.V. Mosby, 1976)

dence of acetabular loosening at 10-year follow-up.[30]

Other causes of loosening are felt to be inadequate surface contact between cement and bone, fracture of the cement secondary to areas of weakness caused by entrapment of blood at the time of cement insertion, breakdown of cement medial to the upper third of the prosthesis secondary to failure to remove cancellous bone medial to the calcar, varus positioning of the prosthesis at the time of insertion, and friction between the moving components.[35,82,109,110,160,166,178] Simon and co-workers have found frictional forces generated in total hip prostheses to achieve levels 40 times greater than those in normal joints and suggest that these forces may well be enough to cause late loosening of the acetabular component by fatigue failure.[158] They also describe the phenomenon of "stiction-friction," defined as the temporary increase in friction be-

FIG. 35-25. Femoral loosening. Note the cement fracture proximolaterally, the varus migration, the calcar resorption, and the subsidence.

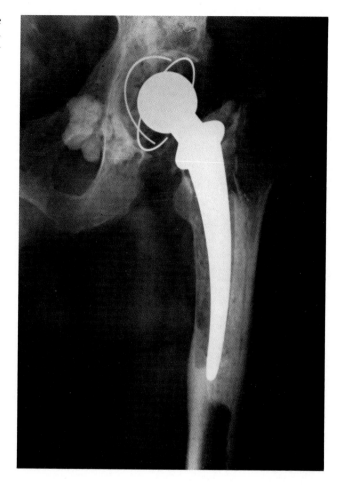

tween the component surfaces that occurs after long periods of standing and high load, during which time the lubricating fluid film is squeezed out.

Swanson and associates note that if both components of a total hip replacement are cobalt-chromium-molybdenum alloy, the particles generated by use will increase the friction to twice that in unworn components, again leading to loosening.[166] This change does not take place when one component is high-density polyethylene and the other stainless steel. Anderson and co-workers and others have pointed out the significant difference in friction demonstrated when both components are metal and when one is metal and the other polyethylene.[2]

Recognition of loosening, particularly in its early stages, is difficult and may be impossible, even with arthrography. Murray and Rodrigo reported on 52 patients with 53 asymptomatic hips, all of whom had arthrography.[125] If entrance of radiopaque dye into the cement–bone interface was defined as evidence of loosening, 12 (22.6%) had findings consistent with loosening. Of 21 patients with 25 painful hips, 11 showed the roentgenographic appearance of loosening, an incidence of 44%. There was no statistically significant difference between the findings of the asymptomatic and symptomatic hips. Only seven of 12 hips explored after arthrogram were, in actual fact, loose. Murray and Rodrigo's conclusion was that contrast medium filling the space between bone and component was not conclusive proof of loosening. Both false negatives and false positives are common.

Feith and colleagues used ^{87m}Sr bone scanning for evaluation of total hip replacements and found that the scan normally returned to normal within 6 months of

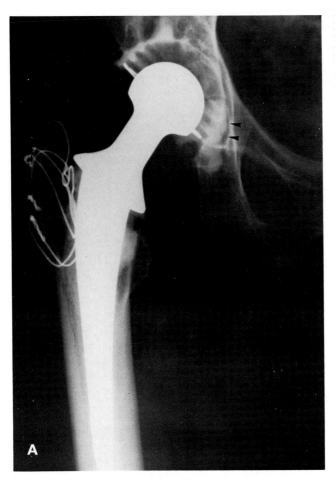

FIG. 35-26. Acetabular loosening. (*A*) Early loosening with tensile failure of cement in zone III. (*B*) Gross loosening with >2 mm of lucency surrounding all of the cement in zones I, II, and III.

surgery.[66] In those hips in which the scan remained abnormal and in which the erythrocyte sedimentation rate was not elevated, six of 22 patients who underwent operation were found to have loosening of one or both components. It would appear that, in the hands of Feith and colleagues, scanning promises to achieve more accurate identification of loosening than does arthrography.

Evidence of a line of demarcation between cement and acetabulum has been suspected to be early evidence of loosening (see Fig. 35-25). DeLee and Charnley, reviewing 155 hips followed for an average of 10.1 years, identified a line of demarcation between bone and cement in 69.5% of patients.[47] Of this group, 13 (9.2%) showed some migration of the acetabular component during this period. Seventy-one percent of patients who developed a line of demar-

cation did so within the first year after surgery. On the average, migration started 5.4 years after surgery. Four of the 13 patients with migration had no clinical problem. DeLee and Charnley concluded that in the majority of patients, demarcation, particularly when seen around the acetabular component, was not associated with symptoms and was not a cause for concern. It became a cause for concern only when the width of the line of demarcation was greater than 1.5 cm.

Salvati and co-workers, reviewing 100 total hip arthroplasties at the Hospital for Special Surgery followed more than 5 years, found a line of demarcation in 100% of 93 hips.[147] In 63 patients, it was 1 mm in width, and in 29 patients, 1 mm to 2 mm. The line was more than 3 mm wide in only one patient, and that patient had late infection with *Staphylococcus aureus.* Asymp-

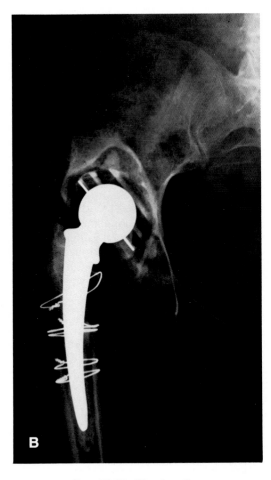

B

FIG. 35-26. (*Continued*)

laboratory study in dogs and has not, to date, been followed by a study in human subjects. Markolf and Amstutz have reported on the use of a plug (either bone or cement) that is inserted prior to final cementing in the distal femoral canal immediately beyond the lowest point of insertion of the femoral stem.[109] This allows for the generation of high pressure at the time of cement and prosthesis insertion. The technique requires filling the cavity from below, proximally. Harris, who has used a similar technique with a cement plug, noted similar favorable findings and also that there was no rise in intramedullary pressure distal to the plug, a phenomenon that should simultaneously reduce the hazards of embolization of fat and marrow.[81] Markolf and Amstutz have also reported on earlier insertion of cement and the use of brief, high-pressure pulses to force the cement more evenly and more completely into the irregularities of the internal surface of the femoral canal.[110] Weinstein and colleagues, as well, have used high-pressure insertion methods to improve fixation.[178] In clinical practice, when bone plugging is used, syringes with long tips must be employed to insert the cement and permit distal-to-proximal filling because the cement cannot be forced down into a closed cylinder. We strongly recommend these cement pressurization techniques to decrease the incidence of component loosening.

Femoral Component Fracture

The fractured femoral stem presents one of the most challenging complications to the surgeon and necessitates revision total hip arthroplasty. The incidence of stem fracture in the literature ranges from 0.23% to 0.67%.[6,22,25,52,75] The largest study, by Chao and Coventry of the Mayo Clinic, quotes an incidence of 0.6%.[25]

Although Chao and Coventry attempted to develop a risk index for prospective analysis of stem fracture, few studies have concentrated on the interrelationship of the multitude of variables connected with this complex problem.

The composite structure formed by femoral bone, methylmethacrylate, and metal endoprosthesis is acted on by numerous forces. Muscle and joint reaction forces apply tensile stresses along the lateral cortex

tomatic lines of demarcation, then, deserve follow-up but are not a cause for great concern unless they increase in width and the joint becomes painful. Marmor pointed out the possibility of confusing a stress fracture of the pubic ramus with loosening; the patient in question showed demarcation, but a few weeks after pain developed, he also showed an undisplaced fracture of the inferior pubic ramus.[113]

Efforts to prevent loosening are aided by careful attention to hemostasis and control of bleeding from bone surfaces before cement is inserted. Cobden and associates have reported on the use of microcrystalline collagen, topical thrombin, and gelatin foam soaked in thrombin to reduce bleeding from the prepared surfaces.[35] Although all of these agents were effective, microcrystalline collagen being the best, Cobden's was a

and compressive stresses medially. Shear forces occur between the conjoint surfaces of the three materials. Failure of one or more of these highly stressed materials may occur between their conjoint surfaces. Also, failure of one or more of these materials may result from the applied forces. Resultant forces on the composite structure depend on the clinical and technical factors.

Certain clinical parameters—age, height, weight, activity level, and osseous quality—are among factors that usually lead to stem loosening and bone resorption.[5,72,79,112] Technical parameters include endoprosthetic design configurations,[6,9,12,32,36,92,128,144] the metals used,[6,8,9,36,75,128,144,149,168] cement quality and distribution about the stem, relative component position, the surgical technique of bone preparation,[6,22,28,36,52,79,144,168] and the technique of cement insertion.

Femoral stem fracture is a complex problem, and a multitude of clinical and technical factors integrate to cause it (Fig. 35-27). The clinical and radiographic experience with this problem at the New England Baptist Hospital demonstrates that the cantilever mode of loosening is the major predisposing factor to stem fracture. When patients with this mode of loosening, weaker stem configurations, and loss of cement and bone support are identified, protection of the hip or prophylactic revision is indicated.

When a patient presents with a fractured femoral stem, revision surgery is indicated. The reader is referred to Scheller and colleagues[150] for a more detailed discussion of the preoperative evaluation and specific techniques for extraction of the retained distal stem fragment.

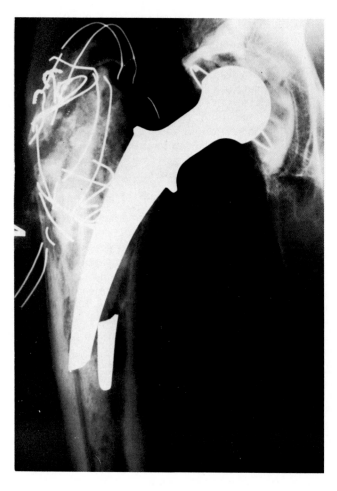

FIG. 35-27. Femoral component fracture is frequently associated with a cantilever mode of loosening. Proximal femoral resorption, cement fracture, use of a varus-designed prosthesis, and weak cross-sectional geometry all increase the stem stress, resulting in fracture.

The basic surgical premises of revision surgery for stem fracture are (1) a thorough preoperative analysis, (2) wide surgical exposure with trochanteric osteotomy, (3) intramedullary drilling and extraction of the distal stem fragment, and (4) reconstruction with a longer, modern-design femoral stem fabricated from a high-strength alloy.

Bone Resorption

Harris and colleagues have reported four cases of extensive localized bone resorption in the proximal femur following total hip replacement.[86] The clinical appearance of each suggested tumor or infection, but none showed either at reoperation. All prostheses were loose. Macrophages, giant cells, and birefringent crystals were present on histologic examination in each instance, but no inflammatory cells. The process appeared benign, patch tests for sensitivity to polymethylmethacrylate and monomer were negative, and one case was bilateral. Fragmentation of the cement was extensive. All were treated by reinsertion, and all have done well. The incidence of this condition at Massachusetts General Hospital was 0.25%. No similar reports have appeared elsewhere to date, although Harris reports that he knows of three others.

Metal Sensitivity

Reports of metal sensitivity as a cause of bone necrosis and loosening of the prosthesis following total joint replacement have been published by Evans and colleagues[62] and by Jones and associates.[92] In reviewing 16 patients with loosening prostheses, Evans and co-workers found cobalt-chromium sensitivity in eight and nickel sensitivity in one. Histologic examination revealed necrosis of bone and soft tissue, obliterative changes in the arterioles, and macrophages and giant cells with birefringent crystals in the soft tissues.

Jones and associates reported on seven cases, six of which were cobalt positive on skin testing but nickel and chromium negative. Five were explored surgically. Presenting symptoms included increasing pain, a feeling of instability within the hip, and, in two, spontaneous dislocation. One showed spontaneous acetabular fracture with bone resorption. Histologic examination revealed nonspecific inflammatory changes and widespread necrosis of bone and adjacent soft tissues. Jones and co-workers recommend patch testing in patients with a history of metal sensitivity. The patch tests are not difficult to perform, and the discs for such testing can be obtained from component manufacturers. When tests for sensitivity to one device are positive, the surgeon can select a device of different material to which the patient is not sensitive.

Fatigue Fracture of the Pelvis

Miller has reported nine instances of late fracture of the acetabulum after total hip replacement.[118] Of these nine, five involved the Ring prosthesis and four the McKee-Farrar. Each had metal-on-metal components; none had metal-on-high-density-polyethylene components. Three of the nine fractures were associated with infection and one with injury. No fracture united, and in each, histologic examination revealed extensive necrotic debris. All of the patients were women. Thermal injury to bone secondary to drilling and cementing was suggested as a possible contributing factor. Along with this, the difference between the elasticity of the bone and that of the cement, and the difference in shock-absorbing qualities between metal and plastic components, were implicated. However, no truly satisfactory explanation for these fractures has been proposed, and there has been no further report in the American literature.

Late Trauma

The hazards of trauma with accompanying femoral or pelvic fracture are no less for the patient who has undergone total hip replacement than for members of the normal population, and perhaps they are greater if the patient's agility has been reduced by age or associated disease. Scott and Turner[154] and McElfresh and Coventry[115] have reported on the management of such fractures in conjunction with total hip replacement. Scott and Turner reviewed a series of 38 traumatic fractures, 13 preoperative, 18 intraoperative, and seven postoperative. Long-stemmed prostheses, with and without long necks, were used in the 31 preoperative and intraoperative fractures.

Traction treatment, with and without bone plates, was used with varying success in the postoperative fractures. Long-stemmed prostheses were inserted when the femoral stem of the prosthesis already in place fractured as well.

McElfresh and Coventry reported on ten patients with 11 fractures, three involving the pubis, six the upper third of the femur, and one a combined acetabular and femoral fracture. Two of the femoral fractures were stress fractures, and all healed with conservative management. McElfresh and Coventry favored conservative management of the shaft fracture by traction, with open reduction only if traction failed. In the management of shaft fractures in which long-stemmed components are employed, Scott and Turner recommend careful preoperative assessment of femoral length to aid in selection of the proper long-stemmed component, preoperative shortening of the stem, and provision for further revision of the stem during the course of the operation, when necessary.[154] They also recommend osteotomy of the greater trochanter, the use of a cement gun to ensure adequate distal extension of the cement, and cooling of the cement before it is inserted to afford a longer working time. Our own experience with long-stemmed prostheses has been totally satisfactory, but we too would recommend careful preoperative roentgenographic assessment of femoral length. Even when this has been done, we have sometimes found it necesary to shorten the prosthesis still more during the course of the operation.

Wear

In the early days of total hip arthroplasty, the problem of wear was a major cause for concern, and rightly so, for it was responsible for the failure of those total joint replacements in which Teflon was used for the socket. To date, however, the wear characteristics of high-density polyethylene have been better than expected. Charnley and Cupic have reported an average wear rate of 0.15 mm per year in patients followed for 10 years.[30] Clarke and colleagues wondered whether wear in total hip arthroplasties could be assessed from roentgenograms and decided that it cannot.[34] In their study the clinical errors associated with

means of measuring wear have been greater than the known wear. They further note that in the 10-year follow-up figures currently available, no socket has been removed because of mechanical wear, and no femoral head has been noted to wear more than halfway through a socket. The authors suggest that wear may be as little as 0.01 mm per year in most patients, or possibly as high as 0.5 mm per year if there is acrylic debris between the femoral and acetabular components.

Looking at the problem of wear in removed McKee-Farrar total hip prostheses, Walker and associates reported on three types of wear:[175] initial surface scratching, formation of a new smooth surface, and pitting on top of the type 2 surface. The maximum depth of wear observed was 1 μm. His observations were based on a specimen removed from a 63-year-old man that had been in place for 3½ years. Walker and co-workers feel that synovial fluid has little effect on wear and that wear in metal-to-metal femoral prostheses will be moderate, although in hinged knees it may be extensive. The consensus seems to be that when no foreign material has become interposed between the bearing surfaces, wear has not been a clinically significant problem to date. Certainly, so far, it is not comparable to the mechanical problems of loosening and stem failure.

Carcinogenesis

Malignant degeneration of the tissues about a total hip arthroplasty has not, to our knowledge, been reported. The follow-up, in terms of numbers of patients, is small, so the problem remains a potential one. In looking at the first 20 failed arthroplasties seen at the Hospital for Special Surgery, Charvosky reported no cell changes in the tissues about the removed prostheses that would suggest a carcinogenic effect in association with the devices in place for 3 years.[33] Final proof of safety of total hip replacement in this regard may be years in coming.

CHOOSING THE IDEAL DEVICE

What is the best device for total hip arthroplasty is still a matter of opinion. Murray and colleagues, comparing functional performances of the McKee-Farrar, Charnley, and Muller total hip replacements, found no group distinctly better or worse.[121] Because of lower friction between the component surfaces and the reduced tendency to loosen, total hip replacements consisting of a metal femoral component and a high-density polyethylene acetabular component fixed in place with cement are currently preferred in the U.S. over devices that are not cemented and over those in which both components are metal. At this time, cemented and noncemented metal femoral components with uncemented acetabular components consisting of a high-density polyethylene lining in a metal socket similar to a Smith-Petersen mold (such as the Bateman and Gilberte prostheses) are still in the early stages of acceptance and follow-up study.

CONCLUSIONS

Although complications associated with total hip arthroplasty are many, their incidence, fortunately, is low; most are remediable, and many are preventable. Few who have experienced the successes of total hip arthroplasty would, in the words of Bonnin, "choose to give it up or return to older methods of management of the painful hip."[10] Let us hope that the continuing experience and contributions of the many physicians who employ this procedure will make the operation ever safer and more successful for our patients.

REFERENCES

1. Amstutz, H.C., and Markolf, K.L.: Design features in total hip replacements. In The Hip: Proceedings of the Second Open Scientific Meeting of The Hip Society, 1974, pp. 111–124. St. Louis, CV Mosby, 1974.
2. Anderson, G.B., Freeman, M.A.R., and Swanson, S.A.W.: Loosening of cemented acetabular cup in total hip replacement. J. Bone Joint Surg., 54B: 590, 1972.
3. Andriacchi, T.P., Galante, J.O., Belytschko, T.B., and Hampton, S.: A stress analysis of the femoral stem in total hip prostheses. J. Bone Joint Surg., 58A:618, 1976.
4. Barton, J.R.: On the treatment of anklylosis by the formation of artificial joints: A new operation, devised and executed by J. Rhea Barton. In Rang, M. (ed.): An Anthology of Orthopedics, pp. 195–202. Edinburgh, E&S Livingston, 1966.
5. Bechenbaugh, R.D., and Ilstrup, D.M.: Looking back at total hip arthroplasty: A review of thirty-three hips four to seven years after surgery with special emphasis on loosening and wear. Presented at the 45th Annual Meeting of the American Academy of Orthopaedic Surgeons, Dallas, February 1978.
6. Bechtol, C.O.: Failure of femoral implant components in total hip replacement operations. Orthop. Rev., 4:23, 1975.
7. Bisla, R.S., Ranawat, C.S., and Inglis, A.E.: Total hip replacement in patients with ankylosing spondylitis with involvement of the hip. J. Bone Joint Surg., 58A:223, 1976.
8. Blacker, G.J., and Charnley, J.: Long-term study of changes in the upper femur after low-friction arthroplasty. Presented at the 44th Annual Meeting of the American Academy of Orthopaedic Surgeons, Las Vegas, February 1977.
9. Blackwell, R.S., and Pilliar, R.M.: Fatigue in a hostile environment. Industr. Research, March 1977, p. 89.
10. Bonnin, J.G.: Complications of arthroplasty of the hip. J. Bone Joint Surg., 54B:576, 1972.
11. Boyd, R.J., Burke, J.F., and Colton, T.: A double-blind clinical trial of prophylactic antibiotics in hip fractures. J. Bone Joint Surg., 55A:1251, 1973.
12. Breed, A.L.: Experimental production of vascular hypotension. Clin. Orthop. Rel. Res., 102:227, 1974.
13. Bronsen, J.L.: Articular interposition of trochanteric wires in a failed total hip replacement. Clin. Orthop. Rel. Res., 121:50, 1976.
14. Brooker, A.F., Bowerman, J.W., Robinson, R.A., and Riley, L.H.: Ectopic ossification following total hip replacement. J. Bone Joint Surg., 55A: 1629, 1973.
15. Buchholz, H.W.: Linische Erfahrungen über die Anwendung von Gentamycin-Polymethylmethacrylat zur Infektionsprophylaxe in der Huftchirurgie und zur Therapie tiefer Infektionen bei der totalen Endoprosthese. In the First International Congress on Prosthetics Techniques and Functional Rehabilitation, pp. 119–135, Vienna, 1973.
16. Buchholz, H.W., Elson, R.A., Engelbrecht, E. et al.: Management of deep infection to total hip replacement. J. Bone Joint Surg., 63B:342, 1981.
17. Burke, J.F.: The effective period of antibiotic action in experimental incisions and dermal lesions in surgery. J. Surg., 50:161, 1961.
18. Burnett, J.W., Gustilo, R.B., Williams, D.N. et al.: Prophylactic antibiotics in hip fractures. J. Bone Joint Surg., 62A:457, 1980.
19. Burton, D.S., and Schurman, D.J.: Hematogenous infection in bilateral total hip arthroplasty: A case report. J. Bone Joint Surg., 57A:1004, 1975.
20. Camer, S.: Surgical complications in revision arthroplasty. In Turner, R.H., and Scheller, A.D. (eds.): Revision Total Hip Arthroplasty, pp. 315–327. New York, Grune & Stratton, 1982.
21. Chapman, M.W., and Hadley, W.K.: The effect of polymethylmethacrylate and antibiotic combinations on bacterial viability. J. Bone Joint Surg., 58A:76, 1976.
22. Carlsson, A.S., Gentz, G.F., and Stenport, J.: Fracture of the femoral prosthesis in total hip

replacement according to Charnley. Acta Orthop. Scand., 48:650, 1977.

23. Casagrande, P.A., and Danahy, P.R.: Delayed sciatic-nerve entrapment following the use of self-curing acrylic. J. Bone Joint Surg., 53A:167, 1971.

24. Chandler, R.W., Dorr, L.D., and Perry, T.: Dislocation following total hip arthroplasty: Function and cost analysis. J. Bone Joint Surg. (in press).

25. Chao, E.Y.S., and Coventry, M.D.: Fracture of the femoral component after total hip replacement: An analysis of fifty-eight cases. J. Bone Joint Surg., 63A:1078, 1981.

26. Charnley, J.: Total hip replacement by low friction arthroplasty. Clin. Orthop. Rel. Res., 72:7, 1970.

27. ———: Long term results of low friction arthroplasty of the hip performed as a primary intervention. J. Bone Joint Surg., 54B:61, 1972.

28. ———: Fracture of femoral prostheses in total hip replacement: A clinical study. Clin. Orthop. Rel. Res., 111:150, 1975.

29. ———: Low-Friction Arthroplasty of the Hip. New York: Springer-Verlag, 1979.

30. Charnley, J., and Cupic, Z.: The nine and ten year results of the low friction arthroplasty of the hip. Clin. Orthop. Rel. Res., 95:11, 1973.

31. Charnley, J., and Eftekhar, N.: Post-operative infection in total prosthetic replacement arthroplasty of the hip joint with special reference to the bacterial content of the air of the operating room. Br. J. Surg., 56:641, 1969.

32. Charnley, J., Follacci, F.M., and Hammond, B.T.: The long-term reaction of bone to self-curing acrylic cement. J. Bone Joint Surg., 50B:882, 1968.

33. Charvosky, C.B., Bullough, P.G., and Wilson, P.D.: Total hip replacement failures. J. Bone Joint Surg., 55A:49, 1973.

34. Clarke, I.C., Black, K., Rennie, C., and Amstutz, H.C.: Can wear in total hip arthroplasties be assessed from radiographs. Clin. Orthop. Rel. Res., 121:126, 1976.

35. Cobden, R.C., Thrasher, E.L., and Harris, W.H.: Topical hemostatic agents to reduce bleeding from cancellous bone. J. Bone Joint Surg., 58A:70, 1976.

36. Collis, D.K.: Femoral stem fracture in total hip replacement. J. Bone Joint Surg., 59A:1033, 1977.

37. Convery, F.R., Gunn, D.R., Hughes, J.D., and Martin, W.E.: The relative safety of polymethylmethacrylate: A controlled clinical study of randomly selected patients treated with Charnley and Ring total hip replacements. J. Bone Joint Surg., 57A:57, 1975.

38. Copher, G.H., and Illingworth, C.R.W.: Mechanism of emptying of the gallbladder and common duct. Surg. Gynecol. Obstet., 46:459, 1928.

39. Couch, N.: Personal communication, 1976.

40. Coventry, M.B.: The treatment of fracture-dislocation of the hip by total hip arthroplasty. J. Bone Joint Surg., 56A:1128, 1974.

41. Coventry, M.B., Beckenbaugh, R.D., Nolan, D.R. et al.: 2012 total hip arthroplasties: A study of postoperative course and early complications. J. Bone Joint Surg., 65A:273, 1974.

42. Coventry, M.B., and Scanlon, P.W.: The use of

radiation to discourage ectopic bone. J. Bone Joint Surg., 63A:201, 1981.

43. Cruess, R.L., Beckel, W.S., and vonKessler, K.L.C.: Infections in total hips secondary to primary source elsewhere. Clin. Orthop. Rel. Res., 106:99, 1975.

44. D'Ambrosia, R., Shoii, H., and Heater, R.: Secondarily infected total joint replacements by hematogenous spread. J. Bone Joint Surg., 58A:450, 1976.

45. Dandy, D.J., and Theodorou, B.D.: The management of local complications of total hip replacement by the McKee-Farrar Technique. J. Bone Joint Surg., 58B:30, 1975.

46. Davis, N.J., Jennings, J.J., and Harris, W.H.: Induced hypotensive anesthesia for total hip replacement. Clin. Orthop. Rel. Res., 101:93, 1974.

47. DeLee, J.G., and Charnley, J.: Radiological evidence of demarcation. Clin. Orthop. Rel. Res., 121:20, 1976.

48. DeLee, J.G., Ferrari, A., and Charnley, J.: Ectopic bone following low friction arthroplasty of the hip. Clin. Orthop. Rel. Res., 121:53, 1976.

49. Denham, R.A.: Hip mechanics. J. Bone Joint Surg., 41B:550, 1959.

50. DiPisa, J.A., Sih, G.S., and Buman, A.T.: The temperature problem at the bone–acrylic cement interface of the total hip replacement. Clin. Orthop. Rel. Res., 121:95, 1976.

51. Downes, E.M.: Late infection after total hip replacement. J. Bone Joint Surg., 59B:42, 1977.

52. Ducheyne, P., Aernoudt, E., and Martens, M. et al.: An analysis of femoral component of Charnley and Charnley-Muller type total hip prostheses. J. Biomed. Mater. Res., 9:199, 1975.

53. Dunn, K.H., and Hess, W.E.: Total hip reconstruction in chronically dislocated hips. J. Bone Joint Surg., 58A:838, 1976.

54. Eftekhar, N.S.: Dislocation and instability complicating low-friction arthroplasty of the hip joint. Clin. Orthop. Rel. Res., 121:120, 1976.

55. ———: Principles of Total Hip Arthroplasty. St. Louis, CV Mosby, 1978.

56. Eftekhar, N.S., and Stinchfield, F.E.: Experience with low friction arthroplasty: A statistical review of early results and complications. Clin. Orthop. Rel. Res., 95:60, 1973.

57. ———: Total replacement of the hip joint by low-friction arthroplasty. Orthop. Clin. North Am., 4(2):483, 1973.

58. Ellis, R.H., and Mulvein, J.: The cardiovascular effects of methylmethacrylate. J. Bone Joint Surg., 56B:59, 1974.

59. English, T.A.: The trochanteric approach to the hip for prosthetic replacement. J. Bone Joint Surg., 57A:1128, 1975.

60. Ericson, V., Lidgreen, L., and Lindberg, L.: Cloxacillin in the prophylaxis of post-operative infections of the hip. J. Bone Joint Surg., 55A:808, 1973.

61. Etienne, A., Cupic, Z., and Charnley, J.: Postoperative dislocation after Charnley low-friction arthroplasty. Clin. Orthop. Rel. Res., 132:19, 1978.

62. Evans, E.M., Freeman, M.A.R., Miller, A.J., and

Vernon-Roberts, B.: Metal sensitivity as a cause of bone necrosis and loosening of the prosthesis in total joint replacement. J. Bone Joint Surg., 56B:626, 1973.

63. Evanski, P.M., and Waugh, T.R.: Total hip replacement with the Charnley prosthesis. Clin. Orthop. Rel. Res., 95:69, 1973.

64. Evarts, C.M., and Feil, E.I.: Thromboembolism after elective surgery of the hip. Orthop. Clin. North Am., 2:167, 1971.

65. Fackler, C.K., and Poss, R.: Dislocation in total hip arthroplasties. Clin. Orthop. Rel. Res., 151:169, 1980.

66. Feith, R., Slooff, T.J.J.H., Kazem, I., and Van Remo, T.J.G.: Strontium ^{87m}Sr bone scanning for the evaluation of total hip replacement. J. Bone Joint Surg., 58B:79, 1976.

67. Finerman, G., Gonick, H.C., Smith, R.K., and Mayfield, J.M.: Diphosphonate treatment of Paget's disease. Clin. Orthop. Rel. Res., 120:115, 1976.

68. Fitzgerald, R.H., Jr., Peterson, L.F.A., Washington, J.A. II et al.: Bacterial colonization of wounds and sepsis in total hip arthroplasty. J. Bone Joint Surg., 55A:1242, 1973.

69. Fleisch, H., Russell, R.G.G., Bisax, S. et al.: The inhibitory effect of phosphonates on the formation of calcium phosphate crystals *in vitro* and on aortic and kidney calcification *in vivo*. Eur. J. Clin. Invest. 1:12, 1970.

70. Fleming, R.E., Michelsen, C.B., and Stinchfield, F.E.: Sciatic paralysis: A complication of bleeding following hip surgery. J. Bone Joint Surg., 61A:37, 1979.

71. Fogelberg, E.V., Zitamann, E.K., and Stinchfield, F.E.: Prophylactic penicillin in orthopaedic surgery. J. Bone Joint Surg., 52A:95, 1970.

72. Fornasier, V.L., and Cameron, H.U.: The femoral stem–cement interface in total hip replacement. Clin. Orthop. Rel. Res., 116:249, 1976.

73. Fremont-Smith, P.: Antibiotic management of the septic total hip replacement: A therapeutic trial. In The Hip: Proceedings of the Third Open Meeting of The Hip Society, p. 301. St. Louis, CV Mosby, 1974.

74. ————: Sepsis and total hip replacement. In The Hip: Proceedings of the Second Open Scientific Meeting of The Hip Society, pp. 301–308. St. Louis, CV Mosby, 1974.

75. Galante, J.O., Rostoker, W., and Doyle, J.M.: Failed femoral stems in total hip prostheses: A report of six cases. J. Bone Joint Surg., 57A:230, 1975.

76. Glenn, F.: Acute cholecystitis following the surgical treatment of unrelated disease. Ann. Surg., 126:477, 1947.

77. Glenn, F., and Wartz, G.E.: Acute cholecystitis following the surgical treatment of unrelated disease. Surg. Gynecol. Obstet., 102:145, 1956.

78. Greenwald, A.S., and Nelson, C.L.: Biomechanics of the reconstructed hip. Orthop. Clin. North Am., 4:435, 1973.

79. Gruen, T.S., McNeice, G.M., and Amstutz, H.C.: Modes of failure of cemented stem type femoral components—a radiographic analysis of loosening. Clin. Orthop. Rel. Res., 141:17, 1979.

80. Hallel, T., Salvati, E.A., and Botero, P.M.: Polymethylmethacrylate in the knee. J. Bone Joint Surg., 58A:556, 1976.

81. Harris, W.H.: Personal communication.

82. Harris, W.H.: A new approach to total hip replacement without osteotomy of the greater trochanter. Clin. Orthop. Rel. Res., 106:19, 1975.

83. Harris, W.H.: Total hip replacement for congenital dysplasia of the hip: Technique. In The Hip: Proceedings of the Second Open Scientific Meeting of the Hip Society, pp. 251–265. St. Louis, CV Mosby, 1974.

84. Harris, W.H., Salzman, E.W., Athanasoulis, C. et al.: Comparison of warfarin, low molecular weight dextran, aspirin and subcutaneous heparin in prevention of venous thromboembolism following total hip arthroplasty. J. Bone Joint Surg., 56A:1552, 1974.

85. Harris, W.H., Salzman, E.W., and DeSanctis, R.W.: The prevention of thromboembolic disease by prophylactic anticoagulation. J. Bone Joint Surg., 49A:81, 1967.

86. Harris, W.H., Shiller, A.L., Scholler, J.M. et al.: Extensive localized bone resorption in the femur following total hip replacement. J. Bone Joint Surg., 58A:612, 1976.

87. Hoffman, E.: Acute gangrenous cholecystitis secondary to trauma. Am. J. Surg., 91:288, 1956.

88. Hume, M.: Thromboembolic complications in revision arthroplasty. In Turner, R.H., and Scheller, A.D. (eds.): Revision Total Hip Arthroplasty. New York, Grune & Stratton, 1982.

89. Irvine, R., Johns, B.L., Jr., and Amstutz, H.C.: The relationship of genitourinary tract procedures and deep sepsis after total hip replacement. Surg. Gynecol. Obstet., 139:701, 1974.

90. Jeffries, C.K., Lee, A.J.C., and Ling, R.S.M.: Thermal aspects of self-curing polymethylmethacrylate. J. Bone Joint Surg., 57B:511, 1975.

91. Johanssen, J.E., McBrun, R., Barring, T.W. et al.: Fracture of the ipsilateral femur in patients with total hip replacement. J. Bone Joint Surg., 63A:1435, 1981.

92. Jones, D.A., Lucas, H.K., O'Driscoll, M. et al.: Cobalt toxicity after McKee hip arthroplasty. J. Bone Joint Surg., 57B:289, 1975.

93. Jowsey, J., Coventry, M.B., and Robins, P.R.: Heterotopic ossification: Theoretical consideration, possible etiologic factors and a clinical review of total hip arthroplasty patients exhibiting this phenomenon. In The Hip: Proceedings of the Fifth Open Scientific Meeting of The Hip Society, pp. 210–221. St. Louis, CV Mosby, 1977.

94. Judet, R., Judet, J., and LeTournel, E.: Fractures of the acetabulum: Classification and surgical approaches for open reduction. J. Bone Joint Surg., 46A:1615, 1964.

95. Khan, M.A.A., Bruckenbury, P.H., and Reynolds, I.S.R.: Dislocation following total hip replacement. J. Bone Joint Surg., 63B:214, 1981.

96. Knudson, R.J., and Zuber, W.F.: Acute cholecystitis in the postoperative period. N. Eng. J. Med., 269:289, 1963.

97. Koide, M., Pilon, R.N., VanDam, L., and Lowell, J.D.: Anesthetic experience with total hip replacement. Clin. Orthop. Rel. Res., 99:78, 1974.

98. Laks, H. et al.: Acute hemodilution: Its effect on hemodynamics and oxygen transport in anesthetized man. Ann. Surg., 180:103, 1974.
99. Lawson, N.W., Thompson, D.S., Nelson, C.L. et al.: Sodium nitroprusside-induced hypotension for supine total hip replacement. Anesth. Analg., 55:654, 1976.
100. Lazansky, M.: Complications revisited: The debit side of total hip replacement. Clin. Orthop. Rel. Res., 95:96, 1973.
101. Levin, P.D.: The effectiveness of various antibiotics in methylmethacrylate. J. Bone Joint Surg., 57B:235, 1975.
102. Lewinnik, G.E., Lewis, J.L., Tarr, R. et al.: Dislocations after total hip replacement. Clin. Orthop. Rel. Res., 95:96, 1973.
103. Lidwell, O.M., Lowbury, E.J.L., White, W. et al.: Effect of ultraclean air in operating rooms on deep sepsis in the joint after total hip or knee replacement: A randomized study. Br. Med. J., 285:10, 1982.
104. Lowell, J.D.: Complications of total hip replacement. Instr. Course Lect., 24:209, 1975.
105. ———: Complications of total hip replacement. In The Hip: Proceedings of the Fourth Open Scientific Meeting of The Hip Society, pp. 224–245. St. Louis, CV Mosby, 1976.
106. Lowell, J.D., and Davies, J.A.K.: Bladder fistula following total hip replacement using self-curing acrylic. Clin. Orthop. Rel. Res., 111:131, 1975.
107. Mallory, T.H.: Rupture of the common iliac vein from reaming the acetabulum during total hip replacement: A case report. J. Bone Joint Surg., 54A:276, 1972.
108. ———: Sepsis in total hip arthroplasty following pneumococcosis pneumonia. J. Bone Joint Surg., 55A:1753, 1973.
109. Markolf, K.L., and Amstutz, H.C.: *In vitro* measurement of bone–acrylic interface pressure during femoral compound insulation. Clin. Orthop. Rel. Res., 121:60, 1976.
110. ———: Penetration and flow of acrylic bone cement. Clin. Orthop. Rel. Res., 121:99, 1976.
111. Marks, K.W., Nelson, C.L., and Lautenschlayer, E.P.: Antibiotic impregnated bone cement. J. Bone Joint Surg., 58A:358, 1976.
112. Marmor, L.: Femoral loosening in total hip replacement. Clin. Orthop. Rel. Res., 121:116, 1976.
113. ———: Stress fracture of the pubic ramus simulating a loose total hip replacement. Clin. Orthop. Rel. Res., 121:103, 1976.
114. Matos, M., Amstutz, H.C., and Finerman, G.: Myositis ossificans following total hip replacement. J. Bone Joint Surg., 57A:137, 1975.
115. McElfresh, E.C., and Coventry, M.B.: Femoral and pelvic fractures after total hip arthroplasty. J. Bone Joint Surg., 56A:483, 1974.
116. McKee, G.K., and Chen, S.C.: The statistics of the McKee-Farrar method of total hip replacement. Clin. Orthop. Rel. Res., 95:26, 1974.
117. Miley, G.B., Scheller, A.D., Jr., and Turner, R.H.: Medical and surgical treatment of the septic hip with one-stage revision arthroplasty. Clin. Orthop. Rel. Res., 170:76, October 1982.
118. Miller, A.J.: Late fracture of the acetabulum after total hip replacement. J. Bone Joint Surg., 45B:600, 1972.
119. Moller, K., Steady, H.M. et al.: Blood conservation in revision arthroplasty. In Turner, R.H., and Scheller, A.D. (eds.): Revision Total Hip Arthroplasty, pp. 343–357. New York, Grune & Stratton, 1982.
120. Muller, M.E.: Preservation of septic total hip replacement versus Girdlestone operation. In The Hip: Proceedings of the Second Open Scientific Meeting of The Hip Society. St. Louis, CV Mosby, 1974.
121. Murray, M.P., Gore, D.R., Brewer, B.J. et al.: Comparison of functional performance after McKee-Farrar, Charnley and Muller total hip replacement. Clin. Orthop. Rel. Res., 121:33, 1976.
122. Murray, W.R.: Results in patients with total hip arthroplasty. Clin. Orthop. Rel. Res., 95:80, 1973.
123. ———: Treatment of deep wound infection after total hip arthroplasty. American Academy of Orthopaedic Surgeons Symposium on Osteoarthritis, pp. 123–131. St. Louis, CV Mosby, 1976.
124. ———: Prophylactic use of antibiotic cement. Syllabus of the Second American Orthopaedic Association International Hip Symposium, Boston, 1981.
125. Murray, W.R., and Rodrigo, J.J.: Arthrography for the assessment of pain after total hip replacement. J. Bone Joint Surg., 57A:1060, 1976.
126. Nelson, C.L., Evarts, C.M., Andrish, J., and Marks, K.E.: Infected total hip replacement—results and complications. J. Bone Joint Surg., 57A:1025, 1975.
127. Nelson, C.L., and Schurmann, D.J.: Preventive antibiotics. Instr. Course Lect., 30:1981.
128. Nicholson, O.R.: Failed femoral stems in total hip prostheses. Proceedings of the New Zealand Orthopaedic Association. J. Bone Joint Surg., 58B:262, 1976.
129. Nolan, D.R., Fitzgerald, R.H., Beckenbaugh, R.D., and Coventry, M.B.: Complications of total hip arthroplasty treated by re-operation. J. Bone Joint Surg., 57A:977, 1975.
130. Nollen, A.J.G., and Slooff, T.J.J.H.: Para-articular ossifications after total hip replacement. Acta Orthop. Scand., 44:230, 1973.
131. Oppenheim, W.L., Harley, J.D., and Lippert, F.G. III: Arteriographic measurement of post-operative bleeding following major hip surgery. J. Bone Joint Surg., 58A:127, 1975.
132. Parker, H.B., Wiesman, H.G., Ewald, R.C. et al.: Comparison of preoperative, intraoperative and early postoperative total hip replacements with and without trochanteric osteotomy. Clin. Orthop. Rel. Res., 121:44, 1976.
133. Pellicci, P.M., Salvati, E.A., and Robinson, A.J.: Mechanical failures in total hip replacements requiring re-operation. J. Bone Joint Surg., 61A:28, 1979.
134. Pollard, J.P., Hughes, S.P.F., Scott, J.E. et al.: Antibiotic prophylaxis in total hip replacement. Br. Med. J., 1:707, 1979.

135. Rang, M.: Anthology of Orthopaedics, Part 5, pp. 195–202. Edinburgh, E&S Livingston, 1966.

136. Riegler, H.R., and Harris, C.M.: Heterotopic bone formation after total hip arthroplasty. Clin. Orthop. Rel. Res., 117:209, 1976.

137. Ring, E.J., Athanasoulis, C., Waltman, A.C. et al.: Arteriographic management of hemorrhage following pelvic fracture. Radiology, 109:65, 1973.

138. Ring, E.J., Waltman, A.C., and Athanasoulis, C.: Angiography in pelvic trauma. Surg. Gynecol. Obstet., 139:375, 1974.

139. Ring, P.A.: Total replacement of hip joint: A review of 1000 operations. J. Bone Joint Surg., 56B:44, 1974.

140. Ritter, M.A.: Dislocation and subluxation of the total hip replacement. Clin. Orthop. Rel. Res., 121:92, 1976.

141. ———: A treatment plan for the dislocated total hip replacement. Clin. Orthop. Rel. Res., 153: 153, 1980.

142. ———: Personal communication, 1981.

143. Robertson, R.D.: Noncalculous acute cholecystitis following surgery, trauma and illness. Am. Surgeon, 36:610, 1970.

144. Rostoker, W., Chao, E.Y., and Galante, J.O.: Defects in failed stems of hip prostheses. J. Biomed. Mater. Res., 121:635, 1978.

145. Rubin, R., Salvati, E.A., and Lewis, R.: Infected total hip replacement procedures. Oral Surg., 41: 18, 1976.

146. Salvati, E.A.: Infection complicating total hip replacement. In The Hip: Proceedings of the Fourth Open Scientific Meeting of The Hip Society, pp. 200–218. St. Louis, CV Mosby, 1976.

147. Salvati, E.A., Im, V.S., Aglietti, P., and Wilson, P.D., Jr.: Radiology in total hip replacements. Clin. Orthop. Rel. Res., 121:74, 1976.

148. Salzman, E.W., and Harris, W.H.: Prevention of venous thromboembolism in orthopedic patients. J. Bone Joint Surg., 58A:903, 1976.

149. Scales, J.T.: Fractures of the femoral component—the need for fatigue studies. Presented at the 42nd Annual Meeting of the American Academy of Orthopaedic Surgeons, San Francisco, 1975.

150. Scheller, A.D., Mitchell, S., and Barber, F.C.: Femoral component fracture in revision hip arthroplasty. In Turner, R.H., and Scheller, A.D. (eds.): Revision Total Hip Arthroplasty. New York, Grune & Stratton, 1982.

151. Schurmann, D.J., Hirshman, H.I.P., and Burton, D.P.: Cephalothin and cefamandole penetration into bone, synovial fluid and wound drainage fluid. J. Bone Joint Surg., 62A:981, 1980.

152. Schwegman, C.W., and DeMuth, W.E.: Acute cholecystitis following operation for unrelated disease. Surg. Gynecol. Obstet., 97:167, 1953.

153. Scott, R.D., and Schilz, J.P.: Femoral fracture in revision arthroplasty. In Turner, R.H., and Scheller, A.D. (eds): Revision Total Hip Arthroplasty, pp. 113–139. New York, Grune & Stratton, 1982.

154. Scott, R.D., and Turner, R.H.: Avoiding complications with long stem total hip replacement arthroplasty. J. Bone Joint Surg., 57A:722, 1975.

155. Scott, R.D., Turner, R.H., Leitzes, S., and Aufranc, O.E.: Femoral fractures in conjunction with total hip replacement. J. Bone Joint Surg., 57A:494, 1975.

156. Sellergren, K.R., and Scheller, A.D.: Total hip instability in revision arthroplasty. In Turner, R.H., and Scheller, A.D. (eds.): Revision Total Hip Arthroplasty, pp. 265–288. New York, Grune & Stratton, 1982.

157. Sherr, D.D., and Dodd, T.A.: *In vitro* instability in bacteriological evaluation of the effectiveness of antimicrobial irrigating solutions. J. Bone Joint Surg., 58A:119, 1976.

158. Simon, S.R., Paul, I.L., Rose, R.M., and Radin, E.L.: "Stiction-friction" of total hip protheses and its relationship to loosening. J. Bone Joint Surg., 57A:226, 1975.

159. Slatis, P., Kiviluoto, O., and Santavirta, S.: Ectopic ossification after hip arthroplasty. Ann. Chir. Gynaecol., 67:89, 1978.

160. Spenglar, D.M., Costenbader, M., and Bailey, R.: Fat embolism syndrome following total hip arthroplasty. Clin. Orthop. Rel. Res., 121:105, 1976.

161. Stauffer, R.N., and Sim, R.H.: Total hip arthroplasty in Paget's disease of the hip. J. Bone Joint Surg., 58A:476, 1976.

162. Stern, M.B., and Spiegel, P.: Femoral neuropathy as a complication of anticoagulation therapy. Clin. Orthop. Rel. Res., 106:140, 1975.

163. Stinchfield, F.E.: Editorial comment: Total hip replacement. Clin. Orthop. Rel. Res., 95:2, 1973.

164. Stinchfield, F.E., Bigliana, L.U., Neu, H.C. et al.: Late hematogenous infection of total joint replacement. J. Bone Joint Surg., 62A:1345, 1980.

165. Stinson, J.T., and Scheller, A.D.: Clinical evaluation of the symptomatic total hip replacement. In Turner, R.H., and Scheller, A.D. (eds.): Revision Total Hip Arthroplasty. New York, Grune & Stratton, 1982.

166. Swanson, S.A.V., Freeman, M.A.R., and Heath, J.C.: Laboratory tests on total joint replacement prostheses. J. Bone Joint Surg., 55B:759, 1973.

167. Taylor, M.M., Myers, M.H., and Harvey, J.P.: Intraoperative femur fractures during total hip replacement. Clin. Orthop. Rel. Res., 137:96, 1978.

168. Taylor, R.G.: Pseudarthrosis of the hip joint. J. Bone Joint Surg., 32B:161, 1950.

169. Thompson, J.W., Ferris, P.O., and Baggenstoss, A.A.: Acute cholecystitis complicating operation for other diseases. Ann. Surg., 155:489, 1962.

170. Thompson, R.C., and Culver, J.E.: The role of trochanteric osteotomy in total hip replacement. Clin. Orthop. Rel. Res., 106:102, 1975.

171. Tronzo, R., Kallos, T., and Wycke, J.O.: Elevation of intramedullary pressure when methylmethacrylate is inserted in total hip arthroplasty. J. Bone Joint Surg., 56A:714, 1974.

172. Turner, R.H., and Emerson, R.H.: Femoral revision total hip arthroplasty. In Turner, R.H., and Scheller, A.D. (eds.): Revision Total Hip Arthroplasty, pp. 75–107. New York, Grune & Stratton, 1982.

173. Turner, R.H., Miley, G.B., and Fremont-Smith, P.: Septic total hip replacement and revision arthroplasty. In Turner, R.H., and Scheller, A.D. (eds.): Revision Total Hip Replacement. New York, Grune & Stratton, 1982.

174. Volz, R.G., and Turner, R.H.: Reattachment of the greater trochanter in total hip arthroplasty. J. Bone Joint Surg., 56A:92, 1974.

175. Walker, P.S., Salvati, E., and Hotzler, R.K.: The wear on removed McKee-Farrar total hip prostheses. J. Bone Joint Surg., 56A:92, 1976.

176. Weber, E.R., Daube, J.R., and Coventry, M.: Peripheral neuropathies associated with total hip arthroplasty. J. Bone Joint Surg., 58A:66, 1976.

177. Weber, F.A., and Charnley, J.: A radiological study of fractures of acrylic cement in relation to the stem of a femoral head prosthesis. J. Bone Joint Surg., 57B:197, 1975.

178. Weinstein, A.M., Bingham, D.N., Sauer, B.W., and Lunceford, E.M.: The effect of high pressure insertion and antibiotic inclusions upon the mechanical properties of polymethylmethacrylate. Clin. Orthop. Rel. Res., 121:67, 1976.

179. Welch, R.B., and Charnley, J.: Low friction arthroplasty of the hip in rheumatoid arthritis and ankylosing spondylitis. Clin. Orthop. Rel. Res., 72:22, 1970.

180. Wetzner, S.M., Newberg, A.H., and McKenzie, J.D.: Radiographic evaluation of the symptomatic hip replacement. In Turner, R.H., and Scheller, A.D. (eds.): Revision Total Hip Arthroplasty. New York, Grune & Stratton, 1982.

181. Willerty, H.G., Ludwig, J., and Semlitsch, M.: Reaction of bone to methacrylate after hip arthroplasty: A long term gross light microscopic and scanning electron microscope study. J. Bone Joint Surg., 65A:1368, 1974.

182. Wilson, P.D., Jr., Aglietti, P., and Salvati, E.A.: Subacute sepsis of the hip treated by antibiotics and cemented prosthesis. J. Bone Joint Surg., 56A:879, 1974.

183. Wilson, P.D., Jr., Amstutz, H.C., Czeriecki, A. et al.: Total hip replacement by acrylic cement. J. Bone Joint Surg., 54A:207, 1972.

184. Winegarner, F.G., and Jackson, G.F.: Post-traumatic acalculous cholecystitis: A highly lethal complication. J. Trauma, 116:567, 1971.

185. Woo, R.G., and Morrey, D.F.: Dislocations after total hip arthroplasty. J. Bone Joint Surg., 65A(9): 1295, 1982.

36 Complications of Total and Partial Arthroplasty in the Knee

William P. Fortune

As we review the first 14 years of total knee arthroplasty and analyze the unacceptable results, we are led to a better understanding of the clinical deformities that present for correction. A more comprehensive understanding of the complex interrelationships among the soft tissue elements about the knee, the material development and design characteristics of the prostheses, and the improvements in surgical technique and postoperative management have combined to allow better surgical care.

The indications and contraindications for total knee surgery are now well established, particularly with regard to the two main areas of knee arthroplasty: surface replacement (as represented by the least constrained types of systems) and that of the linked or articulated prosthesis (represented by those systems requiring some type of inherent connection between the articulating components).[9,47,94,108] The first group, that employing unlinked surface replacement systems, comprises approximately 80% to 85% of all implanted total knee arthroplasties. Within this group, approximately 50% of the systems involve cruciate-sacrificing prostheses, and the balance involve cruciate-retaining prostheses.[60,101,103] Currently, the 15% to 20% of knees requiring a linked system are repaired with either the spherocentric or the kinematic rotating hinge prostheses. These devices are used primarily in salvage procedures in patients in whom significant loss of bone substance and soft tissue laxity are present.

The question of cruciate-retaining versus cruciate-sacrificing systems is unanswered at this time.[47,101] So far, the results do not offer any conclusive evidence on the efficacy of retention or removal. The era of biologic fixation is now upon us. The preliminary information appears to support this approach. However, as with the antecedent three generations of total knee arthroplasties, the indications for knee replacement surgery will become broadened and modified with time.

An attempt has been made in the second edition of this volume to add, at appropriate places within the body of this chapter, pertinent material from the literature and personal experience that will make it current with our present knowledge and the state of the art.

HISTORICAL BACKGROUND

The dawn of replacement arthroplasty came in 1891, in Berlin, when Thermistocles Gluck constructed an ivory ball-and-socket hip joint and attempted to achieve fixation with an adhesive material composed of colophony, pumice powder, and plaster of paris.[38] He is therefore considered to be the pioneer of total joint replacement using a luting agent for cement fixation. The problem of biologic tolerance of metallic substances, coupled with the need for adequate fixation, led early investigators trying to solve the problem of the arthritic knee to use the hinge for motion and medullary stems for fixation.

Walldius, in 1951, was the first to replace the tibiofemoral joint with an acrylic–metallic hinge prosthesis, which was subsequently modified to an entirely metal-to-metal prosthesis made of cobalt, chromium, and molybdenum alloy.[110] In 1952 Sir Herbert Seddon implanted the first Stanmore knee prosthesis in a patient with hydatid disease of the lower third of the femur.[92] In 1954 Shiers reported his first experiences with his original hinge prosthesis for severe arthritis of the knee.[96]

The early successes with these and other

hinged prosthetic implants led to improvements and refinements, but the hinge linkage caused impingement of the components (bone and soft tissues) because the normal polycentric action was replaced with a malpositioned single axis.

In 1958 Charnley, encouraged by Smith, introduced methyl methacrylate to the orthopaedic surgical world. The polymeric, self-curing acrylic cement acted as a mechanical filler or luting agent to hold an implanted prosthesis in position while dispersing mechanical stresses over a wider area.[17,18] In 1968 Gunston, using the acrylic cement, implanted the first condylar resurfacing system and thereby opened the "era of unlinked knee arthroplasty."[39]

The concept of condylar replacement allows for the duplication of anatomical knee relationships and the reestablishment of a more nearly normal polycentric action. The more closely the normal rotation, rocking, and gliding motions of the knee are reproduced by the unlinked system, the greater is the chance for maintaining proper tension in all of the complex ligament and soft tissue structures. To have full motion with stability the ligaments and supporting soft tissue structures must maintain a proper length–tension relationship. The recognition of this important principle of total knee replacement will prevent untimely problems and complications.

GENERAL OVERVIEW OF VARIOUS PROSTHESES

In 1984 I grouped the most commonly used systems available at that time into unlinked and linked groups.[30] The reason for this arrangement was, quite simply, to facilitate the choice of the most appropriate system for the particular knee problem at hand.

Total Knee Systems—1984

Unlinked
  Unicompartmental
    Unicondylar
    Modified Gunston
    Marmor
    Oxford

Unlinked (continued)
  Bicompartmental
    Cruciate-retaining
      Duopatellar
      Kinematic
      Anametric
      PCA
    Cruciate-sacrificing
      Total condylar
      ICLH
      Variable-axis
    Cruciate-substituting
      Kinematic stabilizer
      Total condylar III
Linked
  Modified hinge
    Kinematic rotating hinge
  Condylar-load-bearing intercondylar stabilizing mechanism
    Spherocentric

The unlinked group is divided into those systems that can resurface a single compartment and those that are designed for bicompartmental replacement (two-piece, metal–plastic condylar units). The indications for unicompartmental replacement are quite limited and still controversial. However, it is generally agreed that angular and flexion deformities of not more than 10° to 15° can be corrected with these systems.

When bicompartmental replacement is considered, the degree of deformity, bone loss, and soft tissue contractures must be critically evaluated prior to selecting a prosthetic system.

The obvious problem arises when a system that employs four separate components is considered. The chance of error in positioning increases. As the degree of deformity increases, systems that offer more stability must be used. As a result of this consideration, I further divided the bicompartmental group into three subgroups. The first group includes systems that allow close-to-normal knee motion but require good bone stock, ligaments, and muscle control. It is generally agreed that these systems should be used in knees in which the angular and flexion deformities do not exceed 20°. This group includes the duopatellar (duocondylar) system.[86]

When stability is of greater concern, the systems that have more inherent stability within their bearing surfaces should be considered. Condylar metal-to-plastic replacement prostheses, such as the total condylar (Hospital for Special Surgery), possess this quality. In my opinion, these systems should be considered when angular deformities greater than 20° to 25° are present and when flexion deformities of similar magnitudes are present.

All of these prostheses have been used successfully to correct severe angular and flexion deformities—some on the order of 50° valgus, 35° varus, and 70° flexion.

The great value of these systems is that they allow for the reestablishment of the proper tension–length relationship of the soft tissue elements of the knee to bone and still maintain polycentric action. However, a great deal of experience and clinical judgment are required for their proper and optimal use, and correct patient selection is absolutely critical.

The indications for linked prostheses are, in my view, changing as we gain more experience with the more stable metal-to-plastic condylar systems. I believe, however, that the GUEPAR prosthesis is the most desirable of the hinge prostheses now available.

The prostheses that employ condylar load bearing with some form of intercondylar stabilizing mechanism[74,109] may, in my opinion, replace the need for a hinge prosthesis. However, the problems of bone removal and fixation that have plagued the Walldius and other hinges may also detract from the use of some of these systems. An example is the spherocentric system, which requires massive reaming of the distal femur. My experience with this system is limited, but to date it has been satisfactory over a 10-year period. The linked systems nonetheless offer a salvage arthroplasty for those knees that are devoid of all ligament control and have substantial bone loss.

Our experience now spans 33 years with the hinge, 16 years with the Gunston (polycentric), and 14 years with some of the two-piece, metal-to-plastic condylar units, such as the geometric, UCI, duocondylar, and Freeman-Swanson. During this time, thousands of patients have realized benefits from these advancements, but problems and complications continue to frustrate our attempt to realize a successful result for all patients.

Many complications can be avoided by careful planning and attention to detail, while other problems seem to persist no matter how diligent the surgeon and his team are in trying to prevent them. In reviewing the literature and analyzing the results of our own experience, it becomes clear that several factors are important in the manifestation of complications of total knee arthroplasty.

Causes of Complications in Total Knee Arthroplasty

Time relationship to surgery
Previous surgical procedures
Soft tissue problems
Metabolic problems
Patient selection
Prosthesis selection
Errors of insertion technique
Deficiencies of prosthesis design
Hard tissue (bone) problems
Failure of the prosthesis
Failure of cement–bone fixation

Arden, reporting in 1974 on 160 patients who had undergone Shiers hinge knee arthroplasties, divided his complications into early and late.[5] Though this is accepted as the proper method of reporting problems, it also has some logic other than the obvious time sequence that attends the recognition of complications. The majority of early complications are usually related to soft tissue manifestations. Though some late complications are related to soft tissue, they are primarily associated with bone, cement, and prosthesis failures. I have therefore attempted in this review to summarize these complications from this perspective.

EARLY SOFT TISSUE COMPLICATIONS OF TOTAL KNEE ARTHROPLASTY

Infection

Infection is probably the most feared complication to any surgeon, and even more so to the surgeon who attempts arthroplastic replacement of a knee. Walldius reported on his first 51 patients in 1957; eight patients developed infections, one died of septicemia, one required an amputation, and six required arthrodesis following infection (a 15.5% infection rate).[110] His report in 1960 reviewed a total of 93 patients, and the rate of infection was still alarming.[111] Jones reported in 1971 on his first 80 Walldius hinge arthroplasties; eight patients required removal of the prosthesis and arthrodesis for infection.[50] He reported one more infection after reviewing 120 knees, giving a 7.5% rate of primary deep infections.[51] Arden reported a 3.5% infection rate in 148 patients with 192 Shiers knee arthroplasties.[4,5]

Witvoët and co-workers reviewed 210 GUEPAR prostheses and found a 5% deep infection rate.[118] In seven cases revision was done immediately with irrigation, debridement, and synovectomy, where indicated. Four of the seven were salvaged, and three went to fusion. In two cases arthrodesis was performed immediately. One patient had a fistula with an associated loose prosthesis and required a revision with complete salvage. All of the patients were placed on appropriate antibiotics and remained on them until the wounds and the sedimentation rates returned to normal.

Ranawat, reviewing 415 total knee arthroplasties of different types, found a 1.4% combined immediate and delayed deep infection rate. However, a review by Ranawat of 233 total condylar arthroplasties showed an early infection rate of 0.5%, and only two of 233 patients developed late deep infections. He also reported a 12% deep infection rate in the GUEPAR group.*

Lynch reported in 1974 on a review of 117 total knee replacements (polycentric, geometric, and Walldius) and encountered one infection, which was recognized within 2 weeks of surgery. It was debrided without further evidence of infection.[64] Freeman and co-workers had only one infection in their first 34 procedures, which resulted from delayed wound healing and required removal of the prosthesis.[36] Bryan and colleagues, reporting on the first 450 polycen-

tric knee arthroplasties at the Mayo Clinic, had six deep infections (0.01%).[14]

Coventry's group reported no deep infections in their first 261 cases.[23] However, Petty and co-workers reviewed 1045 patients followed longer than 1 year at the Mayo Clinic and found a 2.3% incidence of deep infection and a 0.02% incidence of superficial infection. Five of these involved geometric prostheses.[82]

In reviewing our first 120 unlinked arthroplasties at The George Washington University Hospital, we have had two deep infections. One required removal of the prosthesis and fusion; the other was salvaged after debridement, irrigation, and appropriate long-term antibiotic therapy.

Waugh found a deep infection rate of only 1% in his first 185 UCI total knee arthroplasties and suggested that the mean operating time of 80 minutes might be an important factor.[113] Siegal reviewed 260 Sledge prostheses ("St. Georg" design) and reexamined 192 patients.[99] There were two infections, both salvaged after reoperation and the addition of gentamicin to the Palacos cement. The addition of powdered antibiotic to methylmethacrylate may prove efficacious in the treatment of the infected total knee arthroplasty.[70]

Since the incidence of deep infection is still quite significant in many large series, we have developed a protocol based to some degree on our early experience with total hip replacement. The skin is washed three times a day for 48 hours prior to surgery with either povidone-iodine (Betadine) or pHisohex solution. The skin is shaved 2 hours before the procedure and only when necessary. Appropriate antibiotic prophylaxis is begun the evening before surgery, given during the procedure, and for 3 to 5 days after surgery. Opening and closing cultures are obtained, and the wound is irrigated periodically with a total of 3 liters of a bacitracin-polymyxin solution.[93] Care is taken not to traumatize the tissues, especially the skin, particularly with retractors and forceps. Traffic in and out of the operating room is controlled, though we do not use any special clean-airflow system. Postoperatively, the dressing and drains are changed at 48 hours, and povidone-iodine-soaked dressings are applied

---

* Ranawat, C.S.: Personal communication, May 1976.

for as long as there is serous drainage from the suture line or drain holes. This is done by sterile-gloved technique.

It does appear that the incidence of deep wound infection is less with the condylar metal-to-plastic systems, and this is no doubt related to alteration in our surgical procedures and the use of prophylactic antibiotics, wound lavage, and some type of environmental control. However, I believe that when early deep sepsis is noted within the first few weeks, vigorous surgical and medical efforts are indicated to attempt to save the arthroplasty. The experience now being recorded in the literature will substantiate this approach, which is similar to the action taken to salvage early infected total hip arthroplasties.

If infection persists or recurs after one attempt to salvage the arthroplasty, arthrodesis with either a Roger Anderson or a Charnley compression device is recommended, after debridement of the bone ends. Use of compression plates is not recommended.

Insall and colleagues, in reviewing the 1970s literature on total knee arthroplasties, reviewed 140 deep infections after 2997 total knee arthroplasties.[46,48] The recorded infection rate ranged from 0% to 23%, with an average of 5%. After salvage procedures in the 140 patients with an infected total knee arthroplasty, the prosthesis was retained in 49 (35%), removed from 65 (46%), and reimplanted in 11 (8%). Amputation was carried out in seven (5%), and eight (6%) patients died. As more total knee arthroplasties are performed, the number of deep infections can be expected to increase, even though the overall infection rate may be declining. Salvage of any joint, but particularly the infected total knee arthroplasty, will be a difficult problem at best. It is the conclusion of many authors that implantation of another prosthesis and treatment of infection of a total knee arthroplasty must be done with significant caution. Salvati and co-workers compared the infection rate after 3175 total hip and total knee replacements performed with and without the horizontal unidirectional filtered airflow system.[91] These authors found a reduction of the infection rate after total hip replacement from 1.4% to 0.9%

and an increase in the infection rate after total knee replacement from 1.4% to 3.9% when patients were operated on in filtered laminar airflow operating rooms. They found that this pattern was statistically significant and was believed to be due to the position of the operating team and of the wound with respect to the airflow. Prospectively accumulated factors (such as the experience of the surgeon, the duration of the surgery, the diagnosis, and the patient's age), as well as retrospectively accumulated factors (such as predisposing conditions of the patient), did not explain the observed patterns of infection. It was the feeling of the authors that during total knee replacement, members of the surgical team inevitably stand between the source of the horizontal laminar airflow and the open wound, whereas during total hip replacement, the procedure does not require the surgical team to come between the source of the laminar flow and the wound.

Rand and Bryan retrospectively reviewed the results of 14 patients in whom salvage of an acutely infected total knee arthroplasty was attempted by the implantation of a new prosthesis within 2 weeks of removal of the infected one.[15,87] Salvage was successful in six of the seven patients with low-virulence infections, but in only two of the seven patients with high-virulence infections. Of the eight patients for whom the result was a functioning prosthesis, two had significant restriction of motion, and one had moderate pain. If these three patients were eliminated from the analysis, the overall success rate was found to be only 35% (five of 14 patients). It was the conclusion of the authors that implantation of another prosthesis for the treatment of infection of a total knee arthroplasty should be done with great caution, as mentioned above, preferably when the infection has been caused by a low-grade organism and after a wait of longer than 2 weeks.

Insall and associates, reporting on their experience with two-stage reimplantation for the salvage of infected total knee arthroplasty, found that 11 two-stage reimplantations to salvage 11 infected total knee arthroplasties were evaluated after an average follow-up of 34 months. The staged procedures included removal of all of the components of the prosthesis and all ce- ment, then 6 weeks of parenteral antibiotic therapy (monitored by maintaining serum bactericidal levels at a peak dilution of 1:8), and, finally, reimplantation with a total condylar prosthesis. All antibiotics were discontinued after reimplantation. At follow-up, no patient had had a recurrence of the original infection, but one had a hematogenous infection with a different organism secondary to an infected bunion. The results after reimplantation were rated excellent in five knees, good in four, and fair in two. Weakness of the extensor mech- anism with an extension lag was the most common complication. It is my belief that antibiotic therapy alone is not adequate for the management of an infection around a prosthesis. The method that the authors describe appears to be effective, but it is costly and time consuming. The surgical procedures and medical management are technically difficult. Often, special equip- ment and custom-made prostheses may be required. As the authors point out, there are no shortcuts. Moreover, it is well known from experimental data that total joint re- placement employing polymethylmethac- rylate may very well impair local defense mechanisms and decrease the vitality of the surrounding tissues and their ability to de- fend against infection. The successful sal- vage of a total knee presents a major chal- lenge to the surgical team, and vigorous surgical and medical efforts are required to save the arthroplasty.

In reviewing their first 84 spherocentric arthroplasties, Matthews and Kaufer had a deep infection rate of 3.7%, which is com- parable to reported infection rates for sur- face arthroplasties and much superior to those reported for conventional hinge prostheses.[54,73] However, the authors point out that when deep infection occurs, it is a very serious complication in the linked sys- tem because of the extent of bone loss and foreign material present. All three patients with deep infections had their prostheses removed. One died, and one required an amputation to control the sepsis. Brause has pointed out that the hematogenous route is responsible for approximately 40% of the infections in major total joint re- placements.[12] Because an infection is cata-

strophic, prevention of the septic process is of considerable importance. Any possible cause of bacteremia with prosthetic joints should be avoided, and prophylactic anti- biotics must be administered in anticipation of bacteremic events.

Complications of Salvage Arthrodesis

In reporting on 23 primary knee ar- throdeses in patients with rheumatoid ar- thritis, Conaty observed that "no patient was truly unhappy with his arthrodesed knee and two patients expressed enthusiasm with the result." This tempered enthusiasm is reiterated by the experience of other authors reviewing knee arthrodesis in a similar patient population.[104,107] As a result of general dissatisfaction in terms of achieving fusion and the functional results once fusion is achieved, alternatives to ar- throdesis are often sought by the patient. Although a successful arthrodesis is fre- quently associated with significant func- tional improvement, adults with polyartic- ular disease often lack adaptability and compensation in adjacent joints. Attempts at arthrodesis require a significant amount of tenacity on the part of the patient and of the surgeon.

Although arthrodesis produces excellent stability, failure of arthrodesis following the removal of an infected total knee prosthesis has been reported to be on the order of at least 50% of cases. One significant func- tional problem with arthrodesis is the handicap that it produces when the knee is fused in complete extension.

The alternative to arthrodesis in the event of a failed total knee arthroplasty is resection arthroplasty, in which there is complete removal of the prosthesis–cement composite without an attempt to obtain arthrodesis.

Kaufer and Matthews reported on pa- tients in whom infected spherocentric knees were treated by debridement and removal of the prosthesis with no attempt at ar- throdesis.[53] The initial experience is quite meager; however, it includes a series of 20 resection arthroplasties in which the major- ity of patients were left with a functional extremity, good stability, and no arthrodesis.

Stulberg feels that there may be a role for the salvage of a failed total knee arthro- plasty in patients with polyarticular rheumatoid arthritis or in patients who require limited ambulation.[104]

To obtain function with a resection arthroplasty, a rather extended period of immobilization in a long leg cast or cast brace of 6 to 9 months following a resection arthroplasty is required to achieve strong fibrous ankylosis. Many patients with multiple joint involvement, particularly patients with rheumatoid arthritis who have compromised upper extremities, find this an unsuitable alternative to failed total knee arthroplasty. Many of these patients have significant loss in bone stock and attenuated soft tissue elements about the knee, and these factors tend to make the limb flail and unsuitable for weight bearing.[107]

In Kaufer and Matthews' experience with 20 patients who had undergone resection arthroplasty and were followed for more than 2 years, 80% were free of drainage at 1 year, while 20% had persistent intermittent drainage.[53] Fifteen of the 20 patients (75%) were reported to be satisfied with the functional results of the resection arthroplasty.

Superficial Skin Necrosis and Wound Dehiscence

In our 1973 report we found two superficial skin sloughs; one required a split graft, and one had a partial wound dehiscence.[31] At that time, we were using a standard medial parapatellar incision. Since then, a straight incision has been used, and we have not had any early or late local skin problems. This incision is almost midpatellar. Arden reported a 9.5% incidence with the Shiers prosthesis. However, he is now using a straight incision and avoids undermining the skin.[5]

Witvoët reported seven wound disruptions or secondary necroses in his initial series, and these were usually associated with patellectomy.[118] Skin necrosis and delayed healing increase the risk of infection, and the final range of motion is often suboptimal.

Walldius reported two cases of skin necrosis in his early series.[110] The initial 261 cases reported by the combined geometric group had three with wound dehiscence requiring knee fusion.[22] Many patients have had multiple surgical procedures on the knee, and these factors predispose the wound to poor healing, skin sloughs, and frank dehiscence.

Superficial skin necrosis was recorded in four patients in the early polycentric group at the Mayo Clinic. All had had previous cortisone treatments. To avoid this complication Bryan and co-workers recommend an almost straight incision.[14]

Hemorrhage and Hematoma

Hemorrhage and hematoma may lead to a deep infection, particularly if large. Many surgeons with extensive experience feel that the tourniquet should be released prior to closure and that all prominent bleeding points should be controlled. The major sources of bleeding in our experience are the raw cancellous bone surfaces, the base of the resected synovium, and especially the genicular vessels, particularly the lateral genicular artery.

A belo-pack drainage system with two drains is used routinely; the average drainage volume over a 48-hour period is approximately 300 ml (a range of 200 ml to 500 ml). The maximum drainage has been 1200 ml to 1500 ml, in three patients (two men with degenerative arthritis and one woman with rheumatoid disease). Each one drained approximately 1000 ml during the first 24 hours. We have seen one hematoma (in 120 patients) that required drainage; the patient's 48-hour drainage was 200 ml. However, approximately 500 ml of clot was removed subsequently without further complication. It has been our practice to release the tourniquet and obtain complete hemostasis prior to closure. We have not had any late bleeding problems related either to the procedure or to anticoagulation therapy.

Arden found that 18 of 160 patients (8%) had postoperative hematomas and suggested that the clots be evacuated.[4,5] Siegal, in his series of 260 Sledge prostheses, found it necessary to evacuate one postsurgical hematoma.[99]

Thrombophlebitis and Pulmonary Embolism

Thrombophlebitis and pulmonary embolism, a serious and life-threatening complication of venous thromboembolic disease, has been a concern to all orthopaedic surgeons. It is a common complication of many surgical procedures and injuries. Harris and colleagues, Evarts and Feil, and others have contributed a great deal of information to the world literature with regard to this problem as it relates to special surgical procedures about the hip.[28,43,44]

In a study of patients undergoing total knee surgery Lynch found a 48% incidence of silent phlebothrombosis.* Ranawat found that in his group of preoperative patients examined by venography the incidence of silent phlebothrombosis ranged from 40% to 50%.† Harris found that thrombi often form in the thigh without an associated calf thrombus and that 51 of 56 episodes of thromboembolic disease were clinically silent at the time of detection.[43,44]

The incidence of fatal pulmonary emboli is approximately 2% of patients undergoing elective hip surgery. Lynch found that the most common complication in his initial series of 117 total knee arthroplasties was thromboembolic disease.[64] The incidence of thrombophlebitis was 40% and pulmonary embolism 12%. In the first 14 patients in whom no specific prophylaxis was used, five had clinically evident thrombophlebitis, three had pulmonary emboli, and two died of the emboli. Ranawat reported nine cases of nonfatal pulmonary embolism in 233 cases of total condylar knee arthroplasties performed in patients on some form of prophylactic anticoagulation therapy. He also reported three fatal pulmonary emboli in a previous group not treated prophylactically.†

Brady and Garber had one nonfatal pulmonary embolus in 20 patients who had had Shiers hinge prostheses implanted.[11] Coventry and co-workers reported two patients having thromboembolic disease in their first 261 geometric knee arthroplasties.[23] One patient had a nonfatal pulmonary embolism, and another was reported with a femoral thrombophlebitis. The authors felt that their low incidence may be accounted for by the fact that they start the patients on early motion and ambulation. They do not use routine anticoagulants.

---

* Lynch, J.A.: Personal communication, September 1973.
† Ranawat, C.S.: Personal communication, May 1976.

Arden found only a 5% incidence of deep vein thrombosis (11 in 160) and suggested that his patients, most of whom had rheumatoid arthritis, were less likely to develop deep venous thromboembolic problems.[5] However, he reported two cases of fatal pulmonary embolism.[5] Freeman reported one nonfatal pulmonary embolus.[37] Witvoët and co-workers reported no thromboembolic problems in their 210 cases of GUEPAR arthroplasties.[118] Bryan's group had three patients develop thrombophlebitis within the first 10 days after surgery.[14] Two had previously had phlebitis. These authors used anticoagulants only in patients with a previous history of phlebitis, embolism, or varicosities. Three other patients with no history of pulmonary embolism had nonfatal pulmonary emboli within the first 11 days after surgery. (One had had a previous episode of phlebitis.[14]) Freeman and associates had two cases of deep venous thrombosis without embolization.[36] We have had one fatal case of pulmonary embolism in 120 cases.[31]

It is my feeling, as well as others', that all patients undergoing total knee surgery should be placed on some prophylactic anticoagulation program (*e.g.*, warfarin, aspirin, or low-molecular-weight dextran) to prevent postoperative venous thromboembolism.[33,64,78,85]

Stulberg and colleagues examined the data on 517 patients for a total of 638 total knee replacements, in which all of the patients had postoperative venograms and 475 had postoperative perfusion scans.[103] Forty-nine patients inadvertently did not receive prophylaxis, and in 41 of them (84%) ipsilateral deep vein thrombosis developed. The incidence of ipsilateral thrombosis was 57% in the 468 patients who did receive some form of prophylaxis. Ipsilateral thrombosis in the popliteal veins or thigh was seen in 11% of the patients with unilateral total knee replacement, and contralateral thrombosis was noted in 3%. Bilateral total knee replacements were associated with 58% incidence of ipsilateral deep vein thrombosis in the calf and a 14% incidence in the thigh. Pulmonary embolism was diagnosed clinically in nine patients (1.7%) but was suggested on perfusion lung scans in 39 patients (7%). Twelve patients (2.3%) received formal anticoagulant therapy, and in no patient was the pulmonary embolism fatal. The authors did not identify any specific population. In the view of the authors, no one prophylactic regimen proved to be more effective than any other. However, they felt that some specific prophylactic measure should be part of the management of patients undergoing total knee replacement.

Lotke and associates reviewed 175 patients who had undergone total knee surgery and who had been examined postoperatively by venography, plethysmography, fibrinogen scans, and ventilation-perfusion lung scans.[63] The authors found that 126 (72%) of the patients had small or large clots in the calf and that only 49 (28%) had no thrombi. Seventy-one (41%) of the patients had small thrombi on the calf, and 55 (31%) had large thrombi in the calf. Six patients had thrombi in the thigh, all of which were associated with large thrombi in the calf. In only two patients, however, did clinically recognized pulmonary emboli develop, one in the group of patients without known thrombi and the other in a patient with a large iliofemoral thrombus. The ventilation-perfusion scans showed six asymptomatic pulmonary emboli that were not associated with the presence of either large or small thrombi in the calf. The fibrinogen scans that were done in the postoperative period were capable of revealing large, but not small, thrombi in the calf. The preoperative plethysmography did not aid in determining in which patients a large thrombus of the calf was likely to develop. This has been my experience with this investigative tool as well. The results of this study confirm that there is a high (72%) possibility of the development of deep venous thrombosis after total knee replacement. They also suggest that most of these thrombi are located in the calf and that there is a low risk of development of clinically important emboli. Because there are significant risks associated with postoperative anticoagulation therapy after total knee replacement, the authors suggest that full therapeutic anticoagulation be deferred for patients who have thrombi in the calf and that it be considered only for those who have thrombi in the thigh. It is their feeling that all patients should be treated with prophylactic anticoagulants to prevent

thromboembolic phenomenon. We are now in the process of evaluating a platelet-tagged ^{111}In study in which all patients are evaluated preoperatively and then at 3 to 5 days postoperatively. All patients in whom there is a suspicion of intraluminal thrombosis are then further evaluated by venography. This approach may help solve some of the problems associated with venography in evaluating patients for thromboembolic disease.

Protocol for Prevention of Venous Thromboembolic Complications

1. Preoperative plethysmograph and Doppler studies are performed.
2. The involved leg is elevated for at least 8 to 10 minutes during the draping and is not exsanguinated mechanically. (I feel that this prevents loosening of any quiet thrombi, and the operative field is quite bloodless.)
3. Patients with a history of phlebitis are started on warfarin therapy the evening prior to surgery and managed in the manner outlined by Harris and colleagues.[44]
4. All other patients are placed on aspirin before surgery, a minimum of 600 mg. Postoperatively, the patients are given 600 mg twice a day orally, or a similar dose by rectum if they are unable to take oral medication. This routine is followed for approximately 7 to 10 days, until the patient is fully active.
5. The foot of the bed is maintained at a 45° angle, and patients wear support stockings.
6. Active exercise, particularly ankle and foot motion, is encouraged. Leg lifting is begun the evening of surgery.
7. Patients are allowed out of bed, usually on the second postoperative day; they walk at least twice, and more if they can.

Arterial Occlusion

Arden reported a patient's developing "white foot" bilaterally, which was relieved by splitting the plasters and flexing the knees.[5] Robson and co-workers reported an interesting case of popliteal artery occlusion following a Shiers total knee replacement and patellectomy in a patient who had had an ankylosed knee at 52° of flexion.[90] Following arthroplasty the pulses became occluded and the foot cold and white upon knee extension; with the knee in flexion the signs disappeared and the pulses returned. Following arteriography, a release of the musculofascial structures in the popliteal area and division of branches of the artery (without exposure of the joint) were performed successfully, and the patient gained full extension without loss of the pulses. A search of the literature has not yielded any specific reported injuries to either the popliteal or anterior tibial arteries directly related to the surgical procedure. However, I have had one case of an acute popliteal artery occlusion occurring on the ninth day following a duocondylar arthroplasty.

The patient was a 55-year-old, slightly obese businessman who had severe gonarthrosis of the right knee. The surgical procedure and postoperative course were routine; all postoperative laboratory studies and roentgenograms were essentially normal. On the ninth postoperative day, after performing his flexion and extension exercises, the patient complained of pain in the popliteal region and heaviness in his foot and leg. He was seen by the House Officer a few hours after the onset of symptoms and was found to have diminished dorsalis pedis and posterior tibial pulses, which had been recorded as normal prior to surgery. The symptoms subsided within 6 hours, and the pulses returned fully. The following morning, on day 10, the symptoms had returned, and the pulses were now obliterated. A vascular surgeon performed an arteriogram using the contralateral femoral artery and found a complete occlusion of the popliteal artery proximal to its division. The patient underwent arteriotomy and thrombectomy, which resulted in relief of pain, increased warmth and color to the foot, and weak return of pulses. He had been placed on heparin therapy.

Six hours later he was returned to surgery for thrombectomy of the contralateral side secondary to an intimal tear from the previous arteriogram. Following these procedures, he was placed on massive doses of heparin and rapidly developed a heparin-induced thrombocytopenia, with platelet levels falling to 50,000. Complete dehiscence of the inguinal wounds followed, and

there was partial superficial separation of the knee wound. The hematologist managed the thrombocytopenia with large doses of corticosteroids, and the heparin was discontinued. Gradually, over the next 4 weeks the patient's hematologic status returned to normal, and the wounds healed without infection. At the time of this writing, he is 9 years postsurgery, is fully employed, and has a range of motion from 0° to 100° without significant discomfort. The arteriogram did not show any abnormalities of the arterial lining.

Peroneal Nerve Injury

Peroneal nerve injury following total knee surgery is not unknown. This complication is often found in patients who have had severe flexion and valgus deformities. Many surgeons feel that it is related to some traction phenomenon rather than to specific localized injury to the nerve during the procedure.[5,14,23,100,118] It is often a complication of an improperly applied dressing and plaster. Coventry and co-workers had three cases that were attributed to the dressings and possibly to a Thomas splint. All patients were reported to be recovering.[23] Brady and Garber had one case of peroneal palsy that recovered in 9 weeks and was associated with pistoning or axle slide of the tibial part of a Shiers-hinge prosthesis.[11] Lynch had three palsies in his patients; two recovered, and one is permanent.[64] Freeman and co-workers reported two cases in their early series with the "roller-in-trough" condylar replacement; both recovered.[36] Others have also reported this complication.

In our series we have had two peroneal palsies that returned to normal.[31] One patient, 2 years prior to a geometric arthroplasty, sustained a severe lateral tibial plateau fracture and had a transient peroneal nerve palsy at the time. Following the arthroplasty, the patient's peroneal nerve function was normal in the recovery room. However, when rounds were made 5 hours later, the nerve function was absent. The dressing was split to the skin immediately, and within 2 minutes the function returned, only to disappear again overnight. Nevertheless, the peroneal function gradually returned almost to normal over the next 9 weeks. The patient also had to have a hematoma evacuated, and though his function is good he still has some pain, and the result is only fair.

It has been our experience that the bed position may be instrumental in producing pressure over the fibular head, particularly in the recovery room. We therefore place a roll under the trochanter and use a boot with a bar to prevent external rotation of the hip. In one series there were three patients with peroneal nerve palsy, one with bilateral palsy; all recovered except one, who still had some slight sensory deficit after 2 years.[5]

We have found that if the peroneal palsy persists, a very lightweight, vacuum-formed, polypropylene ankle–foot orthosis, which can be slipped into the shoe and held around the calf with a Velcro strap, works quite well in footdrop problems with other etiologies.

Hypotension and Operative Collapse

Though hypotension and operative collapse are well known to be associated with total hip arthroplasty, they are relatively rare during total knee replacement procedures. It appears that the highest incidence of intraoperative hypotension and collapse is associated with hinge prostheses, in which the tibial and femoral medullary canals must be reamed to considerable distances, thereby requiring more acrylic cement for fixation.[61]

Witvoët and co-workers reported eight serious cases of operative collapse in 210 procedures, and he attributed the complication to massive release of the polymerizing monomer during tourniquet release. One of these patients died during resuscitation efforts; seven recovered.[118]

We have noted transient hypotension when, prior to cementing, the tourniquet is released for 10 minutes because the procedure has reached 2 hours of tourniquet time. Of course, this phenomenon is well known to be secondary to the release of some of the lactic acid products and substances that accumulate during the anaerobic phase of tourniquet control. Therefore, we follow basically the same protocol for knees as for our total hip replacements: the patient is well oxygenated for a minimum

of 10 minutes before the tourniquet is released, by maintaining him on a minimum of 50% oxygen concentration, and in any questionable situation the concentration is increased. A normal volumetric state is maintained, and the hemoglobin is held at 12 mg/100 ml or above.

Fat Embolism

Fat embolism is not a common sequela of total knee replacement surgery. However, it has been reported to be associated with hinge arthroplasties when large amounts of intramedullary fat are seen at operation. Arden reported two cases of fat embolism, one of which proved fatal.[4,5] Bain reported two cases, one of which was fatal.[7] He also described three other cases with Rolson and suggested using thin plastic catheters to decompress the medullary cavities during insertion of cement and the prosthesis.[7] Two cases were reported by Freeman; both patients had severe cerebral involvement but recovered with immediate intensive care and treatment.[37] In April 1976 Bilsa and co-workers reported a case of fat embolization that occurred in a 58-year-old patient with rheumatoid arthritis who had undergone bilateral GUEPAR total knee arthroplasties at one operation under spinal anesthesia. The patient developed diffuse cerebral dysfunction (documented by EEG) associated with the fat embolism, which did not improve over the ensuing months, though the immediate sequelae of fat embolism disappeared and the wounds healed *per primam.*[10]

Witvoët and co-workers carry out suctioning procedures and temporarily drain the medullary canals before cementing the prosthesis in place. They have not had any known cases of fat embolism.[118] To date, I have been unable to document any recorded cases of fat embolism in the unlinked plastic-to-metal condylar systems.

Fat embolization is a rare sequela to resurfacing total knee replacement surgery. It is a well recognized complication following total hip arthroplasty and has been reported by Bisla and colleagues[10] in a patient undergoing bilateral hinge prosthetic replacement. Stulberg and co-workers did not have any cases of fat embolism syndrome in a large series of total condylar prosthetic arthroplasties, which included 37 bilateral cases.[103] However, Lachiewicz and Ranawat reported two cases of fat embolism syndrome following total knee arthroplasty in which total condylar prostheses were employed.[59] In both cases, bilateral total knee arthroplasty had been performed under general anesthesia.

Fat embolization is probably much more common than we suspect, and it is my feeling that surgical teams should maintain a high index of suspicion in patients who have slight changes in their vital signs following surgical procedures and in anyone whose affect may be altered within the first 24 to 36 hours following these procedures.

Corticosteroid Shock

Corticosteroid collapse has been reported in patients undergoing total knee replacement, sometimes with fatal results.[5] Since a large percentage of patients who undergo elective total knee surgery have been on corticosteroid therapy, it is important that this aspect of preoperative planning be considered. Our general protocol, which is modified as needed with the consulting internist, is as follows: 100 mg of hydrocortisone parenterally on the evening before surgery, then usually 200 mg on the day of the procedure, under control of the anesthesiologist. Following surgery, 100 mg to 200 mg is given the next day. The dosage is gradually decreased over the next 4 to 7 days, and the patient is then placed back on his daily preoperative maintenance dose. ACTH is used, but infrequently.

Drug Fever

Although drug fever is not referred to specifically in the literature of orthopaedic surgery, many surgeons who deal primarily with joint replacement procedures are faced with this frustrating dilemma because of the routine prophylactic use of various antibiotics. In our series of 120 operations we have had six cases of drug fever. Five patients were on sodium cephalothin, and one patient, who was allergic to penicillin, was on erythromycin. In two of these cases, the patients developed the characteristic spiking, fever, and laboratory changes, with elevated SGOT, SGPT, LDH, alkaline phosphatase, and bilirubin. It was felt by

our infectious-disease and gastroenterology consultants that these represented cholestatic allergic hepatitis. One patient developed hepatomegaly and frank icterus that gradually subsided. It is known that erythromycin is excreted via the liver in the bile. Fortunately, all sequelae cleared, and the arthroplasties were not adversely affected.

Patellar Tendon Complications and Extensor Lag

Complications related to the patellar tendon are also not unknown in association with total knee arthroplasties. Patellar tendon avulsions during and after surgery are uncommon, but they do occur.

We have had one patient who had a nylon arthroplasty converted to a geometric prosthesis.[31] At the time of surgery, the substance of the tendon was tissue-paper thin, and although the insertion was removed along with a piece of bone and reinserted with a staple, it ruptured when flexion exercises were begun 10 days after the procedure. However, the patient can walk without aids and has a geometric prosthesis on the opposite side; she has bilateral total hip prostheses, but she cannot ascend or descend stairs unassisted and has active extension only to 35°. Figure 36-1, A, shows the very high riding patella. Figure 36-1, B, shows the patella in its normal position following repair of the ligament; at the same time, a total hip replacement was done on the contralateral side. The patient now has an active range of motion from 5° to 95°.

Jackson and Elson found two instances in which the patellar insertions were avulsed following surgical removal (Fig. 36-2).[49] Extensor lag has been observed by many surgeons and is usually attributed to attenuation of the soft tissue structures, quadriceps muscle weakness, and a relative lengthening of the quadriceps mechanism following arthroplasty.[5,20,37,40,51,98] Walldius has advocated an incision through the patella so that it might be excised in part to take up the slack.[110] Most surgeons find that this is unnecessary and only complicates the procedure further. Phillips had to revise the quadriceps mechanism in patients who had severe lag following patellectomy in association with Shiers arthroplasty.[83]

FIG. 36-1. (*A*) Staples were used for initial fixation of a patellar tendon avulsion. (*B*) Three wires were inserted through osteoporotic bone for fixation in a patellar tendon repair. Good healing and function resulted.

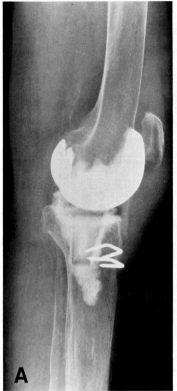
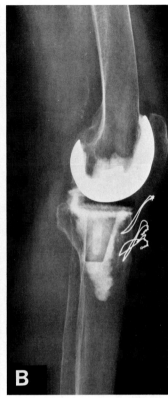

In Freeman and Swanson's initial group of 34 operations, they had eight cases of extensor tendon necrosis. Seven were associated with patellectomy at arthroplasty. One had a supracondylar femoral fracture at surgery; secondary sepsis occurred and the arthroplasty was lost.[36] However, in their second series of 35 operations, patellectomy was not done; instead, they performed "patellaplasty." In three knees the tibial tubercle was detached and reattached with a single screw. One became loose and was reattached, with satisfactory function. Since their early reports, Freeman and others have used polyethylene patellar prostheses, which are discussed later in this chapter.

We have found that when the tissues are attenuated or when there is need for exposure, it is necessary to release the patellar tendon insertion. We use one or two staples to reattach the tendon and its bone insertion under an osteoperiosteal flap. There were three patellar tendon avulsions in our early cases, and we now follow this procedure when there is any question about exposure. In all but one case this has not caused us to modify our postoperative management significantly.

Mazas reviewed the first 112 GUEPAR arthroplasties and found three avulsions that had occurred during attempts to dislocate the patella for exposure in flexion.[75] Convery and Beber suggest that extensor lag may be treated by a tibial tubercleplasty by using part of the resected bone.[20]

It is known that by elevating the tendon insertion anteriorly by 1 cm, the compression forces upon the patella can be decreased by 25% to 33%.[8,55,69] It may be that the improvement in function in these patients is related to a decrease in pain associated with an intact arthritic patellofemoral joint.

Scott and colleagues have pointed out that patellar stress fractures associated with patellar resurfacing have, in their experience, occurred most frequently in the osteoarthritic patient.[95] They note that the patient with rheumatoid arthritis and osteo-

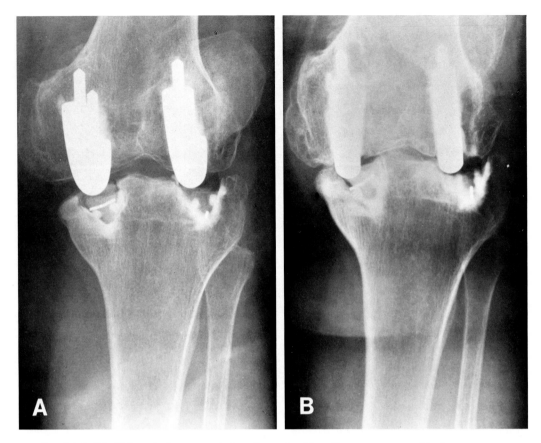

FIG. 36-2. (*A*) Although the varus deformity and subluxation were present before surgery, they were not corrected. (*B*) Consequently, there was further subluxation of the tibia and frank dislocation and loosening of the medial tibial prosthesis.

porosis *should* be more susceptible to this complication, but the osteoarthritic patient appears to be more vulnerable because more force is being generated across the joint with greater use. The authors note that Cybex testing has shown that patients with a duopatellar prosthesis tend to have a stronger quadriceps moment if they do not have a patellar prosthesis. There appears to be a high incidence of patellar stress fractures associated with duopatellar prostheses as compared with total condylar prostheses. The average clinical range of motion with a posterior cruciate–retaining prosthesis, such as the duopatellar, is approximately 10° to 15° greater than that of the more constrained total condylar prosthesis. This motion allows more function on stair climbing and arising from a sitting position, with

greater force generated across the patellofemoral joint. Andriacchi and associates have pointed out that in their study, patients with the less constrained posterior cruciate–retaining designs of total knee replacement had a more nearly normal gait during stair climbing than did patients with more constrained, cruciate-sacrificing designs.[3]

To avoid stress fractures, a minimal amount of patellar articular surface should be resected, and the peripheral cortex of both the medial and lateral facets should be preserved. Many authors have pointed out that smaller fixation lugs reduce the incidence of stress fracture by preserving more of the patellar bone stock.[19,95] In many instances of stress fracture, if the patella is undisplaced, it can be treated in the conventional fashion, restricting flexion and using some type of cylindrical plaster. In those instances in which open reduction is required, removal of the prosthesis and fragments, leaving the quadriceps mechanism intact and retaining part of the patella, has given excellent function and relief of pain.

Complications of Patellectomy–Arthroplasty

Patellectomy–arthroplasty is discussed in greater detail later in this chapter. I believe, however, that it is timely to note at this point that this procedure should be discouraged in knee replacement surgery.[36,56]

Early Minimal Motion

In our early series, patients did not begin active flexion exercises until 10 to 12 days after surgery because of our fear of wound complications. However, we found that the flexion range was less than 80° in many of these patients. As our experience increased, we found that our concern had been overemphasized, and we began a more vigorous program of postoperative exercises that includes the following:

Splinting and Early Motion. After the drains are pulled and the dressing changed at 48 hours, the leg is placed in a removable splint with Velcro straps, and active-assistive flexion and extension exercises are begun.

Ambulation. The patient is ambulatory on the second or third postoperative day.

Exercise. A knee exercise program is begun on day four or day five from the overhead frame, and the patient is allowed to sit on the edge of the bed with the feet dangling, in an attempt to gain 90° of motion without force.

Continuous Passive Motion

Coutts has shown that by using continuous passive motion, patients who have undergone total knee replacement have had significant short-term salutary effects.[21] These seem to be related to improvement in control of postoperative edema, wound healing, and venous pressure, and thereby the reduction of venostasis. Coutts has also pointed out that the range of motion experienced by patients who have been placed in these machines appears to be enhanced compared with that of a control group in

which the standard postoperative regimen was followed.

It has been my experience that continued passive motion does have a significant beneficial effect in preventing postoperative venostasis and improving wound healing. Whether the eventual improvement in joint motion will be significantly increased is difficult to assess at this point. One practical problem that I have noted in the use of these machines is the development by many patients of an extensor deficit because the machine may not allow the patient to come into complete extension on each cycle. There may also be a concomitant decrease in quadriceps control. I believe that these two facets must be looked for. I do not feel that they are a major impediment to the use of this equipment, but the increase in the extensor lag associated with a deficit in extension (which I think can be enhanced by this machine) should be looked for and prevented by the surgical team.

Manipulation. If the patient is unable to obtain 70° to 80° of flexion by the eighth or ninth postoperative day, the knee is manipulated, gently, with the patient in bed under pentathol anesthesia. This procedure is similar to others described in the literature.[14,23]

Fox and Poss found that of 23% of a series of knees undergoing total knee replacement manipulated 2 weeks postoperatively to increase flexion, an immediate increase in flexion was noted from a mean of 71° to a mean of 108°.[32] By 1 week after manipulation, the mean flexion was reduced to 88°. By 1 year postoperatively, the manipulated knees were found to have a range of motion similar to that of their nonmanipulated counterparts.

The authors point out that such factors as preoperative flexion and diagnosis appear to be the major determinants of ultimate flexion and that these seem to offset the temporarily increased flexion afforded by manipulation. They also point out that the primary reason for manipulation is to facilitate the postoperative rehabilitation program for patients with painful, limited motion of the knee. I agree that routine manipulation after total knee replacement for the purpose of improving ultimate flexion is unjustifiable. However, if the patient is progressing in an unsatisfactory fashion with significant restriction in motion at 1 week, manipulation is indicated.

EARLY BONE AND HARDWARE COMPLICATIONS

Inappropriate Selection of Prosthesis

It was estimated that by the middle of 1974, there were approximately 300 different knee prosthesis systems commercially available around the world. Since then, more have been added. Many of these systems are original in thought and design; others are modifications of existing systems. I believe that the real problem for the practicing orthopaedic surgeon, who may not be exposed to a significant number of degenerative knee problems, is to find some realistic guide for the selection of a prosthesis. The best prosthetic system is one that will solve the patient's problem in a fashion that will give a satisfactory result without significant complications related to the system itself.

During the past 12 years, enough experience has been gained with a number of the condylar prostheses to give us a much clearer picture of what makes a patient a good candidate for these devices.

When considering arthroplastic replacement of the tibiofemoral joint or total knee replacement (patellofemoral arthroplasty), one must carefully consider the following factors:

The degree of angular deformity (valgus or varus) present

The degree of flexion contracture present

The status of the medial and lateral collateral ligaments. This consideration must also include the status of capsular contracture and, on the lateral side of the knee, the status of the iliotibial band.

Angular deformity. Is it fixed, or can it be corrected passively to neutral?

Bone loss from the tibia and femur. Riley has pointed out that if less than 2 cm of bone (measured vertically) is present, this should be considered minimal loss.[89] Minimal subchondral bone loss permits the use of any type of nonhinged or hinged unit. However, Riley has pointed out that moderate subchondral bone loss (*i.e.*, more than a total of 2 cm) is felt to

jeopardize a good result with such systems as the polycentric and UCI.

Muscle power and joint control. If the muscles about the knee are atrophic and fibrotic, the arthroplasty will fail no matter how perfectly it is implanted.

Patient selection. Convery and Beber have noted the need for willingness on the part of the patient to endure significant postoperative pain, to participate in a vigorous postoperative program, and to accept a slow but steady improvement in function.[20]

These factors, of course, depend in large measure on the preoperative planning and preparation that is done with the patient by the surgeon and other members of the team.

The need for a comprehensive clinical evaluation procedure is important, and I believe one of the most thoroughly worked out approaches to date is the UCLA proformas, which provide the parameters relevant to preoperative and postoperative anatomical and functional analysis.[2]

Using the criteria listed above, I have found that in replacement arthroplasty of the tibiofemoral joint, at least three systems should be available for use:

A condylar metal–plastic system that will resurface the joint with minimal bone resection in a knee in which the anatomical structures are almost normal and there exists an angular or flexion deformity of no more than 20°

A condylar metal–plastic system that can be used in knees that have essentially normal medial and lateral ligament structures but have instability owing to bone loss and cruciate destruction. These systems require more bone resection but have more stability designed into the bearing surfaces.

A linked system for pure salvage of the knee that has no ligament control and severe bone loss

The size of the patient and the available implant sizes must be considered. Unfortunately, most knee replacement systems have been designed for the so-called average person. Mensch and Amstutz pointed out that when additional sizes and shapes are added to the original design, there is often less than optimal functional increment.[77] They were able to delineate morphology and the size range needed by making comparable anatomical measurements from 30 cadavers and 53 other human knees. When they studied the dimension-equivalent measurements from nine available knee replacement units and compared them with measurements from their cadavers and roentgenograms, they found discrepancies in three areas: (1) Most of the existing sizes of knee units are designed for the smaller-sized patient. (2) The depth of the tibial plateau may be too small to accommodate its prosthesis, since the lateral tibial plateau is shallower than the medial side by an average of 3 mm. Because the prostheses are available in only one size, this requires a compromise at both ends of the scale. They also pointed out that even two or three sizes may not be sufficient for reasonable reproduction of the anatomy for the unlinked condylar units. (3) Several of the hinge units have prominent areas that can cause subcutaneous or skin pressure.

As a result of these considerations, a great deal of time and effort should be invested in preoperative planning when knee replacement is contemplated. This approach, coupled with a careful clinical evaluation of the patient's needs, will lead to consistent selection of the proper prosthesis. For accurate measurement it is important

to have precise, standing roentgenograms that have been corrected for magnification errors. The normograms developed by Mensch and Amstutz will be a great help in choosing the proper size prosthesis when graded prostheses become available.

It has been our experience that the inappropriateness of our selections has been illustrated by the postoperative complications. These have been, by and large, associated with inadequate evaluation of the quality and amount of bone loss, the angular and flexion deformities, and the character of the collateral ligament structures once deformities were corrected at surgery. Two problems are presented for illustration.

Problem 1 is that of a patient with severe bilateral arthrosis, loss of bone stock of the medial tibial plateau, significant varus deformity, and marked subluxation of the femur on the tibia (see Fig. 36-2). The subluxation and varus deformities were not corrected initially (see Fig. 36-2, *B*), resulting in increased concentration of forces on the medial components and a complication by fracture of the attenuated medial tibial cortex.

Problem 2 is that of an elderly woman (Fig. 36-3, *A*) with severe degenerative arthrosis, angular deformity, and instability. After correction of the deformity and implantation of the prosthesis, gross

FIG. 36-3. (*A*) Preoperative view shows valgus deformity. Medial instability was evident at surgery. (*B*) Correction was attempted by advancing the medial collateral ligament and fixing it with a staple, but this effort failed.

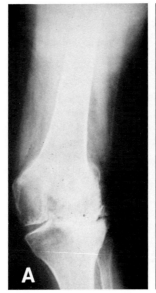 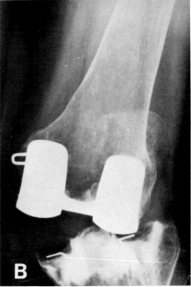

laxity of the medial collateral ligament was noted. The ligament was advanced proximally and fixed with a staple. Post-operatively the limb was placed in a plaster cylinder for 3 weeks. Figure 36-3, *B*, shows a recurrence of the deformity associated with gross medial instability.

These cases illustrate the need for more careful planning and evaluation preoperatively and the obvious need to have more than one system readily available in the operating room so that the deformities can be adequately corrected and stability achieved.

Technical Errors

Technical error is a common reason for complications and subsequent failure. Mal-alignment of the prosthetic components in any of three planes may cause poor load distribution and a mechanical overloading with resulting fracture, fragmentation, or loosening. The cause may be inappropriate selection of a prosthesis, as discussed previously, or malpositioning of the appropriate prosthesis. Three very common errors, pointed out by Stauffer, are as follows:[102]

Failure to correct the tibiofemoral mechanical axis to normal in the frontal plane (i.e., persistent varus or abnormal valgus deformity), causing overloading of either medial or lateral components

Tilting of the tibial components in the sagittal plane, which results in excessive loading anteriorly or posteriorly. The tibial tilt of the tibial prosthetic component and the proximal tibia must be considered relative to the weight line and its association to the floor reaction force.

Using a knee-joint simulator (which flexes and extends a prosthetic knee system with forces similar to those resulting from quadriceps activity) cycled at a rate corresponding to normal human locomotion, Murray found that a bicompartmental prosthesis (geometric) failed after 4.5 million cycles.[79] The failure occurred by loosening of the tibial component, initially anteriorly. Analysis of the failure indicated that tibial fixation is the weak point in this design, and Murray suggested that the anterior portion be anchored, if possible, against cortical bone.

Because of the variations in the proximal tibia, particularly with regard to tilt, it is important, I believe, to seat the tibial component in such a fashion as to obviate this possible complication. We instruct all of our patients to use chairs with armrests when sitting down or arising, so as to decrease the concentration of forces on the tibial components. We hope that this will add to the longevity of the components.

The use of a four-component prosthesis (such as the monocompartmental system) increases the technical demands and thus the possibilities for malalignment and complications.

Nogi and co-workers found that in static tests of polycentric and geometric systems, there were no femoral component failures.[80] They pointed out that one major factor in the failure of the knee replacements tested was improper distribution of load, particularly through the bone–cement interface. They felt that the low modulus of elasticity of the polyethylene tibial components concentrates rather than distributes the load over a given area. The high stress concentration imparted by the polyethylene on low-strength cancellous bone leads to loosening and displacement of the tibial component, so failure was most pronounced in the smaller tibial tracks of the polycentric prosthesis.

Paul has determined that the lateral compartment force is greater than the medial compartment force only early in the stance phase and that throughout the majority of the stance phase, when flexion of the knee is occurring, the medial compartment force exceeds the lateral compartment force.[81] Table 36-1 shows knee joint forces expressed as multiples of body weight, as determined by Paul. This author also points out that, based on analytical gait studies of patients with varus, valgus, and flexion deformities, the greater the deformity angle, the greater will be the offset for the line of action-resultant force from the joint capsule (and, therefore, the greater the joint force).

McGrouther reported on gait studies of a patient who had undergone a Charnley low-friction arthroplasty.[65] He showed that prior to surgery, the position of the line of action of the resultant tibiofemoral joint force was in the lateral compartment and afterward was in the more normal medial

Table 36-1. Knee Joint Forces Expressed as Multiples of Body Weight

ACTIVITY	NO. OF TESTS	FORCE ON TIBIOFEMORAL JOINT (× BODY WEIGHT)	FORCE ON PATELLOFEMORAL JOINT (× BODY WEIGHT)	TORQUE ABOUT TIBIAL AXIS* (Nm, × BODY WEIGHT)
Level walking	22	2.8	0.6	18
Fast level walking	6	4.3	1.5	
Ascending stairs	7	4.4	1.8	33
Descending stairs	6	4.9	2.9	21
Ramp ascent	8	3.7	1.6	30
Ramp descent	8	4.4	2.6	22

* Based on a restricted number of tests

compartment, which corresponded in this instance to the reduction in the antalgic gait pattern.

Incomplete Correction of External Rotation Deformity

External rotation contracture, which is often present with a valgus and flexion deformity, is a difficult problem and must be recognized as such. An inappropriate attempt to correct this can result in subluxation or dislocation. Albright and Brand reported seeing a patient who had received a geometric prosthesis in an attempt to correct a rotational deformity; owing to the abnormal stresses placed on the prosthesis, it failed.[1] Ranawat feels that condylar prostheses do not have sufficient stability to hold the correction necessary for this problem and therefore recommends a linked system.[85]

Reverse Insertion of the Prosthetic Component

Thompson reported an unusual surgical failure in a patient who had had the femoral component of a geometric prosthesis inserted in the reverse position.[106] In addition, a large amount of cement was noted in the posterior compartment of the tibial component. Because it was painful, the arthroplasty was subsequently revised to a fusion. Swanson suggested that the Freeman-Swanson procedure was designed to be as automatic as possible with regard to insertional technique; however, he noted that it could not be made entirely foolproof, because, in reviewing the cases done at Lon-

don Hospital between April 1970 and September 1974, he found that two prostheses had been inserted in reverse fashion.[105]

Anteroposterior Subluxation of the Knee Related to the Length and Size of the Monocompartmental Components

Convery and Beber reported an instance of anterior subluxation of the tibia on extension, which was corrected by replacement of the lateral aspect of a polycentric prosthesis with one that was longer and extended farther posteriorly.[20]

Instability and Dislocation

Bryan and co-workers reported six anterior subluxations of the tibia on the femur.[14] Two knees were reoperated on, and the new, larger femoral components were reset anteriorly, which corrected the subluxations. One knee, an early neuropathic arthroplasty, was arthrodesed. Three were pain free in braces. Some authors have reported medial-lateral subluxation, especially in patients with rheumatoid arthritis following bicompartmental replacement with monocompartmental prostheses.

Instability. In our series of geometric arthroplasties, two patients had sufficient laxity and instability to require external bracing. This laxity was not enough to cause frank dislocation, but it did cause marked valgus instability. There have been other patients in this group and in our duopatellar and total condylar groups who have had 1+ (out of 4) medial or lateral instability that did not pose any serious functional problem during heel strike or foot flat. In many instances the anterior cruciate ligament can be sacrificed without loss of stability. Murray does this procedure routinely.* The posterior cruciate is important to knee stability and should be retained whenever possible; however, many patients without posterior cruciates who have had geometric, Freeman-Swanson, or total condylar prostheses do not dislocate their tibia posteriorly on the femur.[86] In most instances the minimally unstable knee will tighten with time, particularly as quadriceps and hamstring strength increase. Some authors feel that if the collateral ligaments are badly attenuated and an unlinked system is used, reconstruction can be performed later. Coventry and co-workers reported three patients who had enough instability to require bracing.[23]

Dislocation. Dislocation, although rare, does occur and has been reported. Bryan and colleagues reported one.[14] Coventry and colleagues reviewed 261 patients with a total of 317 geometric knee prostheses and found three who had tibiofemoral dislocation.[23] Two patients developed enough quadriceps strength to prevent this complication from recurring, while the third, a patient with a Charcot knee, subsequently required arthrodesis. When this is recognized early, use of a cast for 3 to 6 weeks may help prevent a chronic problem. Another group reported two dislocations of geometric prostheses in patients with contralateral knee fusions.

Fracture of the Medial or Lateral Tibial Cortex

Fracture of the medial or lateral tibial cortex is not unknown and has been reported by many authors. We have found that in patients with substantial loss of bone, particularly the medial tibial plateau with associated osteoporosis, it is very easy to fracture the only supporting buttress remaining in this area. Many times so much bone substance is missing that the fin, particularly of the geometric design, rests against the flare. We have not, to our knowledge, had any frank fractures, but

---

* Murray, D.G.: Personal communication, September 1974.

we have roentgenographic evidence of one undisplaced fracture.

Stauffer feels that there may be factors inherent in the design of the prostheses that could be modified to reduce this complication.[102] He and his associates have been working on a three-dimensional photoclastic study to define a configuration that produces the best stress concentration pattern on the underlying bone. Energy absorption at the interface is also an important consideration, they point out.

Excess Posterior Cement

Excessive cement in the posterior joint space can be a cause of rapid prosthesis wear, pain, and mechanical block to knee flexion.[106]

In our initial geometric series we cemented in the femoral prosthesis first and then the tibial component in an attempt to maintain pressure on the tibial prosthesis. However, we found that we were having problems removing excess cement, particularly behind the tibial prosthesis. On two occasions the tibial prosthesis was loosened during this maneuver and had to be recemented. We now cement the tibial prosthesis first under compression and have had fewer problems with removing the excess cement.

Excess Cement at the Periphery of the Components

It is not uncommon to see cement protruding at the margin of the prosthesis. Particles of cement can and do break off and may be responsible for accelerated abrasive wear of the plastic tibial prosthesis.[36] After 8 months of wear in a study of a geometric prosthesis *in vitro*, Reckling found significant wear and deformation of the polyethylene tibial component where it had been in contact with excess cement or free cement particles, but there was no significant wear of the femoral component.[88]

It should be pointed out here that when hemiarthroplasties are performed or separate tibial components are used to resurface both compartments, the cement keyholes should be divergent and ought to extend to the anterior and posterior cortices for improved fixation. It is imperative that all excess cement be meticulously removed from the periphery of the components and that the joint and soft tissue be flushed of all free particles. This is especially important with new patellar prostheses.

Ipsilateral Dislocation of a Total Hip Prosthesis

Though it is uncommon, ipsilateral dislocation of a total hip prosthesis has been known to occur. It has been suggested that when multiple joint replacements are planned, hip replacement should be carried out first. The rationale is quite obvious. There is a great deal of manipulation of the leg and knee during total hip replacement, which might loosen or fracture a knee arthroplasty. Also, from a rehabilitative viewpoint, if there are significant hip and knee contractures, the hip contracture should be corrected first so that adequate knee extension can be gained. However, when total knee surgery is performed on the same side as a total hip arthroplasty, great care must be taken to protect the hip from dislocation, component loosening, or femoral fracture. Thus far in our series of combined hip and knee procedures, we have not encountered this complication.

Penetration of the Femoral Shaft by the Prosthesis

The complication of femoral shaft penetration by the stem of the hinge prosthesis has been reported. As with femoral head prostheses, penetration may be difficult to detect clinically. Habermann and colleagues reported one case in which visual inspection after insertion failed to reveal the complication.[40] Roentgenograms revealed the complication, which was later corrected. Wilson reported two cases of femoral penetrations that did not affect the final result.[116,117] Phillips also reported a case of a Shiers arthroplasty (Fig. 36-4) that penetrated the anterior femoral cortex, leaving a mass on the thigh, which apparently was not revised; despite all, a good functional result was achieved.[83] Shiers has also had similar complications of femoral shaft penetration.[96,98] The motion of the femoral stem can erode the cortex. Perforation of the anterior aspect of a tibia by a Shiers prosthesis has been reported, and Freeman

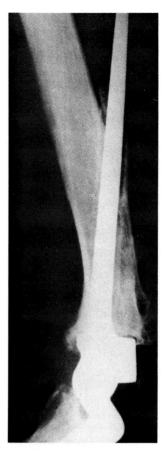

FIG. 36-4. The Shiers prosthesis has penetrated the anterior femoral cortex.

found three cases of tibial stem penetration with Walldius hinge arthroplasties, but evidently they made no difference to the end result.[37]

Complications of Migration and Settling

Phillips has pointed out that in the elderly patient, especially the elderly woman with rheumatoid arthritis, bone atrophy is often prominent.[83] He found that despite the presence of cement, both femoral and tibial components in three knee arthroplasties sank into the medullary canals. It seems obvious to assume that this complication will eventually lead to restricted knee motion and friction. The anteroposterior film showed components sinking into the medullary canal of the femur (Fig. 36-5). This has, as yet, not been as significant a problem

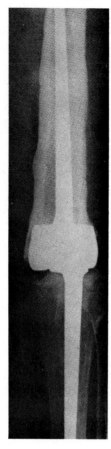

FIG. 36-5. A hinge prosthesis is settling into the femur as a result of bone resorption.

with the two-piece metal-to-plastic condylar systems, though it has been reported as a complication.

LATE SOFT TISSUE COMPLICATIONS

Late Infection

Bain reviewed 100 hinge arthroplasties at 3 years and found seven deep infections developing late; three occurred within 6 months of surgery, and the other four took more than 2 years to develop.[7] One patient had bilateral knee infection. Six of the seven patients were on systemic corticosteroids, and all had severe rheumatoid arthritis. The prostheses were removed in all cases. This late deep infection rate (7%) is alarming; however, Bain suggests that since

he began using topical antibiotic therapy during surgery, the rate of early infection, at least, has been radically reduced, and it is hoped that the rate of late sepsis will be similarly affected.

Freeman found two late cases in 80 hinge tibiofemoral replacements, and one developed 4 years after surgery.[37] Arden found a 1.6% rate in his series, and Jones reported a 2.5% late rate.[5,50,51] Petty and co-workers found that four of 21 deep infections in 1045 metal-to-plastic condylar arthroplasties appeared between 1 and 2 years postoperatively.[82] Witvoët had five cases of late deep infection (2.4%) in the initial GUEPAR series.[118] Waugh had no reported instances of late deep infections in the initial 185 UCI arthroplasties.[114]

Our series to date has not produced any spontaneous late deep infections; the longest follow-up is more than 5 years. However, we have had one case of a chronic late infection in a young woman who had a vague history of bilateral knee problems, beginning at about 10 or 12 years of age. She underwent a metal-to-plastic condylar replacement at another medical center and did well during the initial postoperative period of 4 to 6 months. Then she began having pain, particularly in the patellar region, and was treated with multiple injections of cortisone into the knee. Aspirations were negative for bacterial growth, and arthrography was also negative. When she was seen initially in our department, she was found to have only 20° of motion (from 15° to 35°), and the joint was swollen. At surgery she was found to have 300 ml of loculated, watery, purulent material that subsequently tested positive for tuberculosis. The prosthetic components had been removed at the exploration. She was started on triple-therapy medication and 2 months later returned to surgery, during which bone resection and a Charnley compression arthrodesis were carried out. She now has 7 cm of shortening and an essentially stable, fibrous, nonpainful arthrodesis. Her other knee is painful and has marked deformity.

Amputation

After fatal septicemia, amputation is probably the second most catastrophic complication of knee replacement procedures. Wigren reported three in 15 Walldius prostheses over 9 years.*

In 1972, Arden and Ansell reported their experience with hinge knee replacement surgery on 19 knees in patients with Still's disease whose average age was 25 years.[6] Amputations had to be performed on three patients, or approximately 16% of the group.

Walldius and others have reported this complication as well.[83,98,111,112] To date I have been unable to find any recorded cases of amputation secondary to the complication of deep infection in metal–plastic condylar systems or in any of the linked condylar-loading–intercondylar-stabilizing systems.

It has been observed by many that infections may be most common in patients with rheumatoid arthritis and in patients who have had previous knee operations. Petty found that in these patients the highest incidence of positive cultures (60%) was obtained at the time of metal–plastic condylar arthroplasty; by contrast, only 16% of other patients had positive cultures.[82] They found that five knees later became infected with the same organism that had been cultured at the time of total knee arthroplasty. This group suggests that all patients with positive cultures should be treated with oral antibiotics for a period of 6 weeks postoperatively.

Late Skin Necrosis

A late skin necrosis developed 3 years after a successful Shiers hinge arthroplasty.[83] A necrotic area developed following a fall. At surgery the prosthesis was loose in the femur, and there was a large mass of grey fibrin arising from the medullary cavity of the femur. It had eroded through the quadriceps tendon and finally caused necrosis of the overlying skin. The patient underwent arthrodesis.

Complications Related to the Patellar Mechanism

Quadriceps Tendon Rupture. Arden had six cases (3%) in which the quadriceps tendon ruptured, in most instances, 3 to 4

---

* Wigren, A.: Personal communication, June 1976.

years after operation.[5] One case followed a fall, but the others resulted from wear of the quadriceps by the exposed metal. These were repaired surgically but with less than satisfactory results.

One patient in Lynch's initial series who had had a patellectomy sustained a rupture of the quadriceps mechanism associated with a fistula.[64] Tendon repair and excision of the fistula were performed, and the wounds healed without infection, but quadriceps function has been incomplete.

Brady and Bain have each had one case of late patellar tendon rupture that was repaired; one was complicated by a skin slough that finally healed without infection.[7,11]

Patellofemoral Pain. It has been suggested that patellofemoral pain can be due to one of the following three reasons:

Subluxation or dislocation of the patella or malalignment between the prosthesis and the quadriceps mechanism. Such malalignment can be caused by improper insertion of the prosthesis in the coronal plane. The lateral structures of the mechanism may be tight. If they are not released at surgery, malalignment of the patella to the prosthesis will result, and if there is any external rotation deformity of the tibia, the alignment will be further distorted.[85]

Incongruity of the patellofemoral joint at the junction of the bone and the anterior margin of the prosthetic component

Symptoms arising from an arthritic patellofemoral joint

Ranawat noted that in a follow-up study of 85 unicondylar and duocondylar prostheses, 30% or more of the patients had patellofemoral joint symptoms.[85] In Lynch's group the most frequently experienced pain was in the patella.[64]

Traditionally the surgical treatment for patellofemoral pain has been patellectomy. However, the sequelae of patellectomy in association with tibiofemoral replacement have been significant. In our series the incidence of significantly painful patellofemoral joints is 10% to 15%, and it appears that as the length of our follow-up increases, the incidence of symptomatic patellofemoral joints is likewise increasing.

This dilemma was pointed out by Lynch as illustrated by a patient treated for severe bilateral tricompartmental gonarthroses.[64] A patellectomy was performed in one knee but not in the other. Postoperatively the patellectomized knee was the more comfortable. However, strength was deficient. It was the author's opinion that patellectomy in conjunction with total knee replacement should be discouraged.

When they compared patients' normal knees with their opposite knees after total patellectomy, Kettelkamp and co-workers found a 49% decrease in quadriceps strength.[56] Activities such as going up and down stairs, which require the use of the loaded knee in a flexed position, were adversely affected in patients with patellofemoral arthritis associated with quadriceps weakness. The authors felt that this was primarily the result of associated pain rather than a mechanical effect due to loss of patellar substance secondary to the degenerative process. It was their opinion that to obtain maximal benefit from knee replacement arthroplasty, the pain associated with patellofemoral arthritis must be decreased while the moment arm of the quadriceps is retained. In their opinion, replacement prosthetic patelloplasty appears to offer the best solution.

A number of centers have now had extensive experience with a polyethylene surface cemented to the articular area of the patella. Groenweld has had success using this with various hinge prostheses.* Ranawat reported no patellar prosthesis loosening since he and his colleagues began resurfacing the patella at the Hospital for Special Surgery 10 years ago.

Our experience is quite limited. We have experience with 70 patellar prostheses in duopatellar or total condylar units without any mechanical problems; however, our follow-up is only a little more than 24 months. In one patient we resurfaced the patella with a McKeever prosthesis 1 year after a geometric arthroplasty (Fig. 36-6).[36,42] There was only moderate improvement in her symptoms and function; however, the prosthetic components did not show any

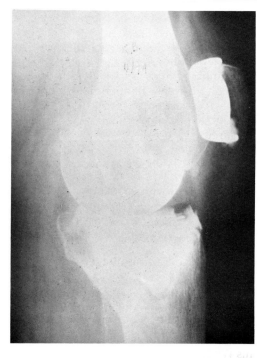

FIG. 36-6. A McKeever patellar prosthesis was used to resurface the patella.

abnormal wear and remained firmly fixed. We have not used patellectomy as a treatment for knees that have tibiofemoral arthroplasties.

Patellar Subluxation and Dislocation. Subluxation of the patella is not an uncommon problem and has been alluded to earlier. Frank lateral dislocation has been infrequently noted in the literature. Witvoët found a 7% incidence in the first 210 GUEPAR-hinge arthroplasties.[118] Eleven dislocations occurred when flexion exceeded 90°. Eight required transposition of the tibial tuberosity with satisfactory results. The remaining three were scheduled for repair. There were four subluxations, none of which was operated on.

Mazas suggested that the design of the GUEPAR, which helps to reestablish the normal valgus position of the knee, may contribute to this complication.[25] He suggested strongly that the patella must sit well on the prosthetic trochlear shield and track in neutral on the prosthesis to 90° or beyond. He recommends that if the patella has a tendency to dislocate, lateral retinac-

---

* Groenweld: Personal communication, May 1976.

ular release, plication of the medial retinacula, and transplantation of the tibial tuberosity, if necessary, be performed. He pointed out once again that marked valgus deformities with associated flexion contractures and external rotation deformities frequently have contractures of the lateral patellar retinacular structures and have to be surgically corrected. It is my belief that this correction must be made no matter what system is used for knee replacement surgery.

LATE COMPLICATIONS OF PROSTHESIS AND CEMENT FAILURE

Prosthesis Loosening in Linked Systems

The Walldius, Stanmore, and Shiers hinge prostheses were originally designed to be used without a luting agent. Jones pointed out that after 5 years, some radiologic evidence of loosening could be found in all of his Walldius patients but that unless clinical evidence of loosening was present, function was not affected.[51,57] Only five of 120 patients had clinical loosening, though function remained reasonably good in walking. Based on his early experience with 30 Walldius hinge arthroplasties followed an average of 3 years, Wilson supports Jones' observations.[116]

Bain noted that one fact has not been explained: loosening of the prosthesis, which allows considerable rocking, is rarely painful when the prosthesis is not cemented but is extremely painful when cement is used.[7] Reviewing 100 cemented Walldius prostheses at 3 years, he found that five were loose. In those reexplored, the loosening was between the cement and the bone and not between the prosthesis and the cement. Freeman reported a similar experience.[37]

Arden found that there was loosening in 14 of his 192 Shiers arthroplasties in which cement fixation had been used (7.3%).[5] Four patients did not consider the pain severe enough to warrant further surgery, but ten did. All of these prostheses were loose, and nine new prostheses were inserted. In the tenth case, the prosthesis was removed, and an arthrodesis was attempted because of large masses of grey fibrous

tissue present everywhere around the joint. In an early review of 210 GUEPAR cases, Witvoët found four cases of aseptic loosening.[118] Two cases appeared to be loose on roentgenograms but were asymptomatic. The other two had clinical symptoms. One was a Charcot joint that was subsequently arthrodesed; the other had a new prosthesis inserted.

It would appear from these experiences that loosening of the prosthesis stem in hinge systems inserted without cement has not, in and of itself, constituted a complication that functionally affects the majority of patients. On the other hand, the combination of cement, long stems, and rigid hinges does seem to place the patient at a higher risk of symptomatic loosening.

To date, I have been unable to find any reports of significant clinical loosening in the condylar load–bearing units with intercondylar stabilizing mechanisms. Matthews' series of spherocentric arthroplasties has, so far, been free of this problem.*

Prosthesis Loosening in Unlinked Systems

The exact incidence of loosening depends on the defining criteria and specifically on two factors. These factors are directly interrelated. One is the design of the prosthesis; the second the bone–cement junction.

The contours of the femoral condyles have a progressively decreasing radius of curvature, and this varies also with respect to medial and lateral condyles. The rotatory, rolling, and sliding motions of the femur relative to the tibia, or vice versa, are governed not only by the surface geometry of these bones but also by the spatial arrangements of ligaments and tendons across the knee joint. It has been suggested that systems that do not provide a changing radius of curvature may provide a constraint to knee kinematics, thereby causing increased ligament tensile forces, abnormal shear, and compressive loading, which could result in loosening of the prosthesis, particularly the tibial component.[80]

It has been reported by Stauffer in a comparative study that the incidence of

---

* Matthews, L.S.: Personal communication, May 1976.

clinically important loosening of a group of polycentric total knee arthroplasties was 0.84%, and in a similar group of geometric knee arthroplasties it was 2.4%.[102] He suggested that "slop" in the polycentric system allowed more rotation (thereby decreasing abnormal soft tissue tensile forces) and that any rotation of the more concentric, "tight" geometric components in a transverse plane would seem to be possible only through a "camming apart" mechanism that ultimately caused increased torque to be transmitted to the prosthesis–cement–bone junction.

It has also been noted that this "camming apart" action may occur when full extension has not been achieved. Full extension must be obtained by removing adequate bone from either the femur (preferably) or the tibia and by stripping, and if necessary incising, the posterior capsule so that it does not restrict knee motion, thereby acting like a hinge during extension. If this occurs, particularly with a system that has a constant radius of curvature in place, it may allow the compressive forces generated to be translated more readily into forces that will actually tend to tilt the tibial prosthesis, thereby loosening it.

Ranawat found that incidences of radiolucency around the tibial plateau were 70% with the unicondylar system, 50% with the duocondylar, and 80% with the geometric prosthesis.[85] He was not sure of the significance of these observations but felt that definite indications of failure of the cement–bone junction are progressive radiolucency, increased or recurrent deformity with instability, and unexplained pain.

Skolnick and colleagues reviewed 119 geometric arthroplasties having a minimum follow-up of 2 years and found an 8.4% incidence of loosening in all tibial units.[100] Matthews has found a loosening rate of approximately 8% of the tibial components in 200 geometric arthroplasties, some of which required conversion to spherocentric arthroplasties.* Others have reported late loosening that has been related to defects in the prosthesis design, malpositioning, and inadequate preparation of the tibial surface to receive the cement. Waugh (as well as others) feels that it is imperative to

make sure that the tibial surface is as dry as possible before cement is inserted.

Insertion of the cement under pressure is essential for proper fixation. Markolf and others have pointed out that effective fixation of prosthetic components with acrylic cement is achieved by penetration and flow of the cement into the interstices of the cancellous bone.[70] The depth of penetration is a function of the pressure generated at the bone–cement interface, the time over which the pressure pulse is applied, and the stage of polymerization of the cement. He found that 80% to 90% of the cement penetration into cavities occurred within 2 to 4 seconds of pressure application, and he therefore recommended a rapid thrust of the prosthesis into the bone site, associated with early cement insertion. He also pointed out that lamination of the cement significantly reduces the tensile strength, which may ultimately lead to complications and failure. The use of a Water Pic to clean the cancellous bed and early insertion of the cement under pressure will enhance the cement–bone bond.

Cold-Flow Deformation of the Polyethylene Prosthesis

Prosthetic devices of the kind that do not permit rotation in extension have been found on removal to show deformation of the polyethylene to accommodate this rotation.[113] The cold-flow characteristics of polyethylene are well known and may affect the wear characteristics if the prosthesis is malpositioned or used inappropriately. Figure 36-7 shows plastic deformation and tibial component loosening in an obese patient over a 2-year period.

Marker Migration

Marker migration has been reported, particularly with the early geometric tibial prosthesis when the wire was not inserted into the polyethylene and bent at a right angle.[23]

Bolt Extrusion

In Arden's series of Shiers hinge arthroplasties, four bolt extrusions were reported.[4,5] One case had to be completely revised, and the other three were success-

---

* Matthews, L.S.: Personal communication, May 1976.

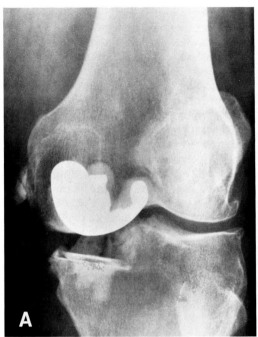
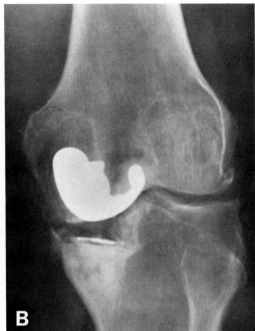

FIG. 36-7. (A) Early postoperative standing roentgenogram of a unicondylar implant. (B) Two years later, the implant shows plastic deformation, and the components have loosened.

fully replaced using two small lateral incisions to reinsert the bolt. Only two regained good function, and one had a persistent sinus. Though this complication is rare, it does occur. To date we know of no such episodes with the GUEPAR system; however, the ring spring–bolt retainer may easily be displaced.

Fracture of the Prosthesis

Fracture of the prosthesis has been observed by a number of authors. Shiers and Jones reported instances of Walldius femoral stem breakage and one early prosthesis in which there was a Teflon roller.[51,96–98] During the past few years the Herbert prosthesis has had significant failures due to fatigue fractures at the stem–prosthesis junction. The Letournel-Lagrange ("LL") prosthesis sustained fatigue fractures at the junction of the tibial stem.[61] Modifications have been made, and no further fractures have been recorded. As of this time there have been no reported instances of metal failure in the unlinked systems.

Mendes and associates reported fracture of a metal tray in a total knee prosthesis.[76] The metal tray used in this instance was made of a cast cobalt-chromium-molybdenum alloy, which is characterized by limited ductility and is therefore prone to brittle fracture. In this instance, there was no significant damage to the plastic insert other than some small indentation caused by the fractured tray. It was the conclusion of Mendes and co-workers that the metallurgical faults and the inadequate cement technique used in this particular case caused the metal tray fracture and loosening of the component. They point out that improvement in the design and structure of the tray and a better method to compensate for bony defects may prevent further occurrences of this complication.

Shaft Fracture

Fractures are most commonly associated with hinge prostheses and usually occur in the shaft at the tip of the medullary stem.[5,37,49,83,117] The majority of these fractures will heal when treated by the usual closed methods, and unless the prosthesis

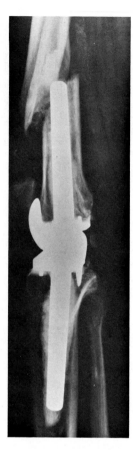

FIG. 36-8. A healing femoral fracture that occurred at the tip of the femoral stem.

is loose, it does not require modification (Fig. 36-8).

A number of supracondylar femoral fractures have occurred in the presence of condylar prostheses and have, by and large, been treated successfully by skeletal traction, cylindrical plaster casting, or fracture bracing. However, in some instances the fractures have been opened and internally fixed (Fig. 36-9). If the prosthesis has been loosened, it is probably wiser to revise it after the fracture has healed.

Metal Sensitivity, Osteolysis, and Arthroplasty Failure

Evans and colleagues reported a series of problems in total knee arthroplasties from which, after thorough investigation, they concluded that the failures were due to osteolysis and loss of bone stock.[27]

It was postulated that the release of metal from the prosthesis in metal-sensitive patients causes obliterative changes in the blood vessels supplying bone into which the prosthesis is implanted and thereby leads to bone death, fibrous replacement, fatigue fracture, and ultimately, prosthesis loosening. Metallic constituents of cobalt-chromium and of stainless steel can be detected in surrounding tissues 4 to 6 months after implantation.

Once the bond between the acrylic and the bone has failed, the acrylic must move relative to the bone, and it seems reasonable to suppose that in so doing acrylic becomes abraded, producing a sterile semi-fluid necrotic mass around the prosthesis. Sometimes a fistulous tract may develop, requiring removal of the prosthesis.

Evans and associates suggest patch-testing all prospective total joint replacement patients. If the patient is sensitive to cobalt, a stainless steel prosthesis may be used; if sensitive to nickel, a cobalt-chromium alloy without nickel may be used. They also suggest patch-testing patients in whom prosthesis loosening associated with some bone loss on the side of the metallic implant occurs. Brown and co-workers, reporting on sensitivity to metal as a possible cause of sterile loosening after cobalt-chromium total hip arthroplasty, noted that lymphokine assays were done for migration inhibition factor and blastogenic stimulation factors.[13] These are the most sensitive tests for determining whether a process of loosening is in fact directly related to metal sensitivity. They found that the patch tests for sensitivity to chromium-nickel-cobalt and methylmethacrylate monomer were uniformly negative in all of their studies and stated that if the lymphokine assay is positive, the extent of the migration of the cells is 80% or less of that found in the control group. Their review of the assay for blastogenic stimulation factor was positive in only one patient out of 20. In this patient the test was positive in the middle dilutions only, and total stimulated counts were barely above the normal range.

If a patient is sensitive to the metals used, removal of the prosthesis is indicated, and revision can be considered only if the new prosthesis is free of the sensitizing

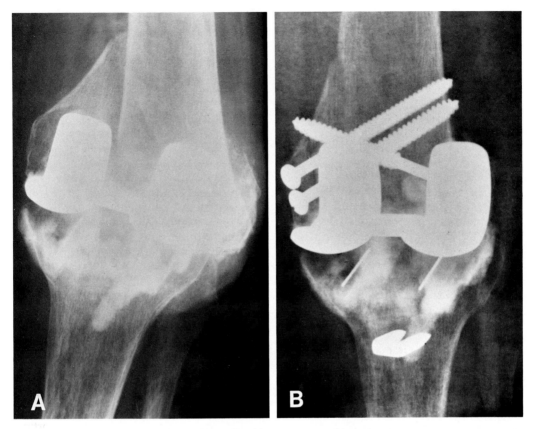

Fig. 36-9. (*A*) A patient who had a geometric prosthesis sustained a supracondylar femoral fracture. (*B*) After open reduction and internal fixation the components were found firmly fixed to the bone.

metallic element. The production of necrotic debris may be regarded as being due to infection, even though no pathogenic organism is cultured, but in reality it is probably due to metal sensitivity. It is also possible that this necrotic metal-sensitive debris may become infected secondarily, so that even in some infected joints the failure may be due primarily to metal sensitivity. Wigren and Fischer reported the development of a cobalt sensitivity in a patient 1 year after insertion of a Walldius implant.[115]

Pain of Undetermined Cause

Bain reported that in a series of patients with hinge prostheses, pain was often present along the medial side of the joint, and he presumed that the synovial lining or capsule was being impinged by the hinge.[7] In our series of nonhinged prostheses in

which the patella has been resurfaced, a number of patients have complained of pain along the incision site many months after arthroplasty. In the majority of instances these symptoms are greatly relieved by a short course of antiinflammatory medication. We are not sure, but we feel that this pain may be related to traction on the scar and adjacent tissues.

Complications of Arthroplasties Other Than Total Knee Replacement

The metal hemiarthroplasties of Mc-Keever and MacIntosh, introduced in the early 1960s, brought to many patients, as did the cup arthroplasty for the hip, relief of pain and considerable improvement in function during the years prior to the use of plastic and cement.[66,68] Fixation of these flat hemispherical objects was a significant

problem, somewhat more with the Mac-
Intosh than with the McKeever, and the
components tended to move, tilt, angulate,
migrate, and dislocate. Where there was
considerable bone loss or angulation, adequate connection of the deformities could
not be achieved. Therefore, it was impossible to obtain optimal tension on the capsular and ligamentous tissues to secure
intrinsic stability, which further created
abnormal motion, resulting in the eventual
loosening and migration of these tibial plateau prostheses.

In most instances these metallic objects
were articulating against cartilage of poor
quality or directly against subchondral bone,
so the relief of pain was less than that
which we have come to expect from the
replacement of both sides of the tibiofemoral joint. The most extensive review of
patients following implantation of McKeever
and MacIntosh prostheses was reported by
Potter and co-workers.[84] They reported only
56% good and excellent ratings in their
rheumatoid group, with an increase to 62%
for the same rating when the results of the

osteoarthritic group were added. Kay and
Martins, in a smaller series, reported less
than 50% good results with plateau
prostheses.[55] Figure 36-10, *A*, shows a cemented, painful McKeever prosthesis with
varus deformity and bone loss of the medial
tibial plateau. Figure 36-10, *B*, demonstrates
the correction of the varus deformity by
revision with a duopatellar system and
heavy metal mesh to reinforce the cement
on the area of the medial tibial plateau.

Jones, Aufranc, and Kermond introduced
their femoral mold prosthesis, and although
fixation was not the problem as with the
tibial plateau prostheses, nevertheless the
problem of metal against suboptimal cartilage and/or bone eventually required the
conversion of some of these to either hinge
systems or to the newer metal–plastic
prostheses because of increasing pain and
loss of motion.

Probably the most extensively used
interposition arthroplasty performed in
this country using material other than
metal was that introduced by Potter and
Kuhns.[57,58] They used a thin sheet of nylon

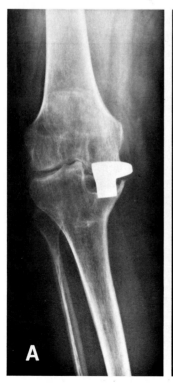
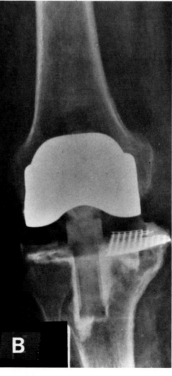

FIG. 36-10. (*A*) Roentgenogram
of a painful McKeever prosthesis. (*B*) The varus deformity
was corrected with a Duopatellar system and heavy metal
mesh to reinforce the cement
and disperse the weight-bearing force over the ostoporotic
medial tibial plateau.

that was secured to the molded end of the femur with staples or sutures. This procedure required a high degree of surgical skill and attention to detail to mold and then mate the convex surface of the femur to the concavity developed in the tibia. Nevertheless, in many patients with severe deformities and pain the results were quite gratifying. However, the postoperative course was more extended, and the majority of knees required routine manipulation, unlike other procedures.

In a review of a series at our institution it was found that these knee arthroplasties by and large became more stable with time but also tended to lose functional motion. As this occurred, pain became an increasing factor once again, resulting in revision to total knee arthroplasties in some instances.

The patellofemoral joint has witnessed such procedures as bony forage of the patella and femoral condyles, soft tissue interposition patellar arthroplasty, McKeever patellar prosthesis,[74] and patellectomy, alone or in combination with various forms of incomplete tibiofemoral arthroplasty, without any method proving superior.

Hanslik reported a review of 62 patients of a total of 78 McKeever patellar arthroplasties performed in conjunction with high tibial osteotomy, which he was able to follow for 1 to 4 years.[42] Though the author concluded that the patellar prosthesis was of help, it appears from these data that many patients still had significant pain related to the patellofemoral articulation. The problem of a metallic object articulating against poor cartilage or bone again becomes a major factor preventing complete relief of pain and requiring replacement arthroplasty.

There have been reports of the use of a high-density polyethylene patellar prosthesis alone for the treatment of patellofemoral arthrosis. Although the data are incomplete, it would appear that this approach will require further surgical revision and modification and should not be considered as a primary method of surgical treatment for this problem.

Potter, after an extensive review of the literature, indicated that in the past 100 years, operative attempts at restoring function and relieving pain in arthritic knee joints have had only partial success. Most large series of various types of knee arthroplasties rated less than 50% of their patients as having good results. It appears, therefore, that a significant number of patients require revision to total knee arthroplasty.

Total knee replacement surgery has made considerable progress over the past 13 years. Second-generation systems incorporating new and improved design features are now available. However, the problems are far from solved, and considerable research—both basic and clinical—is still necessary before this area of reconstructive surgery is stabilized.

Principles of Revision Surgery for Failed Total Knee Arthroplasty

The goal of any revision surgery is basically to improve function. This is realized by the relief of pain, restoration of stability, and restoration of good joint control and motion.[5,7,20,43] The preparation for revision surgery is fundamentally much more complex than that required for initial arthroplasty. Once the reasons for failure are defined, a clear plan can be designed to correct the problem. The ^{99}Tc and gallium scans used for routine evaluation are found to be useful, as are WBC ^{111}In-labeled scans. Aspiration of the joint may or may not be helpful. The amount of bone loss should be estimated as accurately as possible, and these estimations are made primarily on the plain films on long, standing cassettes.

Any attempt at revision would be unwise without having the appropriate size prosthesis for revision.[46] There are enough systems presently available that have sufficient inherent thickness to allow for loss of bone substance without necessitating further bone resection or requiring the surgeon to make up for the defect with bone grafts or composites of methylmethacrylate, mesh, and scaffolding metals.

All soft tissues and scar must be removed completely down to clear bone. One of the major problems of revision surgery is the reflection of the quadriceps patellar mechanism. In many instances the quadriceps mechanism is so scarred and attenuated that a Z-plasty of the quadriceps mechanism is often preferable to reflecting the patellar tendon at its insertion. It should be remembered that when the patellar quadriceps mechanism is again reduced anteriorly, there may be enough adhesions present to prevent full flexion. Once exposure is adequate, *great care must be exercised in preserving all possible bone during the removal and preparation for the revision.* All fibrous tissue must be removed so that the remaining bony geometry is clear and uncovered by any soft tissue elements.

I feel that the least constrained type of prosthesis possible should be employed in any type of total knee arthroplasty, particularly in revision surgery. In the vast majority of patients requiring revision total knee arthroplasty, the replacement prosthesis can be the most unconstrained prosthesis available, whether it is a variant of the cruciate-substituting total condylar such as that represented by the kinematic stabilizer or the total condylar knee. These bearing surfaces allow for the lowest forces on the prosthesis–cement–bone interface. Alignment is critical in revision surgery, and special attention must be given to this facet of surgery. The principles of soft tissue release and soft tissue rebalancing during closure are, obviously, critical in revision surgery, and these principles must be adhered to meticulously. It must be pointed out once again that the major reasons for most failures are technical error.[5,6] The factors that control these technical considerations are the ligamentous and soft tissue constraints about the knee and the mechanical support of the components, particularly with regard to the tibial component in the subchondral cancellous complex. The osteotomy cuts must be accurate and must position the prosthesis at the proper angles to realize the optimal anatomical and mechanical alignment. Patellar alignment must be such that there is no tendency to subluxation or dislocation. The "rule of no-thumb tracking" of the patella before closure must be scrupulously adhered to.

I feel that the indications for hinge prostheses are practically nonexistent. If a hinge of any type is indicated, it is my preference to consider the kinematic rotating hinge as the salvage procedure if no other system can provide the stability and integ-

rity required for the revision surgery. It is also my opinion that the results of revision surgery can be and are nearly as good as those from primary surgery. In a series reported by Insall, 89% were rated good or excellent at follow-up.[46] In his series, extensor mechanism problems were more common in the revision group, and this can be well understood when one considers the restriction scarring that is seen with previous surgery. The revision cases may not show the level of pain relief obtained in primary operations. There also appears to be a higher incidence of radiolucent lines in revision surgery, which can be demonstrated even in immediate postoperative x-rays. Lotke has pointed out that when patients having undergone total condylar knee arthroplasty are followed for periods of time, most radiolucent lines do not seem to correlate with clinical results.[62] He suggested, however, that radiolucent lines that are wide and global seem to have clinical significance. He pointed out that thin radiolucent lines generally prove to be clinically insignificant owing to varying radiographic techniques and positioning. In revision surgery the lines appear to be broader, but the important factor is an increase in the width of radiolucency with time. If no increase in radiolucency occurs, the lines may be considered a radiographic finding that does not have any significant clinical importance.

Biologic Ingrowth

Freeman and co-workers have pointed out that an appropriately designed implant can be fixed without cement to accurately prepared bone surfaces to obtain short-term results comparable to those of cemented fixation.[34,35] The unchanging appearance of the roentgenograms suggests that these results may be maintained in the long term. If these conclusions are valid, the authors state, polymethylmethacrylate may be thought of as an alternative in joint arthroplasty. Thus, theoretically, inert materials (*e.g.*, carbon) can be interfaced directly with a skeleton. Since the authors have achieved interlock with viable bone without relying on bone ingrowth, these materials need not be porous. It is strongly suspected (but as yet unsupported by data) that adequate fixation can be obtained without relying even on the authors' relatively unsophisticated thinned peg, provided that: (1) the overall shape of the implant achieves interlock on the gross scale, with acceptably low sheer stresses at the interface and (2) the surgical technique achieves a correctly positioned implant applied to accurately cut bone surfaces. However, if for any reason accurate bone cuts cannot be achieved, the authors advocate the use of polymethylmethacrylate for fixation. Since January 1979, the results of the Freeman-Samuelson prosthesis with regard to fixation of the tibiofemoral and patellar components with bone fixation pegs have not revealed any component loosening.[35] An increase in the density of the bone interdigitation with the bone fixation peg was believed to be present in 15 of 21 knees, a finding similar to that reported in previous reviews of cementless tibial components. The authors point out that since that time, the tibial component of the ICLH compartmental knee prosthesis has been fixed without cement using a bone fixation peg similar to that on the ICLH total knee tibial component.

Hungerford and Kenna,[45] reporting preliminary results of implanting a total knee prosthesis with a porous coating without cement in 41 patients (46 knees) and following these up for 4 to 25 months, found that there were no clinical interface failures. They found that radiographs showed that an intimate contact between bone and prosthesis was maintained for as long as 2 years. The authors feel that instrumentation is particularly critical to cementless application but also to total knee arthroplasty. They feel that an anatomic, minimally constrained resurfacing design has, in their experience, proven to be successful in the short term and justifies continuation of clinical investigation of cementless total knee arthroplasty. The authors point out that there are certain advantages to avoiding the use of cement, even if the results are only clinically comparable. Without cement, there is a reduction in operating time of approximately 20 to 30 minutes. Without cement, there is no acrylic debris to hasten wear on the polyethylene component. In the event of revision without cement, a maximum of bone stock will be preserved. The authors point out that proper functioning of the posterior cruciate requires accurate component positioning, since this system requires posterior cruciate retention. Component malpositioning, which might be tolerated in the system that sacrifices the posterior cruciate, may result in premature tightening of the posterior cruciate, which would restrict flexion.

It appears that prosthesis design is intimately related to function, and this appears to be dramatically borne out by the experience of Hungerford and Kenna, who remind us once again that the most minimally constrained system is the most successful with regard to the variations in modular elasticity of the implant at the bone interface. Therefore, it appears that the success of any knee arthroplasty in which surfaces that allow for biologic ingrowth are used requires that the bearing surfaces be the most unconstrained available. Freeman and associates believe that immediate osseointegration provides several advantages over techniques requiring polymethylmethacrylate or relying on biologic ingrowth but feel that several requirements must be met[35]:

There must be sufficient bone–implant interface strength to allow further rehabilitation of the patient, just as with implants restabilized with polymethylmethacrylate. This advantage is not seen in implants relying solely on bone ingrowth, they point out.

This immediate strength must not deteriorate with time; the integration system must demonstrate long-term high fatigue strength, and the bone–implant interface must be biologically stable. The material of the implant interface must be well tolerated by bones; ideally, it must not elicit a macrophage response.

Actual intraoperative implantation must not be excessively demanding, yet surface preparation must be exact, or nearly so.

Bone resection requirements must be minimal and certainly must not exceed those for cemented implants.

The method of integration must be such that in the event of failure, removing the implant does not destroy a large amount of bone and thus render implantation virtually impossible.

Freeman and associates feel that immediate fixation by interdigitation between the living skeleton and the implant can be (and has been) achieved, and they feel that such a technique may have a substantial future. However, it must be recognized that the experiences of Hungerford and Kenna with the knee and of Engh and Lunceford with the hip appear to show that the results of using porous surfaces for biologic ingrowth produce the same results that can be achieved with immediate interlock.[26,45] I wish only to point out the differences and similarities in the experiences of these investigators; only with time will these fixation methods be proven.

REFERENCES

1. Albright, J.P., and Brand, R.A.: The relationship of geometric total knee prosthesis placement to failure. National Academy of Sciences Report V 101(134) P-350 and SRS-500-75-0001 and HEW 105-76-4103: 239–246, September 1974.
2. Amstutz, H.R., and Finerman, G.A.M.: Knee joint replacement—development and evaluation. Clin. Orthop., 94:24, 1973.
3. Andriacchi, T.P., Galante, J.O., and Fermier, R.W.: The influence of total knee-replacement design on walking and stair climbing. J. Bone Joint Surg., 64A:1328, 1982.
4. Arden, G.P.: Total knee replacement. Clin. Orthop., 94:92, 1973.
5. ———: Complications of total knee replacement and their treatment. In The Knee Joint. International Congress Series, No. 324: 221–227. Amsterdam, Excerpta Medica, 1974.
6. Arden, G.P., and Ansell, B.M.: Surgical management of juvenile chronic polyarthritis. J. Bone Joint Surg., 54B:169, 1972.
7. Bain, A.M.: Replacement of the knee joint with the Walldius prosthesis using cement fixation. Clin. Orthop., 94:65, 1973.
8. Bandi, W., and Brennwald, J.: The significance of femoropatellar pressure in the pathogenesis and treatment of chondromalacia patellae and femoropatellar arthrosis. In The Knee Joint. International Congress Series, No. 324, pp. 63–68. Amsterdam, Excerpta Medica, 1974.
9. Bartel, D.L., Burstein, A.H., Santavicca, B.A., and Insall, J.N.: Performance of the tibial component in total knee replacement: Conventional and revision designs. J. Bone Joint Surg., 64A:1026, 1982.
10. Bisla, R.S., Inglia, A.E., and Lewis, R.J.: Fat

11. embolism following bilateral total knee replacement with the GUEPAR Prosthesis: A case report. Clin. Orthop., 115:130, 1976.
11. Brady, T.A., and Garber, J.N.: Knee joint replacement using Shiers knee hinge. J. Bone Joint Surg., 56A:1610, 1974.
12. Brause, B.D.: Infected total knee replacement: Diagnostic, therapeutic and prophylactic considerations. Orthop. Clin. North Am., 13:245, 1982.
13. Brown, G.C., Lockshin, M.D., Salvati, E.A., and Bullough, P.G.: Sensitivity to metal as a possible cause of sterile loosening after cobalt–chromium total hip replacement arthroplasty. J. Bone Joint Surg., 59A:164, 1977.
14. Bryan, R.S., Peterson, L.F.A., and Combs, J.J.: Polycentric knee arthroplasty: A preliminary report of postoperative complications in 450 knees. Clin. Orthop., 94:148, 1973.
15. Bryan, R.S., and Rand, J.A.: Revision total knee arthroplasty. Clin. Orthop., 170:116, 1982.
16. Cameron, H.U., and Hunter, G.A.: Failure in total knee arthroplasty: Mechanisms, revisions, and results. Clin. Orthop., 170:141, 1982.
17. Charnley, J.: Anchorage of femoral head to the shaft of the femur. J. Bone Joint Surg., 42:28, 1960.
18. ———: Acrylate cement in orthopaedic surgery. London, E&S Livingstone, 1970.
19. Clayton, M.L., and Thirupathi, R.: Patellar complications after total condylar arthroplasty. Clin. Orthop., 170:152, 1982.
20. Convery, F.R., and Beber, C.A.: Total knee arthroplasty: Indications, evaluation and postoperative management. Clin. Orthop., 94:42, 1973.
21. Coutts, R.D.: Use of continuous passive motion in the postoperative management of patients undergoing total knee arthroplasty. Report before the Orthopaedic Research Association Meeting, 1982.
22. Coventry, M.B., Finerman, G.A.M., Riley, L.H. et al.: A new geometric knee for total knee arthroplasty. Clin. Orthop., 83:157, 1972.
23. Coventry, M.B., Upshaw, J.E., Riley, L.H. et al.: Geometric total knee arthroplasty. II. Patient data and complications. Clin. Orthop., 94:177, 1973.
24. Cracchiolo, A.: Polycentric knee arthroplasty using tibial prosthetic units of a variable height. Clin. Orthop., 94:140, 1973.
25. Crawford, W.J., Hillman, F., and Charnley, J.: A clinical trial of prophylactic anticoagulation therapy in elective hip surgery. Internal publication No. 14. Wiggam, England, Centre for Hip Surgery, Wrightington Hospital, May 1968.
26. Engh, C.A.: Hip arthroplasty with a Moore prosthesis with porous coating: A five year study. Clin. Orthop., 176:52, 1983.
27. Evans, E.M., Freeman, M.A.R., Miller, A.J., and Vernon-Roberts, B.: Metal sensitivity as a cause of bone necrosis and loosening of the prosthesis in total joint replacement. J. Bone Joint Surg., 56B:626, 1974.
28. Evarts, C.M., and Feil, E.J.: Prevention of thromboembolic disease after elective surgery of the hip. J. Bone Joint Surg., 53A:1271, 1971.

29. Ewald, F.C.: Metal-to-plastic total knee replacement. Orthop. Clin. North Am., 6:811, 1975.
30. Fortune, W.P.: A general overview of various total knee prostheses—their relative indications. Report N.A.S., V 101(134) P-350, SRS-500-75-0001 and HEW 105-76-4103: 215–224, September 1974.
31. Fortune, W.P., and Adams, J.P.: Geometric total knee arthroplasties: A report of fifty cases. In The Knee Joint. International Congress Series, No. 324, pp. 251–260. Amsterdam, Excerpta Medica, 1974.
32. Fox, J.L., and Poss, R.: The role of manipulation following total knee replacements. J. Bone Joint Surg., 63A:357, 1981.
33. Freeman, M.A.R.: Total replacement of the knee. Orthop. Rev., 3:2, 1974.
34. Freeman, M.A.R., Blaha, J.D., Bradley, G.W., and Insler, H.P.: Cementless fixation of ICLH tibial component. Orthop. Clin. North Am., 13:141, 1982.
35. Freeman, M.A.R., McLeod, H.C., and Levai, J.-P.: Cementless fixation of prosthetic components in total arthroplasty of the knee and hip. Clin. Orthop., 196:88, 1983.
36. Freeman, M.A.R., Swanson, S.A.V., and Todd, R.C.: Total replacement of the knee using the Freeman-Swanson knee prosthesis. Clin. Orthop., 94:153, 1973.
37. Freeman, P.A.: Walldius arthroplasty—a review of 80 cases. Clin. Orthop., 94:85, 1973.
38. Gluck, T.: Referat über die durch das moderne chirugische Experiment. Arch. Klin. Chir., 41:186, 1891.
39. Gunston, F.H.: Polycentric knee arthroplasty. J. Bone Joint Surg., 53B:272, 1971.
40. Habermann, E.T., Deutsch, S.D., and Rovere, G.D.: Knee arthroplasty with the use of the Walldius total knee prosthesis. Clin. Orthop., 94:72, 1973.
41. Hanslik, L.: First experience on knee joint replacement using the Young hinged prosthesis combined with a modification on the McKeever patella prosthesis. Clin. Orthop., 94:115, 1973.
42. ———: McKeever patellar prosthesis combined with high tibial osteotomy. In The Knee Joint. International Congress Series, No. 324, p. 267. Amsterdam, Excerpta Medica, 1974.
43. Harris, W.H., Salzman, E.W., and DeSanctis, R.W.: The prevention of thromboembolic disease by prophylactic anticoagulation: A controlled study in elective hip surgery. J. Bone Joint Surg., 49A:81, 1967.
44. Harris, W.H., et al.: Comparison of warfarin, low-molecular-weight dextran, aspirin, and subcutaneous heparin in prevention of venous thromboembolism following total hip replacement. J. Bone Joint Surg., 56A:1552, 1974.
45. Hungerford, V.S., and Kenna, R.V.: Preliminary experience with a total knee prosthesis with porous coating used without cement. Clin. Orthop., 196:95, 1983.
46. Insall, J.N., and Dethmers, V.A.: Revision of total knee arthroplasty. Clin Orthop., 170:123, 1982.
47. Insall, J.N., Lachiewicz, P.F., and Burstein, A.H.: The posterior stabilized condylar prosthesis: A modification of the total condylar design. Two to four-year clinical experience. J. Bone Joint Surg., 64A:1317, 1982.
48. Insall, J.N., Thompson, F.M., and Brause, B.D.: Two-stage reimplantation for the salvage of infected total knee arthroplasty. J. Bone Joint Surg., 65A:1087, 1983.
49. Jackson, J.P., and Elson, R.A.: Evaluation of the Walldius and other prostheses for knee arthroplasty. Clin. Orthop., 94:104, 1973.
50. Jones, G.B.: Walldius arthroplasty of the knee. J. Bone Joint Surg., 52B:390, 1970.
51. ———: The Walldius hinge. Clin. Orthop., 94:50, 1973.
52. Kaufer, H.: Mechanical function of the patella. J. Bone Joint Surg., 53A:1551, 1971.
53. Kaufer, H., and Matthews, L.S.: Resection arthroplasty for salvage of infected total knee arthroplasty. Instr. Course Lect., 1984.
54. ———: Spherocentric arthroplasty of the knee: Clinical experience with an average four-year follow-up. J. Bone Joint Surg., 63A:545, 1981.
55. Kay, N.R.M., and Martins, H.D.: The MacIntosh tibial plateau hemiprosthesis for the rheumatoid knee. J. Bone Joint Surg., 54B:256, 1972.
56. Kettelkamp, D.B., Thompson, C., Stauffer, R. et al.: Mechanical and functional role of the patella. Report N.A.S., V 101(134) P-350, SRS-500-75-0001 and HEW 105-76-4103: 279–292, 1974.
57. Kuhns, J.G., and Potter, T.A.: Nylon arthroplasty of the knee joint in chronic arthritis. Surg. Gynecol. Obstet., 91:351, 1950.
58. ———: Problems of the knee joint in rheumatoid arthritis of the knee. Curr. Prac. Orthop. Surg., 2:65, 1963.
59. Lachiewicz, P.F., and Ranawat, C.S.: Fat embolization syndrome following bilateral total knee replacement with total condylar prostheses: Report of two cases. Clin. Orthop., 160:106, 1981.
60. Laskin, R.S.: Total condylar knee replacement in rheumatoid arthritis: A review of 117 knees. J. Bone Joint Surg., 63A:29, 1981.
61. Letournel, E., and Lagrange, J.: Total knee replacement with the "LL" type prosthesis. Clin. Orthop., 94:249, 1973.
62. Lotke, P.A.: Long-term results after total condylar knee replacement: Significance of radiolucent lines. Presented at the Annual Meeting of the American Academy of Orthopaedic Surgeons, Atlanta, February 1984.
63. Lotke, P.A., Ecker, M.L., Alavi, A., and Berkowitz, H.: Indications for the treatment of deep venous thrombosis following total knee replacement. J. Bone Joint Surg., 66A:202, 1984.
64. Lynch, J.A.: Total knee replacement arthroplasty. In The Knee Joint. International Congress Series, No. 324, p. 271. Amsterdam, Excerpta Medica, 1974.
65. McGrouther, D.A.: Load actions transmitted at the knee of arthritic patients. Symposium, Total Knee Replacement, Inst. Mech. Eng., London, 1974.

66. MacIntosh, D.C., and Hunter, G.A.: The use of the hemiarthroplasty prosthesis for advanced osteoarthritis and rheumatoid arthritis of the knee. J. Bone Joint Surg., 54B:244, 1972.

67. McKeever, D.C.: Patellar prosthesis. J. Bone Joint Surg., 37A:1074, 1955.

68. ———: Tibial plateau prosthesis. Clin. Orthop., 18:86, 1960.

69. Maquet, P., Simonte, J., and DeMarchin, P.: Reduction of femoropatellar pressure with bone block under patellar ligament. Rev. Chir. Orthop., 5:111, 1967.

70. Markolf, K.L.: Optimization of prosthetics cementing technique—rheological and mechanical considerations. Report N.A.S., V 101(134) P-350, SRS-500-75-0001 and HEW 105-76-4103: 139–142, September 1974.

71. Marks, K.E., Nelson, C.L., and Lautenschlager, E.P.: Antibiotic-impregnated acrylic bone cement. J. Bone Joint Surg., 58A:358, 1976.

72. Marmor, L.: The modular knee. Clin. Orthop., 94:242, 1973.

73. Matthews, L.S., and Kaufer, H.: The spherocentric knee: A perspective on seven years of clinical experience. Orthop. Clin. North Am., 13:173, 1982.

74. Matthews, L.S., Sonstegard, D.A., and Kaufer, H.: The spherocentric knee. Clin. Orthop., 94:234, 1973.

75. Mazas, F.B., and GUEPAR Group: GUEPAR total knee prosthesis. Clin. Orthop., 94:211, 1973.

76. Mendes, D.G., Brandon, D., Galor, L., and Roffman, M.: Breakage of the metal tray in total knee replacement. Orthopaedics, 7(5):860, 1984.

77. Mensch, J.S., and Amstutz, H.C.: Knee morphology as a guide to knee replacement. Clin. Orthop., 112:231, 1975.

78. Milicic, M.: Early experience with polycentric and geometric implants—indications for total knee replacement. In The Knee Joint. International Congress Series, No. 234, p. 277. Amsterdam, Excerpta Medica, 1974.

79. Murray, D.G.: Laboratory studies—prosthetics testing. Report N.A.S., V 101(134) P-350, SRS-500-75-0001 and HEW 105-76-4103: 113–116. September 1974.

80. Nogi, J., Caldwell, J.W., Kauzlarich, J.J., and Thompson, R.C.: Static testing on two nonhinged total knee replacements. Report N.A.S., V 101(134) P-350, SRS-500-75-0001 and HEW 105-76-4103: 103–112, September 1974.

81. Paul, J.P.: Gait laboratory. Report N.A.S., V 101(134) P-350, SRS-500-75-0001 and HEW 105-76-4103: 173–183, September 1974.

82. Petty, W., Bryan, R.S., Coventry, M.B., and Peterson, L.F.A.: Infection after total knee arthroplasty. Orthop. Clin. North Am., 6:1005, 1975.

83. Phillips, R.S.: Shiers alloplasty of the knee. Clin. Orthop., 94:122, 1973.

84. Potter, T.A., Weinfeld, M.S., and Thomas, W.H.: Arthroplasty of the knee in rheumatoid arthritis and osteoarthritis. J. Bone Joint Surg., 54A:1, 1972.

85. Ranawat, C.S.: Problems and failures in total-

knee arthroplasty. Report N.A.S., V 101(134) P-350, SRS-500-75-0001 and HEW 105-76-4103: 247–262, September 1974.

86. Ranawat, C.S., and Shine, J.J.: Duocondylar total knee arthroplasty. Clin. Orthop., 94:185, 1973.

87. Rand, J.A., and Bryan, R.S.: Reimplantation for the salvage of an infected total knee arthroplasty. J. Bone Joint Surg., 65A:1081, 1983.

88. Reckling, F.W.: Details of studies of an ex-vivo geometric total knee prosthesis. J. Bone Joint Surg., 56A:1302, 1974.

89. Riley, L.H., Jr.: Factors which may influence the indications for use of several prosthetic devices for replacement of the femoral-tibial joint. Report N.A.S., V 101(134) P-350, SRS-500-75-0001 and HEW 105-76-4103: 225–230, September 1974.

90. Robson, L.J., Walls, C.E., and Swanson, A.B.: Popliteal artery obstruction following Shiers total knee replacement. Clin. Orthop., 109:130, 1975.

91. Salvati, E.A., Robinson, R.P., Zeno, S.M. et al.: Infection rates after 3,175 total hip and total knee replacements performed with and without a horizontal unidirectional filtered air-flow system. J. Bone Joint Surg., 64A:532, 1982.

92. Scales, J.T., and Lettin, A.W.F.: The Stanmore hinged total knee replacement. In The Knee Joint. International Congress Series, No. 324, p. 284. Amsterdam, Excerpta Medica, 1974.

93. Scheer, D.D., Dodd, T.A., and Buckingham, W.W., Jr.: Prophylactic use of topical antibiotic irrigation in uninfected surgical wounds: A microbiological evaluation. J. Bone Joint Surg., 54A:634, 1972.

94. Scott, R.D., and Santore, R.F.: Unicondylar–unicompartmental replacement for osteoarthritis of the knee. J. Bone Joint Surg., 63A:536, 1981.

95. Scott, R.D., Turoff, N., and Ewald, F.C.: Stress fracture of the patella following duopatellar total knee arthroplasty with patellar resurfacing. Clin. Orthop., 170:147, 1982.

96. Shiers, L.G.P.: Arthroplasty of the knee: Preliminary report on a new method. J. Bone Joint Surg., 36B:553, 1954.

97. ———: Arthroplasty of the knee: Interim report. J. Bone Joint Surg., 42B:31, 1960.

98. ———: Hinge arthroplasty of the knee. J. Bone Joint Surg., 47B:506, 1965.

99. Siegal, A.: Experiences with the Sledge prosthesis ("St. Georg" design). In The Knee Joint. International Congress Series, No. 324, p. 300. Amsterdam, Excerpta Medica, 1974.

100. Skolnick, M.D., Coventry, M.B., and Ilstrup, D.M.: Geometric total knee arthroplasty: A 2-year follow-up study. J. Bone Joint Surg. 58A:749, 1976.

101. Sledge, C.B., and Walker, P.S.: Total knee arthroplasty in rheumatoid arthritis. Clin. Orthop., 182:127, 1984.

102. Stauffer, R.N.: Reasons for failure of total-knee arthroplasty. Report N.A.S., V 101(134) P-350, SRS-500-75-0001 and HEW 105-76-4103: 273, September 1974.

103. Stulberg, B.N., Insall, J.N., Williams, G.W., and Ghelman, B.: Deep-vein thrombosis following total knee replacement: An analysis of 638 arthroplasties. J. Bone Joint Surg., 66A:194, 1984.

104. Stulberg, S.D.: Arthrodesis in failed total knee replacements. Orthop. Clin. North Am., 13:213, 1982.

105. Swanson, S.A.V.: Reason for failure. Report N.A.S., V 101(134) P-350, SRS-500-75-0001 and HEW 105-76-4103: 273, September 1974.

106. Thompson, R.C., Jr.: Clinical failure in geometric knee prosthesis. Report N.A.S., V 101(134) P-350, SRS-500-75-0001 and HEW 105-76-4103: 263, September 1974.

107. Thornhill, T.S., Dalziel, R.W., and Sledge, C.B.: Alternatives to arthrodesis for the failed total knee arthroplasty. Clin. Orthop., 170:131, 1982.

108. Walker, P.S., Greene, D., Reilly, D. et al.: Fixation of tibial components of knee prostheses. J. Bone Joint Surg., 63A:258, 1981.

109. Walker, P.S., and Shoji, H.: Development of a stabilizing knee prosthesis employing physiologic principles. Clin. Orthop., 94:222, 1973.

110. Walldius, B.: Arthroplasty of the knee using an endoprosthesis. Acta Orthop. Scand., 24:43, 1957.

111. ———: Arthroplasty of the knee using an endoprosthesis. Acta Orthop. Scand., 30:137, 1960.

112. ———: Prosthetic replacement of the knee joint. J. Bone Joint Surg., 50B:221, 1968.

113. Waugh, T.R.: Reasons for failure of the U.C.I. prosthesis. Report N.A.S., V 101(134) P-350, SRS-500-75-0001 and HEW 105-76-4103: 235, September 1974.

114. Waugh, T.R., Smith, R.C., Orofino, C.F., and Anzel, S.M.: Total knee replacement. Clin. Orthop., 94:196, 1973.

115. Wigren, A., and Fischer, T.: Kobalt-allergische Reaktion (metallose) nach kniegelenks-Arthroplastik mit Walldius-Prosthese. Z. Orthop., 113:273, 1975.

116. Wilson, F.C.: Total replacement of the knee in rheumatoid arthritis: A prospective study of the results of treatment with the Walldius prosthesis. J. Bone Joint Surg., 54A:1429, 1972.

117. ———: Total replacement of the knee in rheumatoid arthritis. Part II of a prospective study, Clin. Orthop., 94:58, 1973.

118. Witvoët, J., and GUEPAR Group: GUEPAR total knee prosthesis. In The Knee Joint. International Congress Series, No. 324, p. 305. Amsterdam, Excerpta Medica, 1974.

37 Complications of Total Joint Replacement of the Ankle

St. Elmo Newton III

Ankle fusion has been the traditional treatment for painful and debilitating diseases and injuries of the ankle. But ankle fusion has traditionally had several disadvantages and a high complication rate,[8] as well as a variable fusion rate. Sacrificing ankle motion to relieve pain puts greater stress on the knee and midtarsal joints,[1] and if these joints are diseased, the pain in them might be increased by ankle fusion. Painful degenerative changes frequently occur in the midtarsal region after ankle fusion even in the absence of preexisting disease.

Encouraged by the good results of total hip replacement and total knee replacement, several innovative orthopaedic surgeons began to replace ankle joints in the early 1970s (Fig. 37-1). Over the past 10 years, many other orthopaedic centers have used their designs in an attempt to relieve pain and preserve motion in the ankle joint.

While at first the enthusiasm for ankle replacement arthroplasty ran very high,

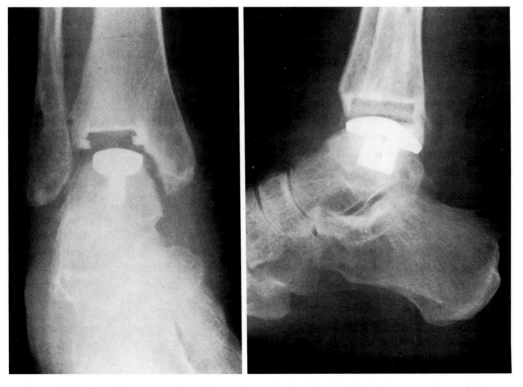

Fig. 37-1. The Newton total ankle replacement in place. Note the separation of the talomalleolar space on the AP view caused by distraction of the ankle during fitting and insertion of the prosthesis.

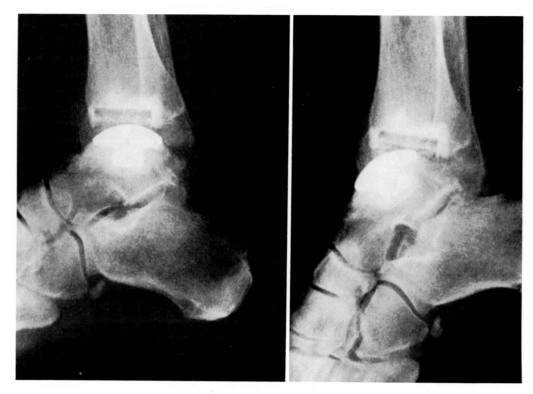

Fig. 37-2. Flexion and extension measured as tibiopedal total motion average 25° (from 5° dorsiflexion to 20° plantar flexion) in the series using the Newton prosthesis.

with early results showing preservation of motion (Fig. 37-2), good pain relief, and a reasonable activity level,[10,11] later, long–term reports[5,13] showed an increasing complication rate. However, the pendulum is now swinging back toward ankle fusion as the treatment of choice for these same painful and debilitating ankle conditions.[6,13,16]

THE ROLE OF CONSTRAINT

Basically, ankle implants can be divided into constrained types (those that attempt to replace the function of ankle ligaments and joint stability) and nonconstrained types (those that depend on reasonably normal ankle anatomy and joint stability with normal ligaments for their function). In the former group are such prostheses as the con-axial, Mayo, ICLH, and Conoidal. In the latter group are such prostheses as the TPR, Smith, and Newton. Some prostheses are designed to allow the freedom of motion of a multiple-axis prosthesis and yet in

some way make up for the lack of ligamentous stability. These would include such prostheses as the Oregon and the St. George-Buchholz.

As might be expected, certain mechanical properties and modes of failure might be expected from each group of prostheses. Those prostheses that are most constrained and have more intrinsic stability transfer larger forces to the fixation interface and are more likely to become loose at the bone–cement junction.[4] On the other hand, those prostheses with the least restraint transfer less force to the bone–cement junction and are less likely to show loosening. These same prostheses, however, are intrinsically less stable and are more likely to show subluxation as a postoperative complication (Figs. 37-3 through 37-5).[3]

BONE REMOVAL

The amount of bone removed for prosthetic implant is also variable with the prosthesis used and might be expected to

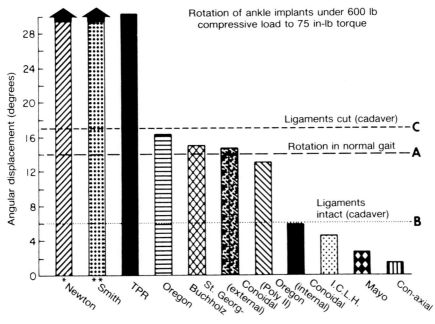

FIG. 37-3. Rotational tests demonstrate that the more constrained prostheses allow less rotational motion (Courtesy of the Cleveland Clinic Foundation, Biomechanics Laboratory)

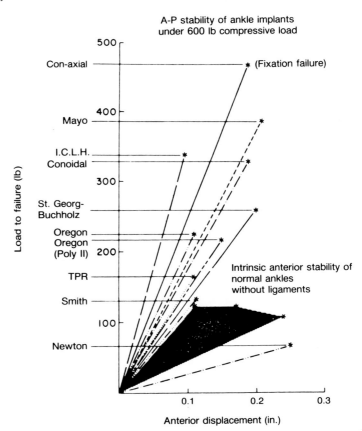

FIG. 37-4. Measurements of anterior-posterior stability demonstrate that the less constrained prostheses have a greater propensity for anterior displacement. (Courtesy of the Cleveland Clinic Foundation, Biomechanics Laboratory)

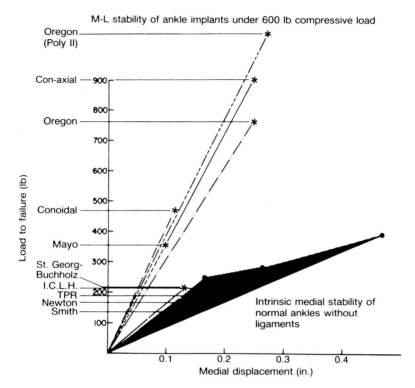

FIG. 37-5. Measurements of medial-lateral displacement demonstrate that more constrained prostheses have less displacement. (Courtesy of the Cleveland Clinic Foundation, Biomechanics Laboratory)

be of importance should complications occur and fusion become necessary. One prosthesis requires no resection of the talus and minimal resection of the tibia,[12] while others require a rather generous resection of both areas. It is advantageous to remove the least amount of bone possible.

THE ROLE OF FUSION IN FAILED ARTHROPLASTY

The published investigations have shown good success in obtaining fusion in failed ankles.[13,15] Those ankles that required minimal bone resection for prosthesis implant have been fused by direct apposition with an external compression device (Fig. 37-6). Those that require a large amount of bone resection have been fused successfully with interposition iliac crest grafts (Fig. 37-7)

and external compression devices. The desired position of fusion is slight dorsiflexion in both men and women to allow a more nearly normal gait.

Complications and/or failure have been multiple and have been reported to be as high as 72% with the ICLH prosthesis (Fig. 37-8)[7] and 41% with the Mayo prosthesis.[14] The types of complications vary with the type of prosthesis used and the center where it was inserted.

CONTRAINDICATIONS TO ANKLE REPLACEMENT

Most authors agree that ankle fusion is in general the treatment of choice for the isolated, painful, arthritic ankle joint with normal midtarsal joints. There is also agreement that the prosthesis should not be

FIG. 37-6. (A) Postoperative AP x-ray demonstrates the technique of fusion by direct apposition without bone grafts using Charnley compression clamps and a vertical Steinmann pin through the os calcis into the tibia, holding the foot in slight dorsiflexion, the desired position for fusion. (B) Postfusion lateral x-ray demonstrates solid ankle fusion following failed total ankle arthroplasty with the foot displaced posteriorly.

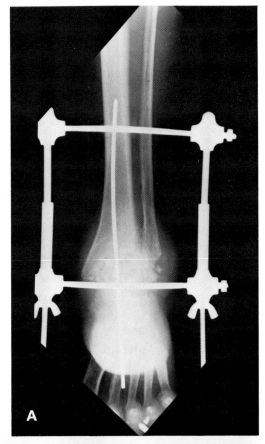

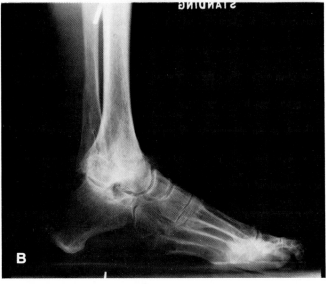

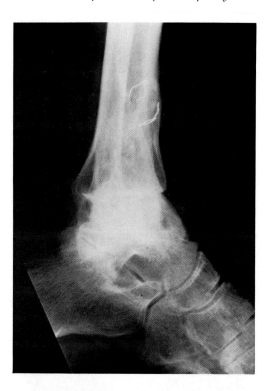

FIG. 37-7. Interposition full-thickness vertical iliac crest grafting can be used for fusion following failure of a total ankle prosthesis that requires removal of large amounts of bone.

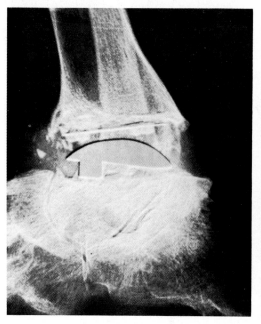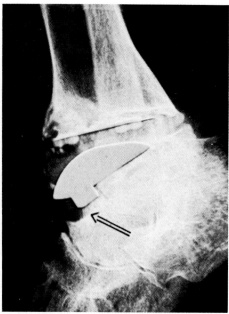

FIG. 37-8. Lateral views of an ICLH ankle joint arthroplasty 30 months postoperatively show loosening of the talar component visible at active flexion and extension. Note the zone between the prosthesis and the talus appearing in plantar flexion (*arrow*). (Herberts, P.: Endoprosthetic arthroplasty of the ankle joint: Clinical and radiological follow-up. Acta Orthop. Scand., 53[4]:687, 1982)

FIG. 37-9. (*A*) AP and lateral x-rays of ankle pseudarthrosis after three attempts at arthrodesis. Note the absence of the lateral malleolus, now recognized as a contraindication to ankle arthroplasty. (*B*) After total ankle arthroplasty, the ankle had residual lateral pain owing to instability and loosening of the prosthesis. The prosthetic components were removed, and arthrodesis was performed. (Stauffer, R.N.: Total ankle joint replacement. Arch. Surg., 112: 1105, 1977. Copyright © 1977, American Medical Association)

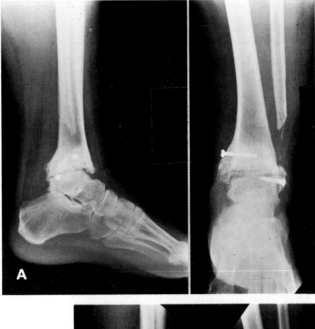

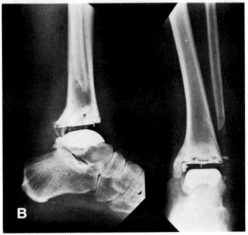

inserted into young, high-demand osteoarthritic patients with a high activity level. The two authors who commented on attempted ankle replacement in failed ankle fusions (Fig. 37-9) both recommend against further attempts because of consistent failure.[13,16] Avascular necrosis of the talus is also a contraindication to ankle replacement because of continuing collapse of the talus and loosening of the talar component (Fig. 37-10).[13] The best results reported were in osteoarthritics, patients more than 60 years

of age with low activity levels, and rheumatoid arthritics. One author noted a high failure rate in rheumatoid arthritics being treated with prednisone.[13] His long-term complications included loose prostheses and stress fractures of the malleoli up to 2 years postoperatively (Fig. 37-11), as well as one wound dehiscence 3 weeks postoperatively, resulting in a deep infection requiring fusion.

Although rheumatoid arthritic patients generally scored lower on the ankle rating

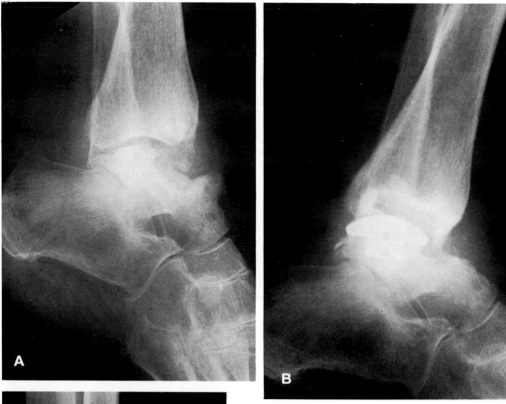

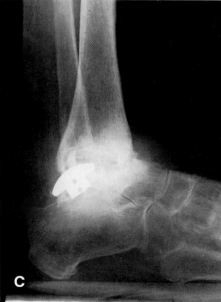

FIG. 37-10. (*A*) Preoperative lateral x-ray of the ankle shows avascular necrosis of the talus with a large anterior defect. (*B*) Immediate postoperative lateral x-ray of the same necrotic ankle shows the talar unit in a satisfactory position. It is placed more posterior than usual because of the large anterior talar defect. (*C*) Lateral x-ray of the same ankle shows that further collapse of the talus caused the talar unit to be extruded from the talus and forced posteriorly into the soft tissues. (Interestingly, this patient denies any pain in her ankle.)

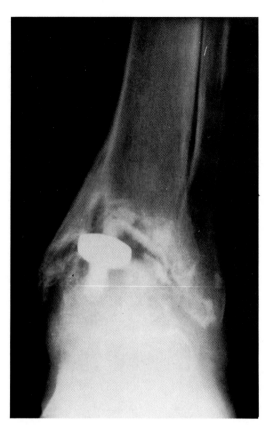

FIG. 37-11. AP x-ray of a total ankle prosthesis in a patient with rheumatoid arthritis on high-dose, long-term prednisone. This patient developed a stress fracture of her medial malleolus approximately 2 years following her ankle replacement. The fracture was asymptomatic and manifested clinically only by swelling in the ankle. After the fracture healed, the ankle remained asymptomatic, apparently owing to the euphoria that accompanies high-dose, long-term corticosteroid intake.

scale postoperatively than did osteoarthritics, they were nonetheless much improved, and it was often their other joint involvement that caused their scores to be low. Revision of failed ankle implants is possible, but one author reports a 76% failure rate in revision arthroplasties.[9] Fusion is the proper treatment for failed total ankle replacements in most cases.

SPECIFIC COMPLICATIONS

Delayed Wound Healing

Delayed wound healing is a frequently reported complication in most series, ranging from 5% to 20% of cases. The skin over the anterior ankle seems prone to skin necrosis, particularly in rheumatoid arthritics when prolonged pressure is applied by retractors. Two techniques to reduce the incidence of skin necrosis in this region are (1) making the skin incision longer and (2) avoiding the use of retractors on the skin, using them only on the deep tissue. Should skin necrosis occur, debridement, administration of proper antibiotics, immobilization, and sometimes skin grafting are necessary for proper wound healing.

Infection

Deep infection has been reported in 2% to 10% of cases and can be a devastating complication. Although it is sometimes possible to rescue a deep joint infection by vigorous antibiotic therapy, immobilization, debridement, and sometimes prosthesis removal, more often a deep infection ends with ankle fusion, and occasionally with amputation.

Amputation

Amputation need not be considered a complication of total joint replacement: sometimes it is simply the last method of relieving pain for some ankle problems that cannot be solved by joint implant or a joint fusion (Fig. 37-12). Some authors reporting on large series of ankle fusions noted a surprising number of amputations as their final treatment.[8] Perhaps amputation should be the primary treatment for some of the limbs that we try to salvage by joint replacement or fusion. One series of joint replacement had a 6% amputation rate.[13]

Ankle Fusion

Ankle fusion, likewise, need not be considered a complication of ankle replacement: it is simply the means to salvage a failed case. Ankle fusion has been necessary in 10% to 20% of the reported series. It is

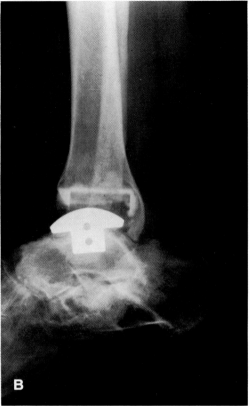

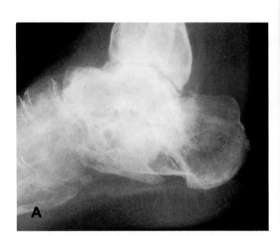

FIG. 37-12. (*A*) Preoperative lateral ankle x-ray shows severe damage of the ankle, subtalar, and midtarsal joints following a compound fracture-dislocation 4 years preoperatively. (*B*) Two years following joint replacement, spontaneous recurrence of a prior calcaneal infection resulted in amputation of this limb. Such severely injured feet might be better treated by earlier amputation instead of prolonged attempts to save a barely functional foot.

likely that as the follow-up in the series gets longer, the incidence of fusion will increase, since the failure rate seems to increase with time. The technique of fusion (Fig. 37-13) employed successfully in my center has been to use Charnley compression external pin fixation and a vertical pin through the os calcis into the tibia, with or without iliac bone grafts, depending on the prosthesis removed and its resulting bone defect.

As with all new types of prostheses, there is a learning curve that must be endured. Malalignment and/or malpositioning is likely to occur early in any large series.

Medial Malleolar Fracture

Fracture of the malleolus during insertion of the prosthesis has been reported with four different types of prostheses—the ICLH, Mayo, Buchholz, and Smith (Fig. 37-14)—though it is likely to have occurred in other smaller, unreported series with other types of prostheses. Fracture, which usually occurs in the medial malleolus, is the result of being too vigorous with bone removal or trying to use too large a prosthesis. Using a smaller prosthesis and being more delicate during bone removal have resolved this problem. This complication should decrease

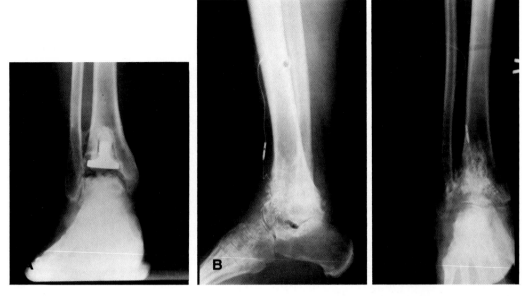

FIG. 37-13. (*A*) AP right ankle x-ray shows a loose tibial Smith-type ankle prosthesis causing symptoms of pain and swelling. (*B*) Six months after removal of the Smith prosthesis and Charnley compression fusion using an iliac bone graft and an implantable electrical bone growth stimulator, the ankle is fused and asymptomatic. The battery pack for the stimulator has not been yet removed.

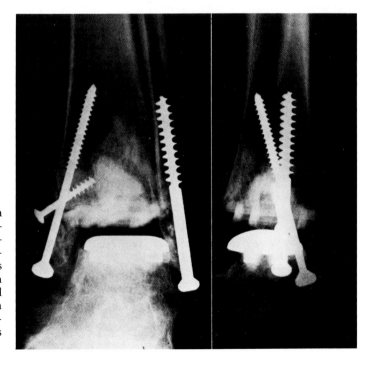

FIG. 37-14. X-rays show a fracture of the medial malleolus that occurred during insertion of the Buchholz ankle replacement. The malleolus has been stabilized by the insertion of two screws. The lateral malleolar screw is for fixation of the fibular osteotomy necessary for insertion of this prosthesis.

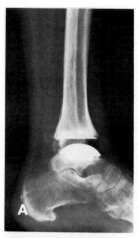
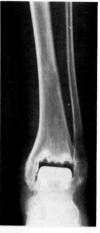
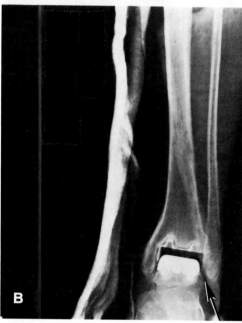

FIG. 37-15. (*A*) AP and lateral x-rays of a patient with persistent anterolateral ankle pain due to residual talofibular impingement following insertion of a Mayo prosthesis. (*B*) After surgical excision of the talofibular impingement (*arrow*), symptoms were relieved. The incidence of impingement syndrome can be reduced significantly by distraction of the foot and ankle during fitting and insertion of the prosthesis. (*B*, Stauffer, R.N.: Total ankle joint replacement. Arch. Surg., 112: 1105, 1977. Copyright © 1977, American Medical Association)

as the learning curve progresses. One surgeon (Buchholz), early in his experience, transfixed the medial malleolus with a screw during the creation of the tibial defect.

Heterotopic Bone Formation

Heterotopic bone formation has been reported by some authors[2,16] and is probably related to the type of bone preparation necessary for prosthesis implantation, since those prostheses that require the least amount of bone removal and bone preparation seem to have no heterotopic bone formation. The overall incidence of this complication is approximately 4%.[2]

Impingement

Impingement of the talomalleolar joint is a common complication in some series.[16] Lateral impingements have been treated successfully by a medial heel wedge, local corticosteroid injections, and sometimes surgery to remove the impinging bone (Fig. 37-15). Medial impingement has been treated with the lateral heel wedge and similar surgical or injection treatment. Lateral impingement seems more common, and this complication has been reported by at least four authors. Distraction of the ankle during fitting and insertion of the prosthesis as recommended by one author seems to prevent this complication.[12]

Peroneal Tendinitis

Transient peroneal tendinitis has frequently been present[2] and has been treated with anti-inflammatory drugs, immobilization, lateral heel wedges, and occasionally surgical decompression. Because the ankle is a small joint with limited posterior access (with the prosthesis in place it is impossible to visualize the posterior joint), excess cement in the back of the joint sometimes becomes a problem. Ideally, by proper application of the cement, excess methylmethacrylate in the back of the joint can be prevented. From a practical point of view, it is often impossible to prevent cement from going into the back of the joint. A large bolus of hard methylmethacrylate in the posterior joint will block ankle flexion. Therefore, it is important to compress this

FIG. 37-16. Preoperative ankle instability greater than 20° precludes a good result even if ankle replacement is combined with ligament reconstruction. This type of ankle should be treated with ankle fusion.

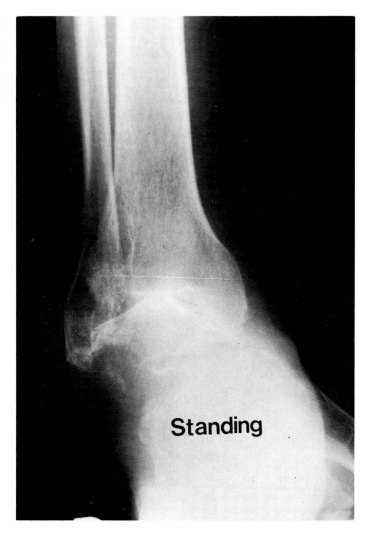

Standing

cement while it is still in a doughy stage by flexing and extending the ankle a few times before the cement hardens. With this maneuver, any cement in the back of the joint will be in such a configuration that it will not block flexion. Should a large bolus of cement be formed that does block flexion, it can be removed surgically from a posterior approach.

Instability

Subluxation of the prosthesis and instability seem to be associated more commonly with those prostheses that have the least inherent stability. One author found that every ankle with preoperative instability had postoperative instability. This same study showed that every ankle with preoperative varus or valgus deformity of the talus greater than 20° resulted in failure of the prosthesis secondary to subluxation and continuing pain (Fig. 37-16). From this experience it was determined that talar tilt greater than 20° is a contraindication to ankle replacement, even if accompanied by a lateral Watson-Jones tenodesis.[13] Stress films should be taken preoperatively if there is any question of instability.

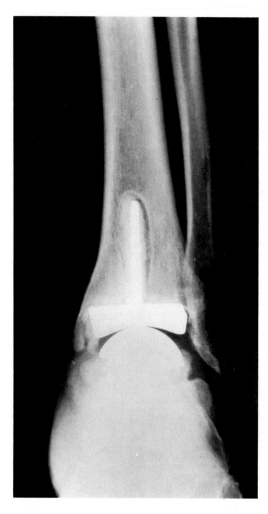

FIG. 37-17. A radiolucent line is visible around the tibial component of this UCLA prosthesis.

and will eventually cause failure. Other authors have noted that a thin radiolucent zone around a prosthesis may remain unchanged for many years. One large series found no correlation between symptoms and the presence of radiolucent lines.[13] Many of the pain-free ankles had radiolucent zones, and some of the painful ankles did not. Although some of the radiolucent zones increased in width and the prosthesis eventually became loose, others stayed the same over several years. In one series, arthrograms of the ankles with radiolucent lines failed to show a loose prosthesis in most cases (Fig. 37-18). Increasing width of a radiolucent zone, or a radiolucent zone greater than 2 mm in thickness, most likely indicates a loose prosthesis. Certainly any shift in position of a component indicates loosening.

Loosening

Loosening of the prosthesis with or without migration of the prosthetic components has been a cause of failure in as low as 6.9% of cases with the Mayo prosthesis to as high as 72% for an ICLH series.[7] Those prostheses requiring large resections of the talus more often have migration of the talar unit (Fig. 37-19). A loose prosthesis, however, does not always indicate a painful joint. One study documented loose prostheses that were asymptomatic in a patient with osteoarthritis and a low-demand job, a patient with rheumatoid arthritis on prednisone therapy, and a patient with avascular necrosis of the talus.[13]

Radiolucent Lines

Radiolucent lines around the prosthetic components (Fig. 37-17) are the most frequently seen complication after ankle replacement—as high as 88% in one reported series.[3] The significance of the radiolucent lines is not clearly understood. Microscopically, these are thin layers of fibrous tissue at the bone–cement interface. The cause of the fibrous reaction has not yet been fully explained. Some authors have speculated that it indicates loosening of the prosthesis

EVALUATION OF RESULTS

Generally, authors have considered ankle replacement to be a success if (1) the patient had little or no pain and was satisfied with the prosthesis (2) there was no evidence of loosening or malpositioning of the prosthesis, and (3) additional surgery was not required. Using these criteria, authors are reporting success in 60% to 70% of their cases in their early results, though the good result rate is likely to decrease as time passes. The normal exposure of the ankle

FIG. 37-18. Arthrogram of an ankle with radiolucent lines around the tibial component failed to show communication of the dye with the radiolucent line. This arthrogram, however, does show communication of the ankle joint with the peroneal tendon sheath, the subtalar joint, and the talonavicular joint, a fairly common occurrence.

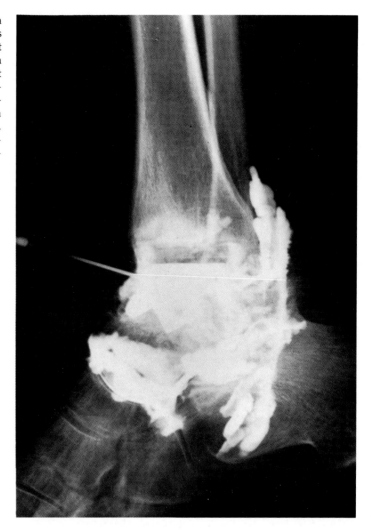

to high stresses five times body weight[14] will likely contribute to the increasing failure rate.

Recent gait studies have demonstrated weakness of plantar flexion and abnormal gait patterns in patients having undergone total ankle arthroplasty and have demonstrated satisfactory gait patterns in patients having undergone ankle fusion who subsequently wore appropriate shoes[3] with raised heels if necessary. The best gait in either sex is seen with the ankle fused in slight dorsiflexion.

CONTRAINDICATIONS

Ankle replacement has certain contraindications. As a general rule it should not be performed in young osteoarthritics, particularly those with a high-demand job or

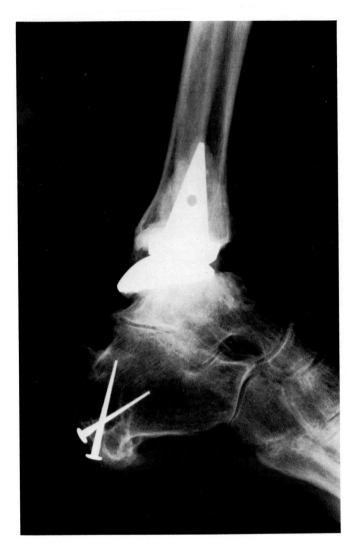

FIG. 37-19. Lateral ankle x-ray with a UCLA prosthesis shows migration of the talar component, indicating component loosening.

avocation. Total ankle arthroplasty is contraindicated in single-joint osteoarthritics with normal midtarsal joints and in patients with failed ankle fusions (Fig. 37-20), avascular necrosis of the talus, unstable ankle ligaments with talar tilt of 20° or greater (see Fig. 37-16), or any significant distortion of normal anatomy (Figs. 37-21 and 37-22).[13]

There remains a place for ankle replacement arthroplasty in osteoarthritics over 60 years of age, particularly those with abnormal midtarsal joints, and in rheumatoid arthritics, particularly those not on long-term prednisone therapy. Ankle fusion, however, remains the treatment of choice in most cases of painful, debilitated arthritic ankle joints.

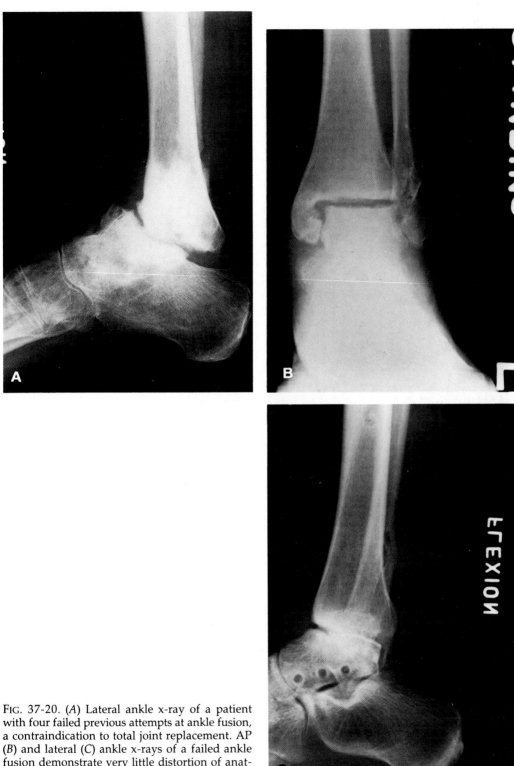

FIG. 37-20. (A) Lateral ankle x-ray of a patient with four failed previous attempts at ankle fusion, a contraindication to total joint replacement. AP (B) and lateral (C) ankle x-rays of a failed ankle fusion demonstrate very little distortion of anatomy, yet attempts at ankle replacement in this type of ankle have also been unsuccessful.

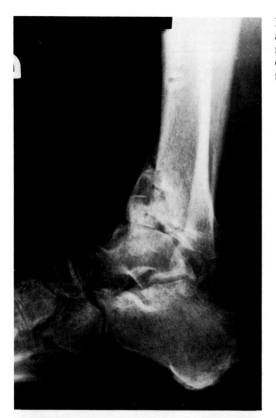

FIG. 37-21. Lateral ankle x-ray 2 years following a fracture of the anterior tibial plafond with malunion. This gross distortion of normal anatomy precludes a satisfactory result from ankle replacement.

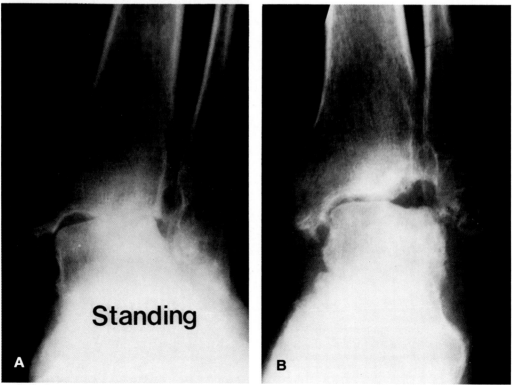

Standing

A

B

FIG. 37-22. (*A*) AP standing x-ray of a rheumatoid arthritic ankle being treated with high-dose corticosteroids shows a 20° valgus deformity of the talus. (*B*) Varus stress film of this same ankle shows significant erosion of the opposing surfaces of the lateral tibia and talus and the distal fibula. Significant distortion of normal anatomy such as this precludes a satisfactory result from ankle replacement.

REFERENCES

1. Anderson, K.J.: Personal communication.
2. Buechel, F.F., and Weiss, A.B.: Post-operative complications of 293 total ankle arthroplasties. Personal communication.
3. Demottaz, J.D. et al.: Clinical study of total ankle replacement with gait analysis: A preliminary report. J. Bone Joint Surg., 61A:976, 1979.
4. Greenwald, A.S., Matejczyk, M.C., and Black, J.Z.: Ankle joint mechanics and implant evaluation. Biomechanics Laboratories, Cleveland Clinic Foundation, personal communication.
5. Groth, H.E.: The Oregon ankle: A total ankle designed to replace all three articular surfaces. Orthop. Trans., 1:86, 1977.
6. Groth, H.E.: Personal communication.
7. Herberts, P.: Endoprosthetic arthroplasty of the ankle joint: Clinical and radiological follow-up. Acta Orthop. Scand., 53:687, 1982.
8. Johnson, E.W., Jr., and Boseker, E.H.: Arthrodesis of the ankle. Arch. Surg., 97:766, 1968.
9. Murray, W.R.: Total ankle arthoplasty: A joint too far. J. Bone Joint Surg., 63B:459, 1981.
10. Newton, S.E.: Total ankle replacement: An alternative to ankle fusion. J. Bone Joint Surg., 57A:1033, 1975.
11. Newton, S.E.: Total ankle replacement arthroplasty: An alternative to ankle fusion. Presented at the 42nd Annual Meeting of the American Academy of Orthopaedic Surgeons, San Francisco, 1975.
12. Newton, S.E.: An artificial ankle joint. Clin. Orthop., 142:141, 1979.
13. Newton, S.E.: Total ankle arthroplasty: Clinical study of fifty cases. J. Bone Joint Surg., 64A:104, 1982.
14. Stauffer, R.N.: Force and motion analysis of the normal, diseased and prosthetic ankle joint. Clin. Orthop., 127:189, 1977.
15. Stauffer, R.N.: Salvage of painful total ankle arthroplasty. Clin. Orthop., 170:184, 1982.
16. Stauffer, R.N., and Segal, N.M.: Total ankle arthroplasty: Four years experience. Clin. Orthop., 160:217, 1981.

Part Four

COMPLICATIONS OF RECONSTRUCTIVE SURGERY OTHER THAN ARTHROPLASTY

38 Complications of Surgery on Muscles, Fasciae, Tendons, Tendon Sheaths, Ligaments, and Bursae

Donald A. Nagel and John J. Csongradi

A successful surgeon must be an optimist and be able to convey optimism and enthusiasm to patients. Optimists do not like to consider complications, yet we have found the systematic review of complications on our orthopaedic service a valuable learning experience. Considering all of the complications (which occur in approximately 5% of the procedures on our service) tempers enthusiasm, producing a more thoughtful surgeon whose optimism is realistic.

After the surgeon involved presents each complication at a monthly conference, we try to reach a consensus about the cause: an error in judgement, an error in technique, or the patient's disease process. Although most complications are the results of errors of commission, we must also consider errors of omission.

ERRORS IN JUDGMENT

Possible Complicating Factors Related to Patient Selection

Poor Patient Motivation. Every surgeon comes to realize that there is more to consider before undertaking a surgical procedure than the patient's desire to have the surgery done and the surgeon's technical ability to do the procedure. Many reconstructive procedures, such as tendon transfers, require the patient's working against a certain amount of pain to achieve the desired result, and the patient who is unable to do this may be worse after the procedure than before. To evaluate the patient's motivation and cooperation, we have found it helpful to prescribe a set of exercises or a weight-reduction program on the patient's first visit. If the patient will not follow these instructions, we have a good indication that he may not follow instructions after surgery, and in these circumstances we do not do an elective procedure that requires much patient cooperation.

Inadequate Local Condition of the Proposed Site of Surgery. Deficiencies of skin, tendon, muscle, or nervous system may lead to complications. Trying to make a silk purse out of a sow's ear is an error in judgment. Examples include a major reconstructive surgical procedure for a hand with absent stereognosis when the other hand is normal, or attempting tendon grafting under split-thickness skin grafts.

Pathology Proximal or Distal to the Proposed Site of Surgery. Failure to consider the condition of an extremity proximal and distal to the site of proposed surgery can lead to complications, particularly if more surgery is planned at another time in one of these areas. Doing a Steindler flexorplasty to improve elbow function after transfer of a wrist flexor to finger extensors could result in unbalanced fingers.

Mistaken patient identity is not common, but it does occur. Constant vigilance must be maintained to prevent patients from receiving mismatched blood, performing an operation on the wrong extremity, or even operating on the wrong patient.

Choice of Surgical Procedure

It requires considerable judgment to select which among the available procedures for a given condition is best for the patient.

Different surgeons may recommend different procedures for a given patient, since their experience has been different. Sometimes no procedure is adequate, and a new procedure must be devised. Here the risks are great.

Possible Complications of Choosing the Wrong Operative Site

Recurrence of Tennis Elbow After Surgery. In a study of 84 of the world's most proficient tennis players, Priest and associates[31] found that 37% had major elbow symptoms related to playing tennis. The symptoms were more common on the medial side of the elbow for men and were associated with radiographic changes of soft tissue ossification, spurring at muscle and ligament attachments, and intra-articular bone fragments. The symptoms and radiographic changes were undoubtedly due to overuse and were treated with local and systemic anti-inflammatory drugs, heat and cold, ultrasound, massage, rest, various types of external bands, equipment changes, and changes of strokes. Many patients who are not tennis players also develop symptoms of medial and lateral epicondylitis and are treated in a similar way. Those who do not respond to these forms of treatment may undergo surgical treatment. The most common complication of this surgery we have seen is that the patient's symptoms persist or recur following surgery. This may be because the patient's symptoms were from entrapment of the radial nerve, which was not released, or from radiohumeral arthritis that could not be relieved. Operations for pain relief are not always successful, and an axillary brachial plexus nerve block should precede surgical treatment if the cause of the symptoms is at all in doubt. Such a block should differentiate a central type of pain, which cannot be helped by peripheral surgery, from a more distal type of pain, which may be helped. The error in judgment here is in doing the surgery at the wrong place, or in choosing to operate in the first place.

Recurrence of Baker's Cyst Following Surgical Excision. Baker recognized the connection between synovial cysts in the back of the knee and disease in the knee joint when he wrote his classic article on the subject in 1877.[1] This association is clearly demonstrated when a Baker's cyst recurs after surgical excision because the disease in the knee joint has not been controlled. We have seen such recurrences associated with degenerative arthritis and with unrecognized reticulum cell sarcoma in and near the joint. The surgeon should look carefully for disease within the knee joint before undertaking the excision of a Baker's cyst. By treating the basic disease, the need for surgery may be less and recurrences fewer.

Recurrence of Pain Following Release for Nerve Entrapment. Erroneous localization of a peripheral nerve entrapment may lead to decompression at the wrong site. Entrapment of the ulnar nerve at the wrist may masquerade as ulnar nerve compression at the elbow, and the nerve may be transposed without resolution of symptoms. The surgeon treating such problems must take exceptional care to localize the lesion by means of history, examination, and electrodiagnostic techniques.

Errors of Omission (Not Operating When We Should)

Very unexpectedly, a patient who needs immediate surgery may present at the most inopportune time. Yet the surgeon must be alert, make the proper diagnosis, and do the proper surgery if serious complications are to be prevented. Occasionally, even with adequate, timely surgery, complications do occur, and the surgeon's hope is to lessen the severity of the complications and to save the patient's life.

Vascular Injury. Insidious posttraumatic or postoperative limb ischemia may force amputation. An intimal tear in a vessel may not be suspected at the initial examination but can produce vascular compromise later. The unconscious patient should be watched carefully. Of particular concern is the patient with torn ligaments secondary to dislocation of the knee. Kennedy noted that involvement of associated vessels or nerves occurred in more than 50% of 22 dislocations.[15] In a patient with multiple injuries it is possible for the ligamentous injury and the arterial injuries to be missed initially; when this happens, valuable time is lost. Most surgeons believe that once the absence of pulse is noted, it is a waste of time to do sympathetic blocks. It is better to get an arteriogram and, if indicated, undertake definitive surgery immediately.

Another serious error in judgment is failure to recognize (and correct) a surgically produced vascular injury. The popliteal artery is occasionally injured during meniscectomy, and this complication may not be recognized as the leg is rendered ischemic by an Esmarch bandage and a pneumatic tourniquet. We prefer to deflate and remove the tourniquet before closing the wound so that all arterial bleeding can be identified and controlled. If the patient develops severe pain and swelling postoperatively, the complication of bleeding into the wound should be considered and appropriate action taken.

Compartment Syndromes. Increasing attention has been paid to the occurrence of various compartment syndromes since the classic article by Richard von Volkmann in 1881, wherein he set forth his reasons for believing that the paralysis and contracture of limbs "too tightly bandaged" were due to ischemic changes of muscles.[36] Jepson is credited with being the first to show in experimental animals the limbs of which were rendered ischemic that contractures could be prevented or minimized if surgical drainage was instituted.[14] Other animals treated similarly except for the surgical drainage developed edema of the extremity, and one was "left with a deformity typical of ischemic contracture and similar to that in man."

In 1945, Horn published an article on "acute ischemia of the anterior tibial muscle" during marching.[10] He noted that "the histological changes in the affected muscles are identical to those occurring in Volkmann's ischemia." Mavor[24] and Leach and co-workers[18] noted that the condition could be chronic as well as acute.

An excellent review of compartmental syndromes edited by Matsen and Clawson presents further causes for this syndrome: prolonged limb compression, complications of the Hauser procedure, complications of trauma, and peripheral vascular surgery.[22]

Still another article, by Sirbu and colleagues, reports ischemic necrosis occurring after the repair of a small hernia of the fascia of the anterior compartment.[33] It is helpful to realize that compartment syndromes are caused by anything that (1) reduces the compartment size (tight casts or bandages, closure of fascial defects, etc.) or (2) increases the compartmental contents (blood from vascular injury or osteotomy; edema following ischemia, burns, snake bites, trauma, exercise, venous obstruction, or the nephrotic syndrome; muscle hypertrophy; or extraneous fluid from infiltrated infusion).

Detailed discussions of the causes, prevention, diagnosis, and treatment of compartment syndromes may be found in a recent monograph by Mubarak and Hargens.[26]

Signs and Symptoms. The classic quintet of pain, paresthesia, pallor, paralysis, and pulselessness is not always present.

Pain is the most consistent sign, but because compartment syndromes are frequently associated with painful conditions (crush injuries, recovery from surgery, etc.), this symptom may be camouflaged with analgesics. Greater tenderness over the compartment than over the bone is an important sign. If pain increases with stable fracture fixation, one should also be more suspicious of ischemia.

Paresthesia (usually burning or prickling) may occur early or late in compartment syndrome.

Pallor may or may not be present. Occasionally the hand or foot has an erythematous or a cyanotic tinge. Neither pallor nor cyanosis should be considered essential for the diagnosis of compartment syndrome.

Paralysis may be due to the patient's fear of the severe pain caused by the active or passive stretch of ischemic muscles, or it may be the result of true motor loss. Motor function is the first nerve function to be lost when a limb is rendered ischemic.

Pulses distal to the involved compartment are frequently normal. More than one patient has developed contractures when his physician put off decompression of the involved compartment because there were good peripheral pulses. It is helpful to remember that arteriolar pressure is lower than arterial pressure.

Onset. The time for the development of signs and symptoms varies with different causes and different patients. Therefore, repeated examinations with careful documentation are indicated for patients at risk. If there is any suspicion of the diagnosis of a compartment syndrome, the cast or dressings should be removed, and the suspected compartment should be palpated and any tenderness or tenseness noted. Occasionally there is swelling over the involved compartment. Specialized neurologic examination techniques, such as two-point discrimination and light touch tests, are said to be better than the response to pinprick test. It should also be noted that in the anterior compartment syndrome of the lower extremity, only the deep peroneal nerve is involved, and therefore the only change in the sensory examination will be found in the web space between the great toe and the next toe. If there is muscular weakness, pressure measurements in the involved compartment should be done.

Measurements. Because the diagnosis of compartment syndrome has been so difficult to make on clinical grounds alone, Whitesides and colleagues have advocated the use of a simple pressure-measuring device consisting of a needle and plastic tubing filled with saline solution and air attached to a mercury manometer (Fig. 38-1).[37] Laboratory and clinical experience has led these authors to believe that "there is inadequate perfusion and relative ischemia when the tissue pressure within a closed compartment rises to within 10 to 30 mm Hg of the patient's diastolic blood pressure." Fasciotomy is, therefore, usually indicated when the tissue pressure rises to 40 torr to 50 torr in a patient with a diastolic blood pressure of 70 torr who has any of the signs or symptoms of a compartment syndrome.

The development of newer techniques utilizing the wick catheter of Mubarak and co-workers[27] and the slit catheter developed by Rorabeck and colleagues[32] allows continuous measurement of tissue fluid pressure without injection or infusion of saline solution. Although these techniques offer significant advantages, they require specialized equipment that may not be immediately

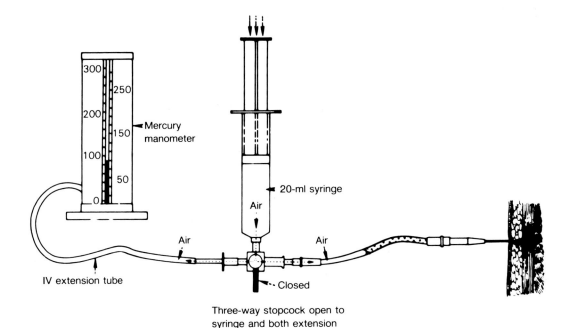

FIG. 38-1. A device for measuring compartment pressures, made up of materials present in most hospitals, has been advocated by Whitesides. (Whitesides, T.C. et al.: Tissue pressure measurements as a determinant for the need of fasciotomy. Clin. Orthop., 113: 43, 1975)

available in all situations. Animal and clinical studies using these techniques have led Mubarak and co-workers to recommend decompressive fasciotomy when the tissue pressure is above 30 torr and the patient has clinical evidence of a compartment syndrome.

Treatment. The extremity should have all circumferential dressings removed and be kept at the same level as the patient. Most physicians now feel that the use of sympathetic blocks should be abandoned. This procedure takes valuable preoperative time and seems to have little influence on arterial spasm. However, it may be indicated after a fasciotomy to help improve collateral circulation.

Since the experimental work of Jepson, the treatment of choice for compartment syndromes has been decompression.[14] The problem is that usually the surgical procedure is not carried out until the damage has been done. In reviewing the literature of anterior compartment syndrome, Bradley noted that only 13% of the patients recovered full function following fasciotomy after they had developed complete footdrop.[2] McQuillan and Nolan reported that a delay of 2 to 3 days was the cause of failure after operation for ischemia of a limb.[20] Matsen and Clawson felt that compartment syndromes lasting longer than 12 hours will probably result in permanent defects, no matter what the subsequent treatment.[22] Of course, decompression fasciotomy after 12 hours may still be indicated. On the other hand, fasciotomy alone will not correct the condition caused by a laceration or thrombus of an artery and subsequent muscle swelling. If fasciotomy does not immediately improve the compartment syndrome, the arterial supply should be evaluated further. Arteriography may be indicated.

Whether one does a subcutaneous fasciotomy, fasciotomy through limited or extensive skin incisions, or fasciotomy by resection of the fibula is a matter of surgical choice. Certainly many surgeons agree that for multiple compartment syndromes of the lower leg, fasciotomy by resection of the mid-fibula and its periosteum is the treatment of choice. The intact fibula, however, does lend stability to the lower leg when the tibia is broken, and the fibula should not be removed unnecessarily. Patman recommends fasciotomy through limited skin incisions for most conditions requiring fasciotomy.[29] This operation is short and cosmetically more acceptable, and infection is less likely. Patman notes, however, that if there is any doubt about the adequacy of this procedure, skin incisions should be extended. Matsen recommends that patients with compartment syndromes be watched closely for myoglobinuria.[21] This is particularly important in crush injuries. If myoglobinuria develops, a high output of alkaline urine should be maintained while one watches for renal failure.

Again, the major complication of surgery for compartment syndrome that we have seen has been necrosis and infection of necrotic muscle because the surgery was done too late and debridement of the necrotic muscles was inadequate.

Infections

Gas Gangrene. The complication of clostridial gas gangrene is uncommon in the United States but still occurs.[5] In our latest case the infection started at a venipuncture site and spread rapidly through the entire upper extremity. Although a forequarter amputation was done within 12 hours of onset, the patient died. Early recognition, vigorous debridement or ablation, and administration of appropriate antibiotic drugs remains the treatment of choice for clostridial myositis. Nonclostridial gas gangrene is probably more common than clostridial gas gangrene, and its course is usually not as fulminating.[3]

Synergistic Necrotizing Cellulitis. Do not wait too long to amputate the extremity with synergistic necrotizing cellulitis.[34] We have seen one case in which the skin of the extremity was alive and well, while underneath all was dead. Septic emboli to the lungs were the cause of this patient's death.

ERRORS IN TECHNIQUE (OOPS!)

Surgery is still an art and a craft that has a scientific basis. Faulty application of basic principles, as well as inappropriate manual procedures, can end in disaster.

Improper Identification of Anatomical Structures

The classic example of improper identification of anatomical structures is the use of the median nerve (mistaken for the palmaris longus) as a tendon transfer.

Complications of Skin Incisions

Occasionally skin incisions are placed improperly, and extensive undermining is necessary to do the surgery. This can lead to fat necrosis or even skin loss. Tight closure of extremity incisions is prone to produce complications if bleeding occurs in the wound. Closing contaminated wounds leads to disaster in some cases.

In recent years, it seems, patients are more upset by having an area of numbness postoperatively than were patients in previous years. If it is impossible to do an operation without cutting a sensory nerve (as it may be in doing a Smith-Petersen approach to the hip that puts the lateral femoral cutaneous nerve in jeopardy), the patient should be informed of this preoperatively. The same might be said about doing a meniscectomy, in which the infrapatellar branch of the saphenous nerve might be damaged, or a pesplasty, in which the main saphenous nerve might be cut. A particularly troublesome neuroma is that caused by damage to the superficial radial nerve following the release of the first dorsal compartment containing the extensor pollicis brevis and the abductor pollicis longus as treatment for de Quervain's disease. Generally, we prefer longitudinal incisions in the limbs; but, in this case, to prevent the formation of this neuroma we make a transverse incision of the skin and then dissect longitudinally in the subcutaneous tissue, being careful to protect all branches of the radial nerve. After releasing the first dorsal compartment of the wrist, attention to the nerves is again necessary for suture closure. Once a neuroma has occurred, injection with lidocaine and use of early motion may help, but the most effective treatment we have found is to section the nerve proximally and place the severed proximal end of the nerve in soft tissue, where it will be protected from irritation when the neuroma reforms. In the words of Arnold Henry, "let us respect cutaneous nerves."[9]

PROBLEMS ENCOUNTERED IN SPECIFIC TISSUES

Muscles

Weakness Following Repairs. Avulsions of muscles, although rare, do occur and occasionally require surgery. Weakness may result from failure to recognize or treat these injuries. A tear of the gastrocnemius at the musculotendinous junction is generally treated by immobilization with the foot in equinus. If the tear is treated surgically and the repair is not protected, the sutures may pull out, resulting in weakness. Likewise, a complete tear of the rectus femoris, usually repaired surgically, should be protected with a single hip spica. Partial tears of muscles, such as a tear of the quadriceps, may result in the formation of ectopic calcification in the hematoma. We recommend that if resection of this calcification is undertaken, it should be postponed until it is fully mature.

Repair during surgical exposure that has required transection of a muscle (such as the deltoid or the vastus medialis) has frequently resulted in weakness. Again, the muscles may not have been adequately reapproximated, or sutures may have pulled out during early mobilization. When taking down the deltoid, we have found it helpful to take a strip of bone from the clavicle and the acromion that remains attached to the muscle. This technique allows firm approximation of the muscle, and the bony healing produces a strong ultimate repair. In parapatellar incisions we leave a strip of tendon attached to the patella and the muscle, allowing a firm repair.

As noted previously, weakness may be seen with compartment syndromes, but it may also result from unrecognized denervation of the muscle at the time of the injury.

Complications Following Myotomy. Hip adductor myotomies have been fraught with complications such as hematoma and infection. Hemostasis is very important in this procedure, and accordingly, we prefer an open approach. The origins of the adductor longus and gracilis are tendinous, and the transection should be done through this portion. The origins of the adductor magnus and brevis and the pectineus are muscular, and when transecting these we have used a cutting electrocautery and then paid particular attention to hemostasis before closing the wounds. Finally, we believe that suction drainage is important in preventing complications in this area. The suction drain will not work unless there is a tight closure of the skin and subcutaneous layers.

Another problem seen with hip adductor myotomies is occasional imbalance because of the overpull of the hip abductors. This type of surgical procedure is frequently done in people with cerebral palsy, and in this type of patient it is important to assess all of the muscles about the hip before any surgical procedure is undertaken. A new approach to this assessment is to have the patient evaluated in a gait analysis laboratory where simultaneous electromyographic studies are taken during walking.[30]

If myotomies are being done to correct contracture, it is important to correct the contracture slowly to prevent stretching of nerves and arteries in the area, producing nerve palsies and vascular complications. Adequate postoperative splinting and protection are very important.

Complications Following Transposition. Failure to achieve expected function has occurred with the use of the pectoralis major for elbow flexion, the latissimus dorsi for elbow extension, the iliopsoas for hip abduction (as described by Sharrard and Mustard), and the posterior tibial muscle through the interosseous membrane for dorsiflexion of the foot. These problems may be due to necrosis of the muscle because of failure to adequately dissect and remove from pressure the arterial supply and venous drainage. If the nerve is stretched, neither it nor the transposed muscle will function. The muscle may be placed in too much or too little tension, and therefore it will have poor strength. The muscle must be placed so that it is pulling in a straight line rather than around a corner. Finally, there can be adherence and scarring-down of the muscle because of postoperative hemorrhage. Attention to

the details of these procedures should help decrease the number of complications.

Complications Following Biopsy. When one is doing a surgical procedure to diagnose a soft tissue mass, the possibility of sarcoma should be considered and the biopsy placed so that a subsequent *en bloc* excision of the biopsy site and malignant tumor can be performed. An incisional biopsy is best if there is a question about the tumor's being a sarcoma, since this technique involves less local tumor spillage than does an excisional biopsy. A limb salvage procedure is more likely to be successful if the operating surgeon is certain about the location of the original lesion. An excisional biopsy around the pseudocapsule of a sarcoma is likely to lead to recurrence if that is the only procedure done. Occasionally an improperly placed biopsy makes a limb salvage procedure impossible or increases the morbidity of an amputation. An example is a biopsy site through the buttock of a sarcoma, which may preclude a limb-saving local pelvic resection or require an anterior flap for a hemipelvectomy.

Tendons

Improper Fixation. Tendons may pull out if they are inadequately fixed or if the extremity is not properly immobilized for at least 6 weeks after surgery. In general, we prefer the pullout wire technique.

Tendon Ruptures Associated With Corticosteroid Therapy. Tendons do rupture occasionally following corticosteroid injections for tendinitis and in patients receiving systemic corticosteroids.[12] This may be from necrosis of the tendons when corticosteroids are injected under pressure, or it may be that the corticosteroids stop the healing process of a partially torn tendon, and the patient who is relieved of symptoms continues to overuse the tendons, causing a complete tear.[35]

It has been our experience that tendon ruptures following corticosteroid injections and in patients receiving systemic corticosteroids do not heal as quickly or as well as most other tendon ruptures. For this reason we take extra care when treating such conditions. If the tendon is ruptured at the point of injection, this area is resected prior to repair, and we try to reinforce the repair. The tendon repair is protected longer with external support than would normally be the case. In this way we have been able to prevent rerupture.

Weakness and Rerupture Following Repair of Rotator Cuff Injuries.   The anatomist Monro illustrated a tear of the rotator cuff in 1788.[25] Since then there have been repeated reports that this condition is present in at least 30% of rotator cuffs of cadavers over the age of 65 years; however, the diagnosis is relatively uncommon as a clinical entity. Codman explained the clinical syndrome of a rotator cuff tear as the sudden onset of pain in the shoulder of a patient over 40 years of age either following lifting a heavy weight with the arms or falling on arms or shoulder.[6] Physical examination reveals limited active elevation of the arm but full passive range of motion of the glenohumeral joint. Roentgenograms rule out calcific deposits and fractures of the greater tuberosity as causes for these symptoms. The classic picture is indeed rare, in our experience, but many patients who complain only of pain, having no symptoms of weakness and no history of injury, are frequently found to have a rotator cuff tear when an arthrogram is done. Codman recommended early surgery for the patient with a rotator cuff tear, but more recently, McLaughlin and Asherman have recommended waiting at least 3 weeks before surgery, except in the case of massive tears.[6,19] Many of their patients became asymptomatic and regained range of motion spontaneously, and therefore they felt that immediate surgery was contraindicated in all but the most severe cases. Most of the patients that we have seen have responded to conservative treatment with the arm in a sling for 3 weeks and then gradual return of motion using, first, pendulum exercises, then wall-climbing exercises and, finally, resistive exercises. Not all patients recover with this conservative program; under these circumstances we recommend an arthrogram to confirm the diagnosis. If the arthrogram shows a tear, we recommend repair of the rotator cuff without resection of the acromion. In the past, resection of the acromion has resulted in weakness of the deltoid because of our inability to reattach the origin of the deltoid adequately following removal of all or part of the acromion. Neer[28] has emphasized that total resection of the acromion is unnecessary, and he advocates an anterior acromioplasty, which we have used recently with good results. Wolfgang advocated the use of the long head of the biceps tendon in the repair of some rotator cuff injuries.[38] Again, the complications of shoulder weakness and rerupture of the rotator cuff have been diminished by the use of the Neer approach and the use of the long head of the biceps tendon for massive tears of the rotator cuff.

Weakness Following Biceps Tendon Rupture.   The long head of the biceps tendon contributes to the rotator cuff, and rupture of this tendon may occur by itself or in association with other portions of the rotator cuff. The diagnosis is easily made by observing the bulging of the biceps muscle on the involved side. Surgery is not always indicated for tears of the long head, since the short head of the biceps remains attached to the coracoid process, and patients usually regain normal strength with exercise. If the patient desires surgery for cosmetic reasons, the tendon of the long head is sutured into the bicipital groove of the humeral head.

Tears of the distal end of the biceps should be surgically repaired. Our experience with patients in whom this was not done indicates that elbow flexion is weak, and the patient may also develop pain in his elbow and forearm from entrapment of the median nerve in reparative tissue coming from the ruptured distal end of the biceps tendon.

Weakness Following Achilles Tendon Rupture.   Reviewing several series, Lea and Smith noted one major complication for every 5.8 surgical repairs of ruptured Achilles tendons.[17] Complications included infections, necrosis of overlying skin, draining fistulas, adhesions of tendon to skin, rerupture, thrombosis and pulmonary embolism, and sensory loss. They therefore advised the closed treatment of this condition with a short leg cast with the foot in an equinus position for 8 weeks. Complications from the cast treatment alone, however, include rerupture of the Achilles tendon and, in some cases, weakness. Inglis and co-workers noted that patients treated surgically had greater strength, power, and endurance of the repaired tendon than did those treated nonsurgically.[11] We therefore recommend surgical repair for the young athlete, and also for tendon ruptures that are the result of injections, with emphasis on reinforcement of the suture line, repair of the tendon sheath, and immobilization for at least 8 weeks. For older patients (particularly lawyers!) we advise the closed cast treatment, with cast removal at 8 weeks and protection with an elevated heel for at least another month.

Tendon Sheaths

Complications Following Repair. Tendon sheaths have occasionally not received the attention they deserve and have not been repaired following injuries. This is frequently seen in skiing injuries, when the peroneal tendons have slipped forward, causing irritation as they glide over the distal end of the fibula rather than behind it. Eckert and Davis described this condition and their results with surgical repair.[7] On the other hand, overzealous repair of tendon sheaths can produce tendon restriction and avascularity if the repair is too tight. Following surgical exposure, skin adhesions to the Achilles tendon occur if there has been failure to close the tendon sheath surrounding it.

Complications Following Release. De Quervain's disease is a fairly common problem with a number of complications. In the section on skin incisions we have noted our preference for a transverse incision. Another complication with de Quervain's disease is the persistence of its symptoms following release of the first dorsal compartment. Occasionally the abductor pollicis longus is in a separate compartment from the extensor pollicis brevis, and unless both compartments are released, the patient's symptoms may continue postoperatively.

Release of the flexor tendon sheaths for a trigger finger is usually a very satisfying procedure, but occasionally there has been neurovascular damage or incomplete release of the sheath. Both of these complications can be prevented by a thorough knowledge of the normal anatomy and close attention to any abnormal anatomy that may be encountered during the surgical procedure.

Occasionally, too much of the tendon sheath is removed from the flexor tendons of the fingers following injury in "no-man's land," which results in bow-stringing. If the flexor sheaths have been completely destroyed, it is possible to make a new sling or pulley with the use of tendon or fascial grafts.

Infections and Necrosis. Incomplete, inadequate release of tendon sheaths in which there is infection or failure to drain at all often leads to tendon slough. This same complication can occur from grease-gun injuries, in which grease is injected into the sheath under pressure. In both instances it is important to do an adequate release of the tendon sheaths and debridement, in the hope of maintaining the blood supply to the tendons.

Fasciae

Complications Following Repair. There has been increasing awareness that it is not always necessary to close fascial defects and that in some instances closure can produce serious complications.[18] Further, it has been advocated that the fascia not be closed whenever orthopaedic procedures are undertaken on the tibia, such as following a Hauser procedure or even plating of a fracture. Leaving the fascia open and reapproximating only the subcutaneous tissue and skin helps prevent compartment syndromes.

Complications Following Release. The Yount procedure will not produce the desired results if there is inadequate release of the fascia or if there is improper postoperative fixation of the hips in plaster for an adequate period.

The treatment of Dupuytren's contracture has been fraught with complications, particularly the production of causalgia with extensive fasciectomies. For this reason we do the minimal amount of resection of the palmar fascia to achieve our ends. Dupuytren's contracture can involve the skin as well as the fascia, and occasionally the fascia and the overlying skin must be removed, with placement of a full-thickness skin graft in the defect to prevent or treat a recurrence.[8]

Release of the plantar fascia for treatment of heel spur has produced some unsatisfactory results. This may be because pain is caused by an excessively pronated foot, and surgical release of the plantar fascia is not the way to treat the painful foot.[4] A blind plantar fasciotomy occasionally produces nerve damage and hemorrhage. For resection of nodules of the plantar fascia, we prefer a longitudinal plantar incision in the non-weight-bearing portion of the sole. Inadequate removal usually results in recurrence.

Ligaments

Complications Following Repair. Following injury to the acromioclavicular joint with significant separation, there is a question as to whether surgical repair of the coracoclavicular ligaments should be undertaken. If it is undertaken, the separation may recur because of failure of the fixation device before ligamentous healing can occur. There may also be persistent pain at the acromioclavicular joint because of damage to this joint,[13] and, accordingly, if we do repair an acromioclavicular separation, we prefer to resect the acromioclavicular joint at the same time by removing the distal 1.5 cm of the clavicle.

Unsatisfactory results from Monteggia fractures have occurred when the unrecognized anular ligament is trapped beneath the radial head, preventing adequate reduction. Our procedure of choice in this situation is simply to resect the ligament.

Less than ideal results from repair of the knee ligaments occur when the ligament is damaged and there is a delay in diagnosis. Late repairs and reconstruction of knee ligaments have produced variable results. The use of prostheses and synthetic tissue scaffolds is presently under investigation with promising early results, but in our opinion these techniques should be approached cautiously and studied thoroughly in several centers before becoming standard procedures.

Complications such as instability of the ankle following repair of the deltoid ligament occur because of inadequate exposure of the ligament or inability to approximate the tissues adequately. We prefer, if at all possible, to approximate the torn end to a bony surface for the best type of healing.

Complications Following Release. Patients have occasionally complained of numbness in the palm following release of the flexor retinaculum as treatment for median nerve compression. In some instances this is due to transection of the palmar cutaneous branch of the median nerve, which pierces the deep fascia and crosses the flexor retinaculum, usually on the radial side of the hand. To prevent this complication we try to place our skin incision on the ulnar side of the forearm and to look carefully for all nerves in the dissection through the subcutaneous tissue down to the fascia of the forearm. Our skin incision extends distally into the palm at the base of the thenar eminence until we are sure that the entire transverse carpal ligament has been transected. We have seen patients who have had recurrences of symptoms or inadequate relief of their symptoms, and on reoperation we have found that the ligament had not been completely transected. We feel that it is important to inspect the floor of the canal by gently retracting the flexor tendons so that if there is a bump in this area from a previous injury, it can be resected.

Bursae

The complications we have seen from surgery on bursae have been infection in the operative wound and recurrence of the bursae.

Infections may result from initial failure in diagnosing infection (tuberculosis infection in bursae is occasionally seen in this country), with seeding of infection into the operative wound. It may also occur by hematogenous seeding of a hematoma that may develop in the space left after removal of the bursae. To prevent this complication, we generally use suction drainage as well as sutures to close the dead space left after removal of the bursae.

Recurrence of a bursa after excision may result from failure to diagnose and treat adequately the initial cause of the bursa. Reference has already been made in this chapter to the recurrence of popliteal bursae owing to pathology in the knee joint itself. Another cause of a recurring bursa is the regrowth of an exotosis or bony deformity (such as a hallux valgus), which produces pressure and irritation of the overlying tissue. Failure of patients to protect themselves from repeated trauma may also cause the recurrence of the bursa, as it sometimes does in housemaid's knee or in the olecranon bursa of a tax accountant.

Pressure From Surgical Dressings

Edema distal to an elastic surgical dressing is a fairly common finding that can lead to major complications if not corrected soon enough. The same is certainly true of rigid dressings (casts). Ischemic contractures of the muscles occur following application of dressings and casts that are too tight, as well as following fractures and surgery.

Malposition of a Joint in a Postoperative Dressing

Placing the hand in a position of function is the intent of most surgeons working in this area, but frequently the hand does not end up in the dressing the way the surgeon desires, and the metacarpophalangeal joints are almost straight. If they are held that way too long, contractures occur.

After release of a flexion contracture, holding the joint in forced extension may stretch nerves to the point at which they will no longer function and arteries to the point at which thrombosis results. This is particularly true in the larger joints such as the knee. Placing a joint in flexion after transverse incision across the extensor surface can lead to poor healing of the wound.

COMPLICATIONS OF THE PATIENT'S DISEASE

Some complications occur that we are unable to predict on the basis of our preoperative evaluation (such as infections), but others may be predictable (such as thrombophlebitis in a patient who has had previous thrombophlebitis).

Infections

Proper administration of preoperative antibiotics and wound irrigation will diminish the occurrence of infection, but there are risks from the use of antibiotics. Adherence to aseptic technique and the presence of a clean environment in the operating room may be as important as antibiotics in the prevention of this complication.

Thrombophlebitis

Prophylactic use of heparin, coumadin, aspirin, or low-molecular-weight dextran reduces the occurrence of thrombophlebitis but increases the incidence of wound he-matoma. The decision as to when to use these agents and which one to use is an important one and must be made on an individual-case basis.

Reflex Sympathetic Dystrophy Syndrome

Aching or burning pain, hyperesthesia, hypoesthesia, paresthesia, swelling and stiffness, and in some cases increased sweating occur any time from immediately to 6 months after injury in patients having undergone elective surgical procedures as well as following trauma. The treatment is active physical therapy and the administration of tranquilizers and anti-inflammatory drugs[16] for the early cases with mild symptoms. The use of stellate ganglion blocks on three to five successive days is recommended for more severe cases, and in those patients who have transient—but not permanent—improvement following blocks, cervical sympathectomy is recommended. The majority of patients, but not all, improve with this treatment. Early and aggressive treatment gives the best results.

CONCLUSIONS

There are risks involved whenever a surgical procedure is undertaken. These should be faced squarely by all concerned. By so doing, complications may be kept to a minimum. The patient must have realistic expectations of the outcome of the procedure so that what is perceived as the condition following surgery is in harmony with the expectations. In most situations the rewards from surgery far outweigh the risks.

REFERENCES

1. Baker, W.M.: On the formation of synovial cysts in the leg in connection with disease of the knee joint. St. Bart's Hosp. Rep., 13:245, 1877; 21:177, 1885.
2. Bradley, E.L. III: The anterior tibial compartment syndrome. Surg. Gynecol. Obstet., 136:289, 1973.
3. Bressman, A.M., and Wagner, W.: Nonclostridial gas gangrene. J.A.M.A., 233:958, 1975.
4. Campbell, J.W., and Inman, V.T.: Treatment of plantar fasciitis and calcaneal spurs with U-C-B shoe insert. Clin. Orthop., 103:57, 1974.
5. Caplan, E.S., and Kluge, R.M.: Gas gangrene. Arch. Intern. Med., 136:178, 1976.
6. Codman, E.A.: The Shoulder. Boston, Thomas Todd Co., 1934.
7. Eckert, W.R., and Davis, E.A., Jr.: Acute rupture

of the peroneal retinaculum. J. Bone Joint Surg., 58A:670, 1973.

8. Gonzales, R.L.: Dupuytren's contracture of the fingers. Calif. Med., 115:25, 1971.

9. Henry, A.K.: Extensile Exposure, p. 8. Edinburgh, E&S Livingston, 1966.

10. Horn, E.E.: Acute ischaemia of the anterior tibial muscle and the long extensor muscles of the toes. J. Bone Joint Surg., 27B:615, 1945.

11. Inglis, A.E. et al.: Rupture of tendo Achillis. J. Bone Joint Surg., 58A:990, 1976.

12. Ismail, A.M. et al.: Rupture of patellar ligament after steroid infiltration. J. Bone Joint Surg., 51B:503, 1969.

13. Jacobs, B., and Wade, P.: Acromioclavicular joint injury. J. Bone Joint Surg., 48A:475, 1961.

14. Jepson, P.N.: Ischaemic contracture, experimental study. Ann. Surg 84:785, 1926.

15. Kennedy, J.C.: Complete dislocation of the knee joint. J. Bone Joint Surg., 45A:889, 1963.

16. Kozin, F., McCarty, D.J., Sims, J., and Genant, H.: The reflex sympathetic dystrophy syndrome. I and II. Am. J. Med., 60:321, 1976.

17. Lea, R., and Smith, L.: Nonsurgical treatment of tendo Achillis rupture. J. Bone Joint Surg., 54A:1398, 1972.

18. Leach, R.E. et al.: Anterior tibial compartment syndrome. J. Bone Joint Surg., 49A:451, 1967.

19. McLaughlin, H.L., and Asherman, E.G.: Lesions of the musculotendinous cuff of the shoulder. J. Bone Joint Surg., 33A:76, 1951.

20. McQuillan, W.M., and Nolan, F.: Ischaemia complicating injury. J. Bone Joint Surg., 50B:482, 1968.

21. Matsen, F.A.: Compartment syndrome. Clin. Orthop. Rel. Res., 113:9, 1975.

22. Matsen, F.A., and Clawson, D.K.: Co-guest editors: Compartmental syndromes. Clin. Orthop., 112:1975.

23. ———: The deep posterior compartment syndrome of the leg. J. Bone Joint Surg., 57A:34, 1975.

24. Mavor, G.E.: The anterior tibial syndrome. J. Bone Joint Surg., 38B:513, 1956.

25. Monro, A.: Description of All the Bursae Mucosae of the Human Body. Edinburgh, C. Elliott, 1788.

26. Mubarak, S.J., and Hargens, A.R.: Compartment Syndromes and Volkmann's Contracture. Philadelphia, W.B. Saunders, 1981.

27. Mubarak, S.J., Hargens, A.R., Owen, C.A. et al.: The wick catheter technique for measurement of intramuscular pressure: A new research and clinical tool. J. Bone Joint Surg., 58A:1016, 1976.

28. Neer, C.S.: Anterior acromioplasty for the chronic impingement syndrome in the shoulder. J. Bone Joint Surg., 54A:41, 1972.

29. Patman, R.D.: Compartment syndromes in peripheral vascular surgery. Clin. Orthop., 113:103, 1975.

30. Perry, J. et al.: Electromyography before and after surgery for hip deformity in children with cerebral palsy. J. Bone Joint Surg., 58A:201, 1976.

31. Priest, J.D., Jones, H.H., and Nagel, D.A.: Elbow injuries in highly skilled tennis players. J. Sports Med., 2:137, 1974.

32. Rorabeck, C.H., Castle, G.S., Hardie, R. et al.: Compartmental pressure measurements: An experimental investigation using the slit catheter. J. Trauma, 21:446, 1981.

33. Sirbu, A.B., Murphy, J.J., and White, A.S.: Soft tissue complications of fracture of the leg. Calif. Western Med., 60:53, 1944.

34. Stone, H.H., and Martin, J.D., Jr.: Synergistic necrotizing cellulitis. Ann. Surg., 175:702, 1972.

35. Unverferth, L.J., and Olix, M.L.: The effect of local steroid injections on tendon. J. Bone Joint Surg., 55A:1315, 1973.

36. Volkmann, R.: Die ischaemischen Muskelahmungen und Kontraktruen. Cbl. Chir., 51:801, 1881.

37. Whitesides, T.C. et al.: Tissue pressure measurements as a determinant for the need of fasciotomy. Clin. Orthop., 113:43, 1975.

38. Wolfgang, G.I.: Surgical repair of tears of the rotator cuff of the shoulder. J. Bone Joint Surg., 56A:14, 1974.

39 Complications of Spinal Surgery for Discogenic Disease and Spondylolisthesis

EDWARD H. SIMMONS AND R. GEOFFREY WILBER

For the young orthopaedic surgeon who is starting in practice, for the orthopaedic resident in the course of his training, or even for the established orthopaedic practitioner, awareness of the various complications that may be associated with surgery of the spine is vitally important. A careful and detailed approach is required in the anticipation, prevention, and management of orthopaedic complications that are a part of surgery of the spine for discogenic disease and spondylolisthesis.

COMPLICATIONS RELATED TO INACCURATE PREOPERATIVE ASSESSMENT AND DIAGNOSIS

Undoubtedly the most valuable guide in assessing patients who present with spine pain is a very careful and detailed history, followed by a careful physical examination.[26] Based on an analysis of the failures of surgery for mechanical disability of the spine, the most commonly neglected and inadequate preoperative assessment is a proper history and the evaluation of its significance.

Patients who are to have any benefit from a mechanical surgical procedure on the spine should have a history of fairly typical mechanical pain with or without neurologic involvement, typically aggravated by activity, bending, lifting, prolonged standing and sitting, and probably also by coughing, sneezing, and even straining at stool. This type of pain improves somewhat with rest, mechanical therapy such as a brace support or cervical collar, and traction. If the patient's distress does not respond to any of these measures, it is doubtful that the pain arises from a mechanical dysfunc-tion that might benefit from surgery. In such circumstances, other causes should be considered.

Pain in the back that comes on insidiously in a young adult, is worse in the morning, is associated with stiffness, and perhaps is aggravated by damp weather and improves with activity should alert one to the possibility of ankylosing spondylitis. Usually it can be detected by loss of normal spine mobility, with early changes noted in the sacroiliac joints, anterior squaring of the vertebrae seen in the lateral roentgenograms, and often an elevated erythrocyte sedimentation rate with positive results on HLA-B27 antigen tests. Not infrequently, patients presenting the early manifestations of this disease are treated for mechanical or discogenic low back pain, and on occasion surgery is mistakenly carried out (Fig. 39-1). Symptoms of claudication, including buttock, thigh, and calf pain on ambulation that is made better by rest, is classic for spinal stenosis. Care must be taken with these presenting complaints to rule out symptoms originating from peripheral vascular disease. An assessment of peripheral pulses as well as skin and nail-bed changes is essential.

Pain of neoplastic origin is usually aggravated, or apparently worse, at night after the patient has been lying down for a prolonged interval, and it is frequently relieved by getting up and walking about. Pain that comes on insidiously in an adult over the age of 40 years and is not typical of discogenic disease should always raise suspicion of neoplasm. In this type of patient the prostate should be assessed in the male and the breasts in the female. Erythrocyte sedimentation rate, acid phosphatase

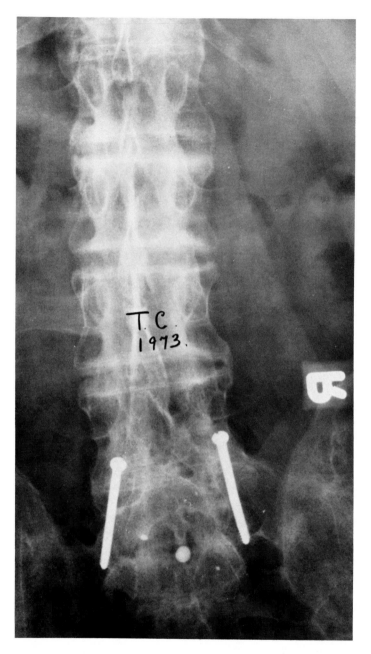

FIG. 39-1. Anteroposterior roentgenogram of the lumbosacral spine of a male patient with ankylosing spondylitis who was referred for osteotomy of the cervical spine. In the early stages of his disease he had undergone lumbosacral arthrodesis for low back pain. Note the fused sacroiliac joints.

levels (in the male), alkaline phosphatase levels, and serum calcium and phosphorus levels are useful adjuncts for screening such patients. If the results of these tests are all normal, it is very unlikely that there is an underlying malignancy of the spine. If there is gross abnormality, further investigation, including bone scans, should be carried out.

It is important to recognize emotional factors and how they can contribute to disability. A purely psychogenic back pain is not too common; however, psychogenic magnification of minor physical complaint out of all proportion is *very* common. The clouding and confusion of the clinical picture by emotional factors can be a trap for the surgeon in assessing the extent of the true physical disability. A patient whose disability has a large psychogenic component compounding a minor complaint will not be cured by operative treatment. Operation on the spine for apparent disc disease should never be undertaken on a desperation basis owing to the apparent failure of all other measures. The indications should be clear cut, the demonstration of obvious physical disability well established, and the emotional reaction of the patient judged to be within normal limits. Otherwise, primary treatment should be directed to the emotional aspects of the problem in conjunction with conservative management of the mechanical disability. Operative treatment should be carried out only when it is evident that the emotional aspects are under satisfactory control.

Gross personality defects should be recognized, when present, because patients with these will not do well with operative treatment alone. An adequate personality inventory may afford valuable insight and help to prognosticate which patients will likely do well following effective surgery for their physical disability. The Minnesota Multiphasic Personality Inventory, as adapted to low back pain, is a valuable test for patients under consideration for operative treatment when personality factors may be involved.[10] We have applied it to patients with discogenic disease of the cervical spine and have found it to be equally valuable for lumbar disc disease. Its preoperative use is recommended.

The importance of financial security, work demands, and litigation settlement are obvious. The significance of each should be carefully evaluated in light of the clinical picture before a final decision is made to undertake surgery. Also it is important to take prior surgical intervention in the spine into consideration when planning future surgical treatment.

A general medical assessment should consider the cardiac and pulmonary status. The possibility of early neuropathy should be raised in patients with paresthesias or burning distress in the lower limbs who are known diabetics or who have a family history of diabetes. Latent diabetes should be ruled out in patients with bizarre symptoms not explained by obvious back pathology. A history of thrombophlebitis or previous embolism should alert the surgeon to the likelihood of this postoperative complication so that prophylactic measures may be instituted. A history of a bleeding tendency or bleeding disorders should point out the risk of this intraoperative and postoperative complication and the need for proper investigation and management.

It is generally considered that a person with a gouty diathesis is likely to develop pseudarthrosis following spinal fusion, and this type of patient should alert one to the increased possibility of that potential complication.

With cervical spine disability, it is important to recognize that not all neurologic signs and symptoms necessarily arise from nerve root compression or injury. There may be a secondary scalenus anterior syndrome associated with spasm of the cervical musculature and the scalenus anterior. With this, the patient frequently complains of numbness and tingling of the little and ring fingers and occasionally part of the long finger. This complaint is commonly unilateral. With pressure on the scalenus anterior at the root of the neck on the asymptomatic side, there is no gross complaint. However, on the symptomatic side, pressure at the attachment of the scalenus anterior to the first rib produces or aggravates the tingling and pain radiating along the ulnar side of the arm and hand. These symptoms are due to lower trunk irritation. It seems evident that division of the scalenus anterior, as has been carried out in the past, is a procedure aimed at a secondary phenomenon and not the primary cause of the disability. It is important to recognize this lower trunk irritation and to realize that it does not represent a disc injury with C7 or C8 nerve root irritation. In a careful review of 221 patients who had been referred because of significant or protracted neck disability following rear-end automobile collisions, 59 were found to have clear-cut signs and symptoms of nerve root irritation. Nine patients presented neurologic symptoms and signs indicative of secondary scalenus anterior syndrome without evidence of nerve root involvement. One of these patients had an associated cervical rib.

Another lesion that may occasionally confuse the neurologic picture is an associated traumatic ulnar nerve neuritis. In a rear-end automobile collision, as the body is thrown forward, certain patients may contuse the forearm against the lower portion of the steering wheel, producing soft tissue injury in the region of the fibrous bridge of origin of the flexor carpi ulnaris. This may give rise to an ulnar nerve entrapment syndrome at this level, producing signs of an ulnar neuritis (Fig. 39-2). This occurs more commonly in women, since they tend to hold the steering wheel with their hands on the upper portion of the wheel, and occasionally it may be of such severity as to require decompression and transposition of the ulnar nerve. The diagnosis is easily made if the possibility is considered. The symptoms are easily reproduced by palpating the swollen ulnar nerve at the level of the fibrous bridge of origin of the flexor carpi ulnaris and rolling it under the examining finger. As Osborne has pointed out, in this lesion the nerve is compressed against a band of fibrous tissue bridging the two heads of the flexor carpi ulnaris.[19] The band is slack in full extension, but as the elbow is flexed, it starts to tighten at 135°. At 90° it becomes quite taut and well defined, diminishing the capacity of the tunnel formed by the band and the joint.

Soft tissue thickening or swelling due to contusion may encroach on the space necessary for the passage of the ulnar nerve beneath the fibrous band. Compression of the nerve against the band is then inevitable in the flexed position, and a conduction block or neuritis develops. In some patients, simple flexion of the elbow causes tingling in the fourth and fifth fingers. Sleeping with the elbow flexed aggravates the condition, and improvement occurs when the patient sleeps with the elbow extended.

Peripheral nerve entrapment syndromes other than cubital tunnel syndrome should also be sought. Lesions in the brachial plexus, the radial nerve in the spiral groove or canal of Frosse, the median nerve at the level of the proximal forearm or carpal

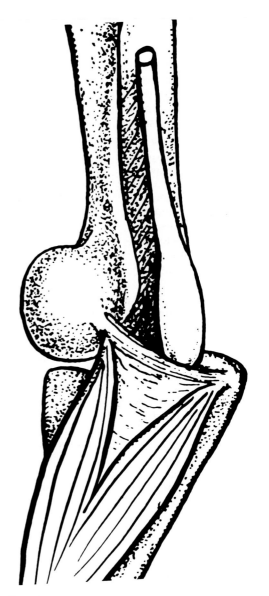

FIG. 39-2. Schematic diagram illustrates how ulnar nerve entrapment produces ulnar nerve neuritis.

tunnel, or the ulnar nerve at the level of Guyon's canal can all mimic some cervical spine–related nerve symptoms. The recording of peripheral nerve conduction times and electromyograms are particularly valuable for confirming and localizing peripheral nerve lesions. These electrical studies offer the advantage of detecting abnormalities when clinical examination is questionable, and they give an objective result that does not require patient cooperation.

The use of electromyography as a routine diagnostic study for both lumbar and cervical discogenic disease has not been reliable in our experience. Its application to lumbar nerve root entrapment and its limitations have been well described by Wilbourn.[35]

COMPLICATIONS RELATED TO ERRORS IN SURGICAL JUDGMENT

There are three essentials for success in the surgical management of patients with discogenic disease of the spine and spondylolisthesis: selection of the right patient, accurate identification of the level or levels involved, and selection of the right operative procedure.

Assuming that the right patient has been selected by careful preoperative assessment and that the nature of the disability has been established, the most likely error in surgical judgment is failure to localize accurately the level or levels responsible for the patient's disability. In many cases the history and physical findings may provide accurate localization. However, there is a very large group of patients with major disability in whom the localization cannot be determined entirely on clinical findings. For them, special diagnostic techniques are indicated to confirm the clinical impression or to localize accurately the area of disability, as well as to evaluate the state of the adjacent areas of the spine.

Good-quality plain radiographs are essential. Excellent definition can be obtained with coned-down views of the affected area. Flexion and extension lateral views offer insight into abnormal motion of involved spinal segments. Three-foot standing anteroposterior and lateral views are important when there is associated spinal deformity. Tomograms should be taken when indicated for the demonstration of congenital anomalies and lesions such as osteoid osteoma. Bone scans are helpful in showing sites of nonunion, neoplasm, or inflammatory disease.

Myelographic techniques are a valuable adjunct to the investigation but certainly not the final word, especially at the L5–S1 level. Iophendylate (Pantopaque) myelographic techniques have had significant favor in the past. However, the unsatisfactory visualization of nerve roots, the higher incidence of arachnoiditis, the need for removal of the dye, and the possible interference with CT scanning of these techniques are major problems with their use. Water-soluble agents, specifically metrizamide, offer many advantages. Metrizamide is an excellent contrast agent that allows visualization of the nerve roots and finer appreciation of detail of the dural canal. It does not have to be removed from the canal, allowing the use of a smaller spinal needle. Another valuable asset is its use in conjunction with CT scanning, which allows in-depth cross-sectional contrast studies never before available. There are concerns about using this material in the cervical spine. (Many complications such as seizure disorders, cerebritis, hallucinations, slurring of speech, and temporary blindness have been reported.) In the hands of a skilled radiographer with good equipment, however, metrizamide CT scanning has proven to be a reliable and safe procedure. The use of phenothiazine derivatives is contraindicated with metrizamide. Given the vast number of patients who have been examined with myelography, the complications have been rather minimal. Infection is always a hazard, but it is rare. Subarachnoid bleeding may induce significant headache, and neck stiffness and dural leaks can give mild discomfort. A very severe but, fortunately, rare complication is that induced by the instillation of the wrong contrast material, for instance, hypaque when an oil-contrast myelogram was intended. This material can be severely toxic and can produce severe neurologic reactions, including convulsions and death.[38] The investigator must always be certain that he has been handed the right contrast material before he injects it.

Intradural venography has its proponents and can act as an adjunct, or even a substitute, for myelography in the lumbar region, particularly if there is a small sac displaced away from the vertebral body. Prior surgery significantly distorts the results of this technique. Its use today lies mainly in the exclusion of malignancy and hemangioma.

We have found discography to be a most reliable diagnostic procedure for determining the symptomatic level in discogenic disease of the cervical, thoracic, and lumbar spine. We have continued to use it in conjunction with myelography, plain radiography, and a very careful clinical assessment.[27] Discography of the spine is valuable in both functional and anatomical assessment. Its value in the cervical spine is largely for functional assessment, in which it is used to reproduce the patient's specific pain pattern on a consistent basis at a particular level. In the lumbar spine it presents an accurate anatomical diagnosis as well as a functional study, indicating a normal disc, a degenerated disc (symptomatic or asymptomatic), or a herniated disc. It is of value in indicating the anatomical state of a disc adjacent to a site proposed for fusion. In a reported study in which success of treatment was accepted as an indication that the right level had been selected, the comparative accuracy of clinical examination alone, routine radiography alone, myelography alone, and discography alone was assessed.[27-29] For patients with cervical disc disease the diagnostic accuracy of the various methods of assessment was clinical examination 43%, routine radiography 46.5%, myelography 45.6%, and discography 91%. For patients with lumbar disc disease the diagnostic accuracy of the various methods of assessment was clinical examination 44.2%, routine radiography 71.5%, myelography 45.6%, and discography 82.2%. When clinical assessment and routine radiography were combined, there was increased accuracy of localization to more than 60%, but discography still remained the most accurate single diagnostic technique. Infection is a rare but potential hazard, and the procedure should be done in a clean diagnostic room using sterile surgical technique. In the senior author's series of 1451 discograms, there was only one disc space infection. It is significant that this occurred at a time when the regular orthopaedic radiology suite was being rebuilt. The discogram was done in a room that was used for other procedures, including barium enemas. The patient developed a febrile reaction indicative of infection. He responded to antibiotic therapy and went on to a spontaneous fusion with relief of his symptoms (the level involved was, fortunately, the symptomatic one) and no late complications.[29]

A common source of error in the interpretation of myelography in the lumbar region is the acceptance of a mild bulge at the L4-5 level as being diagnostic of a symptomatic protrusion at that level in the presence of a small terminal dural sac at L5-S1. Frequently the sac is displaced backward from the disc space at L5-S1 and the vertebral bodies of S1 and L5 to a significant degree, and this may conceal a disc herniation at the L5-S1 level that is the true source of the patient's complaint. The soft, bulgy disc at L4-5 that produces a minimal asymptomatic indentation of the oil column has been called the "sucker disc." The surgeon should not unwittingly fall into this trap, and a discogram is an excellent method of determining whether the L4-5 level is truly abnormal and symptomatic or whether there is, in fact, a concealed symptomatic herniation at L5-S1 (Fig. 39-3). Extradural venography may also be used for this purpose.

CT scanning techniques have been a major advance in imaging the spinal canal.[4,16] The use of high-resolution CT scanning techniques has allowed a new perspective of analyzing spinal pathology. CT scanning is noninvasive and safe. It can be used without contrast material or in combination with water-soluble myelography to enhance the recognition of intradural structures. The use of this modality has markedly increased our understanding of degenerative spine disorders, especially spinal root stenosis and canal configuration (Figs. 39-4 and 39-5). It gives new perspective in demonstrating anatomical change or abnormality, but it does not necessarily establish that the changes are the cause of the patient's symptoms, as can be established with discography. Errors in interpretation can occur, and symptomatic lesions can be missed. Caution should be observed in interpreting these studies because of gantry parallelism, errors in image reconstruction, and cut size. The findings should always be compared with the patient's clinical findings and other

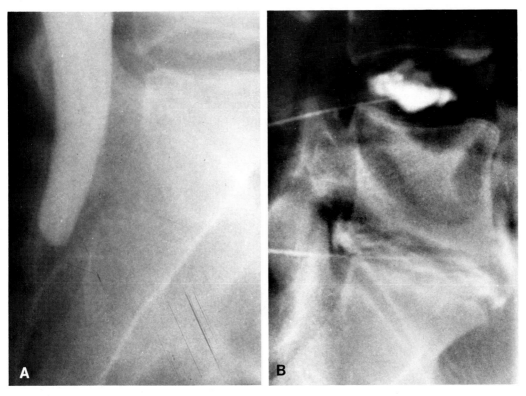

FIG. 39-3. (A) "Negative" lateral myelogram at L5–S1. Note the space between the sacrum and the oil-filled arachnoid sac. (B) Lateral discogram of the same patient shows a normal disc at L4–5, with obvious herniation at L5–S1. Injection at L5–S1 reproduced the patient's typical complaint.

FIG. 39-4. Lumbar CT scan of the mid-body of the lumbar spine shows slowly progressive spinal stenosis. Note the prior posterior fusion mass (*arrowheads*) and the secondary trefoil stenotic changes in the spinal canal with laminar hypertrophy.

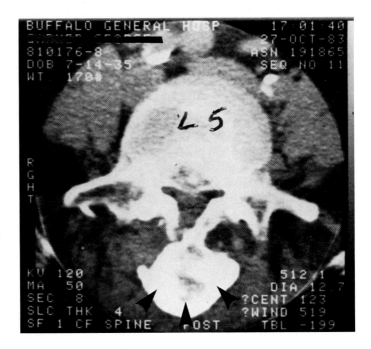

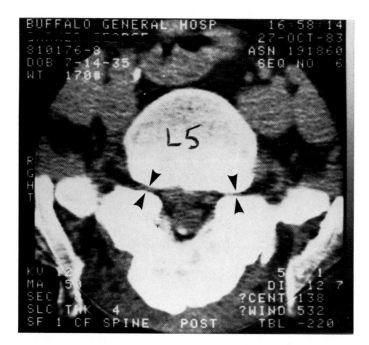

FIG. 39-5. Secondary foraminal and central spinal stenosis in a patient with a prior posterior fusion. This patient's claudication symptoms were relieved after a posterior decompression and "lateral" fusion.

investigations. It is unwise to place sole or undue emphasis on CT scanning in the assessment of painful mechanical spinal disability. The role of this technique in replacing other diagnostic studies has yet to be determined.

Spondylolisthesis has a normal incidence in the population, on the order of 5% to 6%. It may or may not produce back complaints. The radiographic presence of a spondylolisthesis does not necessarily mean that it is causing the symptoms. As a general rule, the younger a person is when mechanical back complaints associated with spondylolisthesis first appear, the more likely it is that the spondylolisthesis is the cause of the complaint. Similarly, the older a patient is when the first symptoms arise, the less likely it is that the spondylolisthesis is the cause. When back complaints first appear after the age of 40 years in a person with spondylolisthesis, it is unlikely that the spondylolisthesis is the source of the complaint, and other causes should be sought, in particular, disc degeneration above the level of the spondylolisthesis.[36] This possibility should be considered in assessing whether a patient's symptoms are from the apparent spondylolisthesis. If the patient is in the discogenic age, it is very

reasonable and wise to confirm that the L4–5 level is normal before carrying out a localized L5 transverse process–sacrum fusion. This can very easily be accomplished by discography at the L4–5 level (Figs. 39-6 and 39-7). Needless to say, the performance of an L5-to-sacrum spinal fusion below a symptomatic degenerative disc at L4–5 will not likely give a satisfactory result. The presence of lytic defects in the pars interarticularis can usually be revealed by good oblique views, coned down if necessary at the L5 level, and tomograms may be used for greater detail if indicated. Also, bone scans will show increased uptake in an area of spondylolysis.

"Pillar" views are frequently of value in the cervical spine in demonstrating an area of previous injury to the cervical "pillars" (Fig. 39-8).[33,34] The demonstration of an area of previous fracture may assist with the localization of a painful level that had its origin in trauma. The right and left oblique and the anteroposterior projections are obtained by placing the patient supine with the head rotated maximally to either the right or left (comparison views should be obtained in all cases). The central ray is directed toward the feet, at an average angle of 35°, centering at the inferior border

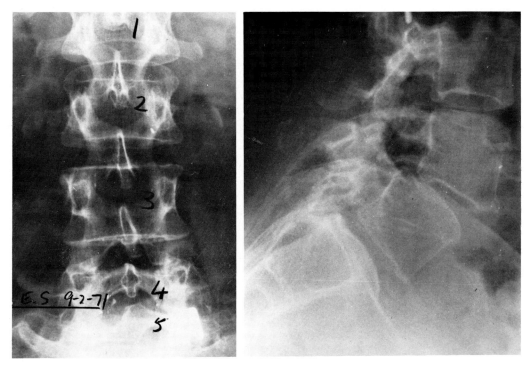

FIG. 39-6. Anteroposterior and lateral roentgenograms of a 50-year-old woman with severe mechanical low back pain and L4–5 spondylolisthesis.

of the thyroid cartilage. The anteroposterior projection is obtained by placing the patient supine with the neck hyperextended in the median sagittal plane. The central ray is directed caudally 20° to 30°, entering at the inferior border of the thyroid cartilage.

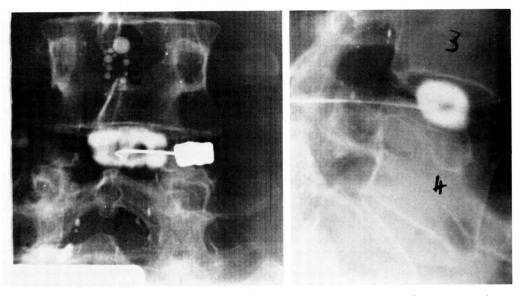

FIG. 39-7. Anteroposterior and lateral lumbar discograms show a normal, asymptomatic L3–4 disc, allowing a successful L4-to-sacrum fusion that produced relief of the patient's complaints.

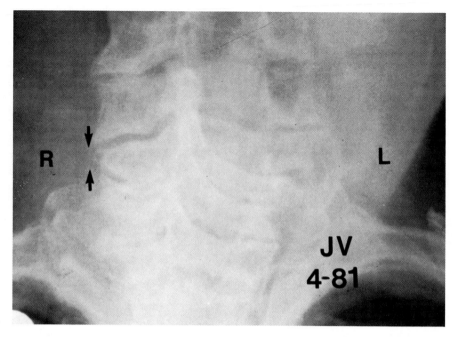

Fig. 39-8. Pillar view of a patient with intractable right-sided neck pain after a prior compression injury. Routine radiographs were entirely normal. Note the compression fracture of the lateral cervical pillars (*arrows*).

COMPLICATIONS RELATED TO TECHNICAL ERRORS AT SURGERY

POSITIONING OF THE PATIENT

One of the essentials for success in surgery of the spine is careful and proper positioning of the patient on the operating table. Failure to do so can seriously compromise a surgical result and may induce various significant complications.

When a posterior approach is being made to the lumbar spine for discogenic disease, it is essential that the field be bloodless. This is impossible if there is pressure on the abdominal cavity, which will direct venous flow through Batson's plexus. Failure to achieve this pressure-free position converts a routine lumbar discotomy from a procedure of simplicity and perfect visualization to a disastrous exercise of fishing in a pool of blood. In the latter circumstance, inadequate visualization may result in failure to recognize fully the extent of the pathology, failure to treat it completely, and increasing the likelihood of iatrogenic neural injury. A position that places no pressure on the abdomen can rarely be achieved with bolsters. A more efficient

support is the MacKay frame, which has lateral supports of adjustable width and curvature.[13] However, the support that combines the utmost in efficiency and simplicity is a Hastings frame, or a modification thereof (Fig. 39-9).[7] In this frame the weight of the patient is taken on the buttocks and the knees, and the abdomen is completely dependent, producing a relatively negative pressure on the vena cava. Anyone who has used other types of supports for positioning and then gone to this type of frame has noted a dramatic difference in the amount of venous bleeding. The lack of blood loss or necessity for transfusion therapy makes it a favorite of any experienced anesthetist. The frame is simply made and adjusted to any conventional operating room table. As the table is tilted, the buttocks come to rest on the support on the frame. The major weight is taken on them, as well as being supported by the femora. The knees should not be excessively flexed, avoiding any pressure on the calves or popliteal areas. It is important that the lateral aspect of the knees be padded and not tightly pressed against the supports of the frame so that pressure on the peroneal

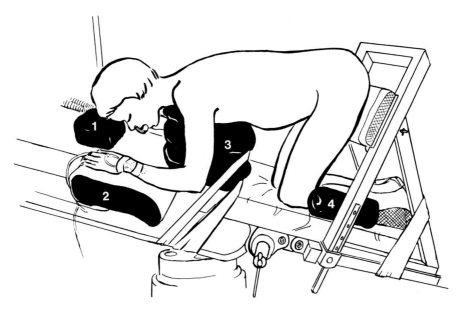

FIG. 39-9. Diagram demonstrates the use of the Hastings frame. Its construction is simple and easily adapted to a conventional operating room table. The frame allows the abdomen to be pendulous without pressure. Cautions for use to be observed include the following: (1) The forehead is supported without pressure on the eyeballs, and without abnormal rotation or extension of the neck. (2) The forearms are supported without pressure on the medial sides of the elbows, avoiding ulnar nerve pressure. (3) The chest is supported well upward, away from the abdomen. (4) The knees are not flexed excessively, avoiding calf pressure. The peroneal nerves are protected by padding from the sides of the frame.

nerve areas is avoided. A support must be placed well upward under the upper chest, and the head and neck should be positioned so that excessive extension and rotation do not occur. This can produce symptoms in an older patient with stiffness due to cervical spondylosis. Abnormal extension and rotation can produce cervical root symptoms and even brachial plexus stretch (Fig. 39-10).

In all surgery on the spine done with the patient prone, strict caution must be observed to be certain that there is no abnormal pressure on the eyes. Sustained pressure on the eyeballs for as little as 2 to 4 minutes can result in blindness. Corneal abrasions should be avoided. Constant attention must be paid by the surgeon and the anesthetist to ensure that the eyes are carefully protected. With the Hastings frame this is fairly easily avoided by using a padded jack support well upward under the chest and the chin. This allows the head to lie in a fairly normal position with a small support under the forehead.

Another matter of constant concern is the avoidance of pressure on the ulnar nerves. In a prone position with the patient resting with the elbows somewhat flexed, certain persons may suffer pressure on the ulnar nerves, particularly those who have a tendency to subluxation of the nerves when the elbows are flexed (approximately 10% of the population). Ideally, the elbows should be free, with no pressure on the medial aspects if the patient is lying prone, the upper extremities being supported by the distal forearms. If attention is not given to this problem, an ulnar neuropathy can be induced, which may become serious enough to require subsequent surgical treatment.

PLACEMENT OF THE INCISION

It is important to center the incision in the operative area. In the lumbar spine it is not uncommon to place the incision too high or too low, requiring later extension

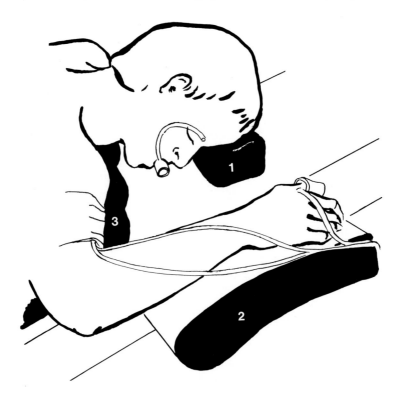

FIG. 39-10. Excessive rotation of the neck. This and hyperextension should be avoided because a prolonged interval in this position can produce cervical root symptoms and even brachial plexus stretch.

and a resulting abnormally long incision. It is essential that the roentgenograms of the patient be in the operating room prior to commencement of the operation. They should be carefully assessed by the surgeon before he undertakes the surgery. The relation of the desired disc space to the level of the iliac crests and the presence of any posterior arch defects in the lumbar and sacral area should be determined. The last spinous interspace should be palpated and correlated with the roentgenograms and the incision planned accordingly. After preliminary exposure, the sacrum should be identified with certainty. The subsequent interspaces can then be identified in relation to it, the presence of the movable interspaces being indicated by the demonstration of movement at each level. In the lumbar area, identification of the level to be treated can usually be done quite satisfactorily in this manner. If there is a question, a lateral x-ray of the lumbar spine may be of value.

In the cervical spine a study of the lateral roentgenogram will indicate the position of the level to be operated in relation to the clavicle and mandible. The cricoid cartilage is usually at the level of the C5–6 disc space. Following exposure of the cervical spine from the anterior approach, a 22-gauge needle should be placed in what is felt to be the appropriate level. Anterior osteophytes can often be a guide in this determination. The position should then be confirmed by a cross-table roentgenogram. When one is approaching the cervical spine posteriorly, the last bifid spinous process of C6 is a valuable localizing level, but even so, it is wise to have a lateral roentgenogram to confirm the operative site.

PENETRATION OF THE SPINAL CANAL

It should be reemphasized that in surgery on the lumbar spine the surgeon should carefully scrutinize the roentgenograms of the lumbar spine before starting his incision. A mental note should be made of the relative width of the interlaminar spaces and the presence of any defect in the posterior arch. In the presence of spina bifida, a large interlaminar space, or deficiencies in the posterior arch of the sacrum, care must be taken to not insert a sharp elevator forcefully through the ligamentum flavum, lest the contents of the spinal canal be damaged. Dissection should be commenced where there is a solid bony posterior arch structure and then extended. A broad elevator is a safer instrument than a sharp-pointed one, which could pass between the posterior arches of adjacent vertebrae. Spondylolisthesis of the type described by Newman as "congenital," with a long, attenuated pars, is frequently associated with spina bifida and posterior arch defects of the sacrum. Special caution should be observed in these circumstances (Fig. 39-11).[17]

If the dissection is carried out on the transverse processes for a posterior intertransverse fusion, care should be taken not to plunge or penetrate between the transverse processes into the retroperitoneal space. The operator should remain posterior to the intertransverse muscles and their fascia. This avoids injury to the large intertransverse vessels, segmental nerves, and great vessels and the development of a significant retroperitoneal hematoma. The transverse process should be identified, and the elevator should be kept in close contact with it. A broad instrument is again advantageous for the initial stripping.

OPERATING ON THE WRONG SIDE OF THE PATIENT

It is important that the surgeon confirm in the operating room the side of the patient on which he wishes to operate if a discotomy is to be done from one approach. It is

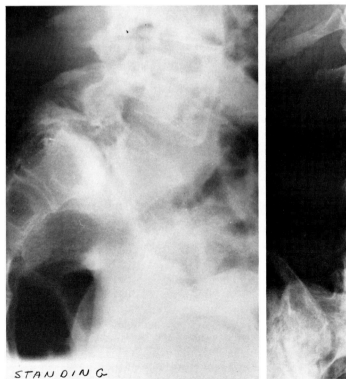
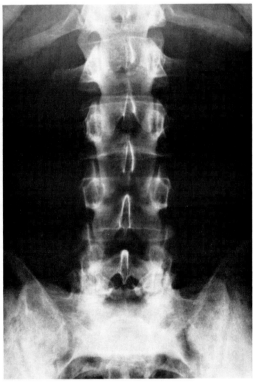

FIG. 39-11. Lateral and anteroposterior roentgenograms of a patient with spondylolisthesis and posterior arch defects of L5 and S1. At operation the sacral defect is often much larger than suspected, and caution must be exercised in the exposure.

important to remember that this will be on the opposite side of the table when the patient has been turned prone. This is a somewhat ridiculous pitfall, but it does occasionally occur.

FAILURE TO RELIEVE ROOT COMPRESSION FOLLOWING LAMINECTOMY OR DISCOTOMY FOR DISC DISEASE

One cause of failure to decompress the root adequately in operation for acute disc herniation is migration of the herniated fragments. In disc rupture following penetration of the anulus, the extruded fragments may track upward or downward deep to the longitudinal ligament and finally herniate at a level above or below the disc space. This can leave a mass of disc tissue lying in the canal above or below the immediate field of exposure between the laminae. When the root is still under tension, the operator must carefully explore to be sure that there is not a significant migration of a fragment above or below that must be removed. Sufficient bone must be removed to allow adequate exposure, and a dural elevator can be passed caudad and cephalad to ensure that there is no remaining disc tissue. A catheter passed upward and downward in the canal can also indicate whether the canal is open and free of encroachment.

Foraminal migration must also be considered and the emergence of the root from the canal examined. Enough bone should be removed to allow adequate examination of the entry of the root into the foramen. A small No. 8 French catheter or an angled dural separator can be passed out of the foramen along the root to test for constriction. If it does not pass easily, further exploration of the root in its canal must be carried out.

In sequestrated disc herniation, it is quite common to find unsuspected fragments extruded upward or downward in the canal and occasionally out along the nerve root into the foramen. These possibilities should be excluded, especially when there is any evidence of residual nerve root tension.

When decompression is carried out in the presence of chronic degenerative changes, the various causes of root entrapment

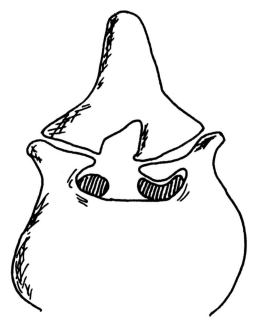

FIG. 39-12. Schematic illustration of subarticular nerve root compression caused by an overhanging osteophyte.

should be considered and treated appropriately. The nerve roots course downward and outward, passing underneath the medial border of the superior articular facets before passing inferolaterally through the foramen. Degeneration with hypertrophy of the superior articular facet may compress the nerve root between the facet and the vertebral body, causing a subarticular entrapment (Fig. 39-12). At exploration the nerve must be followed outward into its foramen to rule out subarticular entrapment. If this is found to be the site of compression, the hypertrophic bone must be removed and the root adequately decompressed. Hemifacetectomy may be required for root decompression.

With advanced intervertebral disc degeneration associated with gross collapse of the disc space, the vertebral bodies approach each other. As the upper vertebral body descends, its pedicle may compress or kink the emerging nerve root to a significant degree, particularly if the collapse is greater on one side (Fig. 39-13). The effect of this pedicular kinking is usually increased by an associated lateral bulge of the disc and collapse of the disc space, the compression

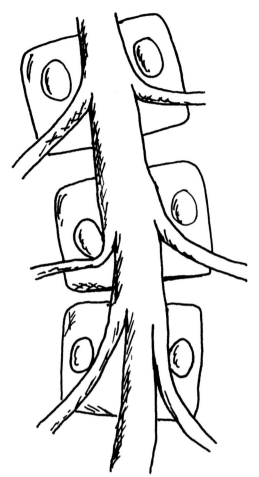

can then be gently removed and the nerve root allowed to slide proximally. This technique avoids undue tension or traction on the root during the decompression.

As the nerve root emerges through its foramen, it lies in close relation to the tip of the superior articular facet of the vertebra below. As the disc space collapses through degeneration, the posterior joints override. This overriding may allow compression of the nerve root by the upward-migrating superior articular facet of the vertebra below, producing foraminal encroachment of the nerve root (Fig. 39-14). Foraminal encroachment caused by overriding of the posterior joints is further accentuated if there is associated osteophytic lipping of the superior articular facet. This possibility of root entrapment and compression in a degenerated, collapsed segment must be considered. The root should be followed outward, and, if this is the site of compression, decompression is carried out, if necessary by superior facetectomy.

The main causes of nerve root compression or entrapment are undoubtedly intraspinal and intraforaminal. However, in rare situations it is possible that extraforaminal compression or irritation may occur. McNab has described extraforaminal entrapment of

FIG. 39-13. Mechanism of pedicular kinking of the nerve root that can occur with asymmetric collapse of the disc space.

occurring between the lateral bulge and the pedicle above. Suspicion of this possibility should be evident preoperatively from an assessment of the anteroposterior roentgenogram showing gross disc collapse, usually asymmetric and greater on the side of the symptoms. For decompression of the nerve root, enough of the pedicle must be removed to leave the nerve root free. To do this without damaging the nerve root, it may be advisable to cut into the pedicle with rongeurs or a power burr above the nerve root, removing a portion of it by commencing proximally and then working distally toward the root so that finally there is only a thin layer of cortex between the root and the area of decompression. This

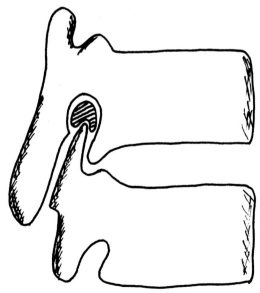

FIG. 39-14. Foraminal encroachment on a nerve root is caused by upward migration of the superior articular facet of the vertebra below.

the L5 nerve root by lateral protrusion of the lumbosacral disc in a cadaveric specimen.[14] He has also described the strong ligamentous band passing from the transverse process of L5 to the body of L5, which lies immediately cephalad to the L5 nerve root as it courses over the ala of the sacrum. He has indicated that with marked narrowing of the lumbosacral disc, this ligament may descend, causing compression of the L5 nerve root.

These lesions justify consideration when, following exposure to decompress an L5 nerve root entrapment, no gross central or foraminal abnormality is found and the nerve root is still under significant tension. The exposure should be continued laterally with examination of the inferior aspect of the transverse process of L5 and release of any obvious ligamentous band. If that is not found to be the cause of the compression and the nerve root is still under tension, exposure can be carried toward the side of the vertebral body.

Lumbar nerve roots may have anomalous origins, or there may be intradural or extradural connections between nerve roots. A recent study shows a 14% incidence of various forms of nerve root anomalies. These anatomical variations may significantly affect level determination, symptoms, and the success rate of surgical decompression.[9]

With spondylolisthesis, pars defects in the lumbar spine can cause significant nerve root compression from impingement of granulation tissue as well as direct nerve root stretch by the slip. This classically involves the L5 nerve root. If there are significant nerve root symptoms at the time of stabilization of a spondylolisthesis, decompression of the involved nerve root may become necessary for relief of symptoms.

OPERATIVE COMPLICATIONS OF LUMBAR DISC REMOVAL

Penetration of the Dura

In opening the spinal canal for lumbar disc removal, one must take care to avoid penetration of the dura. The ligamentum flavum should be exposed and then carefully incised down to its deepest layer. The deepest layer should then be gently incised, or it may be penetrated carefully with a blunt instrument, such as a hemostat, which is spread to increase the size of the opening with less risk of incising the dura. At this stage it is advisable to insert a cottonoid patty to displace the dural sac away from the ligamentum flavum, allowing it to be more safely excised. The patty can then be used to displace the dural sac from the posterior elements as further resection of ligament and bone is carried out. The risk of a dural tear or incision is greater when decompression is carried out for spinal stenosis with marked bony encroachment and thickening of the ligamentum flavum. In these cases the dura is often found to be thin and relatively atrophic and closely applied to the ligamentum flavum. When an incision has been made into the dura, it is advisable, where possible, to repair it. If it is a clean incision or vertical tear, this is usually possible if one uses light, nonirritating 6-0 sutures. To accomplish this, enough bone may have to be removed to allow reasonable exposure of the slit in the dura. When a larger defect is present, a portion of the dorsal fascia may be removed to cover the defect.

Stretching of the Nerve Root

It is important that the nerve root not be stretched unduly in the removal of an extruded disc or in the relief of nerve root entrapment. If the nerve root is under marked tension and is not easily retracted, it should never be pulled forcefully. Sufficient exposure should be carried out to allow visualization of the cause of the nerve root tension. This can then be dealt with, at least partially, to relax the root. Completion of the decompression is then possible without excess traction on the root. Occasionally with a massive extrusion in the axilla of the root, it is not possible or reasonable to try to retract the root medially over it. Adequate exposure should be carried out and the main portion of the extruded mass gently removed from the axilla of the root. The root will then usually be relaxed enough to allow medial retraction without excessive tension.

It is a wise principle for the operator himself to take the responsibility for nerve root retraction. Following exposure of the involved root, it should be freed with a blunt instrument, such as a Howarth elevator or a blunt root hook, and then gently retracted with a Love root retractor. The operator should not delegate this responsibility to an assistant who is not entirely familiar with the varying need for exposure as the decompression is carried out. The nerve root tension can be gauged better by the operator if he retracts the root with his nondominant hand. The surgeon can relax the tension on the root intermittently as the disc-removing forceps are removed from the wound, retracting the root carefully when exposure is required. The assistant should assist with the exposure by controlling the sucker tip to maintain adequate visualization. The synchronized retraction of the root by the operator with one hand and the removal of the disc with the other is less likely to produce undue or excessive traction on the root than is retraction done by an uncoordinated observer across the table. The surgeon constantly knows how much tension is being exerted on the root, and this is his responsibility.

VASCULAR OR VISCERAL INJURY DURING LUMBAR DISC EXCISION

During lumbar disc excision from the posterior approach, the surgeon must be constantly aware of the possibility of anterior penetration of the anulus, allowing vascular or visceral injury. Although relatively uncommon, this penetration results in a high incidence of major, catastrophic complications. The bifurcation of the aorta is usually anterior to the lower border of the L4 vertebral body, approximately 2 cm to the left of the midline (Fig. 39-15). The bifurcation of the vena cava is slightly lower and to the right. The bifurcation of the common iliac artery into the external and internal iliac arteries is usually just lateral to the L5–S1 disc space. The veins tend to lie closer to the vertebrae than do the arteries. The artery that would seem most vulnerable is the common iliac on the left at the L4–5 disc space.

The first major vascular complication of lumbar disc surgery reported in the literature was by Linton and White in 1945.[11] This resulted in an arteriovenous fistula between the inferior vena cava and the right common femoral artery; it was diagnosed and successfully excised surgically 7 months after laminectomy. Vascular injury, when it occurs, is more often sufficient to produce exsanguination if not controlled quickly. This is reflected by the mortality rate reported in the literature (23%–50%).[3,5,8] The surgeon should exercise constant care to try to avoid this complication in lumbar disc

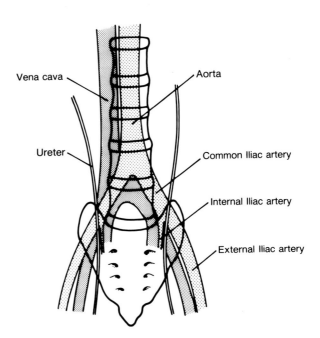

FIG. 39-15. Relationship of the anterior vital structures to the lower lumbar spine. Note the proximity of the ureter, aorta, vena cava, and iliac vessels to the disc spaces. These can easily be injured by passing an instrument through an attenuated anulus.

Vena cava

Aorta

Ureter

Common Iliac artery

Internal Iliac artery

External Iliac artery

excision. After the disc has been exposed with adequate retraction of the nerve root, extruded fragments may be removed, or the longitudinal ligament and anulus may be incised as required. The loose fragments that lie posterior in the disc space should be lifted free with rongeurs without major penetration at that time. Once the posterior portion of the disc space has been evacuated, the rongeur should be angled toward the vertebral plates above and below. The surgeon should be constantly aware of contact with the vertebral bodies by the tip of the rongeurs, carefully extracting all of the disc tissue within the anulus. When exploration of the disc space is carried out, it should be done with the instrument closed. To remove disc fragments, the instrument is opened without any further penetration into the disc. By constantly maintaining contact with the vertebral end-plates, the surgeon usually has good depth perception and an awareness that he is still well within the disc space. When all of the loose disc tissue has been removed, a ring curette can be used to loosen any remaining disc material. This instrument should be inserted carefully without any forceful penetration. Contact should again be made against the vertebral body above and below in the depth of the disc space, and the ring curette should be drawn toward the operator in an anterior-to-posterior direction. Fragments that have been loosened are removed by the rongeurs, with the same technique of vertebral end-plate contact maintained.

Injury to a major vessel is usually indicated by a sudden gush of blood from the depth of the disc space. This is the most important indication and should alert the surgeon to immediate danger. Case reports indicate that in many instances this temporary hemorrhage appears to be controlled or relieved by packing. Consequently, the surgeon is lulled into a false sense of security, and the patient later develops signs of blood loss. When there has been major bleeding from a disc space, the patient should be very carefully monitored, and preparation should be made for an immediate anterior exposure. Time is precious. When major vascular injury has been promptly recognized and an anterior exposure carried out, satisfactory control has usually been possible with the avoidance of fatality. It is a time for decision and action—not wishful thinking or procrastination.

One possible congenital anomaly that may confuse the surgeon attempting an anterior approach to the iliac vessels and make exposure difficult is a horseshoe kidney, which occurs in approximately 1 of every 700 persons. If a mass is found in the area of the apparent bleeding, a horseshoe kidney is a possibility. If present it should be reflected accordingly to allow adequate exposure. We are aware of one fatality that was to some degree the result of confusion and delay in control of the hemorrhage following an anterior approach in the presence of this anomaly.

Injuries to viscera other than the major vessels may occur. Injuries to the ileum and ureters have occurred, requiring appropriate treatment. In one instance described to the senior author, a long, pedunculated structure that proved to be the appendix was drawn into the discectomy wound. It was ligated and transected and the stump returned to the abdominal cavity without apparent subsequent major difficulties to the patient. Despite this isolated success, it is not an approach to be recommended for appendectomy.

Retained Foreign Body

The possibility of a retained surgical foreign body is a complication that may occur with almost any surgical procedure. The use of cottonoid patties in lumbar disc excision helps avoid many complications of dural injury and allows control of bleeding to provide a clearer operative field. These patties are small and may become detached from their strings. Care must be taken to ensure that none is retained in the wound. An accurate count is mandatory. All patties should have radiopaque markers. If there is any question about the count, a roentgenogram can then be taken to document whether one has been retained and to indicate its position.

Larger objects, such as an operative sponge, are less likely to be retained in a discectomy or fusion wound. More commonly they may be left in an iliac crest donor site where the sponge has been used for packing deep in the wound. A thorough search of the wound should be made prior to closure and an accurate sponge count taken. Again, it is advisable to use sponges that have roentgenographically identifiable markers. If there is any question about the count, a radiograph should be taken in the operating room.

The use of a plastic suction drain to evacuate any hematoma during the first 24 to 36 hours following spinal and other orthopaedic procedures has become commonplace. This helps in reducing hematoma formation and postoperative morbidity. When it is used, care must be taken to be certain that the drain is deep in the wound and not caught in the sutures used for closure. Postoperatively, if the drain is found to resist removal, excessive force should not be used; this prevents tube breakage and retention. It is preferable to use a degree of traction for an additional 24 hours. If the drain does not readily free itself by then, the patient must be taken to the operating room for a careful, limited exposure around the drain to release the retaining suture and allow removal.

COMPLICATIONS OF ANTERIOR LUMBAR DISC EXCISION AND FUSION

In anterior lumbar disc excision and fusion, possible complications are often related to the exposure, either retroperitoneally or transperitoneally, including vascular and visceral retraction. Graft ejection and collapse can occur. The incidence of pseudarthrosis in isolated anterior fusions is undoubtedly higher than in comparable posterolateral fusions. This is due to the large area of graft that must be revascularized, the distance between the bony parts that are to be fused, and the distance that the grafts are placed from the axis of minimal motion or "zero velocity."

A significant complication of anterior lumbar disc surgery that must be considered in the male is the possibility of impotence due to damage of the autonomic nerve supply. The superior hypogastric plexus (presacral nerve) lies within the fork of the aorta and ventral to the left common iliac vein, the body of the fifth lumbar vertebra,

and the L5–S1 disc space. It may be damaged during an anterior approach to the lower lumbar spine, particularly at the L5–S1 level. This possibility must be considered when advising men about the alternatives that are available. Significant injury to the autonomic nerve supply is less likely to occur with anterior approaches to the L4–5 disc space. Fortunately, this is the level for which circumferential fusion is occasionally indicated for recurrent pseudarthrosis.

When an anterior approach to the L5–S1 disc space is felt to be indicated, careful infiltration of the prevertebral areolar tissue and retroperitoneal structures with saline solution should be carried out. This distends the tissues to allow easier recognition of the nerve filaments so that they may be avoided or carefully retracted.

COMPLICATIONS RELATED TO THE DONOR SITE

It is a fairly common experience for many patients who have been successfully relieved of their low-back mechanical disability and nerve root problems by effective surgery to have residual complaints related to the iliac donor area. Generally these complaints are only mildly annoying and are associated with occasional ache and tenderness in the scar.

Hematoma formation in the donor wound can be a problem. It is minimized by the use of a suction drain for 24 to 36 hours postoperatively. Care should be taken to control all major bleeding points. A hemostatic agent such as Gelfoam should be used over the raw bone surface to decrease bleeding.

A meticulous closure is important. Dead space should be obliterated and the reflected muscles approximated near their origins. This avoids a long, attenuated scar that would be pulled upon by subsequent muscle action producing distress.

The superficial gluteal nerve crosses the iliac crest about 4 fingerbreadths away from the midline posteriorly. If an incision is made along the iliac crest to obtain the graft, with subsequent division of the superficial gluteal nerve, it may become a later source of pain. In a midline approach to the lower lumbar spine, it is preferable to curve the lower end of the incision laterally. This allows exposure of the posterior superior iliac spine through a midline incision and lessens the possibility of nerve injury. The periosteum should be incised over the posterior superior spine and reflected forward subperiosteally, protecting the nerve.

In those instances in which a gluteal neuroma does occur, the tenderness becomes well localized and may be exquisite. The pain can be temporarily relieved by infiltration of the area with local anesthetic and corticosteroids. If the symptoms and tenderness persist and the complaints are significant, it may become necessary to explore the incision and look for the neuroma. When the neuroma is found, the nerve should be followed proximally, allowing division well above the iliac crest. Any excessive scar should be excised prior to wound closure.

When bone is being taken from the iliac crest with the patient supine for an anterior cervical fusion, the skin incision should be placed well below the crest (approximately 3 cm). The incision is then retracted upward to allow exposure of the crest. One should take care to avoid injury to the lateral cutaneous branch of the subcostal nerve, using subperiosteal dissection. Following removal of the graft, the wound should be closed carefully and the dead space obliterated. Placing the skin incision well below the crest reduces the likelihood of irritation of the scar by tight-fitting clothes and belts.

OPERATIVE COMPLICATIONS OF ANTERIOR CERVICAL DISCECTOMY AND FUSION

The possible operative complications of anterior cervical discectomy and fusion theoretically involve injury to almost every structure in the area. Isolated reported instances confirm this. An awareness of the possible complications, a clear knowledge of the anatomy of the area, and careful technique in reasonable hands should make this an operative procedure of relatively minimal morbidity.

Problems Related to the Incision

Since the incision is placed in an exposed area of the neck, a reasonable cosmetic result is desirable. An ugly scar from a cosmetic standpoint is, to some degree, a complication. The "best" scar is obtained by placing the incision transversely along the line of the skin creases. A subcuticular closure with 3-0 monofilament nylon is used, with the suture removed about 5 days postoperatively. This usually results in a rather insignificant scar, barely discernible from the normal skin creases of the neck.

It is important that the platysma be carefully repaired, as well as the subcutaneous tissues over it. If this is not done, the skin may be stuck to the deep tissues and may pucker with contracture of the platysma. This puckering can be quite evident when the patient smiles or shows some other expression.

After the initial skin incision, the platysma should be delineated and carefully incised. It should then be freed upward and downward from the underlying fascia and muscles. This is easily done with a dry gauze on the operative finger; the flaps are lifted forward as it is cleared. This allows good delineation and mobilization of the ends of the muscle. It can then be easily repaired with care at the end of the procedure.

A transverse incision along the line of the skin creases has proved adequate for operative exposure for all levels of the cervical spine from C2 to T1. However, a vertical incision may occasionally be indicated. This should be closed carefully. It produces a more disfiguring scar than does the transverse incision and is not indicated for routine use. In one early case of the senior author, a keloid developed in a vertical scar in a young woman. This presented a serious problem in management. It would be less of a problem in a transverse scar.

Injury to the Carotid Sheath

In obtaining the exposure, careful dissection should be carried out along the normal tissue planes. Blunt dissection is preferred, avoiding undue bleeding and maintaining a clear exposure. Sharp or prolonged retraction on the carotid sheath and its contents should be avoided to decrease the risk of injury to the vessels or thrombosis.

Injury to the Recurrent Laryngeal Nerve or the Thoracic Lymph Duct

The recurrent laryngeal nerve is slightly more exposed to injury on the right side than on the left. A right-sided approach is not contraindicated if the surgeon exercises proper care. On the left side one must take care to avoid injuring the thoracic lymph duct.

The operator is wise to choose the side of approach with which he feels most comfortable and that he finds easier. The senior author, as a right-handed surgeon, routinely employs a right-sided approach, having used it without major difficulty over the past 25 years.

Injury to the Esophagus and Trachea

The interval between the esophagus, trachea, sternohyoid, and sternothyroid muscles medially and the carotid sheath and sternomastoid laterally is usually the one accepted for anterior approaches to the cervical spine. For caudad exposure the omohyoid may be retracted laterally, or it may be divided and reflected if desired. Blunt dissection carried out in this interval should avoid any significant trauma to the esophagus and trachea. These should be retracted only with a blunt retractor. If a Cloward retractor is used, the smooth blade should be directed toward the esophagus and trachea. The points of the sharp blade should be aimed at the muscle laterally. Undue retraction on the esophagus and trachea should be avoided. Electrocautery injury must also be guarded against. If these guidelines are followed, there should not be a significant incidence of esophageal or tracheal penetration. If esophageal injury with leakage occurs with this procedure, it must be recognized. Esophageal injuries must be repaired at the time of surgery, with placement of a nasogastric tube, adequate wound drainage, and administration of appropriate antibiotics.

Injury to the Vertebral Artery

Injury to the vertebral artery may occur if decompression is carried far laterally, into the area of the vertebral artery canal. As in most vascular penetrations, attempts should be made to control the problem by local packing with thromboplastic agents (*e.g.*, Gelfoam), surgical gauze, and cottonoid patties. If a major laceration with severe hemorrhage occurs, exposure of the artery above and below may be required to control the hemorrhage. Ordinarily the vertebral artery does not enter the spine until the level of the transverse process of C6 (Fig. 39-16). If the area of exposure is in the region of this vertebra, the artery may be exposed below in its free portion and clamped. It will, however, also require proximal control. To do this usually requires a power burr to remove the bone over the anterior aspect of the transverse process. The artery is then exposed at a level above the point of penetration to allow it to be ligated adequately with a metallic clip or suture. If the area of penetration is higher in the spine, it may be necessary to remove the bone over the anterior aspect of the transverse process above and below. Again, a power burr is used, followed by the use of punches to expose the artery in its canal, allowing control above and below. It is important to recognize that retrograde flow can cause significant hemorrhage from above and that control of the vessel proximally and distally to the site of the laceration is required.

Asphyxia due to Lack of Adequate Drainage

It is wise to routinely drain the site of an anterior cervical discectomy and fusion. Prior to closure of the wound, the retractor should be removed. The walls of the wound are then carefully inspected to make certain that there are no uncontrolled bleeding points that were temporarily arrested by the pressure effect of the retractors. These should be adequately controlled. A soft Penrose drain should be used routinely to drain all wounds after anterior cervical discectomy and fusion. The drain is generally removed in 24 hours. There is usually no significant hemorrhage. However, there is occasionally evidence of significant release of liquid blood that has undoubtedly avoided any significant pressure phenom-

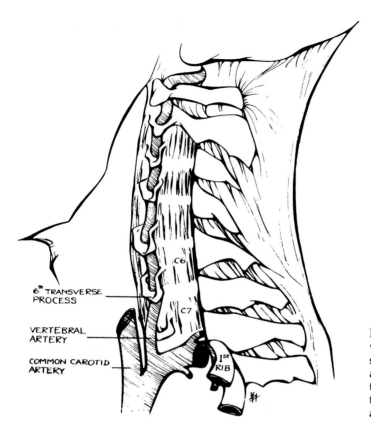

FIG. 39-16. Lateral anatomical view shows the normal passage of the vertebral arteries and veins in front of the transverse process of C7, entering the transverse foramen at C6.

enon. Following removal of the drain, the subcuticular suture is tightened. This does not produce any alteration in or abnormality of the operative scar. The drain is a safety factor. The senior author has knowledge of one fatality caused by asphyxia due to uncontrolled bleeding in a routine anterior cervical procedure performed by a surgeon who routinely did not drain his wounds. It is a simple, but very worthwhile, safety measure.

Faulty Placement of the Anterior Cervical Graft

Placing the Graft Too Far to One Side. In an anterior cervical discectomy and fusion it is important that the graft be placed as close to the midline as possible. When the surgeon approaches the spine, he should identify the lateral landmarks or borders of the cervical spine as visualized from in front. The center point should be identified. The graft site is then cut centered on the midline. This gives better supporting bone on both sides of the graft, as well as above and below, and contributes to its stability. It also decreases the likelihood of vertebral artery injury.

Driving the Graft Too Deep. Strict attention should be given to avoiding excessive posterior placement of the graft. An accurate measurement should be made of the depth of the graft insertion site using a reliable instrument (Fig. 39-17). Where anterior cervical discectomy and fusion is being carried out for painful neck disability or soft tissue disc extrusion, it is not necessary to remove the posterior vertebral cortex of the vertebra at the graft site. This allows reasonable posterior support for the graft and prevents posterior graft extrusion. When the procedure is carried out for cord decompression associated with myelopathy and posterior projecting osteophytes, it is advisable to remove the projecting osteophytes but to leave a rim of normal vertebral cortex above and below in the area of the midportion of the vertebral bodies. This

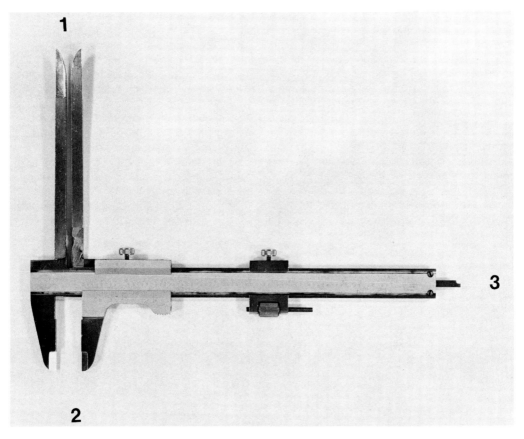

FIG. 39-17. This instrument has been used by the senior author to allow precise measurement of the graft defect and graft. The limbs of the instrument (1) can be inserted and separated to measure the length of the graft with full distraction. The instrument will then be set at 2, showing the length for the graft. To measure the depth, the fine point of the instrument at 3 is inserted into the defect, and the depth is measured by sliding the wider portion against the anterior cortex.

provides some degree of support for the graft. When an accurately measured graft of appropriate size is inserted, it should be carefully tapped into position. When a punch is used for the last portion of the insertion, the graft should be tapped at the margins with a portion of the punch overlapping the normal vertebra above and below. This prevents excessive force directed onto the graft beyond the anterior margin of the normal vertebral bodies. If there is any question about the degree of penetration, the graft should be retracted anteriorly. Traction is applied on the neck to allow this to be done with ease. The graft should likewise be inserted with full distraction applied to the neck so that it can be tapped-

in without excessive difficulty. As the traction is released, the graft is then locked in place.

If it is discovered postoperatively that the graft has been driven too far posteriorly, with cord or nerve root compromise, no attempt should be made to carry out a posterior decompression or laminectomy. The patient should be reoperated on immediately from the anterior approach. The graft is extracted anteriorly to a point at which there is no possibility of cord compression. Although this solution might seem to be just common sense, there are cases on record in which those in charge procrastinated, wasted time in myelography, and carried out futile posterior laminectomy.

Placing the Graft Too Low. A fairly common error in graft placement with both the dowel and the block techniques is to cut the defect for the graft too low. If this is done, the major portion of the graft rests in the inferior vertebra, with little purchase on the superior. This tendency is due to the upward-sloping angle of the disc spaces in the cervical area when viewed from the side (Figs. 39-18 and 39-19). When the site for the dowel graft is centered over the disc space and the drill is directed straight backward, there is a tendency to take more bone out inferiorly than superiorly. This may give inadequate contact above, with a tendency to pseudarthrosis. When fusion is done by the keystone technique, the problem can be handled by merely taking a little more bone from the superior vertebra and inserting a larger graft to give good contact between the vertebral bodies. The Robinson technique, with retained vertebral end-plates, has theoretical disadvantages owing to decreased bone healing, graft stability, and vascular ingrowth.

It is wise to carry out a partial initial removal of the disc so that the operator can orient himself to the alignment of the disc space. This allows accurate centering of the drill for the Cloward graft or the

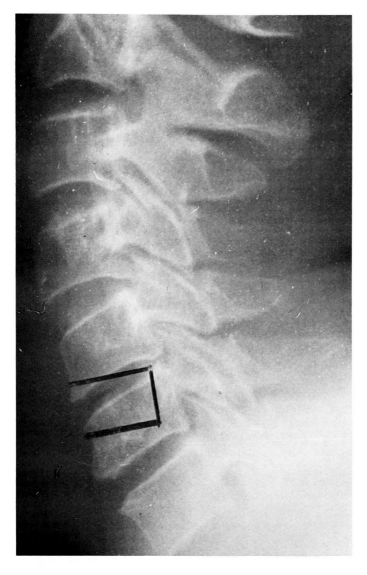

FIG. 39-18. Lateral roentgenogram demonstrates the tendency to place the major portion of the graft site in the inferior vertebra, owing to oblique alignment of the disc spaces.

cutting of a block or keystone graft. Failure to obtain an adequate purchase in the vertebra above may be one of the factors contributing to extrusion (Fig. 39-20).

Graft ejection may occur with all types of anterior cervical discectomy and fusion. It is less likely to occur when the graft is more deeply seated and is closer to the line of "zero velocity." This is at the level of the emerging nerve roots. An attempt should be made to place the graft as far posterior as possible. Ejection is less likely to occur with a block or keystone type of graft inserted with the neck in full distraction. The keystone graft provides inherent stability, with a minimal tendency to extrusion (Fig. 39-21). The amount of bevel does

not have to be extreme and is ideally on the order of 14°. Extrusion of the graft is less likely to occur if it is countersunk 1 mm to 2 mm. When a dowel graft is used, one may undercut the cortices slightly with a small curette. A dowel graft is then shaped slightly shorter than the depth of the defect. This decreases the tendency to extrusion. The extrusion rate in this type of graft is greater than that in the block or keystone types (Figs. 39-22, and 39-23).

Graft and Intervertebral Collapse

When two dowel grafts are placed in succeeding levels with too little bone between, the intervening vertebral body may

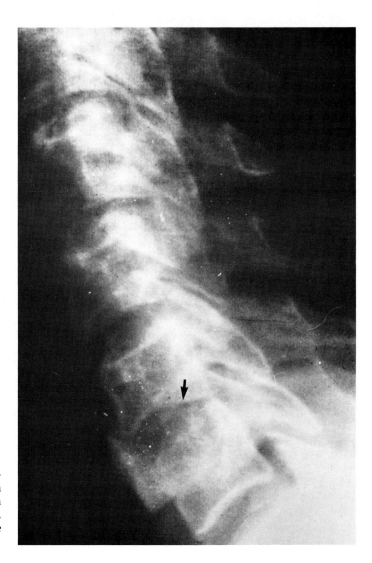

FIG. 39-19. Lateral roentgenogram of a patient with a dowel graft placed mostly in the inferior vertebra (*arrow*), which subsequently became extruded.

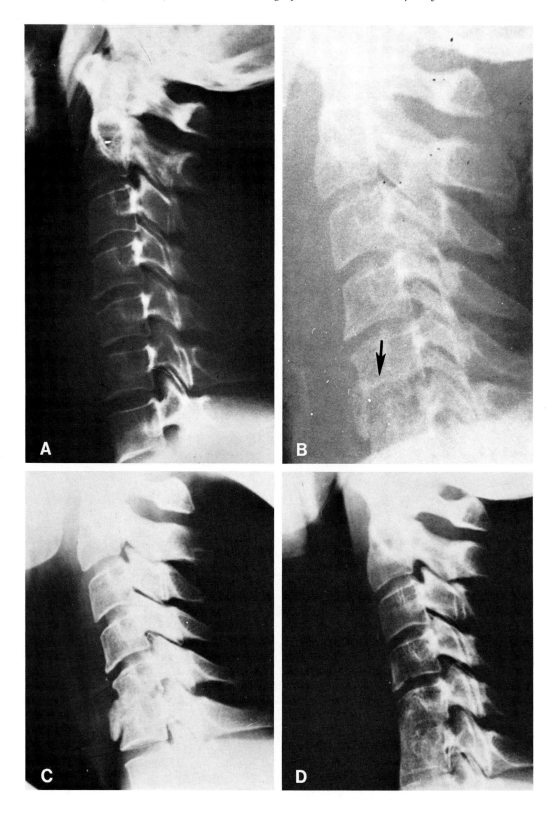

◀ FIG. 39-20. (*A*) Lateral roentgenogram of an orthopaedic surgeon with a C5–6 disc herniation. (*B*) This early postoperative lateral film was made following Cloward C5–6 discectomy and fusion. Note that the graft (*arrow*) is largely in the inferior vertebra, with early extrusion. The patient had increasing C6 root signs and symptoms. (*C*) This later lateral postoperative film of the same patient showed gross collapse of the disc space and extrusion of the graft. The patient was now severely disabled, with gross right C6 root paralysis. (*D*) This postoperative lateral roentgenogram followed revision by the keystone anterior fusion technique. The graft and disc tissue had to be removed at C5–6, and the fusion was extended into C7 to obtain satisfactory purchase below, owing to the low placement of the previous graft in C6. The keystone technique allowed distraction of the operative site and correction of the previous collapse. The patient went on to dramatic relief of the complaint, with full return of function.

collapse. This is presumably due to impaired vascularity, with a tendency to flexion angularity and extrusion. It has been recommended that succeeding grafts be offset slightly so that they are not directly in line with each other. The use of a longer keystone or block type of graft would appear to be advantageous over successive dowel grafts (Fig. 39-24). Alternatively, successive Robinson grafts may be used. Care should be taken to preserve a reasonable portion of the intervening vertebral body.

Pseudarthrosis

The reported incidence of pseudarthrosis ranges from 2% to 21%. A factor that

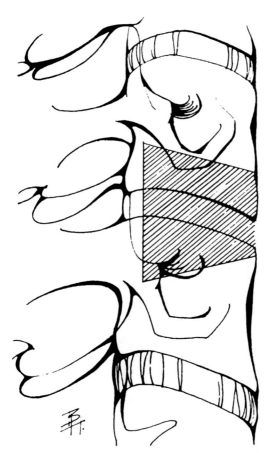

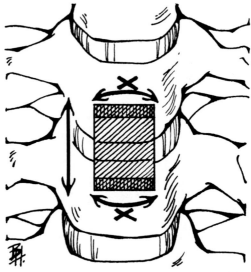

FIG. 39-21. Lateral diagram demonstrates the principle of keystone anterior cervical fusion. The keystone shape allows locking in an excellent bed of vascular bone, with maintenance of distraction and a minimal tendency to ejection.

FIG. 39-22. Anteroposterior diagram illustrates the principle of the keystone block fusion, allowing distraction of the involved disc space with better stability and resistance to lateral bending force.

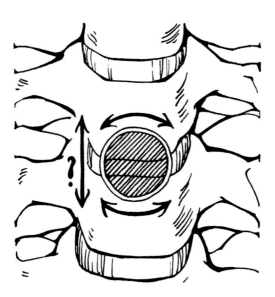

FIG. 39-23. Anteroposterior diagram of a dowel fusion. It is not possible to obtain as much distraction as with a keystone fusion. There is less resistance to lateral bending force and a greater tendency to extrusion.

undoubtedly contributes to pseudarthrosis is the use of heterograft rather than autograft bone. Other factors are the type of graft, its stability, its method of seating, the depth of penetration, the contact of the graft with vascular cancellous bone, and the surface area of the graft for revascularization. It is important that the graft be placed between the two vertebrae with good cancellous bone contact. It should be placed in a stable situation well backward toward the line of "zero velocity." A block rectangular or keystone graft has more inherent stability under side-to-side strain than does a dowel graft. The incidence of fusion appears to be higher if the graft is inserted with the neck distracted, allowing some compression after release of the distraction force.

When pseudarthrosis occurs, it may be the cause of persisting painful complaints. This situation usually responds to a successful posterior fusion. There is usually subsequent healing of the pseudarthrosis, and anterior fusion as well.

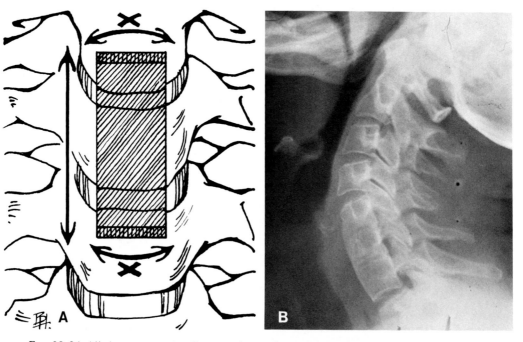

FIG. 39-24. (*A*) Anteroposterior diagram shows the principle of the keystone graft for two-level fusion, allowing distraction of both disc segments. (*B*) Postoperative lateral roentgenogram shows the late result of two-level keystone fusion. Vertebral height has been maintained without collapse of the involved levels.

COMPLICATIONS OF CHEMONUCLEOLYSIS

In applying chemonucleolysis techniques to low back pain, it is important to keep in mind that intervertebral disc herniation is responsible for only a small percentage of low back disability. Again, appropriate clinical assessment is essential in patient selection. A period of conservative management is wise because of the significant number of cases that resolve with conservative management, of which the most important measure is rest.

Other causes of radicular irritation such as spinal stenosis, lateral root and foraminal stenosis, facet impingement, pyriformis syndrome, intraspinal tumor, and spinal arteriovenous malformation must carefully be ruled out. Chemonucleolysis has no place in the treatment of these disorders.

Pretreatment evaluation and patient selection should incorporate the myelogram, CT scan, and discogram as diagnostic modalities when appropriate. The discogram as a part of intradiscal therapy is absolutely mandatory and should always precede the injection.

Since the first reports by Smith on the successful injection of chymopapain,[30] the appeal of injectible agents as an alternative to laminectomy has stimulated many clinical studies.[1,12,15,18,20,23,37] Controversy still surrounds the use of this therapeutic modality, with some question as to its efficacy.[2,22,24] The Food and Drug Administration has recently recognized the potential usefulness of chymopapain, and the substance is currently available for clinical use in the US. Another substance, collagenase, also has proponents for similar use. Both experimental[31] and clinical studies[30,32] suggest its effectiveness in digesting disc material. Collagenase is apparently associated with a much lower incidence of anaphylaxis than that reported for chymopapain. Large clinical studies comparing collagenase with chymopapain in effectiveness are needed.

Chymopapain is an enzyme derived from the papaya plant. Experimental studies have shown epidural animal injection to be safe. In one experimental study,[25] however, epidural injection in rats caused subarachnoid hemorrhage and death. Nonetheless, other investigative trials have failed to duplicate these results. Intrathecal injection causes breakdown of pia-arachnoid capillaries. A large enough dose in animals can cause a rise in cerebrospinal fluid pressure and death. Rydevik[21] studied the effect on rabbit tibial nerve and documented intraneural edema and nerve fiber degeneration. However, this study has been criticized by others. Chymopapain has a direct effect on the capillary wall. Direct intravenous injection in animals causes intra-abdominal and intrapleural hemorrhage and hypocoagulability.

Chymopapain is a antigenic substance that produces a significant incidence of anaphylaxis when injected in humans. A 1.5% incidence of systemic allergic reaction has been reported. There is a higher incidence in females 2.5%. An elevated erythrocyte sedimentation rate and menstruation are increased risk factors. Recent research suggests that pretreatment of patients with cimetidine and diphenhydramine has a protective effect and decreases the severity of anaphylaxis. These are H_2- and H_1-receptor antagonists, respectively. The high incidence of anaphylaxis makes anesthetic support mandatory during chemonucleolysis. Close postinjection monitoring of the patient is also important. There have been no reported cases of anaphylaxis leading to death in procedures done under local anesthesia. We feel that this technique allows early recognition of allergic symptoms without the masking of reactions caused by general anesthesia and allows early treatment.

Candidates for chemonucleolysis should have clear-cut disc protrusion documented by history, physical examinations, and radiologic studies including myelograms, CT scans, and discograms. Patients should have had a prior trial of conservative treatment. Ideal candidates for chemonucleolysis are also ideal candidates for operative disc removal.

Contraindications are

Current or rapidy developing major motor weakness
Disturbance in sphincter function
Excessive spondylosis or spinal stenosis with associated bony spurs
Pregnancy (the teratology of this compound has been inadequately studied)

Allergy to papaya or allergic reaction to a prior chymopapain injection

Evidence of major disc sequestration through the longitudinal ligament with migration of fragments in the canal

A partial contraindication is prior surgery at the symptomatic level.

We feel that chemonucleolysis is best accomplished in a special-procedure room in a radiology specialty suite with the attendance of an anesthesiologist with a full resuscitation cart. Intravenous hydration should be started 12 hours before the procedure. The patient receives cimetidine 300 mg intravenously ever 6 hours and diphenhydramine 25 mg PO every 6 hours for the 24 hours before the injection. Sedatives and analgesia are given prior to the procedure. A 6-inch, 18-gauge needle is passed initially to the level of the disc to be injected. The needle is passed obliquely at 45° to the spine, avoiding all neural elements. Once its position is documented by biplane fluoroscopy, a second, 22-gauge, 8-inch needle is placed through the cannula of the larger needle. The tip of this needle is bent to allow penetration of the disc parallel to the end-plates (Fig. 39-25). Its position is then documented by fluoroscopy, the disc is evaluated by injecting Renografin-60 contrast medium, and a permanent record is made. Usually 15 minutes is allowed to elapse to allow some dissipation of contrast medium before chymopapain injection. Prior to injection the patient is allowed to breathe 100% oxygen. Care must be taken to avoid any moist alcohol on the chymopapain stopper top because residual alcohol could inactivate the enzyme. The injection should be done very slowly, with very careful evaluation of vital signs and patient symptoms. The needles are then removed. The patient is then carefully observed in the recovery room.

At the onset of any systemic manifestation of anaphylaxis, vigorous treatment should be instituted immediately. Epinephrine 1:10,000 should be administered, the airway maintained, and the patient given oxygen. Antihistamines should be given, as well as vasopressor agents as needed.

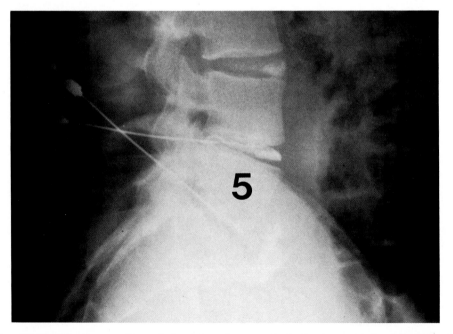

FIG. 39-25. The two-needle technique for chemonucleolysis. A posterolateral approach with 18-gauge, 6-inch needles angled at 45° is used. After this needle is advanced to the level of the disc, a pre-bent 22-gauge, 8-inch needle is passed into the central area of the disc space. A discogram is always done prior to injection of chymopapain.

GENERAL COMPLICATIONS OF MAJOR SURGERY

Pulmonary Complications

When any patient undergoes major surgery, the possibility of chest complications must always be considered. They are more likely to occur in a person who is a chronic smoker or who has preexisting lung disease. It is advisable and reasonable to require any candidate for an elective surgical procedure on the spine to diminish or cease any excessive smoking for an adequate interval preoperatively. This allows time for the chest and lung fields to clear. The patient should be put on pulmonary physiotherapy preoperatively and instructed in postoperative deep-breathing exercises and routine postoperative pulmonary physiotherapy. If attention is constantly paid to these precautions, the incidence of pulmonary complications will be kept at a minimum.

Genitourinary Complications

Although catheter drainage is used routinely for major spinal surgery for the correction of severe deformities, it is not required routinely for lumbar and cervical disc surgery. Catheter drainage should be used only when it is necessary. If that were done, the incidence of catheter irritation and infection would fall. When catheter drainage is required for postoperative retention, meticulous care for asepsis should be used. The use of prophylactic antibiotic agents may be indicated if long-term catheterization is necessary. The patient should be mobilized and the catheter drainage discontinued as soon as possible. A culture of the removed catheter tip is often of value in determining bladder colonization and in guiding antibiotic therapy. Some urologists recommend instillation of an antibiotic, such as neomycin, into the bladder at the time of catheter removal.

Thrombophlebitis and Thromboembolism

The best prophylaxis against thrombophlebitis and thromboembolism is activity, rapid mobilization, and deep-breathing exercises. The patient should be instructed preoperatively by an enthusiastic and intelligent physiotherapist about the importance of early postoperative mobilization. Any fears that the patient may have over activity causing damage to the operative area should be corrected. If the patient understands fully the measures to be adopted postoperatively, and if these have been practiced, he is more likely to do them effectively. For patients at risk or who have a history of thrombophlebitis or embolism, postoperative anticoagulant therapy with heparin or coumadin may be instituted. For those at lesser risk, salicylates are a reasonable alternative.

Infection

Infection is a complication that may accompany major surgery in any area. In lumbar spinal surgery, all of the routine precautions should be used. Laminar air flow in the operative suite is valuable. The wound should be irrigated intermittently with saline solution and an antibiotic agent. All bleeding points should be adequately secured and suction drainage used when there is any indication. Prophylactic antibiotics have a definite place and should be administered prior to commencing the procedure (ideally by the intravenous route) and throughout it. The peak effectiveness is probably obtained from immediately preoperatively until approximately 48 hours postoperatively. Drugs should be used with a reasonably broad spectrum against the common infective agents. Cervical wounds rarely become infected, probably owing to the excellent vascularity of this area. The iliac donor wound is much more likely to become infected. It should be closed carefully to obliterate all dead space, and suction drainage should be used to avoid the development of a hematoma.

When infection does occur and it is felt to be deep seated, it should be recognized early. The patient should be taken to the operating room to have the wound opened and thoroughly lavaged, after which a closed-suction irrigation system is inserted and an antibiotic and Alevaire administered over an adequate interval. When this is done efficiently and early, the results are very satisfactory.

Sewing-in the Drain

One of the problems in wound closures in which suction drainage is used is the possibility of sewing-in the drainage tube. As the wound is closed, the operator should locate very clearly the site of the drainage tube and take care that his closing sutures do not penetrate or encircle the tube so that it may break off during attempts at removal. When the tube is caught in the suture and does not come out easily, traction should be placed on it with a clamp for 24 to 36 hours. If it is not then free, a limited opening of the wound will be required to remove it.

Bleeding

Measures to avoid serious bleeding include preoperative screening for any inherent bleeding tendency, proper positioning of the patient to avoid undue pressure on the vena cava, and finally, to securing all bleeding points adequately. When this is done, there should be no great problems of postoperative bleeding. When hypotensive anesthesia is used with a dry field during the procedure, there may be an increased postoperative bleeding tendency. As a general rule, it is wise to have the patient rest supine following lumbar surgery for a reasonable interval immediately postoperatively to create some pressure effect.

LONG-TERM COMPLICATIONS RELATED TO THE OPERATIVE PROCEDURE OR THE DISABILITY FOR WHICH IT WAS CARRIED OUT

Degeneration at Other Levels Adjacent to the Area of Surgery or in the Same Region

The performance of a solid fusion of one segment of the spine does create some increased stresses and strains at the levels above and below. A not uncommon late complication is recurrent symptoms due to degenerative changes at a level above, below, or near a previous area of fusion. This is not infrequently seen at the L3–4 level above a long-standing fusion from L4 to the sacrum that has been done for degenerative disc disease. Even in patients who have had a "floating" L4–5 fusion, most often the level that later goes on to painful degenerative change is not the L5–S1 segment but the L3–4 level. This is part of the problem of the basic disease that affects

the patient: degenerative disc disease. The patient must be advised that degeneration at adjacent or other levels may occur. Those with discogenic disease should be encouraged to maintain good trunk posture and stay physically fit after surgery on the spine.

Degenerative Changes in Other Areas of the Spine as Part of Degenerative Disc Disease

It is not uncommon for a patient with degenerative disc disease of the lumbar spine to present initially or later with similar problems in the cervical spine, and vice versa. Occasionally patients who had previous disability in their low back or neck requiring surgery return later with painful degenerative changes in the thoracic area. This, however, is relatively uncommon, whereas the association of neck and low back disorders is not.

Of 175 patients who had careful long-term assessment following anterior cervical discectomy and fusion, 102 had some significant complaints related to the low back. In 22 of these patients the low back disability was sufficient to require surgery in that area as well.[28]

Acquired Spondylolysis as a Sequel to Spinal Fusion

Harris and Wiley reported six cases of acquired spondylolysis resulting from the concentration of stresses at the junction of a fused segment of the spine (lumbar and lumbosacral fusion) and the adjacent mobile segments of the spine.[6] The patients were accurately documented from a roentgenographic standpoint, with the pars interarticularis intact prior to the fusion. The acquired spondylolysis was a sequel to a posterior fusion with excessive stresses on the pars interarticularis. Theoretically, this should not occur with a posterolateral intertransverse fusion because the site of the lesion is supported by the uppermost portion of the graft.

Postoperative Spinal Stenosis

Vertebral laminae that are decorticated as a result of operative procedures may subsequently become thickened. If a spinal fusion is carried out in a spine with an already narrowed canal, further narrowing induced by the reaction to operation and fusion may precipitate the symptoms of spinal stenosis. In iatrogenic spinal stenosis the symptoms are usually slow or gradual in onset. The patient presents with a solid spinal fusion that is usually midline and frequently incorporates the L4–5 segment. Examination of the preoperative roentgenograms usually shows radiologic evidence of interlaminar narrowing and the changes that one associates with spinal stenosis. These patients slowly develop the claudicant type of sciatic pain that one associates with root compression secondary to spinal stenosis. They frequently present evidence of impairment of root conduction of more than one segment.

One should consider fusion cautiously in the middle-aged patient and should examine the spine carefully for early evidence of spinal stenosis. If this is suspected and fusion is required, it should be carried out laterally in an intertransverse fashion, with minimal interference with the posterior arch structures.

When gross stenosis occurs with significant symptoms, decompression may be required (see Figs. 39-4 and 39-5).

The "Multi-operated" Back

The avoidance of the "multi-operated" back is of prime importance. To avoid it and to assess the causes of failure that it represents, one must review all of the categories that have been discussed in this chapter. Were there errors in the preoperative assessment and diagnosis? Was the preoperative diagnosis erroneous? Was the wrong level operated on? Has the patient been left with a mechanically unstable spine? Has there been incomplete decompression of the involved nerve roots? Has the surgeon failed to diagnose and recognize the sites of multiple nerve root involvement? The surgeon must consider whether the midline decompression is incomplete. The possibility of extensive peridural fibrosis must also be considered as a cause of the patient's symptoms. This is much more likely to occur when extensive laminectomy has been carried out. Measures to avoid this include insertion of an interposition membrane between the dura and the overlying muscles. Gelfoam has been used routinely, but free fat grafts and dermis have their proponents.

Finally, the surgeon must assess whether the patient with residual physical symptoms has a primary emotional disturbance that is producing major psychogenic magnification, or even whether he may have initially missed the diagnosis of psychogenic regional pain.

To avoid these problems, the surgeon must be certain in his diagnosis and the nature of the patient with whom he is dealing. His judgment must be sound and the need for the operation without question. Finally, he must be certain that his skills and experience are equal to the operative task.

REFERENCES

1. Brown, J.E.: Clinical studies on chemonucleolysis. Clin. Orthop., 67:94, 1969.
2. Brown, M.D., and Daroff, R.B.: The double blind study comparing discase to placebo: An editorial comment. Spine, 2:233, 1977.
3. Connolly, J.F., and Brooks, A.L.: Vascular problems in orthopaedics. Instr. Course Lect., 22:12, 1973.
4. Correra, G.F., Williams, A.L., and Haughton, V.M.: Computed tomography in sciatica. Radiology, 137:433, 1980.
5. Freeman, D.G.: Major vascular complications of lumbar disc surgery. West. J. Surg. Obstet. Gynecol., 69:175, 1961.
6. Harris, R.I., and Wiley, J.J.: Acquired spondylolysis as a sequel to spine fusion. J. Bone Joint Surg., 45A:1159, 1963.
7. Hastings, D.E.: A simple frame for operations on the lumbar spine. Can. J. Surg., 12:251, 1969.
8. Hohf, R.: Arterial injuries occurring during orthopaedic operations. Clin. Orthop., 28:21, 1963.
9. Kadish, L., Simmons, E.H.: Lumbar nerve root anomalies. J. Bone Joint Surg., 66B:411, 1984.
10. Lawlis, G.F., and McCoy, C.E.: Psychologic evaluation: Patients with chronic pain. Orthop. Clin. North Am., 14:527, 1983.
11. Linton, R.R., and White, P.D.: Arterial venous fistula between the right common iliac artery and the inferior vena cava: Report of a case of its occurrence following an operation for a ruptured intervertebral disc with cure by operation. Arch. Surg., 50:6, 1945.
12. McCulloch, J.A.: Chemonucleolysis: Experience with 2000 cases. Clin. Orthop., 146:128, 1980.
13. MacKay, I.: A new frame for the positioning of patients for surgery on the back. Can. Anaesth. Soc. J., 3:279, 1956.
14. McNab, I.: Back Ache. Baltimore, Williams & Wilkins, 1977.
15. McNab, I., McCullough, J.A., Weiner, D.J. et al.: Chemonucleolysis. Can. J. Surg., 14:280, 1971.
16. Meyer, C.A., Haughton, V.M., and Williams, A.L.:

Diagnosis of herniated lumbar disc with computed tomography. N. Engl. J. Med., 301:1166, 1979.

17. Newman, P.H.: Etiology of spondylolisthesis. J. Bone Joint Surg., 45B:39, 1963.

18. Onofrio, B.M.: Injections of chymopapain into intervertebral discs: Preliminary report on 72 patients with symptoms of disc disease. J. Neurosurg., 42:384, 1975.

19. Osborne, G.V.: Ulnar neuritis. Postgrad. Med. J., 35:392, 1959.

20. Parkinson, D., and Shields, C.: Treatment of protruded lumbar intervertebral discs with chymopapain. J. Neurosurg., 39:203, 1973.

21. Rydevik, R. et al.: Effects of chymopapain on nerve tissue: An experimental study on the structure and function of peripheral nerve tissue in rabbits after local application of chymopapain. Spine, 1:137, 1976.

22. Schneider, R.C.: Statement from the American Association of Neurological Surgeons (Position Statement on Chymopapain). J. Neurosurg., 42: 373, 1975.

23. Schoedinger, G.R. III, and Ford, L.T., Jr.: The use of chymopapain in ruptured lumbar discs. South. Med. J., 64:333, 1982.

24. Schwetschenau, P.R., Ramirez, A., Johnston, J. et al.: Double blind evaluation of intradiscal chymopapain for herniated lumbar discs: Early results. J. Neurosurg., 45:622, 1976.

25. Shealy, C.N.: Tissue reactions to chymopapain in cats. J. Neurosurg., 26:327, 1967.

26. Simmons, E.H.: Management of low back pain—the examination. App. Therapy, 8:875, 1966.

27. Simmons, E.H., and Bailey, S.I.: Anterior cervical discectomy and fusion with the keystone technique: A long term evaluation. Presented at the Annual Meeting of the American Academy of Orthopaedic Surgeons, New Orleans, February 1, 1976.

28. Simmons, E.H., and Bhalla, S.K.: Anterior cervical discectomy and fusion: A clinical and biomechanical study with 8-year followup. J. Bone Joint Surg., 51B:225, 1969.

29. Simmons, E.H., and Segil, C.M.: An evaluation of discography in the localization of symptomatic levels in discogenic disease of the spine. Clin. Orthop., 108:57, 1975.

30. Smith, L.: Enzyme dissolution of the nucleus pulposus in humans. J.A.M.A., 187:177, 1964.

31. Stern, W.E., and Coulson, W.F.: Effects of collagenase upon the intervertebral disc in monkeys. J. Neurosurg., 44:32, 1976.

32. Sussman, B.J., Bromley, J.W., and Gomez, J.C.: Injection of collaganese in the treatment of herniated lumbar disc. J.A.M.A., 245:730, 1981.

33. Vines, F.S.: The significance of "occult" fractures of the cervical spine. Am. J. Roentgenol., 107:493, 1969.

34. Weir, D.C.: Roentgen diagnosis of injuries of the cervical spine. Refresher course presented at the Annual Meeting of the Radiological Society of North America, Chicago, 1968.

35. Wilbourn, A.J.: The value and limitations of electromyographic examination. In The Diagnosis of Lumbosacral Radiculopathy Lumbar Disc Disease, pp. 65–109. New York, Raven Press, 1982.

36. Wiltse, L.L., Newman, P.H., and MacNab, I.: Classification of spondylolysis and spondylolisthesis. Clin. Orthop., 117:23, 1976.

37. Wiltse, L.L., Widell, E.H., and Yuan, H.H.: Chymopapain chemonucleolysis in lumbar disc disease. J.A.M.A., 231:474, 1975.

38. Wollin, D.G., Lamon, C.B., Gawley, A.J., and Wortzman, G.: The neurotoxic effect of water soluble contrast media in the spinal canal with emphasis on appropriate management. J. Can. Assoc. Radiol., 19:296, 1967.

40 Complications in the Management of Adult Spinal Deformities

LYLE J. MICHELI AND JOHN E. HALL

The management of spinal deformities, particularly the surgical management, has traditionally been a source of concern for the orthopaedic surgeon. There have been significant differences of opinion on the basic principles and objectives of treatment. In addition, surgical techniques for the treatment of these deformities, particularly those involving instrumentation of the spine, have been technically demanding and hazardous, of particular concern in this age of medicolegal medicine.

It is the purpose of this chapter to review the complications resulting from the treatment of spinal deformities in adults. Lateral deviation of the spine, or scoliosis, is the most common deformity encountered, but it is usually associated with posterior deviation (kyphosis) or anterior deviation (lordosis). Occasionally, kyphosis (particularly in the thoracic region) or lordosis may be the primary deformity to be dealt with, but in general the scoliotic deformities of the spine are the most prevalent and the most difficult to manage. We have included the management of all structural deformities in this review because the basic principles of management of these deformities are similar, and the resultant complications of management are common to all.

In the past 20 years there has been a significant increase in our understanding of the etiology, pathogenesis, and pathophysiology of structural spinal deformities, as well as the development of a number of new techniques to treat these deformities. By and large, attention has been directed toward the detection and management of these deformities in the growing child. Early observers taught that the development and progression of spinal deformities was con-fined to the growing years. Risser and Ferguson, in 1936, stated that "increase in curvature in scoliosis ceases when vertebral growth stops . . . , and the effectiveness of various methods of treating scoliosis must be judged in adolescent patients who have not ceased growing."[103] It is certainly true that most spinal curvatures, of whatever etiology, have their origin and their most rapid progression prior to skeletal maturity.[3,9] In addition, effective correction of spinal curvature with bracing techniques is possible only in the immature spine with residual growth potential.[12,13]

In the adult there are no effective conservative means of correcting or controlling spinal curvature. In addition, a number of observers have noted that significant progression of curvature can occur during the adult years. In 1969, Collis and Ponseti reviewed a group of patients with idiopathic scoliosis not treated surgically, who had been seen in the orthopaedic department of the University of Iowa between 1932 and 1948.[19] They documented significant examples of progression of spinal curvature in patients under their care (Fig. 40-1).[20] Vanderpool and Wynn-Davis reviewed the incidence of scoliosis among the elderly in the Edinburgh area.[109] They found a 6% incidence of scoliosis in patients over 50 years of age. In a similar review done on the same population, children from age 6 months to 18 years showed an incidence 0.6% among boys and 0.3% among girls. They explained this obvious discrepancy by concluding that not only might scoliosis progress in association with aging and thus become detectable, but that a significant number of cases of scoliosis might arise in the adult population.

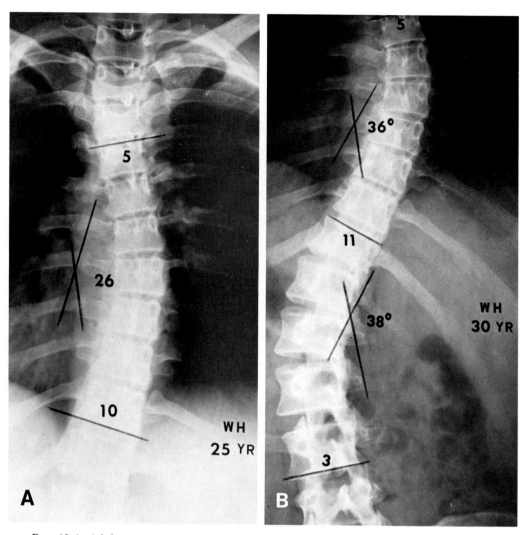

FIG. 40-1. Adult progression of scoliosis. A 65-year-old woman complained of severe, incapacitating back pain and progressive slumping to the right. Roentgenograms of the patient taken earlier were reviewed. (*A*) At age 25 years her right thoracic curvature measured 26°. The lumbar curve is not measurable in this film. (*B*) At age 30 years her right thoracic curve was found to measure 36° and the left thoracolumbar curve 38°. (*C*) Roentgenogram taken at age 61 reveals a double scoliosis curvature, with a right thoracic scoliosis of 51° from T5 to T10 and a left thoracolumbar curve of 65° from T10 to L3. These films document dramatic progression of a benign-looking spinal curvature over a 36-year period. (Courtesy of E. J. Riseborough, M.D.)

In the child and adolescent, techniques used in the management of spinal deformities are directed primarily at preventing any increase in curvature or at stabilizing the spine by bony fusion before further curvature develops.[100] By doing so, it is hoped that further deterioration in cardiorespiratory function secondary to dysfunc-

tion of the deformed thorax and its contents, as well as neurologic dysfunction secondary to mechanical or vascular injury of the spinal cord due to the bony deformity of the spine, may be prevented. In addition, most authors feel that the structurally curved spine, particularly one that results in imbalance of the torso over the pelvis,

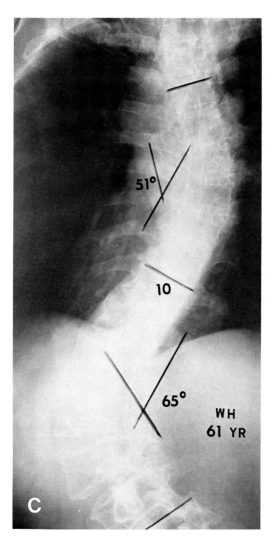

FIG. 40-1. (*Continued*)

eventually results in significant back pain, whether of osteoarthritic or discogenic origin. In the child and the adolescent, then, treatment of spinal deformities is primarily prophylactic. Pain is rarely seen in the young patient with spinal deformity.

In the adult the aims of scoliosis management are similar to those in the child: the prevention of further deterioration of cardipulmonary or neurologic dysfunction. Increasing evidence for progression of scoliotic curvatures in the adult gives this further significance. In addition, however, the scoliosis deformity in the adult is frequently accompanied by significant back pain. Although there is a high incidence of back pain in adults without structural spinal deformity, the back pain associated with spinal deformity is usually disabling and unremitting. In the adult scoliosis patient the prevention or elimination of this back pain has been felt to be one of the major indications for surgical treatment. Finally, the adult with spinal deformity has been found to suffer significant social disability secondary to the cosmetic deformity of the spine.

There is as yet no clear agreement on the extent of the increased morbidity or mortality experienced by the adult scoliotic patient compared with his normal adult counterpart, despite frequent reference to these problems in the literature. In 1968, Nilsonne and Lundgren reviewed a group of patients in Stockholm, Sweden, who had, between 1913 and 1918, been clinically diagnosed as having idiopathic scoliosis.[92] A mortality rate almost twice that of the general population was found, with cardiopulmonary disease the cause of death in two thirds. In addition, 90% of the remaining living patients reported back pain, and 47% were disabled because of their back problems. Seventy percent of the women remained unmarried, which was felt by the authors to be a reflection of the social handicap resulting from their spinal deformity.

Nachemson, in a similar study, reviewed 117 patients with lateral curvature of the spine who had initially been seen in Goteborg, Sweden, between 1927 and 1936.[86] He also found a twofold increase in mortality in this group; the majority died from kyphoscoliotic cardiopathy with cor pulmonale. These patients also appeared to have a significantly limited work capacity, with 22% completely unable to work and none of them remaining engaged in heavy work. Back pain, however, was not felt to be increased in incidence or severity when compared with the general population.

In 1969, Collis and Ponseti reviewed a group of patients with idiopathic scoliosis not treated surgically who had been seen in the orthopaedic department at the University of Iowa between 1932 and 1948.[19,97] They documented substantial progression in the degree of curvature after skeletal maturity, particularly in thoracic curves. However, this progression was not felt to be of clinical significance. They found no increase in mortality in this group and no evidence of cardiopulmonary failure as a cause of death. These patients were not felt to have an increased incidence of back pain compared with the normal population, and the degree of social dysfunction from their deformity was felt to be minimal, with 90% married and most engaged in work. Unfortunately, only 58% of the original patients were available for follow-up, and the possibility of an increased incidence of mortality and morbidity among the nonrespondents must be considered. In 1972, at the Scoliosis Research Society Meeting in Wilmington, Delaware, both John Moe and John Hall presented papers on the treatment of scoliosis.[23,46] In both groups of patients, back pain, usually severe and progressive, was the major complaint, with cosmesis a secondary concern.

More recently, Drummond and associates reviewed a series of adult patients with untreated scoliosis seen as children in three Quebec hospitals. Their results were reported at the 1975 Scoliosis Research Society Meeting in Louisville, Kentucky.[30] These patients were found to be suffering from a disabling disease, with 40% complaining of significant back pain, 24% unemployed, and 69% concerned about their appearance. Of the women, 42% remained unmarried, and of the men 30%. At the same meeting, Coonrad and Feirstein presented a series of 25 adult patients who showed roentgenographic evidence of significant progression of their curvatures during adulthood and presented for treatment because of significant back complaints.[20]

It is the opinion of most observers, then, that scoliosis is a significant, even life-threatening process in the adult, especially if the now well-documented process of adult progression of curvature is added.

Since brace techniques are ineffective in the management of adult spinal deformities, surgery is the primary mode of treatment. The primary objective of surgery in the adult patient is to stabilize the spine to prevent further progression of the deformity or to eliminate the source of back pain, the unbalanced osteoarthritic spine (Fig. 40-2). A number of recent advances in operative and preoperative management of spinal deformities have been found to be particularly useful in adult spinal deformities. The curvatures in the adult are generally more rigid, but at the same time the bone itself is sometimes less strong, limiting the degree of correction obtainable with the more classic techniques of cast correction of the deformity and *in situ* Hibbs fusion.[57] Preoperative, and occasionally postoperative, traction techniques and intraoperative spinal instrumentation techniques are particularly useful in these curves. As will subsequently be noted in detail, the use of these more sophisticated treatment techniques has resulted in a number of complications related specifically to their use.

Techniques of preoperative traction have proven useful in the management of rigid adult spinal curvatures. The use of skeletal traction in the preoperative correction of these deformities has taken two forms. Garrett, Perry, and Nickel first described a system of skeletal traction that used a proximal halo apparatus that was affixed [to the skull by four to eight pins, and distal traction with femoral or tibial Kirschner wires as an adjunct to the management and fusion of severe paralytic spinal curvatures.[42,90] The application of this halo–femoral system of skeletal traction to the preoperative correction of rigid adult curves has been gratifying, particularly because such rigid curves have generally been resistant to treatment by preoperative cast correction or harness traction.

Cotrel and Morel have developed a system of preoperative traction consisting of a head halter specifically designed to apply most of the traction force to the occiput and a well-fitted pelvic band.[21] This Cotrel traction is used to apply both static traction and short, intermittent periods of dynamic traction, with this added force applied by the patient himself by pushing with his legs or pulling with his arms. Various treatment programs using this traction device are now being evaluated. When used over a short period immediately preoperatively, this technique does not appear to improve the rigid adult curve significantly. However,

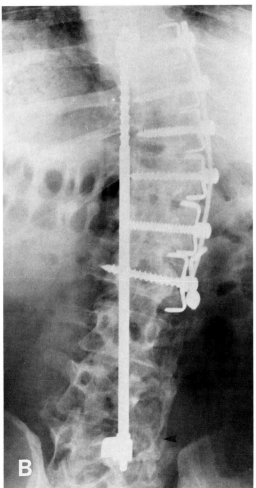

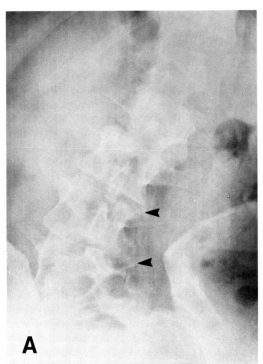

FIG. 40-2. This 26-year-old engineer complained of severe, incapacitating back pain, located in the right lower back, which rendered him unable to work. Roentgenograms revealed a right thoracolumbar scoliosis, which resulted in a significant imbalance to the right, and a lower left lumbosacral curve, with narrowing and degenerative changes in the concavity of this curve (*arrowheads, A*). (*B*) The thoracolumbar curve was corrected and fused with anterior Dwyer instrumentation, with resultant balancing of the torso over the pelvis. Two weeks later, a posterior Harrington fusion was carried out over the extent of both curves to provide added stability.

we have used this apparatus as part of a program of home traction in the adult for a period of 3 to 4 months prior to surgery, and initial results with this long-term program appear more promising.

A further refinement of the halo–femoral traction technique—that of incorporating the halo device into an apparatus employing transfixing pins in the pelvis with rigid distraction rods connecting the cranial halo, the pelvic pins, and the attached hoop—has also been successfully applied to the treatment and preoperative correction of rigid adult curves.[24,58,59] This halo–pelvic traction device was described by DeWald for the management of rigid, primarily paralytic curves and by Hodgson and O'Brien in Hong Kong for the preoperative correction (and in some cases the postoperative stabilization) of the rigid and severe curves often seen in association with tuberculosis of the spine.[24,59,93,94] Using this device, the patient is able to walk about while slow, progressive correction of the spinal deformity is carried out with this apparatus.

In 1962, Paul Harrington described the use of a system of internal distraction and compression rods that were applied to the deformed spine.[50] They were useful as an adjunct in decreasing the degree of curvature at the time of the operation and in maintaining a significant portion of this correction while spinal fusion was being obtained by the use of bone grafts and a Hibbs fusion technique, which had been carried out over the extent of the spinal deformity at the time of surgery. Initially, this apparatus was used in the stabilization and fusion of paralytic curves, particularly those associated with poliomyelitis. The use of Harrington instrumentation found its greatest application, however, in the management of adolescent idiopathic spinal curvatures.

More recently, Harrington instrumentation has been used almost exclusively in the management of adult spinal deformities.[23,65,96] In addition to increasing the final amount of correction obtainable in the adult spine, the use of this apparatus appears to have decreased the incidence of pseudarthrosis following attempts at spinal fusion in the adult. In addition, the internal stabilization provided by the Harrington instrumentation has made it possible to ambulate the adult scoliosis patient early in the postoperative period, particularly with body casts of the Cotrel or Risser types.[68] This has been a particular advantage in the management of the adult scoliosis patient because periods of prolonged recumbency in body casts are poorly tolerated by most adults.[1]

One of the major criticisms of the use of the Harrington instrumentation has been that rapid correction of the spinal deformity is obtained while the patient is under anesthesia.[26] This increases the hazards of undetectable neurologic injury.

In the adult scoliosis patient with a rigid spinal curvature, correction of the curvature has been obtained with preoperative skeletal traction, and the Harrington instrumentation is used only at the time of surgery, simply to stabilize the spine at this degree of previously obtained correction. Use of the system avoids one of the major hazards in the use of Harrington instrumentation.[23,65]

Dwyer has described a technique of spinal instrumentation in which correction of the spinal deformity is obtained by a compression system that is applied to the convex side of the curve.[32–34] An anterior approach to the spine is used, and the intervertebral disc and adjacent bony end-plates are resected across the extent of the curvature from the convex side of the curve.[101] Each vertebral body to be fused is transfixed with a titanium screw, and a braided titanium cable is passed through an eyelet in the head of each screw; this cable is swaged to each screwhead after the vertebral bodies have been approximated by the application of tension to the cable between each adjacent set of screws. This system has the effect of a series of closing wedge-type intervertebral fusions in which the bony elements of the spine are more closely approximated rather than being distracted. The increased degree of correction obtainable with this technique, as well as the increased mechanical stability of these series of anterior interbody fusions, has been used to good effect in adults. Early ambulation in plaster or plastic body jackets following Dwyer instrumentation and fusion has also been used effectively in these adult patients.

A number of specific factors make management of spinal deformities in the adult particularly difficult and vulnerable to complications. These structural deformities are generally more rigid in the adult spine than in the juvenile spine. Attempts to increase the preoperative correction in these rigid curves often require halo–femoral or halo–pelvic skeletal traction, with the further possibility of complications from these techniques alone. The adult patient is, in general, less able to withstand extensive physiological or psychological trauma than is the pediatric patient. As will be noted in further detail subsequently, the potential for hemodynamic shock and cardiovascular arrest and death appears to be significantly higher in the adult than in the child, and techniques of intraoperative and postoperative management must be exacting. The incidence of psychiatric complications from the preoperative traction period and the immediate postoperative period appears to be significantly higher in the adult. In addition, the rate of healing and fusion in the adult is slower than in the child. There is a significantly higher rate of pseudarthrosis following spinal fusion in the adult than in the child. Finally, postoperative plaster immobilization of the adult in body casts, whether he is ambulatory or supine, appears to be associated with increased incidence of skin pressure sores, perhaps reflecting altered subcutaneous fat make-up or altered skin metabolism. In the management of adult spinal deformities, as in the juvenile, attention must also be paid to the cause of the spinal deformity involved, because this can be a factor in the relative incidence and type of complications encountered. The severe collapsing paralytic spine, as seen in the adult with neglected poliomyelitis, is managed with great difficulty, with a significantly higher incidence of instrumentation failure, pseudarthrosis, and cardiorespiratory complications than in the usual idiopathic scoliosis. Significant kyphosis, as seen in neurofibromatosis and certain types of congenital deformities, can present a special threat for the development of paraplegia in association with mechanical elongation while the patient is being treated with skeletal traction or internal instrumentation. The presence of congenital or acquired intervertebral fusions, whether either anterior, lateral, or posterior, is of special concern; they may require separate staged releases if one is to obtain correction and fusion carefully and safely.[67,105]

Finally, the adult patient who has undergone previous attempts at surgical treatment of his scoliosis often presents particularly difficult problems in management. Such patients frequently require staged operative procedures, with osteotomy of previous anterior or posterior fusion masses, removal of previous metallic implants, extended periods of skeletal traction, and both anterior and posterior fusions and instrumentations to correct and stabilize the spine. These salvage procedures have a significantly increased rate of complication, particularly for infection and pseudarthrosis.

COMPLICATIONS OF PREOPERATIVE MANAGEMENT

As we have noted, preoperative skeletal traction is frequently required in the management of adult spinal deformity. Kostuik and co-workers made special note of this in their review of the management of more than 150 adults with scoliosis.[65] Dawson and Moe have also found this useful in the management of certain adults with scoliosis.[23] A number of complications of these traction techniques have been reported, however. In the halo–femoral traction technique the major source of complications has been the halo apparatus. Nickel and associates reviewed the use of the halo apparatus in 174 patients in 1968.[91] The average duration of halo immobilization in these patients was 7 months. Four patients had the halo head ring pull off, with associated excoriations in the margins of the pin tracks, generally due to loosening of one or more pins. There were four significant pin tract infections in these patients, which required surgical debridement and the excision of the drainage tract (Fig. 40-3). It was noted that the loosening of pins with associated superficial infection was a common occurrence that could generally be adequately managed simply by removing the pin and placing it in an adjacent site. One of the patients in this series developed cervical nerve root signs that resolved after release of the traction.

The most serious complication of using the halo apparatus is pin penetration. In 1973 Victor and associates reported in detail on a case of a young girl who had developed a brain abscess secondary to penetration of the halo pin.[111] Prompt recognition and specific treatment resulted in a satisfactory recovery, but the authors recommended careful attention to changes in mental status, headache, and focal neurologic signs as possible signs of intracranial infection. A second case was also mentioned in this report, in which brain abscess developed over a 24-hour period in association with infection at an occipital pin site.

Complications involving the femoral pin sites have been minimal. Several instances of prolonged stiffness of the hips and knees have been noted in adults. These have been

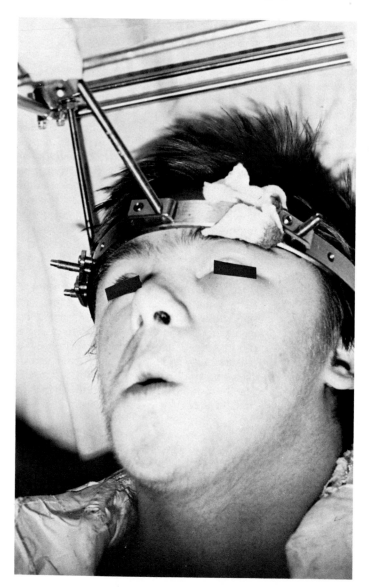

FIG. 40-3. Infection developed at the site of an anterior halo pin, with secondary periorbital swelling. Treatment included pin removal, systemic antibiotic administration, and use of local cleansing and soaks to the pin site. Note that fixation has been transferred to an adjacent pin site.

well managed by physical therapy, although one of our patients took almost a year to regain complete flexion at the knees.

In the halo–pelvic apparatus the patients are subject to the same risk of pin tract problems as in halo–femoral traction. In addition, however, the halo–pelvic traction is often used over prolonged periods of weeks to months, and this results in an increased incidence of pin loosening and superficial infection. A number of complications related to placement of the pelvic pins have also been noted. Occasionally, transient ileus follows the placement of the pelvic pins, secondary to retroperitoneal bleeding. The possibility of transfixion of the abdominal organs due to faulty pelvic pin placement must always be kept in mind. Peritoneal transgression has been seen in at least one case.[93,94]

The amount of force obtainable in both halo–femoral and halo–pelvic traction is significant, and excessive amounts of traction or increases in traction over too short a period can cause injury to neutral elements. Paresis of all of the cranial nerves has been noted. The abducens nerve and oculomotor nerve appear to be most susceptible to this effect. Telfer and associates and Perry have called attention to these complications.[95,107] DeWald and Ray have noted one case of brachial plexus palsy among four patients treated with halo–pelvic traction over prolonged periods.[24] Manning has recorded one case of transient paraparesis in association with halo–pelvic traction and a second case of paraplegia in association with the use of halo–pelvic traction that did not resolve following release of the traction.[76] Both DeWald and O'Brien and colleagues have described cases of cardipulmonary death while using halo–pelvic traction.[24,94] These were patients with severe cardiorespiratory compromise who died while undergoing halo–pelvic stabilization in the postoperative period after spinal surgery.

Treadwell and O'Brien have recently called attention to an unexpected complication of prolonged halo–pelvic traction.[108] They have noted apophyseal joint degenerative changes in the cervical spine in older patients with longer periods of traction. They found the incidence of degenerative changes to be age and time related and recommended that patients over the age of 20 not be immobilized in this apparatus longer than 4 months.

Management

The management of these complications of skeletal traction is relatively straightforward. Once a pin infection of the halo apparatus is evident—and this usually occurs in association with loosening of the pin—the pin must be removed and placed in a new, adjacent site. A culture of the pin and pin site is obtained and topical treatment with warm packs and systemic intravenous antibiotics is begun immediately. Loosening of a pin is generally a prelude to infection, and patients, particularly those sent home with the apparatus, must be warned of this possibility. An infection at the site of a loosened pin can develop rapidly, and periorbital swelling from infections of the frontal pin site can be dramatic. Halo pin site infections must be treated as an emergency because of the potential complications of intracranial sites noted above.

Management of infection at the site of a femoral or pelvic pin is somewhat different. We have successfully managed infection at these sites by simple release of the adjacent skin and soft tissue in the margins of pins to improve drainage from the site. The development of a pin tract infection in these areas seems most often to be related to inadequate drainage about the pin sites. Following this local release, a culture is obtained at the pin site, and a course of specific systemic antibiotics and local heat to the site is begun while the pins remain in place.

Neurapraxic and neurologic complications of these skeletal traction techniques are managed by prompt release of traction and observation for a return to nerve function. The key to the management of these complications is prompt recognition of neurologic deterioration, and nursing personnel should be well versed in the essentials of cranial nerve and peripheral nerve evaluation.[75]

Prevention

Many of the complications of skeletal traction can be prevented with proper placement of the apparatus. The techniques of halo application have been well described by Perry and associates.[90,95] They have carefully detailed the proper placement of the halo apparatus on the skull. This minimizes the possibility of loosening and the associated increased tendency to pin site infection following loosening of the pin. The halo pins are applied with 4 to 5 pounds of torque. A torque screwdriver is used to insert the pins. Nickel and associates recommend tightening the pins to this level for the first 2 days and then leaving them in place without further tightening.[91] In the event that one pin or another becomes too loose in the course of traction or ambulation, it may be tightened to the 5-pound mark, as long as there is no evidence of inflammation or potential sepsis. These loose pin sites should be cultured when a pin is retightened.

The technique for insertion of the pelvic pins has been well detailed by O'Brien and co-workers.[94] They recommend the use of a drilling jig while inserting the pelvic pins to ensure that the abdominal cavity is not violated by misdirection of the pin. As an additional precaution while inserting the pelvic pins, we have made a single transverse incision at the midportion of the pelvic rim carried down subperiosteally over the inner table of the ileum and palpated the inner wall of the ileum as the pin is passed across it. This ensures under direct vision and palpatation that the pin has not been misdirected.

The amount of skeletal traction and the rate of application of the forces placed across the spine are extremely important in the development of complications of traction. Letts and associates and Moe have used a total of 40 pounds of halo–femoral traction as a maximum.[69,81] Beyond this, no further therapeutic effect is evident, and the risks of further traction appear to be prohibitive. Letts has outlined a program in which 2 pounds a day is added over a period of 2 weeks, to a total of 40 pounds of traction, and Moe uses a similar program. Two recent changes in the halo–pelvic apparatus have been instituted to facilitate careful management of the pressure being exerted by the halo–pelvic apparatus and by so doing to prevent the application of excessive forces to the spine. In 1974 Manning described a modified halo–pelvic apparatus that incorporated spring measuring devices in the halo–pelvic uprights.[76] He noted that no further cases of paraparesis resulted once these measuring devices were being used by the spinal service at the Royal National Orthopaedic Hospital in London. In 1975 Gardner and co-workers described the use of electronic load cells incorporated into the distraction bars of the halo–pelvic apparatus.[41] They reported satisfactory results in a number of patients in both Hong Kong and Great Britain using this load-cell device.

O'Brien and colleagues have outlined their routine for preoperative evaluation of the patient about to undergo skeletal traction.[94] Myelography and tomography of the deformed spine are carried out to rule out potential sites of cord compression as trac-

tion is applied. Both Moe and Leatherman have called attention to the hazards of skeletal traction in the presence of kyphotic deformities of the spine, particularly those associated with a posterior-lying hemivertebra.[67,81] O'Brien also recommends obtaining preoperative lateral roentgenograms of the cervical spine to serve as a baseline for the evaluation of subsequent degenerative changes. In addition, a preoperative intravenous pyelogram is obtained in all cases of congenital spinal deformity to rule out anomalies of the genitourinary system, since distraction of a patient with an anomalous genitourinary system might result in disruption or blockage of the ureters.[75,94,96] Pretraction respiratory function tests are also carried out to serve as a baseline in the event of development of respiratory insufficiency in the course of traction.

Prompt recognition of the development of neurologic dysfunction is essential, since it is only by early recognition of cranial and spinal nerve paresis that prompt release of traction can be instituted, with subsequent resolution of symptoms. Daily neurologic examination carried out by the nursing staff or attending physicians must be complete and careful: an early sign, such as an upgoing toe or slight ankle clonus, might indicate cord ischemia.

A routine of daily pin site care must be used to minimize the potential for pin site infection and loosening. It has been our policy to clean the pin sites twice a day with alcohol and to apply a dressing impregnated with povidone-iodine (Betadine) solution. Ointments are not used about the pin sites, since they appear to inhibit drainage and increase the chance of infection.

OPERATIVE AND EARLY POSTOPERATIVE COMPLICATIONS

Paraplegia

The most dreaded complication of spinal surgery of any type is injury to the spinal cord or spinal nerve roots, with secondary loss of function below the site of the lesion. Paraplegia following spinal fusion and instrumentation in adults is, fortunately, a rare occurrence. The Morbidity and Mortality Report of the Scoliosis Research Society for 1973 reported on a total of 2500 patient procedures submitted by the membership that year.[85] Nineteen of these patients developed significant neurologic complications. There were eight cases of postoperative paraplegia. Six of these were associated with Harrington-rod instrumentation, and five of the six were noted in the recovery room. In two of these six patients the rods were removed in an average of 3.5 hours, with complete recovery of neurologic function. Three others had the rods removed from 8 to 9 hours after surgery, with partial recovery. One patient, in whom the rod was not removed, had no recovery of neurologic function. Two paraplegias developed after anterior appraches; one had complete recovery and the other no recovery at all. In 1971 the Morbidity and Mortality Committee of the Scoliosis Research Society reported 86 neurologic complications among 7100 patients treated for scoliosis of all causes.[83] Of these patients, 42 developed paraplegia, either during insertion or following spinal fusion with Harrington instruments. Of these 42, 21 had a partial paraplegia; 67% of these patients recovered completely, and 5% showed no recovery. The remaining 21 patients developed total paraplegia following surgery. Forty-eight percent recovered completely. Thus, there were 18 cases of permanent partial or complete paraplegia among 7100 patients of all ages operated on for scoliosis by this group.

There appear to be two distinct mechanisms responsible for injury to the spinal cord or its elements during the course of corrective spinal surgery. *Direct mechanical damage* to the spinal cord may occur during insertion of the Harrington hooks under the posterior elements of the spinal column, during preparation of the site of fusion by stripping the muscle and ligaments from the lamina, or during the process of decorticating the lamina or resecting the facet joints of the spine. In addition, however, stretching of the spinal column in the course of correction may cause *indirect injury* to the spinal cord by stretching and injuring the blood supply to the cord. In certain cases, as in correction of the spinal deformity following osteotomy of the spine for kyphosis, both of these mechanisms may be responsible for damage to the spinal

cord. A number of authors have called attention to the critical role of the blood supply of the spinal cord in the occurrence of spinal cord injury.[27,62,105] Dommissee has performed a valuable service to all spinal surgeons with his meticulous work on the blood supply of the human spinal cord.[27] This work was prompted by his observation that there was a significantly increased risk of paraplegia in the correction of severe fixed curves in the adult. In 1970 Dommissee and Enstein noted a 6% incidence of paraplegia following the use of Hodgson's circumferential osteotomy in the correction of fixed spinal deformities in adults.[28]

Dommissee's anatomical dissections indicate that there is a "critical zone of the spinal cord" extending from the T4 to T9. The blood supply of the cord in this area is tenuous, with no significant collateral circulation to the cord. It was recommended that great care be taken while operating in this area of the spinal cord, particularly when procedures on both anterior and posterior aspects of the spine are contemplated. Our experience with single-stage procedures that approach both the anterior and posterior aspects of the spinal column has been similar, and we now feel that one should perform staged operations in such cases, at intervals of at least 2 weeks. Leatherman also recommends the use of two- and three-stage procedures in the management of rigid spinal curves requiring osteotomy or vertebral resection.[67]

Keim and Hilal have recommended preoperative thoracic angiograms to assess the blood supply of the spinal cord and have recommended caution in cases in which preoperative angiography indicates limited blood supply to the spinal cord.[62] Criteria for determining sufficient vascularity of the spinal cord by angiographic techniques, however, are not well defined, and this procedure itself carries a significant risk to the patient. It is therefore our feeling that this is rarely indicated in routine preoperative assessment for the feasibility of spinal surgery.

The most practical approach to preventing vascular embarrassment of the spinal cord during the course of spinal surgery appears to be to monitor cord function during the course of surgery. Nash and associates have carried out studies for a number of years using a technique of cortical-evoked potentials, with stimulation of the sciatic nerve distally and the analysis of cortical potentials proximally.[49,88] At the most recent report, this technique was used effectively in 14 patients, in one of whom evidence of an altered cortical-evoked pattern following spinal instrumentation was reversed when the instrumentation was released.

A more pragmatic technique, and one that we have been using on our spinal service for the past 8 years, was presented by Stagnara and associates of Lyon, France, in 1973.[110] With this technique, the patient is awakened intraoperatively during the course of the spinal fusion, following the attainment of maximum distraction with the Harrington instrumentation. The patient is asked to move his legs, and his ability to move both legs and feet is checked. If there is evidence of loss of motor function at that time, instrumentation is removed and distraction discontinued. The authors described the use of this technique in 124 procedures. Loss of motor power was detected in three patients. All of these patients demonstrated return of motor function on the operating table following release of distraction of the spine. In our institution this technique has been used with success in more than 100 cases of distraction-type spinal fusions.[106] There have been no significant complications from the use of this technique, and most patients have no memory of the period of awakening during surgery.

Certain factors tend to increase the possibility of paraplegia or significant spinal cord injury in association with corrective spinal surgery, and particular caution should be used in these cases. Kyphosis in association with scoliosis, particularly in the high thoracic region and secondary to a congenital anomaly of the spine, presents a particular danger of operative paraplegia.[71,81] The presence of congenital anomalies of the spinal column in association with spinal deformity must be carefully ruled out before proceeding with this corrective spinal surgery. Posterior hemivertebrae and diastematomyelia are particularly dangerous when distraction techniques are used to correct spinal deformity. Preoperative myelography should be carried out, and resection of the potential sites of tethering or angulation of the cord elements in the course of spinal correction should be done early as an initial procedure before undertaking the definitive spinal procedure.

Ponte has reported on six transient postoperative paraplegias among 183 patients treated with Harrington-rod distraction and costotransversectomy.[98] Reviewing each of these patients, Ponte noted that they had experienced periods of hypotension during the operative procedure. Postoperative recovery in several of these patients was directly related to rapid fluid and blood replacement, which raised the systemic blood pressure. In several others a combination of release of Harrington-rod distraction plus elevation of the systemic blood pressure also resulted in reversal of the paraplegia. Ponte recommended careful monitoring of blood pressure during the course of the spinal corrective procedure and the avoidance of hypotension in patients undergoing distraction of the spine.

Hemorrhage

Spinal instrumentation and fusion is often accompanied by severe blood loss, and this blood loss appears to be higher in the adult patient undergoing instrumentation and fusion. Because the periosteum is a less definite layer in the adult, maintaining a level of subperiosteal dissection in the adult is significantly more difficult than in the adolescent. In addition, the bone of the adult appears to be more vascular, and more extensive bleeding is noted following decortication. Excessive intraoperative blood loss can result in transient hypotension. As noted above, this may be associated with decreased blood supply to the spinal cord at the time of surgery. In addition, the whole blood that is used to replace this operatively lost blood presents the potential complication of serum hepatitis in 0.5% to 1% of patients.[114]

We have taken a number of steps toward minimizing this blood loss in spinal fusion surgery. The subcutaneous tissue and muscle are routinely infiltrated with a solution of 1/500,000 epinephrine and normal saline solution. In Harrington instrumentation, this infiltration is carried down over the dorsum of all laminae to be involved in the fusion mass, as well as over the iliac crest, which will be the site of donor bone graft. The use of a muscle relaxant during surgery, with relaxation of the diaphragm and the anterior abdominal musculature, prevents a rise in intra-abdominal pressure and helps keep the venous pressure of the torso low.

A specialized scoliosis operating frame that gives adequate support to the anterior chest and pelvis while allowing the abdomen to hang free is used during surgery. This has been demonstrated to decrease operative blood loss in association with scoliosis fusion, owing to lowered central venous pressure and lowered venous pressure in the area of the dorsolumbar spinal vessels.[100]

Certain intraoperative ventilatory techniques have been shown to decrease blood loss.[99] These include controlled hyperventilation in which the arterial PCO_2 is maintained between 25 torr and 30 torr. Resultant alkalosis is felt to decrease blood loss by causing peripheral venous constriction. In addition, the use of negative pressure in the respiratory phase has been used to lower mean intrathoracic pressure and increase venous return. This technique must be used with caution because this negative end-respiratory pressure can result in airway closure and can prevent satisfactory gas exchange. In the patient with significant pulmonary impairment, such techniques should be used only in association with careful arterial blood gas monitoring. We have not used hypotensive anesthesia for scoliosis fusion surgery. The advantages of this technique in decreasing blood loss are well documented in other types of surgery, but the potential danger of spinal cord anoxia in association with this hypotension and distraction techniques to the spine must be considered.

MacEwen and associates have reported the use of autotransfusion in scoliosis surgery.[74] Using this technique, two and sometimes three units of the patient's own blood are withdrawn in the immediate preoperative period, and then replaced at the time of surgery to minimize the possibility of complications in association with donor blood transfusions, including intraoperative allergic blood reaction and hepatitis.[14,114] The duration of corrective spinal surgery appears to be the most significant determinant of total blood loss. Therefore, an accurate and careful subperiosteal dissection of the overlying muscles and soft tissue of the spinal column is the single most important technical factor in minimizing blood loss, with extreme care being taken to remain in the subperiosteal level at each site of dissection. When this is combined with rapid and effective instrumentation techniques carried out by a team of experienced surgeons, blood loss can generally be kept to a minimum in adult scoliosis surgery. Kostuik and associates reported an average blood loss of 1400 ml in their adult patients, and Ponder and co-workers observed an 864-ml average blood replacement for all of their adult scoliosis patients.[65,96]

Infection

One of the major complications of spinal surgery, particularly in adults, is postoperative infection. Deep wound infection in surgery of this extent can be life threatening. Factors that appear to contribute to the incidence of infection in corrective spinal surgery are prolonged surgery, extensive tissue dissection with wide exposure of muscle and partial devitalization of marginal tissues, and implantation of a foreign body in the wound. Moe noted a 2% incidence of infections in spinal fusions prior to the use of instrumentation in his fusions, compared to a 7% rate with the subsequent use of metallic implants.[81] Goldstein had eight deep infections in a series of 295 patients treated with Harrington instrumentation.[44] Kostuik and associates reported an overall infection rate of 8.5% in their adult patients, but only a third of these were deep infections.[65] Several authors have noted the difficulty of making the diagnosis of wound infection following Harrington instrumentation.[64,81] A high index of suspicion is essential. An elevated temperature is common in the early postoperative period after spinal fusion, but persistent elevation of temperature beyond this point or a recurrence of a spiking type of temperature elevation on the second or third postoperative day is reason for concern. If a diagnosis of wound infection is entertained, a series of blood cultures are obtained, and multiple aspirations of the wound are carried out under sterile conditions. The bone graft donor site must also be included in this workup and should be aspirated with a completely separate setup. The appearance of the spinal wound can be quite deceptive; a benign-looking wound can be a site of deep infection, and the diagnosis can be made only with aspirations.

If a diagnosis of wound infection is made, the patient should be taken to the operating room immediately, and an extensive surgical debridement of the operative site should be undertaken. Gaines and associates and Keller and Pappas recommend a similar program for the management of postoperative wound infections.[40,64] Following extensive surgical debridement and removal of all obviously devitalized tissue, the wound is copiously lavaged with saline or antibiotic solution, and the Harrington instrumentation is left in place in the wound. The wound is then closed primarily over large irrigation tubes, which are placed across the entire wound bed. Gaines and co-workers recommend the use of two ingress and two egress tubes and irrigation with a solution of normal saline containing antibiotics at a rate of 1 liter in every 8 hours. The egress tubes are attached to intermittent suction drainage. We now use a variation of this technique in which rapid infusion of 400 ml to 500 ml of normal saline solution containing antibiotics is carried out over a period of approximately 1 hour. Suction is then applied for the next 1 to 2 hours, and the instillation of the irrigating solution is then resumed. This system of closed irrigation has been continued from 4 to 5 days on our patients, the duration depending on the continued patency of the tubes. Intravenous antibiotics of the appropriate spectrum for bacteria present in the wound are used, and the patient is immobilized supine in a plaster cast for the initial postoperative period. Gaines and colleagues have recommended resumption of early ambulation activities in a well-made plaster cast following this program of debridement and lavage; Keller and Pappas have recommended 2 to 3 months of bedrest in plaster immobilization prior to resumption of ambulation.[40,64]

Gaines's group has reported excellent results with this regimen, with no cases of residual infection.[40] Keller and Pappas reviewed six deep wound infections that had occurred in a series of 150 spinal fusions.[64] In three of these six the Harrington instrumentation was removed following debridement of the wound, and all three went on to pseudarthrosis formation and delayed healing. The three patients in whom the immobilization was left in place obtained satisfactory fusion without further drainage. In the event that drainage does develop after deep wound infection, the patient is treated with systemic antibiotics, usually oral, and the rods are left in place until there is evidence of adequate fusion in the operative site. Removal of the Harrington rod and a second local debridement of the wound then usually results in cessation of drainage and clearing of infection.

A program of prophylactic antibiotics is not used at many centers in spinal instrumentation and fusion procedures. Moe reported a drop in his infection rate from 7% to less than 1% with the use of prophylactic antibiotics.[81] Our experiences have been similar, with the infection rate from Harrington instrumentation and spinal fusion dropping from 3.5% to less than 1% with the use of prophylactic antibiotics. Our present regimen for the administration of prophylactic antiobiotics includes the administration of 1 g of oxacillin or cephalothin (Keflin), intramuscularly or intravenously, 1 hour prior to surgery, with a second gram of the antibiotic given intravenously at the time of the skin incision. Antibiotic administration is continued intravenously every 4 hours thereafter, for the first 48 hours postoperatively.

The beneficial effect of local antibiotic irrigation in spinal surgery is uncertain.[7] Several investigators have experimentally demonstrated the beneficial effects of local antibiotic irrigation, and we routinely use antibiotic irrigation containing penicillin or a combination of neomycin and polymyxin in our spinal surgery. A review of all of our cases of spinal surgery over a 3-year period has shown that our infection rate dropped from approximately 1.5% to less than 0.5% after the use of local antibiotic irrigation was instituted.

Experiences with infection following Dwyer instrumentation and fusion have been limited to date. We have had two cases of superficial infection that responded to appropriate antibiotic therapy, but no cases of deep infection in approximately 140 cases. Dwyer and associates presented their experience with three cases of deep infection from a series of 77 Dwyer fusions in Hong Kong.[36] Each of these infections occurred late in the postoperative periods, presenting as a draining sinus or low-grade fever. Removal of instrumentation was carried out as part of the treatment of the paravertebral abscess. In two of the three, loss of correction and pseudarthrosis developed. In the third, posterior Harrington fusion was performed, with correction maintained and fusion obtained. Based on their experiences, the authors recommended the use of prophylactic antibiotics, careful surgical technique, and copious lavage as aids in the prevention of infection. For cases in which infection is detected early they recommended debridement, administration of systemic antibiotics, and retaining the implant. For cases in which infection presents late, with associated paravertebral abscess and the necessity of removing the Dwyer apparatus, they recommend performing early, adjunctive posterior Harrington fusion to maintain correction and ensure fusion.

Cardiorespiratory Complications

Respiratory complications in the surgical management of spinal deformities are a relatively common occurrence. More significantly, these complications appear to be a major contributor to operative mortality in scoliosis surgery. In morbidity and mortality reports from the years 1970 to 1973, the Scoliosis Research Society recorded 75 deaths out of a total of almost 10,000 patients who had received surgical treatment for spinal deformity.[85] Respiratory failure was noted as the cause of death in 21 of these patients and cardiac arrest in 17. Cardiac failure with acute pulmonary edema and pulmonary embolism caused five deaths each.

Postoperative respiratory complications occur relatively often following reconstructive spinal surgery. Most of these patients have some degree of respiratory insufficiency secondary to the primary spinal de-

formity, especially those with thoracic or thoracolumbar scoliosis.[6,10,11,18,104] In addition, the decreased respiratory excursions and chest splinting secondary to the pain from surgery on the thoracic spine can predispose to atelectasis and pneumonitis. Finally, direct injury to the chest cavity can occur in the course of dissection of the thoracic spine. Kostuik and associates reported a 10.2% rate of respiratory complications, including pneumothorax, pneumonia, and atelectasis.[65]

Hemopneumothorax is most often the result of direct injury to the parietal pleura in the course of dissection of the thoracic spine. This usually occurs on the convex side of the curve, where the rotation of the vertebrae and ribs results in posterior displacement of the hemithorax on the convexity, rendering it more easily injured in the course of soft tissue dissection. A high index of suspicion is important, since this complication results in no grave problem if recognized at the time of surgery and treated appropriately. We have heard of several cases of intraoperative tension pneumothorax developing because injury to the pleural cavity was not recognized. If a small rent in the parietal pleura is noted during surgery, we would prefer to perform a primary repair of this lesion while the lung is hyperinflated by the anesthetist to expel air from the pleural cavity. When adequate mechanical repair has been possible, the patient is followed postoperatively with serial chest films. Evidence of significant fluid or air accumulation is then an indication for drainage with a chest tube. Generally, a chest tube placed in the midaxillary line posteriorly is adequate, though occasionally an anterior chest tube for a pneumothorax has been used. If a satisfactory repair of the parietal pleura is not possible at surgery, a chest tube is placed in the pleural cavity at the completion of surgery. We have made it a routine practice to prepare the entire chest and the margins of the thorax prior to surgery, to both anterior axillary lines, and this area is included in the operative draping of the wound to provide ready access to the chest during surgery. Pneumonitis is occasionally seen following scoliosis surgery, and the incidence seems to be higher in adults than in the young.

Splinting of the chest and decreased excursion of breathing are common following surgery on the thoracic spine. Pneumonitis must always be considered a possibility in the differential diagnosis of a persistent postoperative fever. Treatment includes the use of specific antibiotics based on culture of chest secretions, an aggressive program of physical therapy, postural drainage, and coughing exercises.

Atelectasis is also seen in the postoperative period of spinal surgery, most frequently as a cause of an elevated temperature in the first 12 to 24 hours after surgery. It is most effectively treated with physical therapy, blow bottles, and intermittent positive-pressure readings. Persistent atelectasis is an indication for bronchoscopy, but this can usually be avoided by paying careful attention to the details of pulmonary toilet and breathing techniques in the postoperative period.

A number of steps can be taken to help prevent postoperative atelectasis and pneumonitis.[70] Our patients are routinely given instructions for a program of preoperative physical therapy and breathing and coughing exercises, including postural drainage techniques. Preoperatively, intermittent positive-pressure breathing is demonstrated. Each patient is asked to refrain from smoking for a period of at least 2 weeks prior to surgery. The use of these techniques in the immediate postoperative period is facilitated because of patient familiarity and cooperation with them.

In the severely scoliotic patient with significantly depleted respiratory reserve, especially one who has associated paralytic disease with weakening of the chest walls and diaphragm muscles, pulmonary care is a critical part of the surgical and postoperative regimen. In 1957 Nickel and colleagues outlined the protocol used at Ranchos Los Amigos Hospital for undertaking elective spinal surgery in patients with respiratory paralysis or significantly limited breathing capacity:[89] careful preoperative assessment of respiratory capacity, elective preoperative or intraoperative tracheostomy, and careful attention to medical ventilation in the postoperative period. Both Moe and Hall have called attention to an additional aid in the preoperative assessment and care of the

respiratory-crippled patient.[5,81] The use of halo–femoral traction in a certain number of these patients has resulted in significant improvement in respiratory function as these patients underwent progressive correction of their curvatures with traction. Their ability to maintain adequate respiratory function at the completion of halo–femoral traction has been one of the criteria used for the advisability of spinal fusion and corrective surgery. If a patient was able to maintain satisfactory respiratory function with this degree of correction, corrective surgery and fusion were carried out, with assistive respiratory therapy used in the immediate postoperative period.

Gastrointestinal Complications

Ileus is frequently seen in the period after spinal procedures, especially those extending across the thoracolumbar junction into the lumbar area. Usually it can be treated successfully with gastrointestinal suction techniques and avoidance of oral feeding until there is evidence of good bowel function (satisfactory bowel sounds, decreased distention, and hunger). Prolonged ileus can occasionally be a problem. This frequently occurs in association with extensive retroperitoneal bleeding and the formation of wound hematoma. Paralytic ileus is a diagnosis of exclusion, and care must be taken to ensure that other causes of mechanical obstruction of the bowels are not present. It is imperative to wait until there is evidence of satisfactory bowel function before oral feeding is resumed. The use of intravenous hyperalimentation feedings and careful monitoring of metabolic status has proven successful in managing this preoperative complication.

Acute cholecystitis has been seen in a number of our patients in the period immediately following spinal surgery. We have had four patients develop this complication over a 2-year period following corrective surgery for scoliosis or kyphosis. All have been adults. Bunch reported on three patients at the 1975 Scoliosis Research Society Meeting who manifested acute abdominal pain in the early postoperative period after spinal surgery.[16] Each of these patients was explored with the presumptive diagnosis of acute appendicitis, and each was found to have acute cholecystitis as a cause of the pain. Bunch hypothesized that the cause of this acute cholecystitis was injury to the cystic artery due to the stretching of the vasculature of the posterior abdominal wall following intraoperative correction of spinal deformity with Harrington-rod distraction. Acute cholecystitis has frequently been seen in the immediate postoperative period after both major general surgery and trauma. Whether the acute cholecystitis that has been observed following spinal surgery with distraction of the spine is specific to this type of corrective spinal surgery or whether it is a manifestation of the other, more general postoperative occurrence is uncertain. Whatever the explanation, acute cholecystitis must be included in the differential diagnosis of abdominal pain following spinal fusion.

A more specific complication of the treatment of spinal deformity, including spinal instrumentation, is that which has been described by various authors as cast syndrome, or superior mesenteric artery syndrome.[4,17,39] In 1971 Evarts and associates reviewed the literature on vascular compression of the duodenum associated with treatment of scoliosis.[39] This syndrome is felt to be the result of mechanical compression of the third portion of the duodenum by the trunk of the superior mesenteric artery. The causative mechanism appears to be traction applied to the posterior abdominal wall at the time of correction of spinal curvature. This complication has occurred following the application of corrective casts to the spine in both the preoperative and the postoperative periods, following the installation of Harrington-rod distraction alone, and, in at least one instance, after the patient was kept supine prior to beginning skeletal traction. The typical patient is generally thin and asthenic, frequently with a decreased anteroposterior diameter of the chest and torso. The characteristic clinical picture is that of a high intestinal obstruction. When such an obstruction continues unrecognized, severe hypokalemic alkalosis, hypovolemia, and finally even death can be the result. Of the 18 patients reviewed by Evarts and colleagues, one third died of this complication. This condition must always be considered

a possibility in any case of prolonged gastrointestinal dysfunction in the period following spinal surgery. Careful evaluation of the patient with prolonged gastrointestinal dysfunction, especially when associated with vomiting and increased gastric output from the Levine tube suction, must be undertaken. Plain roentgenograms of the abdomen may reveal gastric and duodenal distention. Further evaluation with contrast material, either sodium diatrizoate (Gastrografin) or dilute barium solution, would reveal the obstruction in the third portion of the duodenum. This obstruction is frequently only partial. Abdominal films taken at hourly intervals thereafter frequently show evidence of passage of some contrast material past the point of obstruction.

When the diagnosis is made in the early postoperative period, conservative management is often successful. Nasogastric suction is continued. The patient is placed in the optimal position for drainage of the stomach and duodenum. We often elevate the head of the bed on shock blocks and maintain the patient in the prone or lateral decubitus position, with the left side down if this is possible. In several patients, early cast application and resumption of upright standing has been successful in relieving partial obstruction. Hyperalimentation is a useful adjunct in treating this syndrome. Hardy and co-workers have reported successful conservative treatment of two cases of this syndrome with 3 to 4 weeks of hyperalimentation.[48] In the event that conservative techniques are unsuccessful and metabolic dysfunction, including alkalosis, is evident, surgical intervention is indicated. Duodenojejunostomy has been used successfully in a number of our patients with this syndrome, and this appears to be the procedure of choice. Division of the ligament of Treitz, with mobilization of the third portion of the duodenum, has also been suggested as a possible mode of treatment. This operation was described by Ladd and was used in one of our patients, without success.

There appears to be no effective means of preventing this postoperative complication. It appears to be most important to maintain a high index of suspicion in the postoperative period, particularly in thin, asthenic patients, and to evaluate carefully all patients in whom there is prolonged gastrointestinal dysfunction. With prompt diagnosis, this complication can be satisfactorily managed either by a combination of conservative techniques or by operation.

Certain scoliosis surgeons seem to be under the impression that spinal fusion patients have an excessive incidence of postoperative upper gastrointestinal symptoms.[38] Dickson and associates have noted that 3% to 4% of their patients complained of gastrointestinal symptoms, including hyperacidity, regurgitation, and mild pain.[96] In 1972 these authors took preoperative and postoperative gastrointestinal surveys of 68 patients who underwent spinal fusion and instrumentation.[25] The gastrointestinal pattern was basically unchanged in the postoperative studies, and it was concluded that there was no evidence of an increased incidence of hiatal hernia in postoperative fusion patients.

Genitourinary Complications

Corrective spinal surgery may be associated with genitourinary complications with relative frequency. Injury to the genitourinary system in the course of dissection of the spine is a real possibility because of the proximity of the kidneys and ureters to the retroperitoneal space immediately adjacent to the spinal column. In addition, mechanical correction of severe curves can result in excessive stretching or acute angulation of the genitourinary system, with resultant injury and obstruction.[63] One of two deaths reported by Ponder and associates in their reported series of 132 adults with scoliosis who had been treated with Harrington instrumentation and fusion was associated with an infected hydronephrosis apparently due to ureteral obstruction at the pelvic brim following correction of a 170° thoracolumbar curve to 100°.[96]

McMaster and Silber described a case of hydronephrosis associated with para-ureteral scarring following the extensive retroperitoneal dissection used in the Dwyer instrumentation.[79] Dwyer and colleagues noted one similar case of extensive retroperitoneal fibrosis with resultant ureteral obstruction in their series of 81 Dwyer anterior spinal fusions in Hong Kong.[35] This case also required late reexploration of the retroperitoneal space and release of adhesions.

In addition to possible structural injury to the genitourinary system with the dissection and instrumentation of spinal surgery, urinary tract infections are frequently seen following spinal surgery. Postoperative care and the monitoring of urinary output of the spinal surgery patient frequently require the use of an indwelling urinary catheter for extensive periods. Kostuik and co-workers reported a 15% incidence of urinary tract infection in their adult scoliosis surgery patients, which was the most common complication seen in their series.[65] Ponder and colleagues noted a 6% incidence of acute cystitis following scoliosis surgery in adults.[96]

Careful attention to strict aseptic technique in the introduction of the indwelling catheters can help to reduce the incidence of infection. Use of the indwelling urinary catheter is required for hourly monitoring of urine outputs and specific gravities. Therefore, adjunctive techniques that have been useful in other situations to control urinary tract infections, such as the use of two- or three-way catheters with instillation of antiseptic or antibacterial solutions, are not generally possible. In addition, the use of intermittent straight catheterization under strict aseptic technique by a catheter team, which has resulted in a significant decrease in urinary tract infections in certain other clinical situations such as the care of paraplegics, is also generally not applicable in this circumstance.

Psychiatric Complications

Although psychiatric complications of adult scoliosis management have not previously received attention in the literature, we have often found them to present a formidable problem in both preoperative and postoperative management. We have seen a number of patients develop acute situational psychosis during the period of preoperative skeletal traction, particularly in halo–femoral traction and Stryker frame immobilization. The primary symptoms have been paranoia and depression. Although the manifestations of this acute situational psychosis have often been adequately handled by reassurance and therapeutic sessions of psychotherapy with our consultant clinical psychologist, several patients have had to be treated with psychotropic drugs to maintain an adequate program of therapy.

Acute situational psychosis following surgery is also not uncommon, and again, both clinical psychotherapy and psychotropic drugs have been used to treat these complications. We have had no permanent manifestations of psychotic break or psychiatric deterioration following these procedures, and recovery has generally been prompt following progressive decrease in pain and resumption of walking. Ponder and associates recorded two cases of acute postoperative psychosis in their series of 132 adult patients who had undergone instrumentation and fusion.[96]

It has been our observation that the adult patient is much less tolerant, both physiologically and psychological, of recumbent treatment during the course of correction of scoliosis, whether in traction or cast immobilization, than is the child or adolescent. The use of early ambulation after the surgical treatment of scoliosis has found particular usefulness in the management of the adult scoliosis patient. Initially, the major benefits were thought to be physiological (decreases in the tendency to postoperative thrombophlebitis and cast sores), but we have found that an unexpected advantage of this ambulation has been the restoration and maintenance of psychological stability in a number of our patients.

The acute situational psychosis associated with the treatment of adults by corrective spinal surgery is probably not specific to these techniques, since this has frequently been observed as a phenomenon in the care of the acutely ill adult cardiac patient, particularly in the immediate postoperative period. Factors that apparently contribute to this psychological deterioration include excessive and prolonged pain, high levels of anxiety, sensory deprivation, and decreased periods of sleep because of the extensive nursing care required in the immediate postoperative period.[66]

Thromboembolic Complications

Clinically significant thrombophlebitis and pulmonary emboli have been seen in the management of the adult scoliosis patient, both in the period of preoperative skeletal traction and in the immediate postoperative period. Kostuik and co-workers reported three cases of significant thrombophlebitis and two cases of pulmonary emboli in their series.[65] A review of the management of 52 adult patients who had been operated on over the past 3 years at the Boston Children's Hospital revealed three cases of clinically recognized pulmonary emboli in this population. Other authors who have reviewed their treatment of adult scoliosis have not mentioned this as a recognized complication of their treatment, but the possibility that a number of these have gone unrecognized must be raised.

The relatively high incidence of thromboembolic complications following lower-extremity injuries and lower-extremity corrective surgery in adults is well known.[38,53,80] The incidence of thrombophlebitis has been known to be as high as 30% in patients undergoing corrective hip procedures, and a number of studies indicate that the early formation of thromboembolic foci takes place during the operative period itself. Thromboembolic complications of extensive spinal surgery in adults would also appear to be a significant hazard. The paucity of clinical signs in the thromboembolic process may result in its going unrecognized as a cause of progressive respiratory dysfunction, especially in the scoliosis patient with previously impaired respiratory function.

Treatment of thrombophlebitis in scoliosis patients, especially those who are in the midst of a series of two- or three-staged corrective procedures, can present special difficulties, because often the operative treatment program must be continued and bedrest maintained because of spinal instability. We have used a program of immediate intravenous heparin administration and then begun the patient on a program of oral dicumarol anticoagulation. When adequate therapeutic levels of anticoagulation have been obtained as measured by prothrombin time, the heparin has been discontinued, and dicumarol alone has been used to manage anticoagulation therapy in these patients.

If the diagnosis of thrombophlebitis has been made, serial chest roentgenograms and artifical blood gases are used to rule out pulmonary embolism. Lung scans with radioisotope tracers or pulmonary arteriograms are indicated as an aid in diagnosis if there is a question of pulmonary embolization.

Techniques used in the prevention of thromboembolic complications in adult patients are still only partially successful in the prevention of this dreaded complication. Daily physical therapy is performed on all of our patients who are immobilized at bedrest in traction or in the postoperative period. This includes range-of-motion and muscle-strengthening exercises for both upper and lower extremities. Elastic above-the-knee stockings are used as an adjunct to prevent venous pooling in the lower extremities. We have not undertaken prophylactic anticoagulation in these patients because of the apparent low incidence of thromboembolic complications at present and because of the relatively high rate of complications of the anticoagulation regimens themselves. We have, however, instituted a program of antiplatelet prophylaxis. Patients on prolonged bedrest are administered 300 mg of aspirin three times a day. There is evidence from studies of a number of reconstructive hip procedures that this antiplatelet regimen can result in a decreased incidence of thromboembolic complications in adults.[54]

Complications of Instrumentation

Harrington Instrumentation. A number of complications directly related to the Harrington instrumentation technique have been recorded. The most common problem is loss of seating of the upper hook in the early postoperative period (Fig. 40-4).[43,51] A number of investigators have examined the forces involved in this fixation procedure, and it has been demonstrated that the limiting factor in fixation of the Harrington distraction apparatus is the strength of the bone under which the superior and inferior distraction hooks insert.[37,87,112] Waugh found that the posterior elements of the thoracic vertebrae of the spine, where the upper hook is placed, could withstand from 30,000 to 50,000 pounds of axial force before breaking. The posterior elements of the lumbar vertebrae (where the lower hook is usually placed) could withstand about twice that force. In 1973 Elfstrom and Nachemson described the use of a modified

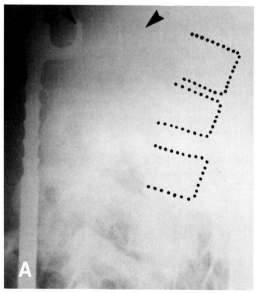 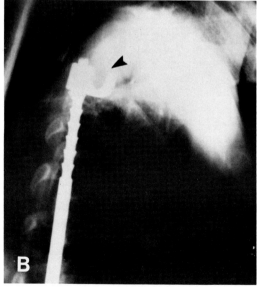

FIG. 40-4. Loss of upper hook fixation in a Harrington instrumentation occurred in the early postoperative period, with excessive pain and a palpable mass in the upper back. The lateral roentgenogram (*A*) reveals the extent of displacement of the hook (*arrowhead*) from the posterior spinal elements. At reoperation (*B*) the hook (*arrowhead*) was moved to the next higher thoracovertebral lamina.

Harrington distraction incorporating a telemetric device in the rod to measure the axial forces along the rod.[37] They found a similar range of limiting forces. They recommended the use of this special rod to determine the amount of force being applied to the bony lamina at the site of hook placement during the course of Harrington-rod surgery to avoid exceeding the limits of bone strength during the procedure.

Although the application of excessive force across the distraction rod may occasionally cause the upper hook to cut out of its fixation site, the more usual cause is probably malpositioning of the upper hook at the time of its insertion. Instead of being passed beneath both cortices of the posterior margin of the vertebral lamina, the distraction hook is passed between the cortices and in the process splits the lamina, with the resultant significantly decreased strength of seating of the hook. This malpositioned hook then breaks through the weakened lamina at the time of initial distraction during surgery or in the early postoperative period.

It has been suggested that the application of excessive force across the distraction rod in the early postoperative period, owing to movement or nursing care of the patient, might be a cause of displacement of the upper hook. Though this might occasionally be a causative factor in association with malplacement of the upper hook, as described above, it would appear to be a rare cause of this complication by itself.[37] The possibility of this displacement can be minimized in the early postoperative period by minimizing the amount of excessive axial loading or pressure applied to the spine. We have routinely used Stryker frame immobilization in this early postoperative period. The patient is kept supine on the Stryker frame for the first 12 hours and then is begun on a program of turning prone on the Stryker frame for 1 hour out of 8 in the early postoperative period. We have noted no significant complications following this treatment regimen and have not felt the need for rigid plaster immobilization in the early postoperative period, except in such instances as when the cooperation of the patient in the early postoperative period could not be guaranteed.

Nachemson and Elfstrom, using the telemetric Harrington rod device, have confirmed the safety of the Stryker frame postoperative regimen.[87]

A second complication of the instrumentation itself has been the excessive length of the proximal tip of the Harrington rod beyond the upper distraction hook. This can be particularly significant in the adult with scoliosis and associated kyphosis, in whom projection of the rod more than 1 inch beyond the distraction hook can result in a significant prominence beneath the skin, which may later require resection of the rod tip or removal of the apparatus.

Pain directly attributable to the Harrington instrumentation is rare. Several patients, however, have complained of a dull ache over the site of the rod in cold weather, and this sensation has been relieved by removal of the metallic implants.

Management of these instrumentation complications is straightforward. In the event of loss of fixation of the upper hook, we have generally performed a second operation 7 to 10 days after the initial surgery, when the clinical status of the patient permits, with reinsertion of the upper distraction hook one spine level proximal or distal to the original site of insertion.

In the case of excessive length of the proximal tip of the rod, this has generally been left untreated in the early postoperative period, unless there is a possibility of migration of the tip through the skin, in which case resection of the tip with a second, more proximal small incision and rod cutters is used. Generally, we have left this untreated in the early postoperative period of cast immobilization, and if it appears to present a problem later, either the rod tip has been resected or the entire rod has been removed when there is evidence of satisfactory fusion.

A third, relatively rare, technical complication of the Harrington instrumentation is slipping of the distraction rod through the upper hook and consequent loss of relative correction. A safeguard against this is placement of a double-looped, tightly affixed coil of 18-gauge stainless steel wire at the notch immediately subjacent to the most proximal notch used or use of a metallic fixation ring at this site.[51]

Prevention of these instrumentation complications requires special attention to the specific details of rod insertion and placement, as described by Harrington, Hall, and Goldstein.[43,46,51] Great care must be taken in placing the upper distraction hook beneath both cortices of the posterior lamina of the thoracic vertebra at the time of hook insertion. In addition, care must be taken to avoid applying excessive distraction force to the apparatus. We obtain our distraction correction by applying manual correction forces to the curvature at the time of placement of the distraction rod. The surgeon applies pressure to the convexity of the curve with his hands while his assistant applies counterpressure at points proximal and distal to the convexity of the curve. The distraction rod is then advanced through the upper hook without the apparatus itself applying excessive force to the bone. Because the use of the telemetric device is not practical in most instances, the surgeon must gain experience in clinically assessing the safest maximal force to be applied across the distraction rod at the hook apparatus, taking into account the relative strength and integrity of bone of the patient on whom he is operating.

The prevention of protrusion of the proximal rod tip is straightforward. Care must be taken at the end of the procedure to palpate this tip beneath the surface of the skin, and if excessive length appears to be present, it is best to cut the proximal rod one notch to its hook fixation using the heavy bolt cutters that should be available during the procedure. Care must be taken at the time of this procedure to ensure that no rotational force is applied to the proximal hook while the rod is being cut, since this can also cause cutting out of the upper hook.

An added technical consideration in the Harrington instrumentation of adults with scoliosis, especially those with associated thoracic kyphosis, is the requirement to bend the distraction rods at the time of placement. The adult spine is more rigid than the child's and more resistant to flattening of the thoracic kyphosis and lumbar lordosis at the time of instrumentation. If the rod is kept straight and an attempt is made to insert it across the kyphoscoliotic

thoracic spine, excessive dorsal force can be applied by the upper distraction hook to the vertebral lamina, with cutting out of the upper hook at the time of placement or soon afterward. Sufficient bending of the distraction rods should be carried out to compensate for the remaining lumbar lordosis and thoracic kyphosis in the spine, but if the bending is excessive, a significant portion of the distractive effect of the rod will be lost. In the adult patient who has had preoperative correction with skeletal traction, this is a less significant consideration because the distraction rod is used more as a spacer to maintain stability of the spine while fusion is taking place than as an actual device to obtain further correction of the spine at the time of surgery.

Dwyer Instrumentation. Instrumentation technique in the Dwyer procedure is also demanding and requires careful attention to detail. In the Dwyer instrumentation, transfixion screws are placed traversely across each vertebral body. Proper direction of these screws is absolutely critical, since maldirection of the screw into the spinal canal can result in serious injury to the spinal cord or cauda equina. Dwyer and Schafer have reported one case of paraplegia related to malposition of the thoracic screw.[34] Screw placement can be aided by placing the tip of the forefinger of one hand on the opposite side of the vertebra and then directing the screw at it. This ensures that the location of the screw tip on the opposite side of the vertebra is known with certainty. Maldirection of the uppermost thoracic screw because of the overhanging rib cage has occasionally been a problem, with the screw angulated in more cephalad than desired, resulting in weak fixation of the screw in the bone. This has been associated with partial pullout and loss of correction at the uppermost interspace in at least two of our patients.

Great care must be taken to avoid applying excessive mechanical force when tension is being applied between two adjacent screwheads and their transfixed vertebral bodies. Correction is obtained gradually by applying force directly to the spine itself and taking up the resultant slack in the cable using the tension device. Failure to do this may result in vertebral body fracture or pulling out of the screw. In the adult spine, especially that with idiopathic curvatures, the quality and strength of the vertebral bodies is generally good, and up to 80 to 100 pounds of force can be applied across each interspace by the Dwyer tension device.

Other Early Complications

A number of relatively unusual complications of spinal correction and fusion have been described. In 1972 Curtis and associates reported two cases of air embolization as a complication of spinal fusion.[22] This occurred during operation and appeared to be associated with entrance of air into the venous system through the paraspinous venous plexus of Batson.[5] Brown and Stelling reported two cases of fat embolism as a complication of scoliosis fusion, one of which resulted in death.[15] They called attention to the fact that scoliosis operations that involve extensive dissection and decortication are analogous in their metabolic effects to the multiple trauma and long-bone fractures that are most commonly the precursors of fat embolism syndrome. In addition, many of the usual complications seen in various types of major surgical procedures are also seen following spinal surgery. These include transfusion reactions, acute gastrointestinal bleeding as a stress reaction in the immediate postoperative period, wound hematoma, and wound dehiscence.

SEGMENTAL SPINAL INSTRUMENTATION

A recent development in spinal instrumentation techniques has been segmental spinal instrumentation, the fixation of individual vertebrae in a fusion site to the longitudinal rods spanning the extent of the fusion. As originally described by Luque in 1977, individual wires were passed beneath the laminae of the vertebrae and affixed to longitudinal rods extending the length of the spine to be stabilized.[72] Luque used longitudinal rods of his own design, "L rods," usually in pairs, contoured to fit both the convexity and concavity of the curve, and each wired to the corresponding lamina at each level.[72,73] The proposed advantage of this technique was that it provides much greater stability of fixation because each vertebra throughout the length of the instrumentation is stabilized, not just the two end vertebrae. As initially conceived by Luque, this obviated the need for both arthrodesis and supplementary external support of the portion of the spine that was instrumented.[72]

Most spinal surgeons, however, have incorporated arthrodesis with the segmental wiring, and many use supplemental bracing, at least for a limited period, following instrumentation and grafting.[2,56] In addition, many now supplement Harrington distraction instrumentation with segmental fixation or use a combination of the two techniques, with a segmentally wired Harrington distraction rod on the convexity of the curve and a contoured, segmentally fixed Luque rod across the concavity (Fig. 40-5).

The major concern in using this technique has been the additional risk of neurologic injury resulting from both the passing of the sublaminar wires and the greater mechanical correction of severe deformity made possible by this mechanically advantageous system, with the additional risk of neurovascular traction or impingement.

The potential for neurologic injury appears to be twofold: at the time of operative instrumentation (usually evident immediately) and later in the postoperative period (as a result of failure to attain union, with associated wire breakage and broken-wire impingement in a neural canal).[8,31,113] Although the potential for a neurologic impingement may be less of a concern in spinal deformity associated with neurologic disorders such as myelomeningocele, cerebral palsy, or poliomyelitis, the risk may be less acceptable in the correction of idiopathic scoliosis. Thompson and associates recently reported a 17% neurologic complication rate in the correction and segmental instrumentation of idiopathic scoliosis, and noted that this must be weighed carefully in the use of segmental instrumentation in such cases.[113]

With respect to late complications following wire breakage, Bernard and co-workers reported five cases of significant wire breakage of a total of 69 cases performed over a 3-year period. In two of these pa-

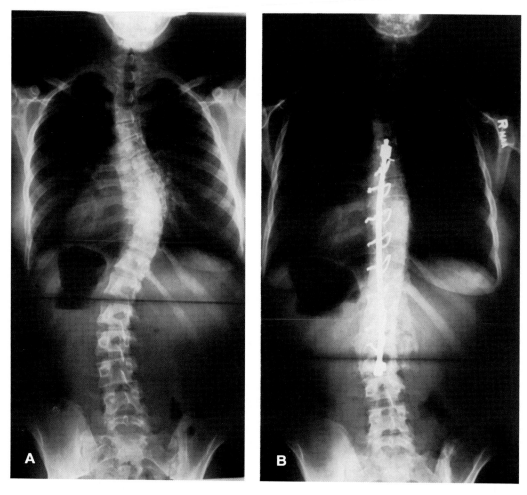

FIG. 40-5. (*A*) Woman with painful dorsolumbar scoliosis. (*B*) The same patient after segmental instrumentation (segmental wiring combined with a Harrington distraction rod on the convexity of the curve).

tients, major complications resulted, necessitating additional surgery.[31]

To circumvent this potential for sublaminar neurologic injury, while still attaining the advantages of segmental instrumentation, Drummond has devised a system of instrumentation through the base of each spinous process—without entering the neural canal.[31] In this system a Harrington rod is used on the concavity of the curve and a contoured Luque (L) rod is used on the convexity, with each, in turn, wired to the respective sides of the spinous process. Although instrumentation failure, including hook dislodgement and wire breakage, were reported in the original series of 40 cases, no neurologic complications were seen.

LATE COMPLICATIONS

Pseudarthrosis

Failure to obtain fusion at one or more levels remains the central problem of all spinal fusion surgery. The ultimate test of any technique or alteration of technique in spinal arthrodesis is the effect that it has on the ability to obtain fusion. The ability of a technique to obtain dramatic correction of a spinal deformity will be lost if it does not also obtain spinal stabilization and fusion. The relatively high rate of pseudarthrosis in adult arthrodesis surgery, when compared with that in adolescents, is probably the most frustrating aspect of adult corrective spinal surgery.

A number of factors seem to influence the relative rate of nonunion. The physiological age of the patient is a critical factor. A number of surgeons have compared their rate of fusion in adults versus adolescents and noted a significant increase in the pseudarthrosis rate in the adult patients. Kostuik and associates have noted a 7% incidence of pseudarthrosis in their adult idiopathic scoliosis patients, compared to less than 1% in their adolescent idiopathic fusion patients.[63] Dawson and colleagues have similarly noted a difference in the rate of pseudarthrosis in adults and adolescents. They found a 27% incidence of pseudarthrosis in adults, while an analogous group of adolescent patients was noted to have a pseudarthrosis rate of only 10%.[23] Ponder

and colleagues noted a pseudarthrosis rate of 6.6% in their Harrington instrumentations and fusions in adults with idiopathic scoliosis. They also called attention to the discrepancy in the rate of union between the adult and adolescent patients.[96]

Even within the adult age group, age appears to remain a factor. Dawson and co-workers reported an overall pseudarthrosis rate of 27% in 82 adult patients. However, the pseudarthrosis rate was 17% in patients under 30 years and 60% in patients between 30 and 40 years of age.[23]

The extent of the arthrodesis and its location in the spinal column also appear to be factors in the relative rate of union. There is a relatively high rate of pseudarthrosis in the thoracolumbar junction from T11 to L1, and again in the area of the lumbosacral junction (Fig. 40-6). As has been noted in bone healing in general, the rate and effectiveness of bone healing is significantly enhanced when the healing

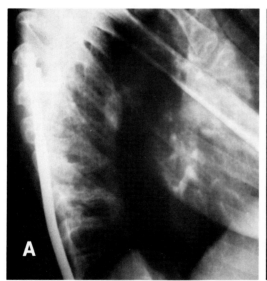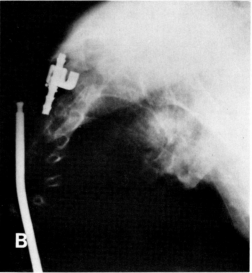

FIG. 40-6. Instrumentation failure. This case of severe kyphoscoliosis in a 36-year-old man was corrected by staged operations of initial anterior release and intervertebral grafting, halo–femoral traction, and second-stage posterior Harrington instrumentation and fusion. (*A*) Lateral radiograph 6 months after operation shows satisfactory correction of the kyphotic deformity. Ten months after the operation, the patient fell while dancing, heard a snap, and noted immediate pain in his upper back. (*B*) The lateral roentgenogram of his spine showed fracture of the Harrington rod and increased kyphotic deformity. Surgical exploration revealed pseudarthrosis at the highest level of fusion, posteriorly. Removal of the broken rod, stabilization, and re-fusion were performed.

site is in mechanical compression; conversely, mechanical distraction at the fusion site is a relatively unfavorable environment for bone healing. Thus, posterior fusion techniques would be expected to be less effective in regions of relative kyphosis when the posterior bone graft is in tension, and anterior spinal fusion techniques would be expected to be less effective in association with lordosis of the spine.

Associated disease processes have also been observed to be a factor in the relative success of arthrodesis in the spine. There is a significantly increased rate of pseudarthrosis in paralytic curves and those associated with congenital defects or neurofibromatosis.[82]

In addition to the physiological factors, various aspects of the arthrodesis technique—including associated instrumentation, techniques of decortication, graft material used, and techniques of postoperative care and immobilization—can affect the rate of fusion. A number of these factors appear to be significant in the relatively increased rate of pseudarthrosis in adults. In addition to the physiologically determined decreased rate and extent of bone healing seen in the adult, the ability to correct and stabilize the spinal deformity mechanically in the adult is often limited owing to the increased rigidity of the curve, and in some instances to the relatively poor quality of the vertebral bone. The resultant inadequate mechanical correction of these spines often results in a relatively unfavorable environment for bony healing. Thus, in the adult with significant thoracic kyphoscoliosis, inadequate correction of the kyphotic deformity can significantly limit the ability to obtain satisfactory posterior arthrodesis.

Harrington Instrumentation. Rates of pseudarthrosis following Harrington rod posterior spinal fusion have varied. Dawson and colleagues noted a 27% pseudarthrosis rate in their series of 82 adult patients with scoliosis of varied origin.[23] Kostuik and co-workers reported a 10% rate of pseudarthrosis overall, with a 7% rate of pseudarthrosis in their adults with idiopathic scoliosis.[65] Ponder and co-workers found a 6.6% pseudarthrosis rate in their series of 132 adult patients with idiopathic scoliosis.[96]

The diagnosis of pseudarthrosis is often difficult. Loss of correction of the spinal arthrodesis is cause for concern (Fig. 40-7). According to Moe, loss of correction of more than 5° at 1 year following fusion must raise suspicion of pseudarthrosis.[81] Initial diagnostic evaluation should include satisfactory anteroposterior, lateral, and oblique roentgenograms of the fusion site. Areas of particular concern are the thoracolumbar junction and the lumbosacral junction. The site of pseudarthrosis can occasionally be seen as a radiolucent line extending across the graft site. In addition, obliteration of facet joints as seen on the oblique views is an important part of the radiologic assessment. Breakage of the Harrington instrumentation is usually an indication of pseudarthrosis of the graft site, particularly when there is resultant overlap of the distraction rod and progressive loss of correction. The recurrence of back pain in association with roentgenographic loss of correction is a clear indication of pseudarthrosis and an indication for reoperation.

Recently, several investigators have suggested the use of bone scans and thermoradiography as adjuncts in the localization of the pseudarthrosis site owing to the increased level of metabolic activity at this site. Initial reports are encouraging, but no large series of patients diagnosed by means of this technique has yet been reported.

A number of authors have recommended routine reexploration of spinal fusion sites at 3 to 6 months following initial surgery.[45,60,73,77] Some earlier studies, which primarily reviewed scoliosis in association with paralytic disease, and in which techniques of fusion did not always include the use of autogenous bone grafts or facet resection, found as high as a 69% rate of pseudarthrosis 6 months after surgery, as determined by surgical exploration in paralytics, and a 58% rate of pseudarthrosis in patients with idiopathic curves.[78] Donaldson and associates reported a 33% incidence of pseudarthrosis as determined by reexploration 6 months following surgery in fusions in which bone-bank bone was used.[29] However, this incidence decreased to 9.9% when autogenous bone grafts were used. Reexploration of certain specific spinal fusion sites at 6 months after surgery, such as in neurofibromatosis and certain types of paralytic curvatures, could be considered.[82] Routine exploration of idiopathic scoliosis fusions is not indicated.

When a diagnosis of pseudarthrosis has been made, surgical reexploration is indicated if there is evidence of significant loss of correction or clinical symptoms. Exposure of the area of pseudarthrosis is carried out, and fibrous tissue in the bony defect is curetted out and removed until margins of satisfactory bleeding bone are obtained. If the degree of curvature is still felt to be satisfactory at this time, a bony fusion is carried out with autogenous bone graft. Decortication of both margins of the pseudarthrosis site is carried out. A Harrington rod may be put in place across the fusion site to maintain stability. This should be a compressive rod if possible.

Occasionally, an excessive amount of correction has been lost, and realignment of the spine is undertaken before re-arthrodesis is undertaken. In this instance, the site of pseudarthrosis is used as a site of osteotomy of the fusion mass. The pseudarthrosis site is widened, and its anterior cortical margins are undercut. Additional osteotomies of the fusion mass are frequently made above and below the pseudarthrosis site to increase the degree of correction obtained. Progressive slow correction is then carried out with skeletal traction, and a second-stage fusion and correction across the pseudarthrosis site is then carried out after a satisfactory mechanical correction has been obtained. The postoperative course is then similar to that for the usual scoliosis fusion, and the same techniques of postoperative immobilization are used to obtain solid bony fusion. Sometimes a second or even a third reexploration and regrafting may be required to obtain solid union.

Preventing pseudarthrosis or decreasing its incidence is possible in a number of ways. Techniques of decortication of the graft bed must be exacting. These depend on careful exposure and soft tissue stripping of the site of bony fusion as a first stage in the operative treatment. Both Moe and Harrington have demonstrated the advantages of including the facet joints in the fusion. A lateral gutter fusion in the lumbar area that includes the transverse processes has been demonstrated to increase significantly the rate of union in this area.

Certain techniques of instrumentation, and the instrumentation itself, appear to have a decreased rate of pseudarthrosis. Early reviews by Risser and others of overall fusion rate found a pseudarthrosis rate of 24% to 40% when instrumentation was not used.[57,102] With the use of Harrington instrumentation, Hall, Moe, and others have noted a significant decrease in the relative rate of pseudarthrosis in similar types of patients.[46,67,68,87]

The use, when possible, of Harrington *compression* instrumentation in cases of thoracic kyphoscoliosis appears to increase the rate of union across this area of the curve. We use the compression apparatus routinely whenever there is sufficient kyphosis in association with the scoliosis to warrant its use. Unfortunately, relative thoracic lordosis is a contraindication to the use of the compressive system. The use of autogenous bone grafts appears to decrease the incidence of nonunion significantly when compared with the use of heterogenous or homologous bone grafts. Cancellous grafts obtained from the ilium have proven ideal. Both rib and tibia have been used as sources of graft material for the spine with satisfactory results.

In 1972 Harrington and Dickson reviewed eight different groups of patients who had undergone Harrington instrumentation by various techniques of instrumentation, grafting, and fusion.[52] By comparing the variations in technique used in three separate groups of patients, the authors demonstrated that the use of Harrington instrumentation, when supplemented by extensive decortication, facet joint resection, and transverse process fusion with cancellous autogenous bone grafts, resulted in a decrease of the pseudarthrosis rate from 33% to less than 1%.

Postoperative immobilization in a well-fitted body cast has become an essential part of the postoperative care of the scoliosis patient. Leider and colleagues reviewed a series of 106 patients who, within 2 weeks of Harrington rod instrumentation and fusion, had walked in a well-fitted Cotrel-type cast.[68] The authors found a pseudar-

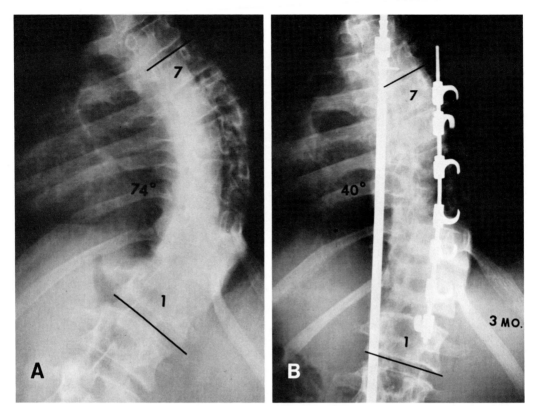

Fig. 40-7. Curve progression, instrument failure, and pseudarthrosis. (A) An 18-year-old man initially presented with an idiopathic thoracolumbar scoliosis measuring 74° from T7 to L1. (B) Posterior spinal fusion with Harrington rod instrumentation was done, and roentgenograms at 3 months after fusion showed correction of his initial curvature to 40°. (C) By 9 months after fusion, 7° of correction had been lost, the curve now measuring 47°. (D) At 1½ years after fusion, the initial curve measured 50°, a total loss of 10° since fusion, but the patient remained asymptomatic, and no further evaluation was carried out. (E) Three years after fusion the patient returned, complaining of intermittent mechanical-type back pain of several months' duration. Roentgenograms revealed further loss of correction to 58°, with fracture of the distraction rod at the thoracolumbar junction. (F) A pseudarthrosis of the fusion mass was seen on oblique views at the site of fracture (*arrowhead*).

throsis rate of 4.7% in these patients. It was their feeling that early postoperative ambulation was a factor in decreasing the rate of pseudarthrosis, owing to both its compressive effect on the spine and the improved metabolic activity of the fusion site. A number of other centers, including our own, have now added early postoperative ambulation in a well-fitted cast to their treatment regimen.

The duration of external immobilization appears to have some relationship to the relative rate of union after fusion. We have routinely immobilized our adolescent sco-

liotics in a Cotrel-type cast for 6 months. In the adult, however, we feel that 9 months of immobilization is indicated. We have often used a plastic body jacket for immobilization in the final 3 months. If, following 9 months of immobilization, there is still a questionable area of fusion on x-ray, this immobilization is carried on to 12 or even 15 months with the plastic body jacket until there is good roentgenographic evidence of union and no evidence of progression of curvature.

Dwyer Instrumentation. The incidence of pseudarthrosis following Dwyer instru-

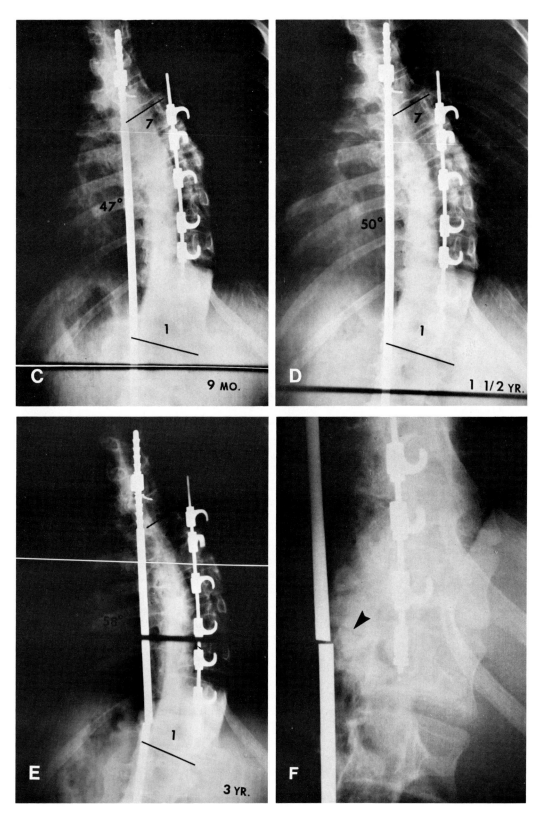

FIG. 40-7. (*Continued*)

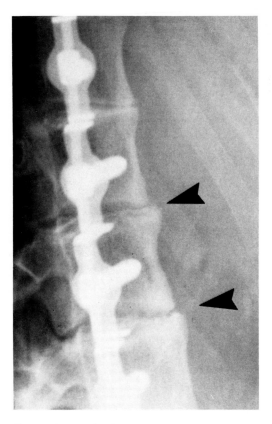

Fig. 40-8. Pseudarthroses are present at the two lowest levels of Dwyer instrumentation (*arrowheads*).

mentation and fusion is higher than was initially expected.[34,35,47] The rigid immobilization of the spine provided by the Dwyer instrumentation was felt to be an important factor in early and rapid union of these spinal fusions. However, in reviewing 78 patients with Dwyer fusion, Hall found a 16.6% incidence of clinically significant pseudarthrosis.[47] These patients had roentgenographic evidence of lack of interbody fusion but no evidence of progression of curvature or symptoms (Fig. 40-8). In 33 patients with idiopathic scoliosis, however, a 6% incidence of pseudarthrosis was found; in the 18 patients with myelodysplasia in this series, a 44% incidence of pseudarthrosis was noted.

Dwyer and colleagues reviewed the late complications of 81 Dwyer anterior spinal fusions performed at the Duchess of Kent Children's Orthopaedic Hospital in Hong Kong. They found a 20% incidence of nonunion overall, with a 21% rate in paralytic curvatures, 15% in idiopathic curvatures, and 22% in a miscellaneous group of curvatures.[35]

Diagnosis of pseudarthrosis after the Dwyer instrumentation is based primarily on roentgenographic assessment. Often, loss of correction is not clinically evident because of the continued stabilization of the level by the Dwyer fixation apparatus. However, with fracture or breakdown of the screw or cable, as observed by x-ray, in association with lack of evidence of bony union across the fusion site, established nonunion is assumed, and loss of correction is usually observed.

Hall[47] and Dwyer[32] agree on the management of nonunions following this procedure. Those that remain clinically quiet without evidence of progression have been followed with periodic roentgenograms. As long as they remain asymptomatic without loss of correction, no further surgery is suggested. In those cases in which the nonunion is clinically significant, posterior fusion *in situ* is carried out across the level of nonunion. If there has been significant loss of correction in association with the nonunion, posterior instrumentation with the Harrington equipment may be carried out.

Prevention of this complication in the Dwyer fusion is still a matter of active investigation. Careful resection of vertebral end-plate and cartilage back to the posterior margins of the vertebral body is a necessity in this technique. We are presently using cut-up portions of the resected rib and cancellous iliac bone grafts as an adjunct, particularly at the end-sites of the fusion area. Postoperative immobilization following Dwyer instrumentation has included ambulation and the use of a body jacket type of cast for a period of 6 months.

The use of anterior fusion with the Dwyer instrumentation and associated posterior Harrington fusion has been successful in a number of special instances, as in patients with dystonia musculorum deformans and certain types of spastic cerebral palsy. In addition, Dwyer[35] has recommended that all curves of paralytic origin have a supplemental posterior spine fusion and instrumentation following the initial anterior spinal instrumentation and fusion, because of the high rate of nonunion seen in these paralytic curves. Use of both anterior and posterior instrumentations and fusions is being replaced by Luque instrumentation, sometimes preceded by an anterior discectomy and fusion—to produce more correction and more certain fusion.

Extension of Curvature Beyond a Preexisting Fusion Site

Another late complication of spinal fusion in adults has been the extension of curvature, either above or below a site of previous fusion. Generally, this is the result of an error in selecting the initial levels of fusion, the result being that a fusion does not extend far enough. In some cases, however, usually in association with paralytic or neuromuscular disease, this progression of curvature is unanticipated.

In general, fusion of scoliosis curves must extend from neutral vertebra above an area of curvature to neutral vertebra below. Many adults with progressive, troublesome spinal deformities have had inadequate spinal fusions as youngsters. In some of these, only one of two structural curves was fused, with resultant progression of the other curve. In others, only part of an associated structural curve was fused, with further progression of this curve, often with the formation of a second structural curve in association with this. Frequently, these cases require posterior osteotomy of the previous fusion mass, a period of skeletal traction, and then re-fusion over the full extent of the spinal deformity.[58,67,105]

Cast Problems

We seem to encounter a significantly increased number of problems related to cast immobilization in adult patients. Pressure sores, in particular, appear to be more common.[1,55] In 1952 Adam made the observation that pressure sores associated with immobilization of adults supine in casts (whom he was treating with osteotomy of the spine for Strümpell-Marie's disease) were his most common and often most significant postoperative complication.[1] He noted that pressure sores developed easily in adults and were in two cases the cause

of death because of the secondary infection and sepsis. It has also been our observation that adults tolerate supine immobilization very poorly following spinal procedures, and the incidence of cast problems and pressure sores with supine immobilization is on the order of 20% to 30%. In addition, we have noted a relatively high incidence of pressure sores even when ambulatory cast immobilization is used postoperatively. The incidence of pressure sores over the sacroiliac margins and residual rib humps has been high and is frequently a cause of readmission. Treatment requires immobilization on a Stryker frame until decubiti heal. Adult male scoliosis patients seem particularly at risk, possibly owing to their small amounts of subcutaneous adipose tissue.

Other Late Complications

Several other late postoperative complications have been noted following the treatment of spinal deformities. We have noted several cases of spondylolisthesis that were previously asymptomatic but became symptomatic with low back pain following spinal fusion for deformity in the more proximal portion of the spinal column. Several patients have complained of pain in the area of the fusion site, despite the absense of pseudarthrosis. This pain has been localized to the site of Harrington rod fixation, and removal of the Harrington rod has resulted in relief of these symptoms. Whether this represents some type of low-grade metal toxicity or allergy to the metals in question is unknown. No unusual tissue reaction or corrosion has been noted about these endoprostheses. Allergy to the metallic endoprosthesis has been reported in a number of patients following total hip replacement.

GENERAL MEASURES TO HELP PREVENT COMPLICATIONS

Careful preoperative evaluation of the adult patient who is to undergo extensive spinal surgery can significantly decrease the incidence of complications in the operative and postoperative periods. Evaluation of cardiorespiratory function is critical. The majority of operative and postoperative deaths in this age group has been attributed to cardiorespiratory failure in poor-risk patients. Pulmonary function tests, including both ventilation and perfusion studies with arterial blood gas studies, should be routine.[89] Mention has already been made of the pulmonary assessment of certain high-risk patients undergoing halo–femoral traction as a means of predicting what their pulmonary function will be in their final, corrected position.

Preoperative physical therapy, including range-of-motion and muscle-strengthening exercises to the extremities, and instructions in breathing exercises are useful. Preoperative psychological evaluation of patients who show tendencies toward aberrant behavior or abnormal mentation can be extremely useful in managing those who develop significant psychological problems in the postoperative period.

The use of prophylactic antibiotics has dramatically decreased the incidence of wound infections in most centers. Careful attention to operating room procedures and limiting the flow of traffic in these extensive procedures is also indicated.

The basic rules of surgical dissection, with attention to tissue planes and with respect for tissue, are important to spinal surgery. With proper care and meticulous surgical technique, freeing of the soft tissues and muscles from the spinal elements in the subperiosteal plane can be carried out with a minimum of bleeding and can help decrease the amount of necrotic tissue in and about the wound. A surgical technique that combines complete exposure of the spine, facet joint resection, careful decortication of the posterior elements of the spine (including the traverse process in the lumbar region), and the use of autogenous bone grafts from properly selected donor sites on the posterior iliac crest will significantly improve the rate of fusion and decrease the possibility of spinal injury.

Postoperative pulmonary care requires careful monitoring of cardiorespiratory function, particularly in the adult patient. Postoperative management includes the monitoring of arterial blood gases, central venous pressure, and hourly urine output and specific gravities. An indwelling arterial blood line is generally used in the first 48 hours after surgery. If there is any question about the respiratory function, a nasotracheal tube is inserted at the end of the procedure, and the patient is maintained on assisted ventilation in the early postoperative period. When there is evidence that he is mechanically able to maintain his pulmonary function, with or without assisted supplemental oxygen therapy, he is progressively weaned from assisted ventilation, and the tube is removed. If he shows continued need for assisted ventilation beyond 5 to 7 days, elective tracheostomy is carried out. We have rarely found it necessary to include preoperative tracheostomy in our regimen, since most of our patients with borderline pulmonary function could be managed successfully with the newer, soft nasotracheal–endotracheal tubes in the immediate postoperative period. Postoperative pulmonary physical therapy, with vibration and deep-breathing techniques as well as the use of blow bottles, has been quite useful in helping eliminate secretions and prevent atelectasis. Our patients are immobilized on Stryker frames for the initial 10 to 14 days postoperatively until plaster casts are applied. This has been useful in preventing skin problems and allows the patient to be turned without applying significant mechanical stress to the spine. The use of postoperative ambulatory plaster immobilization appears to be particularly useful in adults. In addition to decreasing the incidence of pressure sores from the cast, it has rendered the prolonged immobilization required following these procedures if not pleasant, at least tolerable to the adult patient.

REFERENCES

1. Adam, J.C.: Techniques, dangers, and safeguards in osteotomy of the spine. J. Bone Joint Surg., 34B:226, 1952.
2. Allen, B.L., and Ferguson, R.L.: The Galveston technique for L-rod instrumentation of the scoliotic spine. Spine, 7:276, 1982.
3. Arkin, A.M.: The mechanism of the structural changes in scoliosis. J. Bone Joint Surg., 31A:519, 1949.
4. Barner, H.B., and Sherman, D.C.: Vascular compression of the duodenum. Surg. Gynecol. Obstet., 117:103, 1963.
5. Batson, O.V.: The function of the vertebral veins and their role in the spread of metastases. Am. Surg., 112:138, 1940.
6. Bergofsky, E.H., Turino, G.M., and Fishman,

A.P.: Cardio-respiratory failure in kypho-scoliosis. Medicine (Baltimore), 38:263, 1969.

7. Bernard, H.R., and Cole, W.R.: The prophylaxis of surgical infection: The effect of prophylactic antimicrobial drugs on the incidence of infection following potentially contaminated operations. Surgery, 56:151, 1964.

8. Bernard, T.N., Johnston, C.E. II, Roberts, J.M., and Burke, S.W.: Late complications due to wire breakage in segmental spinal instrumentation. J. Bone Joint Surg., 65A:1339, 1983.

9. Bick, E.M.: Vertebral growth: Its relation to spinal abnormalities in children. Clin. Orthop., 21:43, 1961.

10. Bjure, J., Grimby, G., Kasalicky, J. et al.: Respiratory impairment and airway closure in patients with untreated idiopathic scoliosis. Thorax, 23:451, 1970.

11. Block, A.J., McDonnel, J., and Wexler, J.: Cardiopulmonary failure of the hunchback. J.A.M.A., 212:1520, 1970.

12. Blount, W.P.: The principles of treatment according to curve patterns of scoliosis and roundback with the Milwaukee brace. In Postgraduate Course on the Management and Care of the Scoliosis Patient (New York, October 1969). Warsaw, IN, Zimmer, 1969.

13. Blount, W.P., and Bolonski, J.: Physical therapy in the non-operative treatment of scoliosis. Phys. Ther., 47:919, 1967.

14. Broude, A.I.: Transfusion reactions from contaminated blood: Their recognition and treatment. N. Engl. J. Med., 258:1289, 1958.

15. Brown, L.P., and Stelling, F.H.: Fat embolism as a complication of scoliosis fusion. J. Bone Joint Surg., 56A:1764, 1974.

16. Bunch, W.: Cholecystitis following spinal fusion. Presented to the Scoliosis Research Society Meeting, Louisville, 1975.

17. Bunch, W., and Delaney, J.: Scoliosis and acute vascular compression of the duodenum. Surgery, 67:901, 1970.

18. Caro, C.G., and Dubois, A.B.: Pulmonary function in kyphoscoliosis. Thorax, 16:282, 1961.

19. Collis, D.K., and Ponseti, I.V.: Long-term follow-up of patients with idiopathic scoliosis not treated surgically. J. Bone Joint Surg., 51A:425, 1969.

20. Coonrad, R.W., and Feirstein, M.S.: Progression of scoliosis in the adult. Presented to the Scoliosis Research Society Meeting, Louisville, 1975.

21. Cotrel, Y., and Morel, G.: La technique de EDF dans la correction des scoliosis. Rev. Chir. Orthop., 50:59, 1964.

22. Curtis, B.H.: Air embolism as a complication of spine fusion. J. Bone Joint Surg., 54A:201, 1972.

23. Dawson, E.G., Caran, A., and Moe, J.H.: Surgical management of scoliosis in the adult. J. Bone Joint Surg., 55A:437, 1973.

24. DeWald, R.I., and Ray, R.D.: Skeletal traction for the treatment of severe scoliosis. J. Bone Joint Surg., 52A:233, 1970.

25. Dickson, J.H.: Pre-operative and Post-operative evaluation of scoliosis patients for hiatus hernia. J. Bone Joint Surg., 54A:199, 1972.

26. Dolan, J.A., and MacEwen, G.D.: The surgical treatment of scoliosis. Clin. Orthop., 76:125, 1971.

27. Dommissee, G.F.: The blood supply of the human spinal cord: A critical vascular factor in spinal surgery. J. Bone Joint Surg., 56B:225, 1974.

28. Dommissee, G.F., and Enstein, T.B.: Hodgson's circumferential osteotomy in the correction of spinal deformity. J. Bone Joint Surg., 52B:778, 1970.

29. Donaldson, W.F., Wissinger, H.A., and Stone, C.S.: Exploration of scoliosis spine fusions. J. Bone Joint Surg., 51A:205, 1969.

30. Drummond, D.S., Fowles, J.V., Ecuyer, S. et al.: Untreated scoliosis in the adult. Presented to the Scoliosis Research Society Meeting, Louisville, 1975.

31. Drummond, D.S., Keene, J.S., and Breed, A.: The Wisconsin system: A technique of interspinous segmental spinal instrumentation. Contemp. Orthop. 8(6):29, 1984.

32. Dwyer, A.F.: Experience of anterior correction of scoliosis. Clin. Orthop., 93:191, 1973.

33. Dwyer, A.F., Newton, N.C., and Sherwood, A.A.: An anterior approach to scoliosis: A clinical report. Clin. Orthop., 62:192, 1969.

34. Dwyer, A.F., and Schafer, M.F.: Anterior approach to scoliosis. J. Bone Joint Surg., 56B:218, 1974.

35. Dwyer, A.F. et al.: The late complications following Dwyer anterior spinal instrumentation in the management of scoliosis. Presented to the Scoliosis Research Society Meeting, Louisville, 1975.

36. ———: Paravertebral infection following Dwyer anterior spinal instrumentation. Presented to the Scoliosis Research Society Meeting, Louisville, 1975.

37. Elfstrom, D., and Nachemson, A.: Telemetry recordings of forces in the Harrington distraction rod: A method of increasing safety in the operative treatment of scoliosis patients. Clin. Orthop., 93:158, 1973.

38. Evarts, C.M., and Feli, E.J.: Prevention of thromboembolic disease after elective surgery of the hip. J. Bone Joint Surg., 53A:1271, 1971.

39. Evarts, C.M., Winter, R.B., and Hall, J.E.: Vascular compression of the duodenum associated with the treatment of scoliosis. J. Bone Joint Surg., 53A:431, 1971.

40. Gaines, D.L., Moe, J.H., and Bocklage, J.: Management of wound infections following Harrington instruments and spine fusion. J. Bone Joint Surg., 52A:404, 1970.

41. Gardner, A.D.H., O'Brien, J.P., and Hodgson, A.R.: Accurate electronic measurement of the forces applied to the spine with halo–pelvic traction. Presented to the Scoliosis Research Society Meeting, Louisville, 1975.

42. Garrett, A., Nickel, V.L., and Perry, J.: Stabilization of the collapsing spine. J. Bone Joint Surg., 43A:474, 1961.

43. Goldstein, L.A.: The surgical management of scoliosis. Clin Orthop., 35:95, 1964.

44. ———: The surgical treatment of idiopathic scoliosis. Clin Orthop., 83:131, 1973.

45. Graham, J.J.: Pseudarthrosis in scoliosis: Routine exploration of 45 operative cases. J. Bone Joint Surg., 50A:850, 1968.

46. Hall, J.E.: Scoliosis in adults. Presented to the Scoliosis Research Society Meeting, Wilmington, DE, 1972.

47. Hall, J.E., and Grey, J.: Complications in Dwyer

instrumentation and fusion of the spine. J. Bone Joint Surg., 58A:156, 1976.

48. Hardy, J.M., Cooke, R.W., and Einbund, M.: Hyperalimentation in the treatment of "cast syndrome." J. Bone Joint Surg., 54A:200, 1972.
49. Hardy, R.W., Nash, C.L., and Brodkey, J.S.: Follow-up report, experimental and clinical studies in spinal cord monitoring: The effect of pressure, anoxia, and ischemia of spinal cord function. J. Bone Joint Surg., 55A:435, 1973.
50. Harrington, P.R.: Treatment of scoliosis: Correction and internal fixation by spinal instrumentation. J. Bone Joint Surg., 44A:591, 1962.
51. ————: Technical details in relation to the successful use of instrumentation in scoliosis. Orthop. Clin. North Am. 3:49, 1972.
52. Harrington, P.R., and Dickson, J.H.: An eleven-year clinical investigation of Harrington instrumentation: A preliminary report on 578 cases. Clin. Orthop., 93:113, 1973.
53. Harris, W.H., Salzman, E.W., and DeSanctis, R.W.: The prevention of thromboembolic disease by prophylactic anticoagulation: A controlled study in elective hip surgery. J. Bone Joint Surg., 49A:81, 1967.
54. Harris, W.H. et al.: Comparison of warfarin, low-molecular-weight dextran, aspirin, and subcutaneous heparin in prevention of venous thromboembolism following total hip replacement. J. Bone Joint Surg., 56A:1552, 1974.
55. Herbert, J.J.: Vertebral osteotomy for kyphosis, especially in Marie-Strumpell arthritis. J. Bone Joint Surg., 41A:291, 1959.
56. Herring, J.A., and Wenger, D.R.: Segmental spinal instrumentation: A preliminary report of 40 consecutive cases. Spine, 7:285, 1982.
57. Hibbs, R.A.: A report on 59 cases of scoliosis treated by fusion operation. J. Bone Joint Surg., 6:3, 1924.
58. Hodgson, A.R.: Correction of fixed spinal curves: A preliminary communication. J. Bone Joint Surg., 47A:1221, 1965.
59. ————: Halo-pelvic traction. Spectator, 9:171, 1971.
60. Howorth, M.B.: Evaluation of spinal fusion. Ann. Surg., 117:278, 1943.
61. Kassen, N.Y., Graen, J.J., and Frankel, M.: Spinal deformities and esophageal hiatus hernia. Lancet, 1:887, 1965.
62. Keim, H.A., and Hilal, S.K.: Spinal angiography in scoliosis patients. J. Bone Joint Surg., 53A:197, 1971.
63. Keim, H.A., and Weinstein, J.: Acute renal failure: A complication of spinal fusion in the tuck position. J. Bone Joint Surg., 52A:1248, 1970.
64. Keller, R.B., and Pappas, A.M.: Infection after spinal fusion using internal fixation instrumentation. Orthop. Clin. North Am., 3:99, 1972.
65. Kostuik, J.P., Israel, J., and Hall, J.E.: Scoliosis surgery in adults. Clin Orthop., 93:225, 1973.
66. Lazarus, H.R., and Hagens, J.: Prevention of psychosis following open heart surgery. Am. J. Psychiatry, 124:1190, 1968.
67. Leatherman, K.C.: The management of rigid spinal curves. Clin. Orthop., 93:215, 1973.
68. Leider, L.L., Moe, J.H., and Winter, R.B.: Early

ambulation after surgical treatment of idiopathic scoliosis. J. Bone Joint Surg., 55A:1003, 1973.
69. Letts, R.M., Palakar, G., and Bobechoko, W.P.: The temporal effect of preoperative spinal traction in the treatment of scoliosis. J. Bone Joint Surg., 57A:616, 1975.
70. Lindh, M., and Nachemson, A.: The effect of breathing exercises on the vital capacity in patients with scoliosis treated by surgical correction with the Harrington technique. Scand. J. Rehabil. Med., 2:1, 1970.
71. Lonstein, L., Winter, R.B., Moe, J.H., and Chou, S.: Spinal deformity and cord compression. J. Bone Joint Surg., 56A:444, 1974.
72. Luque, E.R.: Treatment of scoliosis without arthrodesis or external support. Orthop. Trans. 1: 37, 1977.
73. ————: The anatomic basis and development of segmental spinal instrumentation. Spine 7:256, 1983.
74. MacEwen, D.G., and Cowell, H.R.: Autogenous transfusion for spinal surgery in children. J. Bone Joint Surg., 56A:440, 1974.
75. MacEwen, D.G., Hardy, J.H., and Winter, R.B.: Evaluation of kidney anomalies in congenital scoliosis. J. Bone Joint Surg., 54A:1451, 1972.
76. Manning, C.: The use of halo–pelvic distraction in preoperative reduction of scoliosis. J. Bone Joint Surg., 56A:440, 1974.
77. Mathews, R.S., and Stelling, F.H.: Second look spinal exploration for scoliosis. J. Bone Joint Surg., 52A:409, 1970.
78. May, V.R., and Mauck, W.R.: A critical analysis of exploration of the spine following spine fusion in the treatment of scoliosis. J. Bone Joint Surg., 50A:850, 1968.
79. McMaster, W.C., and Silber, I.: A urologic complication of Dwyer instrumentation. J. Bone Joint Surg., 57A:710, 1975.
80. Micheli, L.J.: Thromboembolic complications of cast immobilization for injuries in the lower extremities. Clin. Orthop., 108:191, 1975.
81. Moe, J.H.: Complications of scoliosis treatment. Clin. Orthop., 53:21, 1967.
82. ————: Neurofibromatosis and scoliosis. In Postgraduate Course on the Management and Care of the Scoliosis Patient (New York, October 1969). Warsaw, IN, Zimmer, 1969.
83. Morbidity Report. Scoliosis Research Society Meeting, Hartford, September 1971.
84. Morbidity Report. Scoliosis Research Society Meeting, Wilmington, DE, September 1972.
85. Morbidity Report. Scoliosis Research Society Meeting, Gothenburg, Sweden, September 1973.
86. Nachemson, A.: A long term follow-up study of non-treated scoliosis. Acta Orthop. Scand., 39: 466, 1968.
87. Nachemson, A., and Elfstrom, G.: Intra-vital wireless telemetry of axial forces in Harrington instrumentation rods in patients with idiopathic scoliosis. J. Bone Joint Surg., 53A:445, 1971.
88. Nash, C.L., Schatzinger, L., and Lorig, R.: Intra-operative monitoring of spinal cord function during scoliosis spine surgery. J. Bone Joint Surg., 56A:1765, 1974.
89. Nickel, V.L., Affeldt, J.B., Dail, C.W., and Perry,

J.: Elective surgery on patients with respiratory paralysis. J. Bone Joint Surg., 39A:989, 1957.

90. Nickel, V.L., Garrett, A., Perry, J., and Snelson, R.: Application of the halo. Orthop. Pros. Appl. J., 14:81, 1960.

91. Nickel, V.L., Perry, J., Garrett, A., and Heppenstahl, M.: The halo: Analysis of its use on 174 patients. J. Bone Joint Surg. 50A:847, 1968.

92. Nilsonne, J., Lundren, K.: Long term prognosis in idiopathic scoliosis. Acta Orthop. Scand., 39: 456, 1968.

93. O'Brien, J.P., Hodgson, A.R., Smith, T.K., and Yau, A.: Halo-pelvic traction—a preliminary report of external skeletal fixation for correcting deformities and maintaining fixation of the spine. J. Bone Joint Surg., 53B:212, 1971.

94. O'Brien, J.P., Yau, A., and Hodgson, A.R.: Halo-pelvic traction: A technique for severe spinal deformities. Clin. Orthop., 93:179, 1973.

95. Perry, J.: The halo in spinal abnormalities: Practical factors and avoidance of complications. Orthop. Clin. North Am., 3:69, 1972.

96. Ponder, R.C., Dickson, J.H., Harrington, P.R., and Erwin, W.D.: Results of Harrington instrumentation and fusion in the adult idiopathic scoliotic patient. J. Bone Joint Surg., 57A:797, 1975.

97. Ponseti, I.V., and Freidman, B.: Prognosis in idiopathic scoliosis. J. Bone Joint Surg., 32A:381, 1950.

98. Ponte, A.: Post-operative paraplegia due to hypercorrection of scoliosis and drop of blood pressure. J. Bone Joint Surg., 56A:444, 1974.

99. Relton, J.E.S., and Conen, P.: Anesthesia for the surgical correction of scoliosis by the Harrington method in children. Can. Anaesth. Soc. J., 10: 603, 1963.

100. Relton, J.E.S., and Hall, J.E.: An operation frame for spinal fusion. J. Bone Joint Surg., 49B:327, 1967.

101. Riseborough, E.J.: The anterior approach to the axial skeleton. Clin. Orthop., 93:207, 1973.

102. Risser, J.: Scoliosis; past and present. J. Bone Joint Surg., 46A:167, 1964.

103. Risser, J.C., and Ferguson, A.B.: Scoliosis, its prognosis. J. Bone Joint Surg., 18:667, 1936.

104. Shannon, D.C., Kazemi, H., Riseborough, E.J., and Valenca, L.M.: The distribution of abnormal lung function in kyphoscoliosis. J. Bone Joint Surg., 52A:131, 1970.

105. Simmons, E.H.: Observations on the technique and indications for wedge resection of the spine. J. Bone Joint Surg., 50A:847, 1968.

106. Sudhir, K., Smith, R., Hall, J.E., and Hanson, D.: Intra-operative awaking to prevent neurologic sequelae following Harrington fusion. Anaesth. Analg., 1976.

107. Telfer, R.B., Hoyt, W.F., and Schwartz, H.S.: Crossed-eyes in the halo-pelvic traction. Lancet, 2:922, 1971.

108. Treadwell, S.J., and O'Brien, J.P.: Apophyseal joint degeneration in the cervical spine following halo-pelvic distraction. Presented to the Scoliosis Research Society Meeting, Louisville, 1975.

109. Vanderpool, D., and Wynne-Davis, R.: Scoliosis in the elderly. J. Bone Joint Surg., 51A:446, 1969.

110. Vauzelle, C., Stagnara, R., and Jouvinroux, P.: Functional monitoring of spinal cord activity during spinal surgery. Clin. Orthop., 93:173, 1973.

111. Victor, D.I., Bresnan, M.S., and Keller, R.B.: Brain abscess complicating the use of halo traction. J. Bone Joint Surg., 55A:635, 1973.

112. Waugh, T.R.: Intra-vital measurements during instrumentation correction of idiopathic scoliosis. Acta Orthop. Scand. [Suppl.], 93, 1966.

113. Wilber, G.R., Thompson, G.H., Shaffer, J.W. et al.: Spinal cord monitoring and neurologic deficits in segmental instrumentation. Presented at the Annual Meeting of the American Academy of Orthopaedic Surgeons, Anaheim, CA, 1984.

114. Young, L.E.: Complications of blood transfusions. Ann. Intern. Med., 61:136, 1964.

41 Complications and Salvage Procedures in Surgery of the Foot

Charles H. Epps, Jr., and Alfred Kahn III *

Because surgery of the foot is most often performed to correct deformity, to relieve pain, or to improve function, patients who have had successful surgery are usually grateful. When complications develop, the effects are usually devastating: pain or deformity or both. The patient now has pain with each step—a frequent, sometimes constant reminder of the complications— and a concomitant loss of function.

GENERAL CONSIDERATIONS

A thorough examination of the extremity should be performed, which includes vascular and neurological examination, as in any surgical procedure. Any deficiency should be carefully noted in the record so that should complications arise, the new problems can be differentiated from the old.

The surgeon should be alert to the clinical signs of vascular insufficiency that would contraindicate elective surgical procedures. The skin offers definite clues such as the absence of hair and the presence of ulceration, infection, and ischemia to the point of cool skin. Additional signs of vascular insufficiency are absent pulses, intermittent claudication, pain at rest, blanching on elevation, dependent rubor, thickening of the nails, and neuropathy (Fig. 41-1). The diabetic with neuropathy also presents increased risk of failure.[8] Signs that should alert the surgeon are dysesthesia, radicular pain, loss of reflexes and vibratory and position sense, anhydrosis, heavy callus formation over pressure points, trophic ul-

cers, footdrop, atrophy, and the radiographic signs of demineralization, osteolysis, and Charcot's joint (Fig. 41-2).[26]

Generally speaking, we feel that tourniquet control is mandatory. Exceptions to this rule are the elderly or others with compromise of the circulation. If there is any question regarding the status of the circulation, a vascular surgeon should be consulted. Most certainly, with decreased or absent pulses, a tourniquet is contraindicated. Furthermore, the use of local anesthesia, with or without sympathomimetic drugs, is also not recommended in the presence of vascular compromise.

Instrumentation and tissue care are as important in surgery of the foot as they are in surgery of the upper extremity. Only the finest osteotomes, rongeurs, forceps, and other instruments should be used. An atraumatic technique is essential if one hopes for the best results. Skin loss as a result of overzealous retraction is a well-known complication of foot surgery. Incisions should be placed with the greatest of care. With repeat procedures, one may have to alter the planned incision because the skin may be extensively scarred. In these cases one may have to proceed more proximally or distally and then perform a subperiosteal dissection, leaving the skin and the subcutaneous tissues intact, so that the tenuous blood supply that remains is left intact with the subcutaneous tissue. A word of caution: Electrocautery should be used with caution in those areas in which there is poor circulation, or where there has been previous surgery, because in such circumstances the result will be slough of the skin and perhaps of the underlying structures.

The least radical procedure should be

* The authors acknowledge the contributions of the late Nicholas J. Giannestras to this chapter.

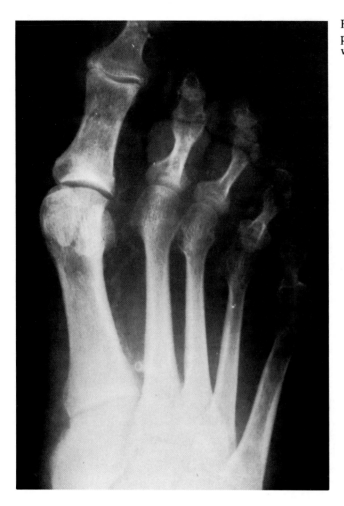

FIG. 41-1. Calcification of the dorsalis pedis artery in a 50-year-old diabetic who presented for a painful bunion.

attempted first. In the foot this means that the surgeon should opt for such procedures as osteotomies and tendon transpositions over those procedures that result in loss of joint motion. Generally speaking, the functional result is much better when joint motion is left intact.

FAILURES RELATED TO STATIC PROBLEMS IN PREADOLESCENTS AND ADOLESCENTS

Surgery for the correction of the symptomatic flatfoot or the severe valgus foot has, in the past, fallen into disrepute because of the failure of the procedure to achieve the desired result. Frequently, the same operation was used for all kinds of flatfoot. There are three joints and four bones in-

volved in the integrity of the longitudinal arch: the talocalcaneal, the talonavicular, and the naviculocuneiform articulations. Flatfoot deformity is the result of malalignment of one, and frequently two, of these joints (*i.e.*, the talocalcaneal, with or without the talonavicular joint, or the naviculocuneiform joint, with or without the talonavicular). Very seldom is the talonavicular joint alone responsible for a valgus foot deformity, and only rarely do all three joints contribute to this type of flatfoot. In a number of instances the hind part of the foot may be in equinus and valgus position, as in the serpentine foot or the congenital rigid flatfoot (talipes equinovalgus), yet the average surgeon performs the same operation with resultant failure; eventually the patient must have a triple arthrodesis.

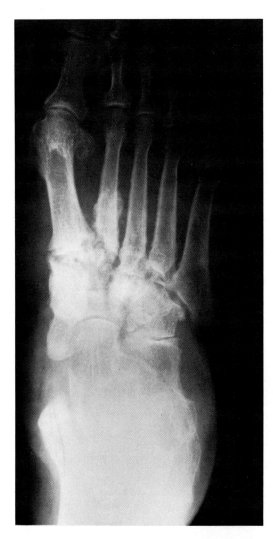

FIG. 41-2. Neuropathic changes in the tarso-metatarsal joints of the right foot of a diabetic who had been on insulin for more than 20 years. The foot was only mildly painful and became asymptomatic with application of an orthosis.

THE PLANOVALGUS FOOT

The Kidner procedure does not correct a true flatfoot, and the Hoke operation is only 50% successful for flatfoot due to a naviculocuneiform sag. The Miller-Durham and Young procedures are more effective for this type of flatfoot, and the modified Grice and Chambers operations give optimal results for the planovalgus foot due to plantar flexion of the talus. Furthermore,

these procedures are effective in patients through the ages of 16 to 18, provided that the foot is flexible. When the foot is rigid, or when no further growth is anticipated, the flatfoot can be corrected and rendered asymptomatic only by triple arthrodesis. Still, it should be kept in mind that triple arthrodesis may salvage a foot, but it will not produce a normal foot. Motion of the peritalar joints is synchronous, and loss of part of this motion places added stress on the remaining joint or joints, including the ankle joint.

Triple Arthrodesis

Performed correctly, the triple arthrodesis offers the best opportunity to obtain correction and to prevent complications.[17,18] The incision avoids the sural nerve and the peroneal tendons and sheaths. Numbness of the lateral aspect of the foot or loss of function of the peroneus longus tendon can lead to additional disability. Vigorous retraction must be avoided to prevent skin damage. Cartilage and subchondral bone are removed from adjacent surfaces of the talocalcaneal, calcaneocuboid, and talonavicular joints. The bases of the wedges are located either medially or laterally to correct either valgus or varus. At the time of stabilization, the joints are aligned with the ankle. The foot should be aligned with the heel in slight valgus position, and under no circumstances should the heel be placed in varus position. Whether staples are used to hold the bony components together depends on the technique and experience of the orthopaedist. One author (C.H.E.) prefers smooth Steinmann pins for fixation. These are removed at the end of six weeks.

Hoke's technique of removing the talar head (Fig. 41-3, *A*), which we prefer, facilitates exposure of the navicular.[17,18] This is accomplished by osteotomizing the talus at the junction of the head and neck and carefully and gently removing the head. After the apposing articular surfaces of the navicular and the talar head have been denuded of all cartilage, the head is wrapped in a sponge moistened with Ringer's solution and set aside until the remaining deformity has been corrected by removal of the necessary bone wedges from the talocalcaneal and calcaneocuboid joints.

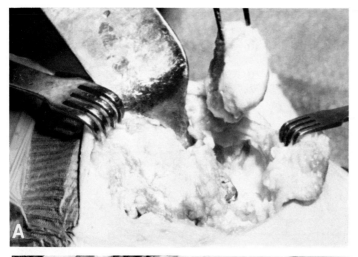

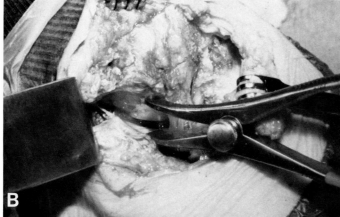

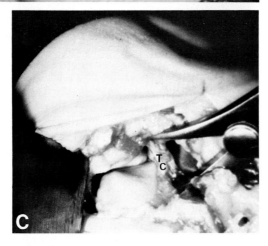

FIG. 41-3. (*A*) The head of the talus is resected, exposing the articular surface of the navicular, thus facilitating excision of the cupped, cartilaginous surface of the navicular. A bone wedge can then be removed, depending on the correction desired. (*B*) A spreader is inserted between the inferior articular surface of the body of the talus and the trochlear surface of the calcaneus. The spreader is placed under the neck of the talus and in front of the articular surface of the calcaneus. Note that a bunion retractor is being used to expose the posterior edge of the talocalcaneal joint. (*C*) Close-up of the talocalcaneal joint and exposure of the interosseous talocalcaneal ligament (*TC*).

After the proper wedges have been removed from the calcaneocuboid joint to correct any cavus or varus deformity of the midpart or forepart of the foot, attention should be turned to the subtalar joint. The valgus or the varus angulation of the hindpart of the foot is controlled by the talocalcaneal articulation. A modified laminar spreader (Fig.

41-3, *B*) is used to distract the talus from the calcaneus, thus facilitating exposure of the distal, middle, and posterior articular facets (Fig. 41-3, *C*). In addition, a Crego retractor can be inserted between the capsule and the talus and navicular laterally and posteriorly to protect the posterior and medial structures overlying the talus. The facets, with the bases of the wedges located either medially or laterally to correct either valgus or varus, are then excised. A curette should be used to remove the articular cartilage from the sustentaculum tali if one is unsure of excising the sustentaculum with an osteotome. The apposing flat bony surfaces of the talus, calcaneus, and cuboid are then approximated. The head of the talus is shaped to fit the defect that remains between the neck of the talus and the navicular, and foot alignment is then tested. In some instances the surgeon may elect to use an additional medial incision to facilitate talonavicular cartilage removal. Occasionally, additional bone may have to be removed to correct some small portion of residual deformity or to ensure congruity of the adjacent bone surfaces. It should not require any particular force to hold the foot in the corrected position (Fig. 41-4).

One of us (C.H.E.) prefers to denude the articular cartilage and to contour the ball-and-socket configuration of the talonavicular joint to produce a better cosmetic effect and to minimize nonunion of the talonavicular joint.

Residual varus angulation of either the heel or the forepart of the foot is not acceptable because with either deformity, as weight is transferred along the lateral border of the heel, the forepart of the foot undergoes increased varus deformity with each step.

Variations in technique are indicated depending on the deformity present and the residual muscle power, as noted above. Calcaneocavus deformities are corrected by removal of a generous wedge from the proximal posterior facet of the calcaneus, together with a dorsal wedge from the head of the talus and navicular. In addition, a Steindler release of the plantar fascia from the calcaneus may be necessary. The cavus is thus corrected, and the forepart of the foot is aligned with the calcaneus. Thus, by taking the appropriate wedges of bone and performing the appropriate soft tissue releases, one can correct almost any deformity in this region of the foot. The Lambrinudi type of triple arthrodesis is indicated in a fixed equinus, flail foot, or dropfoot deformity. For children the period of immobilization is 6 weeks in a non-weight-bearing,

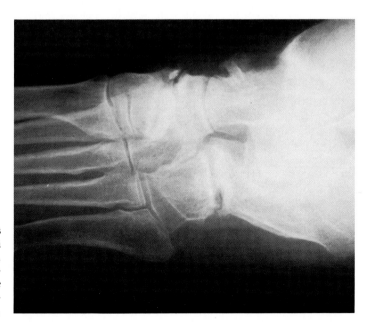

FIG. 41-4. Triple arthrodesis complicated by partial fusion of the calcaneocuboid joint. The surgeon missed the talonavicular joint and fused the medial cuneiform to the navicular. The foot was painful.

below-knee cast or an above-knee cast, depending on the surgeon's choice and 6 weeks in a walking cast. For adults, the period of no weight-bearing should be extended to 8 weeks, followed by 8 weeks' ambulation in a walking cast. The cast should be used to immobilize the foot, *not* to correct it.

When dealing with a symptomatic, plantar-flexed-talus type of flatfoot, one should again try conservative therapy first, depending, of course, on the patient's age. It should be noted that in older children this type of flatfoot is due to inadequate or ineffectual conservative treatment. Failure to recognize and treat it or lack of response to adequate therapy is the case in approximately 35% to 50% of such feet. Complications here may be the result of poor choice of procedure. If the plantar flexion is moderate to severe and the dorsoplantar talonavicular angle is less than 45°, or if the patient is a girl over age 10 years or a boy over age 12 years, surgical correction is indicated. Prior to maturity of the foot, the modified Grice extra-articular arthrodesis—transplantation of the tibialis anterior to the plantar surface of the navicular—is recommended. Care should be exercised to avoid placing the heel into a varus position, since it will lead to further varus deformity as the foot continues to grow. Lengthening of the calcaneus tendon may be necessary, and, if so, it should be carried out 6 to 8 weeks after the arthrodesis has been performed. Failure to recognize a contracted heel cord will leave the patient with equinus deformity of the hindpart of the foot, which will cause failure of the Grice procedure. With failure there remains no alternative but triple arthrodesis, as is the case if treatment is delayed until the foot reaches maturity.

To obviate failures from the Grice-Green extra-articular arthrodesis, Giannestras has recommended the following changes from the classical description. First, a fibular graft is deemed superior to one from the tibia (as described in the original paper). It is obtained by making an incision over the lateral aspect of the leg, directly overlying the fibula approximately 10 cm proximal to the tip of the lateral malleolus. The fibula is exposed subperiosteally between the peroneal and flexor digitorum longus muscles,

and the entire fibula is removed for a distance of not more than 3 cm. The amount of bone removed is dictated, of course, by the size of the foot and the size of the graft required. As long as the periosteum is maintained, the defect will fill in with new bone within a matter of 6 to 9 months. The dissection should be done carefully, since it is possible to injure the superficial peroneal nerve. In bilateral cases, fibular grafts should be taken from each fibula rather than a single long graft from one side. The second deviation from the classical procedure involves sectioning the dorsal talonavicular capsule to facilitate the positioning of the talus on the calcaneus.

A final alteration involves transferring the anterior tibial tendon to the plantar surface of the tarsal navicular. A medial incision is made beginning just proximal to the navicular tubercle and extending distally to the level of the metatarsocuneiform joint. Through this incision the anterior tibial tendon is exposed and detached at the medial plantar aspect of the foot. The tendon sheath is split to the level of the inferior edge of the anterior cruciate ligament. The plantar aspect of the navicular is denuded of soft tissue, and a hole is drilled dorsoplantarly in the middle portion of the navicular just distal to the proximal cortical surface. The hole must be big enough to accept the tendon. A 2-0 chromic suture is passed through the tendon end, the suture is passed through the hold from plantar to dorsal, and the tendon is pulled through from the plantar to the dorsal surface and tied on itself. The tendon should be placed in position under physiological tension. An additional one or two sutures of 2-0 chromic catgut are passed through the edge of the tibialis anterior to the posterior tibial tendon, as the former crosses over the latter just posterior to the navicular tubercle. This dynamic sling thereby corrects the dorsoplantar talonavicular sag (Fig. 41-5). Furthermore, it contributes actively to the maintenance of the new longitudinal arch.

CAVUS DEFORMITIES

For the correction of the cavus deformity to be successful, it is necessary first to establish a diagnosis. Every effort, including

FIG. 41-5. The tibialis anterior is passed through a drill hole in the plantar surface of the navicular.

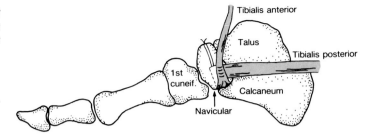

muscle biopsy, should be made to determine the cause of the deformity, since by establishing the cause, the prognosis and thus the therapeutic regimen can be more accurately established.

In mild cases conservative therapy nearly always suffices, but occasionally the Steindler procedure may be required. This is a holding procedure, at best, and will not change the appearance of the foot. Failures in treating these cases are usually related to lack of recognition of the cause and severity of the bony deformity. If the patient is under 18 years of age and the deformity is severe, a vigorous attack should be instituted. The procedure of choice is closed-wedge osteotomy of the calcaneus with careful detachment of the plantar musculature and fascia from the plantar aspect of the calcaneal tuberosity through a lateral incision with or without a dorsal closing wedge of all five metatarsals, depending on the severity of the deformity (Fig. 41-6). In severe cases it may be necessary to perform a triple arthrodesis. This is not a desirable procedure, since it results in rigidity of the hindpart of the foot. Numerous other procedures are cited in the literature, including transfer of the long extensors to the heads of the metatarsals or to the middle cuneiform, transfer of the anterior tibial tendon to the dorsum of the head of the first metatarsal, fusion of the first metatarsocuneiform joint with excision of a dorsal wedge of bone, open wedge osteotomy of the plantar surface of the medial navicular, and the Japas procedure. Each proponent of a recommended operation feels that his is the procedure of choice for correcting the deformity. However, the results of many of these operations are not consistently satisfying. One must evaluate the age of the patient, the standing roentgenograms, and the clinical appearance of the foot before

deciding on the procedure to be used. If the problem is a calcaneocavus deformity, an upward displacement osteotomy of the calcaneus with a Steindler procedure is the operation of choice. If it is a clawfoot deformity and the patient is less than 10 years of age, the transplantation of the long toe extensors to the metatarsal neck or to the middle cuneiform, combined with a Steindler stripping of the plantar fascia, may be a good holding procedure until the bones of the foot mature. If the surgeon does not wish to consider a triple arthrodesis, except as a salvage operation, he can combine the calcaneal osteotomy with dorsal closed wedge osteotomy of the metatar-

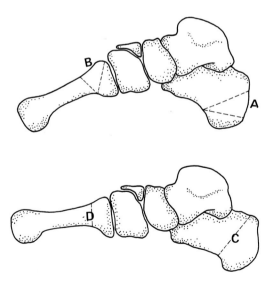

FIG. 41-6. (*A*) Biplanar osteotomy of the calcaneus to correct cavus and varus deformities. (*B*) Dorsal open wedge osteotomy of all five metatarsals. The plantar cortical surface is left intact. (*C*) Closed calcaneal osteotomy. (*D*) With acute hyperextension, the dorsal wedge osteotomy of the metatarsals is closed. Plantar fasciotomy is performed as needed.

sal bases, with or without Steindler stripping. In the event of failure of surgery for the cavus foot, as always, a well-performed triple arthrodesis may be the only means to salvage a foot that is severely deformed in the hind part.

Rarely, when the cavus deformity is produced exclusively by plantar flexion of the first ray, it is preferable to perform either a Jones tenosuspension (a holding procedure) or an osteotomy of the first metatarsal only as a corrective operation after age 14 years. The osteotomy is a closed wedge type, with the base located dorsally. When the tendocalcaneus must be lengthened because of an equinus deformity associated with the pes cavus, it must be performed after all other bony procedures have been accomplished, since if heel cord lengthening is carried out as a first step, the manipulation of the bony components of the foot is more difficult.

CONGENITAL RIGID FLATFOOT

Most investigators report treating congenital rigid flatfoot (variously called congenital convex pes valgus and talipes equinovalgus) successfully only by surgical means. After 6 months of age, surgery is the only alternative. But, if the deformity is attacked at birth, cast correction can be, and is, successful in 50% of patients, and surgical intervention consists only of lengthening the tendocalcaneus with a posterior ankle capsulotomy. A plea for its consideration is made here in the hope of avoiding surgical intervention, if possible. Except when the foot is resistant to this treatment, casting should be the first line of therapy.

Certainly, this type of foot (like the moderately severe to severe plantar-flexed-talus type of flatfoot) is very difficult to correct by any means. It is imperative that the deformity be recognized because the earlier the treatment is instituted, the better the chance for correction. If the child is seen after the age of 6 months, the use of corrective casts is worthless, even in the mildly rigid congenital flatfoot. At this early age the surgical procedure of choice is that advocated by Herndon and Heyman.[15] The Craig procedure can also be used. Any of

these procedures may be performed as early as 6 months to 1 year of age. Detailed accounts of these operations are found in the standard texts, as mentioned previously.

Failure of correction in this type of deformity is not uncommon. The procedure chosen to salvage the foot depends largely on the age of the patient. If the patient is under 8 or 9 years, but over 5, the Grice procedure, with lengthening of the tendocalcaneus, may be used. At times, open reduction of the calcaneocuboid joint is also necessary. A few investigators have advocated this operation for younger children, but we feel that joint changes that occur in Chopart's joint as a result of a subtalar arthrodesis can occur as a result of the Grice procedure as well, and thus might well predispose the child to further problems. Should the Grice procedure be chosen as a means of salvage or as a means of initial treatment, care must be taken to ensure that the heel is not placed in even a minimal amount of varus, which would compound the deformity. In older patients the surgeon must perform a triple arthrodesis with lengthening of the tendocalcaneus and posterior ankle capsulotomy.

Occasionally, after a Heyman-Herndon or Craig operation, the result will be a partial correction of the problems in the hindpart and midpart of the foot, with valgus deformity of the forepart. To avoid a salvage triple arthrodesis, a metatarsal osteotomy can be performed to realign the forepart of the foot.

THE PRONATED FOOT IN THE ADULT

Symptomatic pronated feet in adults are very seldom attacked surgically. In teenagers, prominent navicular tubercles, with or without accessory naviculars, can be symptomatic and do, at times, require surgical intervention. In these cases excision of the accessory navicular (with or without the navicular tubercle) along with transfer of the posterior tibial tendon to the plantar aspect of the navicular (Kidner procedure) is indicated.

In the exceptional case the patient may have reached adulthood with a third-degree pronation that is symptomatic and totally unresponsive to conservative therapy. A triple arthrodesis is the only sound surgical approach to this deformity. At that level, however, before a triple arthrodesis is performed, the patient's foot should be immobilized in a walking cast. If this relieves the patient's foot pain completely, then—and then only—should a triple arthrodesis be considered for a symptomatic adult flatfoot. In performing such a triple arthrodesis, one can fuse the foot *in situ,* which leaves a cosmetically unacceptable foot, or one can so perform the triple arthrodesis as to improve the cosmetic appearance of the foot as well (Fig. 41-7). There are certain extremely rigid flat feet in which cosmetic correction of the foot through a triple arthrodesis cannot be achieved on the first attempt. The patient should be informed of this and of the fact that should he later desire revision to obtain a normal-looking foot rather than severe flatfoot, that can be done. Occasionally, a patient complains of pain at the first tarsometatarsal joint that can definitely be attributed to the abnormal stress placed on this articulation because of a flatfoot deformity. In such instances there is roentgenographic and clinical evidence of a bony prominence dorsally, medially, and plantarly at the first tarsometatarsal joint (Fig. 41-8). The prominence is painful because of shoe pressure on this articulation. In such circumstances, the therapy of choice would be debridement and excision of the bony prominence with arthrodesis of the first tarsometatarsal joint in the neutral position. No attempt should be made to correct the pronated foot through this articulation.

CLUBFOOT

Although the cause of clubfoot remains obscure, problems related to its treatment are ever present and occur under the best of therapeutic programs. Surgical correction of clubfoot is not simple surgery, particularly with the present-day preference for early surgery, even as early as 6 weeks of age. The dissection must be careful, precise, and performed always with fine instruments, often with magnification. The orthopaedist must realize that these tissues can be attacked safely only once. There is only one

golden opportunity for successful surgery—the first time. The object of treatment is a foot that is plantigrade, serviceable, and relatively symptom free. A corrected clubfoot is not a normal foot, and the child should be followed until the twelfth birthday or skeletal maturity.

The classification of the clubfoot deformity is presented in *Foot Disorders—Medical and Surgical Management.*[12] The surgeon will find therein a well-thought-out plan of attack should correction not be obtained with the usual first-line conservative or surgical procedures. By using the classification, one is better able to decide when to operate and how much to do. Repeat procedures should be kept to an absolute minimum. Goldner very properly points out that the most common error in classifying clubfoot is underestimating the degree and extent of contracture involved.*

Preoperatively, the surgeon is obliged to review the patient's history carefully and to perform a very detailed examination—clinical and roentgenographic—of the foot. In this way only can he determine where previous therapeutic attempts failed, whether they were due to unrecognized muscle imbalance, abnormal muscle insertions, ligamentous structures not released previously, or joints that were not properly aligned to begin with.

Often one can be misled into thinking that correction is being achieved by plaster application, because the foot appears to be correcting properly. Imagine the orthopaedist's chagrin when rapid recurrence of the deformity follows as soon as the foot is left out of plaster. He has difficulty understanding the cause of this recurrence when in reality it is because the midtarsal joints were manipulated rather than the talonavicular and talocalcaneal joints, where the pathology exists. Likewise, in the hindpart of the foot, eversion of the mobile pad of the heel may be obtained, with but minimal improvement through the subtalar joint and with actual external rotation of the calcaneus. Occasionally, a foot is seen that appears to have regained extension when, in reality, a false correction has occurred be-

---

* Goldner, L.J.: Personal communication.

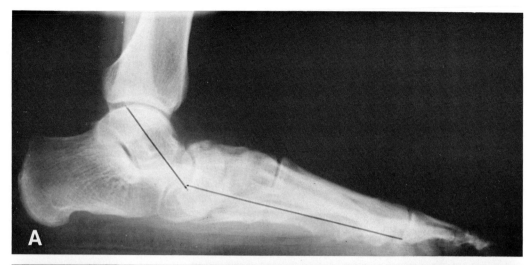

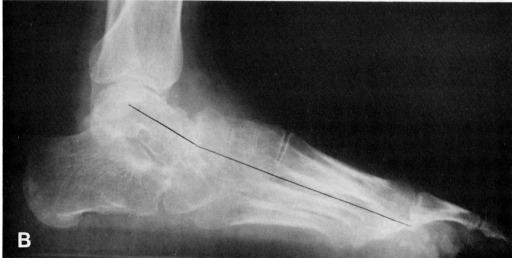

Fig. 41-7. (*A*) Symptomatic flatfoot in a young adult due to unrecognized congenital rigid flatfoot (congenital convex pes valgus). (*B*) Postoperative appearance of the same foot following a Hoke triple arthrodesis. (*C*) Right foot corrected, left foot uncorrected. Note the balance of the right foot.

tween the calcaneus and the midtarsal bone. What appears to be extension is actually motion at the midtarsal joint, the ankle remaining stationary. It is because of problems such as these that Goldner's classification is so useful.[12]

The amount of surgery performed during the first procedure on the clubfoot depends on a number of factors, not the least of which is the experience of the orthopaedic surgeon. If the surgeon is familiar with the clubfoot and the deformity is a mild or moderate one, it may be possible to correct the foot in its entirety in one stage. We feel that correction of the hindpart and midpart of the foot during the first procedure is essential. In this way the talus can be properly positioned in the ankle mortise, and the calcaneus beneath it. This then affords the sound buttress for correcting the tarsometatarsal deformities. The standard operations for correction of the club-

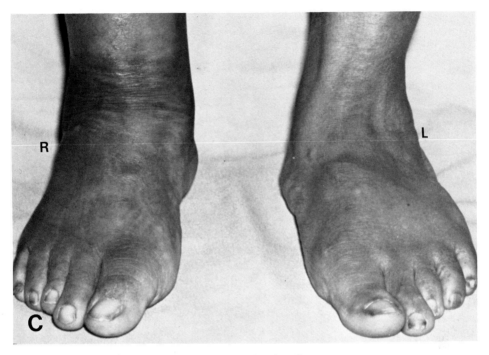

FIG. 41-7. (*Continued*)

foot deformity are available in several texts.[4,6,10,12,19,32,33]

Complications of Clubfoot Surgery

Complications associated with the surgery *per se* are those associated with surgery in orthopaedics in general. However, because of the delicate tissues with which the surgeon deals in this instance, he is obliged to be even more cautious and meticulous than ever. For example, the weight of a large hemostat with a rubber band is enough to damage these tissues. Again, as in other surgery, the tourniquet should be released and all bleeding controlled prior to closure of the soft tissues.

If the skin incision cannot be closed with the foot in the fully corrected position, the skin edges should be carefully repaired, and the foot should be left in a partially corrected position and casted. One week later the cast is removed, and the foot is gently manipulated to achieve as much correction as the skin will allow and then recasted. If another cast change is necessary to effect maximal correction, it should be performed in 5 days. The skin sutures are not removed. In fact, absorbable sutures are recommended, but the suture material should not be catgut. The initial cast should be adequately padded, but not excessively, and if there is any question about the circulation, the cast and padding should be split before the patient leaves the operating room.

Osteonecrosis of the head of the talus or the talar body is not a common complication, although it has been reported, usually in the range of 0.5%. As can be imagined, the complication is much more common with the more severe types of foot disorder, particularly feet in those of Goldner's subgroups 5, 6, 7, and 8.[12] Most authors feel that the complication can be avoided if the surgeon refrains from entering the talocalcaneal joint and the ankle joint simultaneously.

Among the significant complications of talipes equinovarus deformity and its treatment are resistant equinus, rocker-bottom deformity, resistant metatarsus varus, hindfoot varus deformity, and ankle deformity.

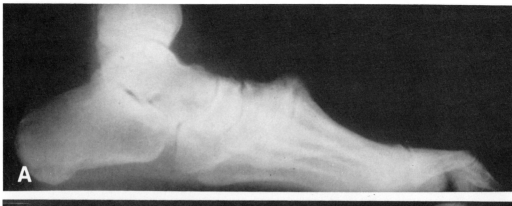

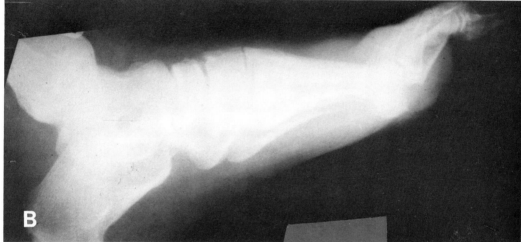

FIG. 41-8. (*A*) Dorsomedial osteophytic prominence of the first tarsometatarsal joint is frequently seen in symptomatic adult flatfeet. (*B*) Postoperative appearance of the same foot following excision of the osteophytic ridge.

Resistant equinus is usually found in the infant whose foot has been corrected except for the equinus deformity. In these cases a lengthening of the calcaneus tendon, with or without posterior ankle capsulotomy, is indicated. Three to 6 months of age is considered to be the optimal time for elective surgery, provided that anesthesia is administered under ideal conditions. Prior to this time, surgical intervention carries an anesthesia risk. Calcaneus tendon lengthening alone is contraindicated when the heel is in fixed varus or rocker-bottom deformity or shows structural alteration of the talus. Cast immobilization should be maintained for a period of at least 3 months postoperatively or after complete correction has been achieved in the less severe types,

with the cast being changed at 4 weeks after surgery and again at 8 weeks. The foot must be kept in a snug, overcorrected position. In Goldner's subgroups 3 and 4, it is recommended that the surgery be performed in two stages unless the surgeon is skilled in clubfoot surgery. The second stage should be carried out not more than 8 weeks after the first stage. Cast immobilization should be maintained for at least 4 to 6 months after the first stage. Under no circumstances should the second stage of the procedure be delayed.

A word of caution regarding complete sectioning of the deltoid ligament: The surgeon must correct the talar position but must not hinge the talus in such a manner as to place the entire hindpart of the foot into valgus position. To do so will lead to a permanent valgus malposition of the hindpart of the foot.

Rocker-bottom deformity can be an iatrogenic complication associated with overzealous manipulation and cast therapy by the orthopaedist. Deformity can be created at the midtarsal or tarsometatarsal joints by attempts to force extension in the presence of a fixed varus deformity of the heel. The varus heel cannot be extended, and, as a result, the extension occurs at either the midtarsal or the tarsometatarsal joints.[32] In the event of a rocker-bottom deformity (Fig. 41-9, *A*), one must first manipulate the foot into a position of flexion and (with lateral roentgenograms) determine whether the deformity has been corrected. The foot is then immobilized in a cast in the equinus position for 6 weeks to allow the tarsometatarsal ligaments to "take up" the slack. Should the heel demonstrate any varus deformity along with the equinus deformity, an incision is made like that for a posteromedial release. Following a tibiotalar capsulotomy and posterior lengthening of the calcaneus tendon, a Kirschner wire is driven through the midportion of the tuberosity of the calcaneus (Fig. 41-9, *B*). Following closure of the incision, downward traction on the wire is applied to correct the equinus position of the calcaneus. If any varus exists, the heel is also manipulated into valgus position. Simultaneously, downward flexion is applied on the midpart and forepart of the foot to correct the rocker-bottom deformity. The varus position of the talus is thus more than adequately corrected. The operator can visualize the exact positions that the various tarsal bones will take. A lateral roentgenogram should be taken at the time of surgery (Fig. 41-9, *C*) and prior to closure of the soft tissues to determine whether all deformity has been corrected. The tourniquet is released. The bleeding is controlled. The soft tissues are closed, the foot is again manipulated into the corrected position, and a plaster cast is applied over adequate padding. The cast should extend from the toes to the knee, with the cast well molded about the heel and the midpart and forepart of the foot and with the wire incorporated in the cast. Immobilization is maintained

for 6 to 8 weeks. Following removal of the cast and wire (Fig. 41-9, *D* and *E*), a walking cast is applied with the foot still held in the corrected position for another 8 weeks.

Resistant Metatarsus Varus. According to Coleman,[4] resistant metatarsus varus is handled best when the hindfoot has already been acceptably corrected. The relationship of the calcaneus and the talus must be correct, or the forefoot procedure will ultimately fail. The most common forefoot deformity is adduction, or varus, either at the midtarsal or tarsometatarsal level. Three types of procedures are designed to achieve correction at this level: metatarsal osteotomy, open wedge osteotomy of the cuneiform bone, and transmetatarsal capsulotomy.

Forefoot correction, when accomplished by metatarsal osteotomy, can be done either by osteotomy of the first metatarsal alone or by osteotomy of all five metatarsals. Coleman has found it rarely necessary to perform more than an open wedge or crescent osteotomy of the first metatarsal. When all five metatarsals require osteotomy to achieve adequate correction, procedures described by Tachdjian[32] or Berman and Gartland[1] can be used after the patient has reached the age of seven years (Fig. 41-10). The surgeon may choose a transverse incision or two longitudinal ones. One longitudinal incision is made between the first and second rays and the other over the fourth ray. Care should be exercised to preserve the superficial veins and the sensory innervation of the dorsum of the foot.

Another procedure that can correct forefoot varus and equinus deformity is that described by Fowler and associates.[11] The (open wedge) osteotomy is made in the medial cuneiform bone and is adjusted to obtain the desired correction. Through a medial incision the abductor hallucis is exposed and a formal radial plantar release is accomplished. The medial cuneiform is exposed subperiosteally and sectioned at its midpoint. The osteotomy is opened as wide as necessary, filled with bone graft (preferably autogenous), and transfixed with a threaded pin that remains in place 6 weeks. After healing, graduated weight bearing is begun, usually in a cast.

The tarsometatarsal capsulotomy de-

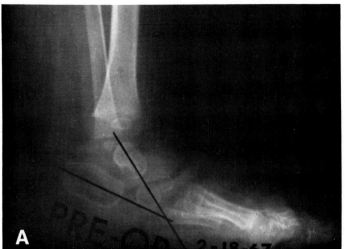

FIG. 41-9. (*A*) Rocker-bottom foot. (*B*) The Kirschner wire is placed through the calcaneus to help correct the rocker bottom. (*C*) Roentgenogram at the time of surgery. (*D* and *E*) Postoperative appearance of the same foot.

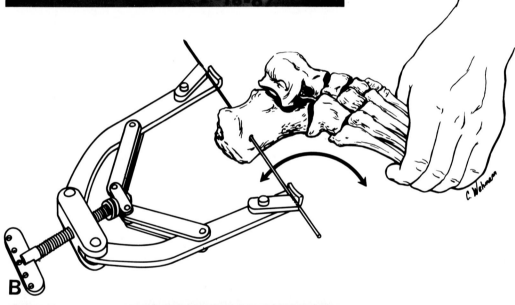

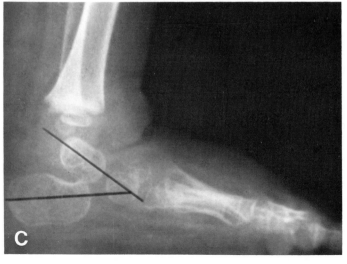

FIG. 41-9. (*Continued*)

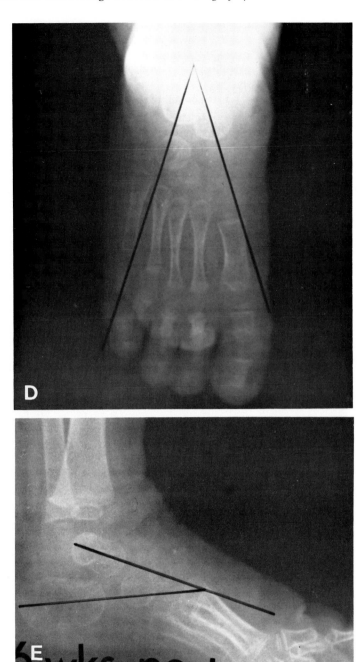

scribed by Herndon and associates[16] was designed to correct residual and resistant adduction of the forefoot. The essence of the procedure is mobilizing the tarsometatarsal joints by severing the tarsometatarsal and intermetatarsal ligaments and joint capsules. The capsular structures must be completely severed dorsally, medially, laterally, and plantarly. It is done through a dorsal transverse incision extending from the base of the first to the base of the fifth. Care must be exercised to preserve the dorsalis pedis artery and vein and cutaneous nerves and veins. It is often necessary to employ internal fixation to maintain correction during the period of immobilization

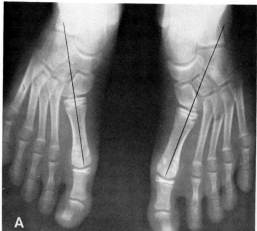

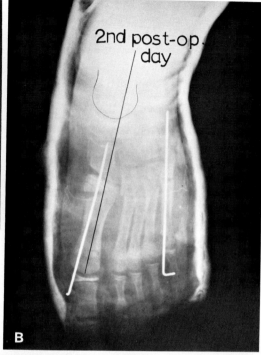

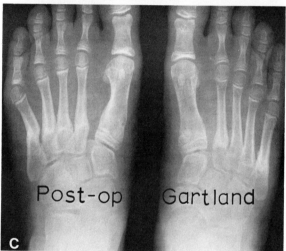

FIG. 41-10. (A) Standing anteroposterior view of metatarsus varus deformity of the forepart of the foot. (B) Immediate postoperative appearance following a Gartland procedure. (C) Same feet 3 months later.

and healing. Corrective casts are maintained for 6 weeks.

Hindfoot varus alignment can be corrected by a lateral displacement osteotomy of the calcaneus.

The varus alignment of the heel can be corrected by a lateral displacement osteotomy of the calcaneus. This procedure does not disturb the relationship of the talocalcaneal and talonavicular joints. Coleman[4] emphasizes that the surgeon should

appreciate that the varus deformity will recur because the osteotomy does not change the direction of growth of the tarsal bones.

The Evans calcaneocuboid arthrodesis has been used for persistent varus deformity of the heel due to "hooking" of the calcaneus.[9] One disadvantage is that one cannot predict the growth of the calcaneus and the cuboid, and therefore one cannot determine the amount of correction possible. The Dwyer[7] operation has also been recommended as a salvage procedure for medial deviation of the calcaneus. However, if the varus deformity of the heel is due to malposition of the articular surface of the talocalcaneal joint, the Dwyer procedure is not as effective as the Evans. Persistent heel deformity and equinus deformity are difficult to correct adequately. If they persist to bone maturity, triple arthrodesis is indicated.

Removal of the talus, or astragalectomy, is a salvage procedure that is used only when all other, less radical procedures have failed to correct the hindfoot deformity. In my personal experience (C.H.E.) astragalectomy has been used only in severe arthrogryposis and myelodysplasia and in one instance of severe scarring due to burns. After removal of the talus it is important to displace the foot posteriorly so that the anterior aspect of the tibia articulates with the navicular and the plafond of the tibia articulates with the superior surface of the calcaneus. The position is maintained by insertion of a Steinmann pin upward through the calcaneus into the tibia.

Triple arthrodesis, described above, is excellent for correction of the residual clubfoot deformities. The result is a serviceable plantigrade foot with retained ankle motion. By employing the Lambrinudi[24] modification, the surgeon can also correct ankle equinus deformity. The major disadvantages are destruction of the hindfoot joints, thus putting more stress on the ankle and the midfoot joints and making the foot slightly smaller.

Ankle Deformity. When the posterior ankle structures are excessively scarred, the foot deformity is not severe enough to justify astragalectomy, and the foot has insufficient skeletal maturity to undergo Lambrinudi triple arthrodesis, closed wedge osteotomy of the distal tibia has been employed. In addition, there is an occasional patient with a significant degree of internal tibial torsion associated with clubfoot. When it can be definitely established both clinically and radiographically that the foot is adequately corrected, the tibial torsion should be corrected. Coleman has performed the procedure at the supramalleolar level of the tibia and higher in the fibula. Threaded transfixion pins are placed above and below the tibial osteotomy site.[4]

The ultimate salvage procedure in the severe uncorrected equinovarus deformity is the Syme amputation. We recommend this procedure only for severe arthrogrypotic clubfoot deformity.

COMPLICATIONS OF TREATMENT OF THE POLIOMYELITIC FOOT

Surgery to correct deformity or to stabilize a paralytic lower extremity requires extremely careful planning, selection of patients and procedures, and timing. Generally, tendon transfers are more successful when bony stabilization of the foot is first carried out. However, there are many instances when the deformity progresses rapidly yet the child's foot is too immature to permit surgery of the osseous structures. In such instances, therefore, tendon transfers are recommended, but they should be delayed until the age of 8 years. Bony procedures should be delayed until the age of 9 to 12 years so as not to disturb bone growth any more than is absolutely necessary. It is to be stressed, however, that each patient's treatment must be individually tailored after very careful analysis of the muscle imbalance of the foot.

A multitude of osseous procedures are described in the literature. The procedures that have the greatest value have been discussed in previous sections and include triple arthrodesis, the Japas procedure,[20] and the Grice-Green operation.[6] The number of tendon transfers encountered in the literature is also numerous. Some of the more common ones are

The Jones suspension procedure for correction of cock-up deformity of the great toe

Dixon and Dively transfers of the extensor hallucis longus to the flexor hallucis longus for cock-up deformity of the great toe

Transplantation of the posterior tibial tendon through the interosseous membrane, combined with transfer of the extensor hallucis longus to the neck of the first metatarsal, with lengthening of the calcaneus tendon for footdrop deformity due to loss of the tibialis anterior muscle

Transfer of both peroneal muscles to the dorsum of the foot, for paralysis of the anterior and posterior tibial muscles

Transfer of the peroneus longus and the tibialis posterior into the calcaneus to correct loss of triceps surae muscle power
Caldwell hemigastrosoleus transfer to the cuneiform for paralyzed foot extensors

It must be kept in mind that the power of the transferred muscle is diminished by a factor of one value by such a procedure. Therefore, a muscle of grade III or lower power should not be used as a transfer to reinforce a weaker muscle. In addition, it is mandatory to have some power in the muscle for which the transfer will be effected. Complications related to these procedures include technical failures in selecting the proper muscle transplant, failures of technique such as skin slough and infection, and finally, improper patient selection. Salvage procedures may include additional tendon transfers and, more commonly, osseous procedures. The pantalar arthrodesis (triple arthrodesis plus tibiotalar arthrodesis) is indicated in the patient with a totally flail foot and ankle.

COMPLICATIONS OF TREATMENT RELATED TO UPPER MOTOR NEURON DISORDERS

The most common disorders of the lower extremity related to cerebrovascular disease are the equinovarus and equinovalgus foot. As in the poliomyelitic foot, the entire trunk must be carefully evaluated, since the disease involves much more than just the terminal aspect of the lower extremity. In this way one can avoid mistaking knee and hip deformities for primary deformities.

Many factors related to the central nervous system can complicate diagnosis and treatment. For example, the overflow phenomenon, in which contraction of one muscle group results from stimulation of another muscle group, may occur. As a result, spasticity may be much worse, particularly when a patient is attempting to perform a task voluntarily. If the patient is examined only at rest and not during voluntary activity, it is quite possible to underestimate the degree of involvement. Furthermore, because of the spasticity present, the results one sees following surgical intervention are not uniform. Other factors

to consider are whether the patient has the necessary intelligence and is capable of cooperating in rehabilitation. Most authors agree that tendon transfers should not be performed in patients who are mentally deficient or unable to cooperate. Surgery in the presence of athetosis is indicated only after extremely careful evaluation of the patient. Surgery may also be indicated for the patient who is wheelchair bound or who cannot be braced. In these cases, cosmesis and custodial care must be considered, but generally speaking, surgery should be reserved for patients who are ambulatory or potentially ambulatory and who have the mental capacity necessary to follow instruction and rehabilitation.

When first-line procedures fail to correct the deformity at hand, the surgeon is left with few alternatives. The triple arthrodesis is the procedure of choice; the only question is, what type of triple should be performed? The standard triple arthrodesis is described above. These patients present a somewhat different problem, however, in that the talus may be fixed in severe equinus. When this is the case, the Lambrinudi triple arthrodesis should be performed. It consists primarily of resection of the anterior dorsal surface of the head of the talus, resection of the anterior portion of the body of the talus and the calcaneus, and upward displacement of the navicular on top of the beak of the talus. Before embarking on a Lambrinudi triple arthrodesis, the inexperienced surgeon is advised to procure a lateral roentgenogram of the foot in the standing position and then make tracings over the talus, calcaneus, navicular, and cuboid. These tracings can be cut out and arranged to simulate the correction that is desired at the operating table. This gives the surgeon a good idea of how much bone must be removed to achieve the desired results.

COMPLICATIONS OF SURGERY OF THE FOREPART OF THE FOOT

HALLUX VALGUS

There are more than 80 bunion procedures currently discussed in the orthopaedic literature.[6,12,13,19,21,22,25,27] Each, undoubtedly, has the potential for complications peculiar to it. It is the purpose of this section, however, to elucidate only the common complications and to present salvage procedures that have been found to be of value. It should be remembered that no single bunion operation is applicable to all bunions at all ages. Selection of the procedure depends on the patient's age, the angle between the first and second metatarsal shafts, and the flexibility of the patient's foot. Each procedure must be further tailored to the problem after careful evaluation of the entire foot, including, of course, the patient's circulatory status. To simply look at a patient's foot and decide on bunion surgery is inadequate preparation for a rather specific procedure. An illustration may be in order: Normally, in a standing anteroposterior roentgenogram of the foot, the angle between the first and second metatarsals is between 8° and 10°, and the angle of the articular surface of the first tarsometatarsal joint with the medial edge of the first cuneiform is between 90° and 105°. The angle between the fourth and fifth metatarsal shafts is between 5° and 8°. In a bunion that is secondary to a splayfoot deformity, the angle between the first and second metatarsals will be upwards of 12°, the angle between the fourth and fifth metatarsals being 10° or more. The angle between the leading edge of the first cuneiform articular surface and the medial cortex is found to be greater than 105°. Obviously, the pathology in this type of bunion is not at the metatarsophalangeal joint; rather, it is a sequela of the angulation found at the tarsometatarsal joints. Surgery directed at the metatarsophalangeal joint would have little hope of success. Figure 41-11 shows the case in point, in which a 17-year-old patient had a splayfoot that went unrecognized. The procedure, a simple bunionectomy, was directed toward the metatarsophalangeal joint, and, of course, the bunion recurred. The lateral displacement of the extensor hallucis brevis and longus must also be evaluated, and bowstringing or displacement is corrected by

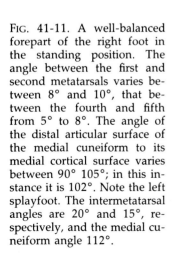

FIG. 41-11. A well-balanced forepart of the right foot in the standing position. The angle between the first and second metatarsals varies between 8° and 10°, that between the fourth and fifth from 5° to 8°. The angle of the distal articular surface of the medial cuneiform to its medial cortical surface varies between 90° 105°; in this instance it is 102°. Note the left splayfoot. The intermetatarsal angles are 20° and 15°, respectively, and the medial cuneiform angle 112°.

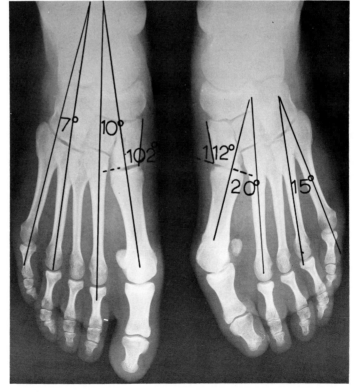

lengthening the longus and tenotomizing the brevis.

The position of the abductor hallucis must be carefully analyzed, since in some patients it will slip plantarward, producing axial rotation of the great toe. Therefore, repositioning of the abductor hallucis is necessary in such cases. The adductor hallucis is frequently contracted and must be tenotomized. The concept of transposing this muscle through or under the first metatarsal shaft and attaching the former to the medial cortex of the latter is fallacious. The adductor hallucis is a rudimentary muscle and does not possess the power to adduct the first metatarsal toward the second. The sesamoids—one or both—should be excised only when symptomatic. The belief that the displaced lateral sesamoid becomes trapped between the first and second metatarsals is unfounded. One has but to look at a cross section of the foot at the capital level to realize that such entrapment is impossible.

Thus, it must be remembered that the bunion deformity is not only the lateral deviation of the great toe on the first metatarsal head, but a combination of deforming factors, all of which must be considered before attempting correction.

General Considerations in Failed Bunion Surgery

When surgery to the great toe has failed to produce the desired result, the operator should carefully investigate the cause of the failure. The worst "solution" is to perform the same procedure, or another one, blithely, without carefully analyzing why the first procedure failed. In our opinion, there are several basic operative procedures that, if carefully evaluated and then performed—with or without some slight modification to fit the particular need or situation—should result in a successful correction of the deformity when initial corrective surgery is attempted. These are Giannestras's modifications of the Lapidus,[12,25] the Silver and Akin procedures,[31] the Mitchell procedure,[5,30] the Keller operation,[12,19] and the chevron operation.[19] Performed carefully, they are successful in a high percentage of patients.

Shortening the first metatarsal to correct a bunion almost invariably either aggravates preexisting metatarsalgia or produces it when it did not previously exist (since, with shortening of the first metatarsal shaft, greater thrust is placed under the second metatarsal head). So further shortening of the first metatarsal by resecting the head to correct previous failure compounds the problem rather than relieving it. Therefore, one axiom of failed bunion surgery is, never shorten the first metatarsal. Preserve all of its length.

Second, one may read that the lateral sesamoid should be excised because it is displaced laterally and is trapped between the first and second metatarsal heads. To begin with, trapping cannot occur; the sesamoid is located plantar to the transverse metatarsal ligament (a very strong structure), which would have to be ruptured before the sesamoid could be trapped. Furthermore, as long as the patient does not complain of pain at the sesamoid-metatarsal joint (and fewer than 1% do) why remove the innocuous, displaced sesamoid? This is unnecessary surgery. Sesamoids should not be removed except when they are symptomatic. If possible, save the first metatarsophalangeal joint while attempting to correct the failure. If, on the other hand, the great toe joint has been destroyed, the only remaining alternative by which the toe can be salvaged—and rendered asymptomatic—is arthrodesis. If arthrodesis is contemplated, the surgeon should make certain that there is at least 5° of flexion motion passively in the interphalangeal joint of the great toe. Furthermore, to achieve the arthrodesis one must resect bone to expose raw surface to raw surface. This will cause further shortening. We prefer to take iliac bone to fill in the defect and regain length in the first ray.

Very often, the bunion will recur because of contracture or lateral displacement of the extensor hallucis longus and brevis tendons at the metatarsophalangeal joint. One can correct much of the deformity in such cases by tenotomizing the brevis and lengthening and repositioning the longus.

Failed surgery of the great toe inevitably leads to complications, which can include circulatory complications with tissue loss, hallux varus, recurrent hallux valgus, hallux hyperextensus, foreign-body reaction to Silastic implants, sesamoid metatarsal malalignment, and metatarsalgia.

In attempting repair of these various complications, one must again take the time to evaluate the deformity carefully and then determine what type of procedure offers the best chances for success. General principles of salvage procedures for failed bunion surgery, before or after, include the following:

The excision of the metatarsal head, as a salvage operation for the failed bunion procedure, is never indicated, nor is it recommended as a primary bunion operation. The correction should be achieved either at the phalanx or through the surrounding soft tissues.

In years past, the Mayo procedure has been used as a primary operation.[28] It became evident that the mechanics of the entire foot were distorted by the loss of the metatarsal head, and as a result the procedure was abandoned.

The metatarsal shaft should not be shortened excessively, either primarily or secondarily, since this inevitably throws more weight on the second metatarsal, resulting in aggravation of a preexisting metatarsalgia or contributing to its development.

CIRCULATORY COMPLICATIONS

We are in complete agreement with Kelikian, who believes that circulatory problems are perhaps the most common complications related to surgery of the foot.[22] Before applying a tourniquet to the lower extremity, one must be certain that the limb can stand the circulatory embarrassment. If the dorsalis pedis and the posterior tibial pulse are not palpable, use of the tourniquet is contraindicated. If surgery is indicated in the face of large- or small-vessel disease, as in diabetics, the surgery should be performed without the tourniquet. Factors that contribute to circulatory insufficiency include the use of local sympathomimetic drugs, overzealous retraction of the soft tissues, too great a correction of the toe, and application of a dressing that is too snug. Figure 41-12 demonstrates what can happen if these precepts are not followed strictly. Generally, in such a situation, one must salvage as much of the toe as possible by covering the area with a split-thickness

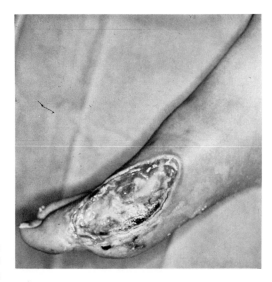

FIG. 41-12. Result of the use of sympathomimetic drugs with local anesthesia for removal of a bunion.

skin graft, later to be covered by a full-thickness graft, depending, of course, on what the patient's particular situation dictates.

HALLUX VARUS

Miller[29] and Hawkins[14] have pointed out that hallux varus deformity may be static or dynamic. The former is the result of initial overcorrection that occurs with the Keller, Silver, Mayo, or other osteotomy procedures (Fig. 41-13). Muscle imbalance is not a feature of this type, and, therefore, malalignment usually corrects itself with time, provided that the capsular structures are not repaired and maintained in the varus position postoperatively. The dynamic deformity, Miller feels, is a result of unopposed abductor hallucis pull following correction of the internal rotation and hallux valgus, with section of the entire conjoint tendon and excision of the lateral sesamoid, so that the abductor is placed in a position that effectively pulls the digit into varus deformity. This is usually a result of the McBride procedure. Hawkins points out that acquired dynamic varus results when the adductor mechanism, consisting of the adductor hallucis and the lateral head of the flexor hallucis brevis, is mistakenly released or tenotomized as a unit.[14] He further

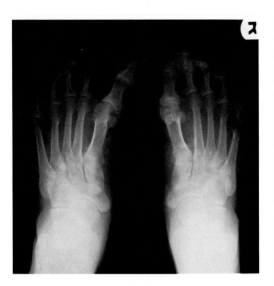

F<small>IG</small>. 41-13. Hallux varus deformity complicating a McBride bunionectomy.

points out that either may be sacrificed alone without producing a varus deformity.

The procedure that Hawkins has described involves excising the scar from the previous bunionectomy, after which a V-shaped incision is made through the capsule, extending into the periosteum along the first metatarsal shaft.[14] This flap is then reflected distally, with its base attached to the phalanx. The medial sesamoid can then be mobilized with its tendon so that it can easily be shifted under the first metatarsal head. The tendon of the abductor hallucis is then separated from the medial sesamoid, as much length being maintained as possible. If necessary, a portion of the tendon of the medial head of the short flexor, along with a strip of periosteum, is taken as the abductor is detached. A second incision is then made between the first and second metatarsal heads. The original surgery is then evaluated to determine whether the capsule has been detached, the adductor hallucis transplanted, or the lateral sesamoid removed, and whether any portion of the conjoint tendon is intact. If possible, any defect in the lateral capsule is repaired, the adductor hallucis tendon then being attached to the stump of the conjoint tendon, which had been previously cut. The abductor hallucis tendon is then drawn through a tunnel between the metatarsal shaft and

the flexor hallucis brevis to the lateral aspect of the first metatarsal. A drill hole is made through the proximal end of the proximal phalanx of the great toe with a small drill. The abductor hallucis tendon is drawn through the drill hole in the proximal phalanx, and the suture, previously placed through the distal end of the abductor hallucis tendon, is tied on the medial aspect of the proximal phalanx. Reinforcing sutures are then placed through the tendon of the abductor hallucis into the remaining lateral capsule of the metatarsophalangeal joint. After closure of the incision, an immobilizing strap is used to maintain the great toe in neutral position or slight abduction. This type of immobilization is then continued for approximately 4 weeks. When using this salvage procedure, the surgeon must forewarn the patient that there will be a further loss of metatarsophalangeal motion.

In a mild hallux varus deformity in a cooperative patient, we have on occasion been able to deal with this complication by taping the overcorrected toe in normal alignment. When such conservative efforts fail—and they usually do—surgical intervention is indicated. Every effort must be made to preserve motion in the first interphalangeal joint whenever possible, particularly if the interphalangeal joint of the great toe has been compromised. However, in certain instances this cannot be accomplished because of the partial or complete resection of the first metatarsal head. In such situations, arthrodesis of the first metatarsophalangeal joint is indicated, provided that there is some passive flexion and extension of the interphalangeal joint of the great toe. If the interphalangeal joint of the great toe is not flexible, a closed wedge osteotomy on the lateral aspect of the proximal phalanx has helped to correct the deformity and at the same time preserve motion at the metatarsophalangeal joint. We have, on occasion, been able to salvage a failed, painful bunion with loss of bone substance, whether from hallux varus or recurrent hallux valgus, by applying skeletal traction to the distal phalanx of the great toe to stretch the tissues and gain as much length and correction as possible. This is accomplished by placing a smooth Kirschner wire transversely through the distal phalanx of the great toe and then applying a distraction force of 3 to 5 pounds of overhead traction for approximately 7 days. Next, very carefully, the pseudarthrotic interspace is dissected open, and an inlay graft of corticocancellous iliac bone is applied. The patient's foot is immobilized in plaster for 12 weeks, bearing no weight for the first 6 (Fig. 41-14). Syndactylizing procedures are used to salvage the adjacent toe deformities.

Kimizuka and Miyanaga[23] reported on five cases of acquired hallux varus after the McBride procedure that were corrected by a combination of lengthening of the extensor hallucis longus tendon, partial proximal phalangectomy of the great toe, and syndactylization between the first and second toes.

RECURRENT HALLUX VALGUS

As noted previously, hallux valgus can occur as a result of improper evaluation of the entire foot. The surgeon should constantly be aware, particularly in young patients, that splaying of the foot may be responsible for a bunion deformity. In these cases, the hallux valgus must be attacked not only at the metatarsophalangeal joint but also in the region of the tarsometatarsal joint. This circumstance would dictate the use of the modified Lapidus[25] procedure or the Giannestras[12] splayfoot operation, depending on the cause of the bunion deformity.

Giannestras's Modification of the Lapidus Procedure

Giannestras's modification of the Lapidus procedure is performed by making a straight longitudinal incision along the medial aspect of the great toe, beginning from the level of the proximal phalanx and extending proximally almost to the naviculocuneiform joint (Fig. 41-15, *A*). The subcutaneous veins are ligated, and the medial cutaneous nerve, frequently seen in the wound, is identified and retracted safely out of the way. The bursa over the bunion is automatically opened, and further dissection is carried out proximally in the same plane. The fascia covering the abductor hallucis muscles is incised longitudinally, just below its insertion along the first metatarsal shaft. The

muscular belly of the abductor hallucis is identified and carefully dissected. Its loose connection to the first metatarsal shaft may easily be separated by blunt dissection. As a rule, the abductor hallucis is found displaced plantarward, blending with the medial belly of the flexor hallucis brevis and acting as a plantar *flexor* of the great toe rather than its abductor. These muscles are gently separated from one another. After the slender tendon of the abductor hallucis has been identified, it is carefully separated from the capsule of the metatarsophalangeal joint, down to its insertion into the base of the proximal phalanx, care being taken not to sever this tendon or to open the joint capsule. The tendon is retracted plantarward, and a V-shaped flap is made in the medial capsule, with its base attached to the proximal phalanx. This flap is usually 2 cm to 3 cm long and 1 cm wide at its base, tapering proximally to the neck and shaft of the first metatarsal. The capsular flap is reflected distally, care being taken to dissect it from the medial aspect of the first metatarsal head, thus preserving its full thickness. The dissection should begin at the metatarsophalangeal joint and extend proximally. The neck of the metatarsal is exposed. The joint is exposed by reflecting the flap distally. The sagittal groove is observed. It runs in a dorsoplantar direction, separating the normal lateral articular cartilaginous surface that remains in contact with the laterally subluxated proximal phalanx from the fibrous degenerated cartilage on the medial part of the head. In cases in which the bunion deformity is severe and long-standing, this groove may be quite deep. The exostosis of the first metatarsal head is excised. The portion removed should include the sagittal groove and the exostosis but none of the normal cartilaginous surface of the head. As a result of this resection, the medial part of the head is in the same plane and is continuous with the cortex of the neck and shaft of the metatarsal. Occasionally, there may be a dorsal prominence on the dorsomedial edge of the first metatarsal head. This too must be excised. When resecting the medial part of the first metatarsal head, only the bone medial to the lateral edge of the sagittal groove is removed. Care should be taken to preserve

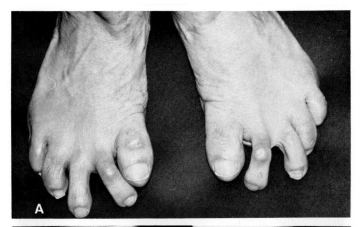

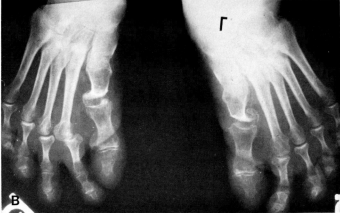

FIG. 41-14. (*A*) Appearance following four different procedures for the correction of bunions. (*B*) Roentgenogram of the same feet. Note the surgical loss of the distal half of each metatarsal, as well as the dislocation of the second metatarsophalangeal joint of each foot. (*C*) After 1 week of traction of the great toe, a substantial portion of the length was regained. (*D*) Postoperative appearance of the left foot following arthrodesis of the great toe and syndactylization of the second toe to the third. (*E*) Postoperative roentgenographic appearance of the same foot.

the rounded shape of the first metatarsal, especially the part covered with normal cartilage (Fig. 41-15, *B*).

Through a 4-cm to 5-cm incision located between the first and second metatarsal heads, the transverse metatarsal ligament is identified and sectioned. The spreader-retractor is inserted, and the adductor hallucis is exposed (Fig. 41-15, *C*). The conjoint tendon is carefully delineated and tenotomized. In addition, if necessary, the lateral capsule is cut transversely to permit correction of the valgus deviation of the great toe. The V-shaped flap of the capsule is next sutured to the fascia, with the toe held in not more than 5° of overcorrection. The plantar and dorsal capsular incisions are similarly closed with several 2-0 chromic catgut sutures, or whatever suitable suture material is preferred. The abductor hallucis belly, together with its tendon, is shifted medially, running now along the medial aspect of the first metatarsal head and neck

instead of plantar to it (Fig. 41-15, *D*). Its action as an abductor is reestablished. The capsular closure should be performed carefully and judiciously. The redundant capsule along both sides of the flap should be excised. The capsule should not be sutured so tight as to cause limitation of motion or overcorrection of the great toe at a later date. A good balance between adduction and abduction, as well as extension and flexion, should be created. If the procedure is carried out adequately, the great toe remains well corrected without any external support.

Next, the metatarsal shaft is grasped with a small Lane bone-holding clamp and derotated, thus correcting the axial rotation of the metatarsal and great toe. With this maneuver the toenail should then face in the proper direction. A sterile gauze bandage is applied tightly across the midmetatarsal region, compressing the forepart of the foot and correcting the varus deviation

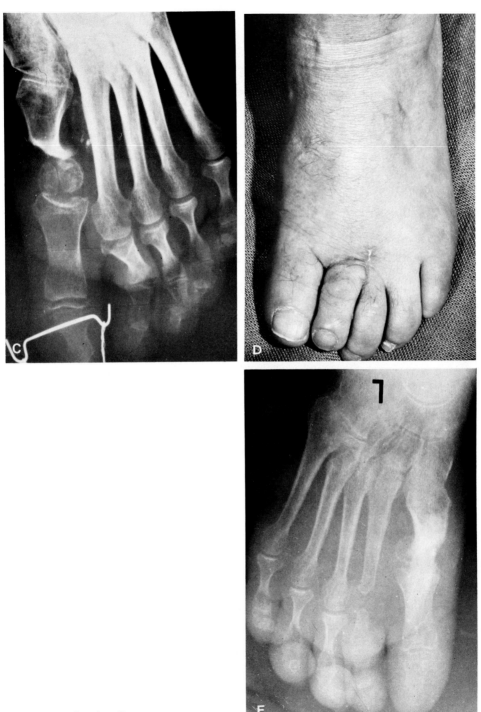

FIG. 41-14. (Continued)

of the first metatarsal. A threaded Kirschner wire, 0.2 cm in diameter, is then driven transversely through the neck of the first metatarsal into and across the shaft of the second metatarsal to maintain the correction. This step plays a dual role. It maintains the correction of the deviation and rotation of the first metatarsal and stabilizes the

(Text continues on page 1278.)

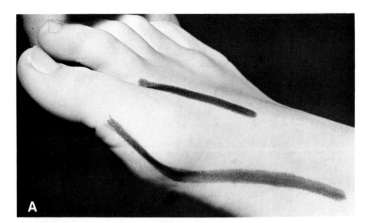

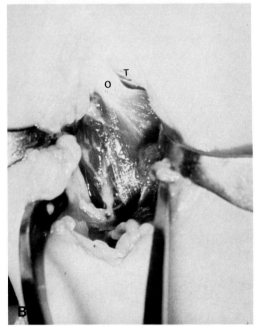

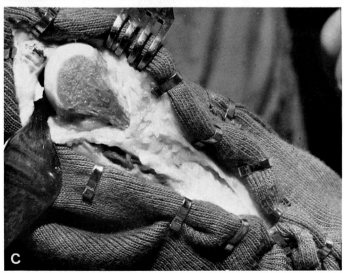

FIG. 41-15. (*A*) Note the shorter incisions (usually 4 cm) between the first and second metatarsal heads to expose the adductor hallucis. A medial incision was made along the first ray from the level of the first metatarsal joint to the middle of the proximal phalanx of the great toe. (*B*) Note the excellent delineation of tendon and the excellent exposure with the use of the previously described spreader. *O*, oblique head of the adductor hallucis; *T*, transverse head of the adductor hallucis. (*C*) The medial bony prominence is excised. The raw bone surface is covered with bone wax to inhibit bleeding and additional bone formation. (*D*) The capsule is closed, and the abductor hallucis tendon (*AH*) is sutured to the medial capsular surface. (*E*) Arthrodesis of the first tarsometatarsal joint with a bone wedge developed from the medial prominence. (*F*) Preoperative appearance of both feet. (*G*) Appearance 15 months later.

FIG. 41-15. (*Continued*)

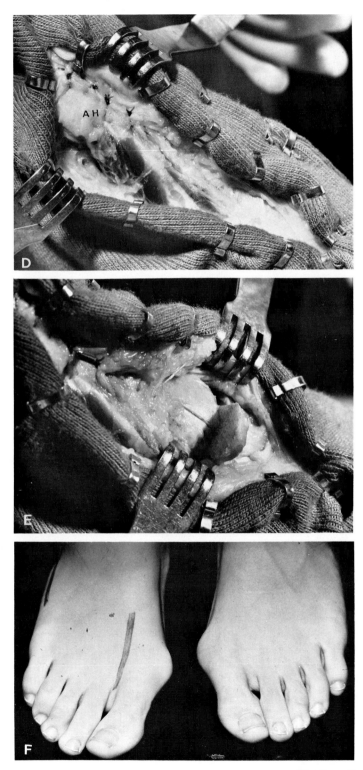

(*Continued*)

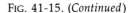

FIG. 41-15. (*Continued*)

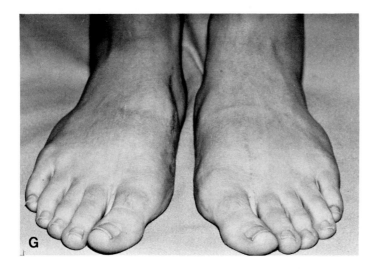

shaft so that resection of the articular cartilage and arthrodesis of the first cuneiform-metatarsal joint are much easier.

The cuneiform-metatarsal joint is approached next. The capsule is reflected from the dorsal, medial, and plantar sides of the articulation and severed transversely on the lateral side. This joint opens automatically. The articular cartilage at the first tarsometatarsal joint is completely excised, care being taken not to injure the metatarsal epiphysis should it be open and active. The previously excised exostosis is then carefully shaped into a wedge and is used to fill the defect created by excision of the cartilage (Fig. 41-15, *E*). After it has been driven into position, the capsule is closed. The circular gauze bandage is released. The Kirschner wire is cut, but the end is left long enough so that it can protrude through a stab wound in the skin.

The length of the extensor hallucis longus and brevis tendons is then carefully inspected with the great toe in full flexion. If they appear to be bow-strung or short, the longus tendon should be lengthened and replaced in its proper position. The extensor hallucis brevis should be concomitantly tenotomized. No subcutaneous sutures are applied. The skin incisions are closed with care. The tourniquet is released and all bleeding controlled. A firm—but not snug—pressure dressing is applied with the great toe held in minimal varus position (not more than 5°). This dressing is left in place for 1 week; at that point it is changed, and

a walking cast is applied. The cast is applied snugly, with the great toe held in minimal, if any, varus position and neutral or slight flexion by wrapping one or two turns of plaster of paris about it and by extending the cast from the tips of the toes to the tibial tubercle. Cast immobilization is maintained for 6 weeks after the operation. On removal of the cast, the sutures and the Kirschner wire are removed. Active weight bearing with crutches is then instituted. No running or jumping is permitted for at least 3 months after the operation. Elastic stockings and loosely fitted sandals are worn for the first 2 to 3 weeks. The patient is then encouraged to wear his regular shoes but with the continued use of an elastic stocking, as long as any foot edema persists. The crutches are discarded at the patient's discretion (Fig. 41-15, *F* and *G*). In adult patients, in whom the first metatarsal epiphysis is closed, an open wedge osteotomy at the base of the first metatarsal is preferred over arthrodesis of the first tarsometatarsal joint.

Butson[3] has reported on a modification of the Lapidus procedure very similar to that of Giannestras, with which 119 operations were performed in 78 patients. Follow-up was between 2 and 16 years, and good or excellent results were reported in 92%.

The Giannestras Splayfoot Operation

The Giannestras splayfoot operation is based in part on the author's modification of the Silver operation.[31] It is performed by making a medial longitudinal incision, beginning at the midshaft level of the proximal phalanx and extending proximally along the medial aspect of the first metatarsal shaft to its base. The skin and subcutaneous fat are carefully reflected, both dorsally and plantarly, to expose the dorsomedial and plantar medial portion of the capsule of the first metatarsophalangeal joint. A second incision, 3 cm to 5 cm in length, is then made on the dorsum of the foot, beginning at the level of the interdigital space between the first and second metatarsal heads. Traction is applied to the corresponding metatarsal necks. The transverse metatarsal ligament is exposed and sectioned transversely. The spreader is applied, and the first and second metatarsal heads are separated. The adductor hallucis communis tendinous insertion is exposed and carefully dissected, and the common tendon is then severed. Next, the medial capsule of the first metatarsophalangeal joint is approached. A V-shaped incision is then made, with the arms of the V beginning at the base of the proximal phalanx. They join 2 cm to 2.5 cm farther down, over the midmedial aspect of the neck of the first metatarsal. The capsule is carefully reflected distally to form a flap of tissue. The medial prominence and the sagittal groove, but none of the metatarsal head adjoining the groove, are removed in the usual manner. The sharp edges of the metatarsal head and neck are smoothed off. The toe is then placed in no more than 5° varus position. The proximal end of the capsular flap is sutured back with 2-0 chromic sutures to the surrounding tissues at a more proximal level so as to maintain the great toe in the minimal varus position. The toe should be carefully placed in neutral position as regards flexion and extension before the plantar and dorsal capsular sutures are placed to secure the flap in the new position. Next, the abductor hallucis is inspected. If it has slipped to the plantar surface of the first metatarsophalangeal joint, it is freed up to the level of its insertion. The musculotendinous junction is brought up to its normal position and sutured to the capsule at the level of the metatarsal neck, thus helping to correct any minimal axial rotation of the great toe. The transposed tendon acts as a tether. One

may wonder about the function of the abductor hallucis following this tendon transposition. With this step, the abductor is prevented from sliding under the metatarsal head and acting as a deforming factor. In its normal position in the adult it has but slight active function.

Next, after making a direct lateral incision over the metatarsophalangeal joint of the fifth ray, the fifth metatarsal bunionette is excised. The subcutaneous tissue and the capsule can be reflected in one unit. The exostosis is then removed, just as in the removal of the medial prominence of the great toe. Both exostoses are preserved in a moist saline dressing.

The next step consists of compressing the forepart of the foot at the midmetatarsal level as strongly as possible with sterile gauze. Any axial deviation of the great toe should be corrected at this time. A heavy, threaded, 2.38-mm Kirschner wire is then driven carefully through the neck of the fifth metatarsal, via the lateral incision, transversely across the forepart of the foot and plantar to the fourth, third, and second metatarsals, to exit through the medial cortex of the neck of the first metatarsal. A guide is used in inserting the Kirschner wire. The wire thus holds the metatarsals in the desired corrected position. The compression bandage is removed. Roentgenograms should be procured to make certain that the proper correction has been achieved. The leading end of the wire is cut just beyond the edge of the medial cortex of the first metatarsal. The proximal end of the wire is allowed to protrude slightly beyond the skin surface laterally through a stab wound. The excess is cut off. Just enough of the wire is allowed to protrude to facilitate its removal after 6 weeks. The operator should not use a power tool to drive in the wire.

The splaying of the first and fifth metatarsals having been overcome, a transverse open wedge osteotomy is performed at the base of the respective metatarsals. The osteotomy should be opened as much as possible, and the defect thus created is filled with bone wedges derived from the previously excised bony prominence. They are firmly impacted into place. The tourniquet is released and bleeding controlled. The three skin incisions are closed with nylon sutures. A firm dressing is applied. On the seventh postoperative day the dressing is changed, and if the incisions are healing well, a short-leg, below-knee walking cast is applied. This cast should be particularly snug about the forepart of the foot. Only a minimal amount of padding should be used. Felt should be placed on each side of the Kirschner wire to prevent pressure on the wire. At the end of 6 weeks, the cast, the Kirschner wire, and the sutures are removed.

If, by some happenstance, on roentgen-ographic examination the osteotomy sites are not healed, another snug cast is applied for 3 to 4 weeks. The patient is instructed in proper heel-to-toe gait following cast removal. Although the feet will be somewhat edematous following this step, the swelling can be controlled by elastic stockings.[12] Figure 41-16 shows the preoperative and postoperative appearance of a left splayfoot that had previously been corrected by simple bunionectomy; hence, the cause of the original deformity had not been carefully analyzed. As a result, the bunion

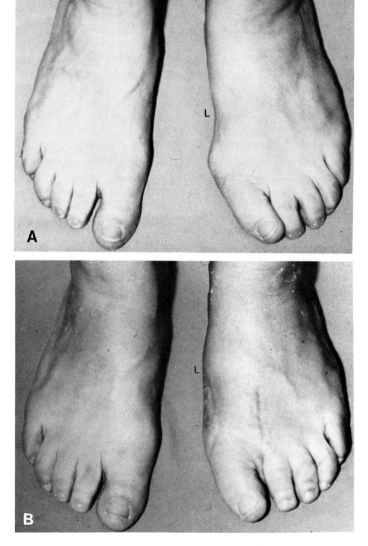

Fig. 41-16. (*A*) Preoperative appearance of left splayfoot. (*B*) Postoperative appearance of the same foot 1 year later.

recurred, and this procedure had to be repeated.

In the older patient in whom bunion surgery has been unsuccessful, it may be possible to obtain a good result using the modified Akin procedure (Fig. 41-17). The incision begins on the lateral side of the great toe and the first metatarsal. The dorsal, lateral, and plantar surfaces of the proximal two thirds of the proximal phalanx are then exposed. A wedge of bone is removed with the base located laterally. This can be performed with a narrow, practically needle-nosed rongeur and should be done approximately 1 cm distal to the metatarsophalangeal joint. The osteotomy is carried up to, but not through, the medial cortex of the phalanx. Under direct visualization, a smooth Kirschner wire is inserted through the distal phalanx and the distal portion of the proximal phalanx. The lateral cortex is broken in a greenstick fracture to realign the great toe in relation to the first metatarsal and to the foot in general. Any axial rotation of the great toe can also be corrected. The osteotomy is then closed, and the wire is driven into the proximal fragment, care being taken not to drive it into the metatarsal head. A Kocher clamp is applied to the wire at its point of exit at the tip of the great toe. The wire is then bent to a right angle just beyond the clamp and cut off, leaving a small stub of the wire just beyond the right-angle bend. This prevents migration of the wire into the toe. At this point the tourniquet is released as usual, and bleeding is controlled. The capsule and skin are then closed, as has been

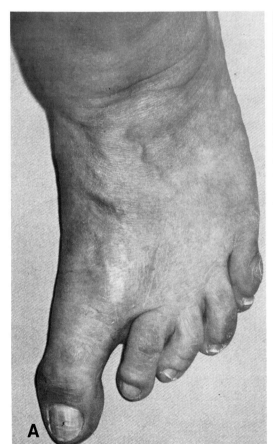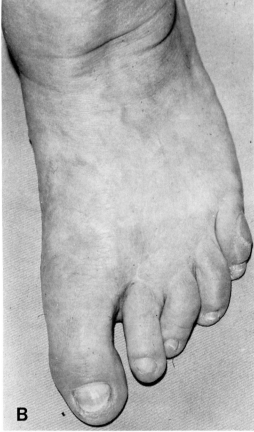

FIG. 41-17. (*A*) A failed McBride procedure with a hallux varus deformity. (*B*) Postoperative appearance of the same foot following lateral closed wedge osteotomy of the proximal phalanx.

described previously. Again, the toe is held in neutral or slight valgus position, and the dressing is not disturbed until the fifth postoperative day, unless there is some contraindication. On the fourth or fifth postoperative day the patient is encouraged to walk in a thong-type sandal or a wooden-soled canvas shoe.

Bishop and colleagues[2] reported on 116 splayfoot operations performed in 72 patients who were followed between 1 and 12 years. Results in 78% of the procedures were good or excellent, while 14% were fair and 8% judged as poor. The poor results (nine feet) were all a result of failures of the osteotomy. Two had infected nonunions, and the remainder had collapse of the bone graft, with recurrence of varus angulation of the first metatarsal. All of these required salvage procedures to correct deformity. Five feet were treated by Akin bunionectomy; the Keller procedure was used in four.

HALLUX HYPEREXTENSUS

Hallux hyperextensus is usually associated with a hallux varus. It is most commonly associated with Keller's bunionectomy. It is likely a result of injury or laceration of the flexor hallucis longus at its insertion into the distal phalanx or to failure of maintenance of the intrinsic muscle insertion. Correction by a soft tissue procedure is occasionally possible in this deformity but is not recommended. This is accomplished by lengthening the long toe extensors and tenotomizing the short extensors. When the deformity is long-standing, the only solution is arthrodesis of the metatarsophalangeal joint.

FOREIGN-BODY REACTION TO SILASTIC IMPLANTS

Swanson has developed a Silastic spacer to be used when performing the Keller procedure. With this spacer it is possible to maintain length of the great toe while preserving painless motion. However, on rare occasions, a patient may develop a foreign-body reaction to this spacer, which then must be removed (Fig. 41-18). Following its removal, the reactive tissues should be cultured and then curetted out. The soft tissue should be closed loosely. The patient

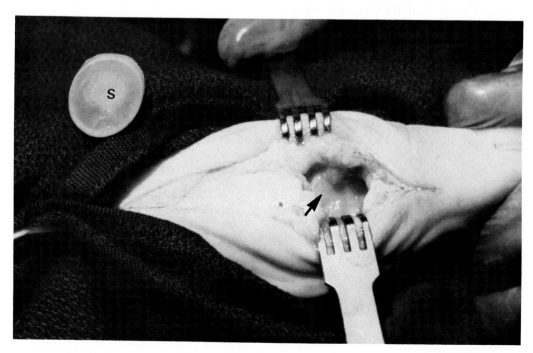

Fig. 41-18. Foreign-body synovitis (*arrow*) due to a Silastic great-toe implant. (*S*, Silastic implant.) There is no evidence of implant failure.

should be placed on a broad-spectrum antibiotic until the report of the culture is received. Should it be negative, the antibiotic can be discontinued. Should the culture be positive, appropriate steps should then be taken to control the infection with antibiotics.

METATARSALGIA

As mentioned previously, metatarsalgia as a result of osteotomy or decapitation of the first metatarsal bone occurs very frequently. There is seldom an indication for osteotomy of the first metatarsal head or neck. When this is done, the remaining metatarsals are placed under abnormal

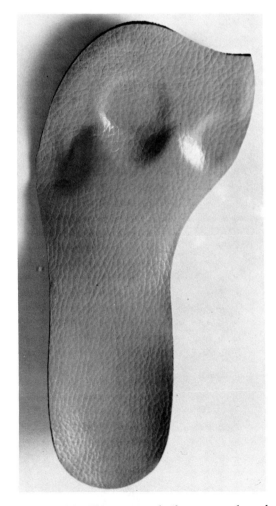

FIG. 41-19. This custom-built comma-shaped metatarsal pad is designed to relieve pressure under the third metatarsal head.

stress, and, almost always, the result is pain under the second and third metatarsal heads.[34] Likewise, osteotomy of the metatarsal, like that described for the Mitchell procedure,[30] can result in dorsal tilt of the distal fragment. The effect is quite similar to that discussed above in that there is abnormal weight bearing in the forepart of the foot, just as if the distal aspect of the metatarsal had been removed. If at all possible in such situations, the treatment should be conservative management with a properly constructed comma-shaped metatarsal pad (Fig. 41-19), to distribute the weight evenly under all of the metatarsal heads. In a fair number of patients, however, conservative management fails because of the development of extremely painful plantar keratoses under the second and/or third metatarsal heads. Resection of the offending metatarsal head is mentioned only to decry its use. We recommend correction of the hammer-toe deformity, which frequently accompanies this problem, along with shortening of the second metatarsal shaft at its base and, if necessary, of the third metatarsal shaft as well. Cast immobilization is unnecessary. The patient should be permitted to walk and to bear full weight as soon as he comfortably can. The patient should be fitted with a wooden-soled canvas shoe.

OTHER PROBLEMS OF THE FOREPART OF THE FOOT

Floppy Toe Syndrome

Resection of the proximal phalanx is a procedure used by some to correct hammer-toe deformities. When performed on the proximal phalanx of the fifth toe, it presents a problem, particularly for women, because the toe catches on sheer hose. Treatment consists of placing a Kirschner wire through the distal aspect of the distal phalanx and applying traction. This pulls the toe into proper alignment, and some of its length is reestablished (Fig. 41-20). After 5 days' traction, syndactylization can then be carried out. Kelikian's technique of syndactylization is applicable in this situation.[22] It is a precise procedure and, if carefully and properly performed, gives excellent results. Performed poorly, it invariably results in additional deformity.

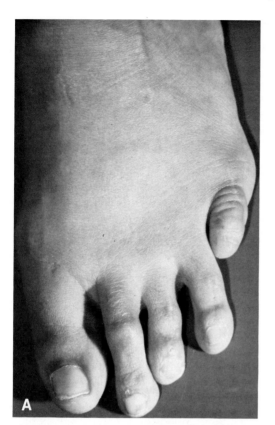

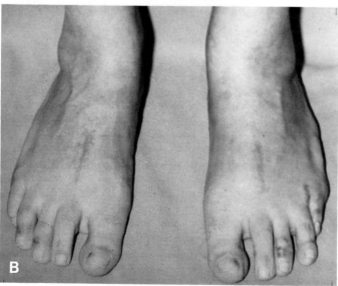

FIG. 41-20. (*A*) Floppy fifth toe following resection of the proximal phalanx to overcome hammer-toe deformity. (*B*) Appearance of the same toe 6 months following syndactylization of the fifth toe to the fourth. Note the gain in length.

Recurrent Hammer-Toe Deformity

Often a patient may have undergone surgery for the correction of hammer-toe deformity with an unsuccessful result. This happens if the surgeon did not carefully study the deforming factors producing the hammer toe and performed only arthrodesis of the proximal interphalangeal joint or resection of the proximal half of the proximal phalanx without taking into consideration any contractures produced by the surrounding soft tissues. Alternately, arthrodesis of the proximal interphalangeal joint may have been carried out, the dislocation of the metatarsophalangeal joint having been either disregarded or "reduced" and realigned by inserting the Kirschner wire through the toe and into the head of the metatarsal. Such a procedure inevitably fails. If the metatarsophalangeal joint is subluxated or dislocated, any attempt at reduction will fail. Furthermore, one will find that the second and/or third toe is now so displaced that it is not in contact with the floor, and the patient's symptoms are worse than they were preoperatively. What to do? Careful evaluation will disclose that the toe is again dislocated in relation to the metatarsal head. The long toe extensors are contracted, as are the capsular structures around the head, and the toe is displaced dorsally. Resection of the metatarsal head will not solve the problem. In fact, it will compound it. The metatarsal heads can be resected for only one indication: disease and deformity, as in rheumatoid arthritis. Complete resection of a normal metatarsal head should never be used to correct a hammer-toe deformity. Such an operation disturbs the weight-bearing mechanics of the forepart of the foot. The salvage procedure of choice is syndactylization to the adjacent normal toe after reestablishing the length of the deformed toe by careful tenotomy of the extensor tendons and complete capsulotomy. The proximal phalanx of the normal toe must not be resected. A Kirschner wire should be driven through the deformed toe and into the head of the metatarsal to maintain alignment, after which syndactylization, as recommended by Kelikian,[22] should be carried out.

Recurrent Symptoms Following Excision of the Plantar Digital Nerves

The vast majority of patients with recurrent symptoms following excision of the plantar digital nerves have had inadequate surgery. *"Office incisions" are to be condemned.* It is inconceivable that proper exposure can be obtained through a 1-cm incision. Many patients who have had this

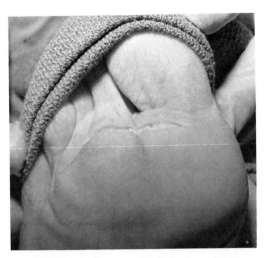

FIG. 41-21. A transverse plantar incision just proximal to the transverse plantar crease permits better exploration of the metatarsal interspaces. The incision is also distal to the metatarsophalangeal joints and avoids the problem of scar formation and pain on weight bearing.

type of incision for the removal of a neuroma have experienced recurrent symptoms. On reexploration of the interspace, one usually finds a neuroma. Occasionally a patient will have metatarsal pain and recurrence of the symptoms of plantar digital neuroma following adequate exploration of the third and fourth interspaces for the plantar digital neuroma. In such instances, reexploration is, of course, indicated. A plantar incision is used (Fig. 41-21), which allows better exploration of the foot. In some instances there is recurrence of the neuroma at the amputation stump and thus recurrence of the symptoms because the nerve had not been sectioned as far proximally as it should have been on the initial surgery (Fig. 41-22). In other instances the resected end of the plantar digital nerve is adherent to one of the metatarsal heads. It must be remembered that referred pain may be the cause of the discomfort. Both neuroma in an adjoining interspace and nerve entrapment have been seen to be the offender in such cases. Entrapment of the medial or lateral plantar nerves can occur in the midplantar region of the foot. A more common finding is a tarsal tunnel syndrome, with entrapment of the posterior

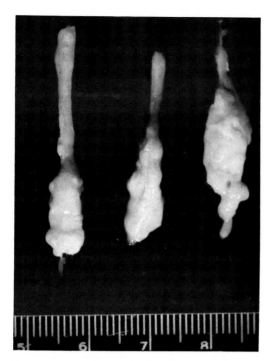

FIG. 41-22. Recurrent amputation neuromas followed resection of symptomatic plantar digital nerves. These can best be removed through a transverse plantar incision.

tibial nerve. These entrapments can be treated conservatively with one or two corticosteroid injections about, but not into, the nerve, with moderate success. However, when this fails and there is evidence of delayed nerve conduction time, decompression is indicated.

Proper Digital Nerve Syndrome

Following bunionectomy or other trauma to the medial aspect of the first ray, patients occasionally develop excruciating pain on the plantar medial aspect of the first metatarsal, just proximal to the head. Discomfort at the site of the surgical incision or at the site of trauma, with hyperesthesia or hypoesthesia and a positive Tinel's sign, is the usual presenting complaint. With post-bunionectomy pain in the metatarsophalangeal joint that is relieved by the injection of 1 ml to 2 ml of lidocaine (Xylocaine) into the proper digital nerve, one should

suspect entrapment of this nerve as the likely cause of the discomfort. Neurolysis or excision of the proper digital nerve is the procedure of choice in these instances.

REFERENCES

1. Berman, A., and Gartland, J.J.: Metatarsal osteotomy for the correction of adduction of the forepart of the foot in children. J. Bone Joint Surg., 53A: 501, 1971.
2. Bishop, J., Kahn, A., and Turba, J.: Surgical correction of the splayfoot: The Giannestras procedure. Clin. Orthop. Rel. Res., 146:234, 1980.
3. Butson, A.R.C.: A modification of the Lapidus operation for hallux valgus. J. Bone Joint Surg., 62B:350, 1980.
4. Coleman, S.S.: Complex Foot Deformities in Children. Philadelphia, Lea & Febiger, 1983.
5. Corless, J.R.: A modification of the Mitchell procedure (abstr.) J. Bone Joint Surg., 58B:138, 1976.
6. Crenshaw, A.H.: Campbell's Operative Orthopaedics. St. Louis, C.V. Mosby, 1971.
7. Dwyer, F.C.: The treatment of relapsed clubfoot by the insertion of a wedge into the calcaneum. J. Bone Joint Surg., 45B:67, 1963.
8. Epps, C.H., Jr.: Amputation of the lower limb. In Evarts, C.McC. (ed.): Surgery of the Musculoskeletal System. New York, Churchill Livingstone, 1983.
9. Evans, D.: Relapsed clubfoot. J. Bone Joint Surg., 43B:722, 1961.
10. Evarts, C.McC., (ed.): Surgery of the Musculoskeletal System, Section 9: The Foot. New York, Churchill Livingstone, 1983.
11. Fowler, S.B., Brooks, A.L., and Parrish, T.F.: The cavovarus foot. Proc. A.A.O.S., J. Bone Joint Surg., 41A:757, 1959.
12. Giannestras, N.J.: Foot Disorders—Medical and Surgical Management. Philadelphia, Lea & Febiger, 1973.
13. Gibson, J., and Piggott, H.: Osteotomy of the neck of the first metatarsal and treatment of hallux valgus. J. Bone Joint Surg., 44:349, 1962.
14. Hawkins, F.B.: Acquired hallux varus: Cause, prevention and correction. Clin. Orthop., 76:169, 1971.
15. Herndon, C.H., and Heyman, C.H.: Congenital convex pes valgus. J. Bone Joint Surg., 45A:413, 1963.
16. Herndon, C.H., Heyman, C.H., and Strong, J.M.: Mobilization of tarsometatarsal and intermetatarsal joints for the correction of resistant adduction. J. Bone Joint Surg., 40A:299, 1958.
17. Hoke, M.: An operation for stabilizing paralytic feet. J. Orthop. Surg., 3:494, 1921.
18. ———: An operation for the correction of extremely relaxed flatfeet. J. Bone Joint Surg., 13: 773, 1931.
19. Jahss, M.H., (ed.): Disorders of the Foot. Philadelphia, W.B. Saunders, 1982.

20. Japas, L.M.: Surgical treatment of pes cavus by tarsal V-osteotomy. J. Bone Joint Surg., 58A:827, 1968.

21. Joplin, R.J.: The proper digital nerve, vitallium stem arthroplasty, and some thoughts about foot surgery in general. Clin. Orthop., 76:199, 1971.

22. Kelikian, H.: Hallux Valgus, Allied Deformities of the Forefoot and Metatarsalgia. Philadelphia, W.B. Saunders, 1965.

23. Kimizuka, M., and Miyanaga, Y.: The treatment of acquired hallux varus after the McBride procedure. J. Foot Surg., 19:135, 1980.

24. Lambrinudi, C.: A method of correcting equinus and calcaneus deformities at the sub-astragaloid joint. Proc. R. Soc. Med., 26:788, 1933.

25. Lapidus, P.W.: Author's bunion operation from 1931 to 1959. Clin. Orthop., 16:119, 1960.

26. Levon, M.E., and O'Neal, L.W., (eds.): The Diabetic Foot. St. Louis, C.V. Mosby, 1977.

27. McKeever, D.C.: Arthrodesis of the first metatarsophalangeal joint for hallux valgus, hallux rigidus, and metatarsus primus varus. J. Bone Joint Surg., 344A:129, 1952.

28. Mayo, C.H.: The surgical treatment of bunions. Ann. Surg., 48:300, 1908.

29. Miller, J.W.: Acquired hallux varus: A preventable and correctable disorder. J. Bone Joint Surg., 57A(8): 183, 1975.

30. Mitchell, C.L., Fleming, J.L., Allan, R. et al.: Osteotomy bunionectomy for hallux valgus. J. Bone Joint Surg., 40A:41, 1958.

31. Silver, D.: The operative treatment of hallux valgus. J. Bone Joint Surg., 5A:225, 1923.

32. Tachdjian, M.O.: Pediatric Orthopaedics. Philadelphia, W.B. Saunders, 1972.

33. Turco, V.J.: Clubfoot. New York, Churchill Livingstone, 1981.

34. Viladot, A.: Metatarsalgia due to biomechanical alterations of the forefoot. Orthop. Clin. North Am., 4:165, 1973.

42 Complications of Arthrodesis Surgery

Peter G. Carnesale and Marcus J. Stewart

Arthrodesis of major peripheral joints is performed infrequently; however, certain conditions, such as joints destroyed by infection and many failed arthroplasties, are still best treated by fusion. It is important for surgeons to know the complications that may be encountered and their preoperative and postoperative management; the knowledge of such complications may also help prevent them.

COMPLICATIONS OF ARTHRODESIS OF THE HIP

INTRAOPERATIVE COMPLICATIONS

Complications of Anesthesia

Arthrodesis of the hip is an extensive operation, usually requiring endotracheal anesthesia and careful attention to fluid and blood replacement. Unusual anesthetic problems, such as malignant hyperthermia and prolonged respiratory hypoventilation following succinylcholine administration and due to pseudocholinesterase deficiency, have occurred. Careful preoperative evaluation of patients undergoing such extensive surgery is required. Acute adrenocorticosteroid insufficiency with attendant vascular collapse may occur when patients on long-term corticosteroid therapy are subjected to general anesthesia without corticosteroid supplementation. Our policy has been to use cortisone acetate, 50 mg to 100 mg intramuscularly every 6 hours, starting 12 to 18 hours before operation, 100 mg of hydrocortisone intravenously during the surgery, and then cortisone acetate over 72 to 96 hours following surgery. This is in addition to the patient's customary dosage.

Complications of the Exposure

Complications of surgical approaches may result from the violation of major blood vessels or nerves. The commonly used exposures for arthrodesis of the hip are anterior, lateral, and posterior. The anterior approach may violate the lateral femoral cutaneous or femoral nerves or vessels. The sciatic nerve may be endangered in the posterior approach, whereas the lateral approach places no important structure in jeopardy. Clearly, an accurate knowledge of and attention to anatomy is indispensable.

Shock (Blood Loss)

Most hip arthrodeses incur blood losses requiring replacement; therefore, adequate provision for replacement should be made prior to surgery. Hemorrhagic shock will occur when blood loss amounts to approximately 15% of total blood volume. Plasma volume averages 40 ml/kg. An accurate estimate of total blood volume can be made with knowledge of the patient's hematocrit. Another useful estimate is that blood volume equals 6% to 8% of the body weight. An average adult male weighing 70 kg has a blood volume of 5000 ml; therefore, shock may be expected to occur with losses of 1200 ml to 1300 ml.[71,72] Accurate monitoring of blood loss during surgery and replacement of such loss should be routine. We replace blood loss with packed red cells supplemented by appropriate volumes of crystalloid solution.

Transfusion Reaction

Immediate transfusion reactions causing urticaria or fever are not uncommon but rarely cause serious problems. Discontinuation of the unit of blood is all that is required. Hemolytic reactions are occasionally due to mismatch of donor and recipient, but more often to misidentification of donor and recipient. If such a reaction occurs under general anesthesia, the result is often a precipitous drop in blood pressure.

Vessel and Nerve Injury

Neural and vascular injuries occasionally occur with the use of internal fixation devices. Careful attention to the length and direction of such devices will prevent this complication. Sciatic nerve injuries have been reported with extra-articular ischiofemoral fusions, especially when the Trumble or Brittain methods are used.

Injury to the Pelvic Viscera

Internal fixation devices crossing the hip joint have, on occasion, perforated the bladder. Early recognition and correction is necessary, and urologic consultation is advisable. Careful attention to the length and direction of the hardware should prevent this complication.

EARLY POSTOPERATIVE COMPLICATIONS

Systemic

Cardiopulmonary. *Pulmonary atelectasis* may occur in the first 24 to 48 hours after surgery and is manifested by fever and diminished breath sounds over a portion of the lung field. Chest roentgenograms are usually unnecessary for diagnosis. Prevention is by deep-breathing exercises. Treatment is by deep breathing, coughing, administration of expectorants, intermittent positive-pressure breathing, and endotracheal suctioning, if necessary.

Pneumonitis, a common sequela of atelectasis, may develop when early recognition and appropriate treatment have not been instituted. Persistent fever, productive cough, rales, and rhonchi occur. Treatment includes the measures mentioned above for atelectasis, plus administration of antibiotics. Sputum investigation by Gram stain, culture, and sensitivity studies should be accomplished.

Pulmonary emboli may occur from 24 hours to 6 weeks postoperatively, but the peak incidence is between 2 and 3 weeks. Debate continues as to prophylactic measures. Aspirin, heparin, low-molecular-weight dextran, warfarin sodium (Couma-

din), exercises, compressive wraps, and elastic stockings have all been widely employed with varying success. It is our opinion that routine use of these agents in young patients (the likely candidates for hip fusion) is not warranted. Many pulmonary emboli are clinically silent, and often the only manifestation is a sudden temperature elevation. However, the sudden onset of chest pain, dyspnea, fever, cough, and hemoptysis is classic. There may be tachycardia, tachypnea, and pleural friction rub; cardiograms and roentgenograms may show changes. There is usually lowering of the arterial oxygen saturation, and the lung scan confirms the diagnosis. The patient should not be moved to the nuclear medicine or the x-ray departments for such investigation until the vital signs are stable and appropriate heparin and oxygen therapy are accomplished. Consultation is advisable.

Postoperative myocardial infarction is uncommon in the young patients who usually undergo arthrodesis. A history of angina pectoris or valvular heart disease would indicate an increased risk, and appropriate preoperative evaluation should be accomplished. When infarction occurs, prompt attention, with appropriate sedation, oxygen therapy, and consultation, is necessary.

Gastrointestinal. *Cast syndrome* results from compression of the third portion of the duodenum by the overlying superior mesenteric artery and the celiac plexus.[45,70,86] This has occurred in patients placed in spica casts following arthrodesis. Persistent nausea and vomiting associated with abdominal pain occurs in the early postoperative period. Treatment consists of turning the patient prone and to the right lateral decubitus position, splitting the cast, windowing the abdominal area, or removing the cast completely. Nasogastric suction and intravenous alimentation may become necessary. The consultation of an abdominal surgeon should be requested if symptoms persist. Gastrojejunostomy has occasionally been necessary, and an occasional death has been reported.

Intestinal ileus and gastric dilatation occur as the result of autonomic dysfunction, probably secondary to retroperitoneal hematoma. Abdominal distention, diminished peristalsis associated with nausea, and vomiting may occur. Treatment is by withholding all oral intake, administering intravenous alimentation, applying nasogastric suction, and using autonomic drugs such as neostygmine (Prostigimin).

Stress ulcer may follow arthrodesis of the hip, and massive gastrointestinal bleeding may result. Appropriate modifications of the diet, the use of antacids and sedation, and nasogastric suction are usually necessary. Consultation is advisable.

Acute postoperative cholecystitis has occurred following arthrodesis of the hip. It may or may not be associated with a history of previous gallbladder disturbances. Fever, abdominal pain, nausea, vomiting, and tenderness in the right upper quadrant are usually present. Jaundice may occur. Early recognition and treatment with elimination of all oral intake, intravenous alimentation, antibiotic administration, and consultation with an abdominal surgeon are indicated.

Intestinal obstruction has followed arthrodesis of the hip and is usually associated with a history of previous abdominal surgery. Danger signs are the lack of flatus, abdominal distention, hyperactive abdominal bowel sounds, and colicky abdominal pain with nausea and vomiting. Treatment is stopping all oral intake, nasogastric suction, intravenous alimentation, and consultation with an abdominal surgeon.

Constipation is a common problem of hospitalized patients and is compounded by inactivity, bland hospital food, and analgesic medication. Treatment includes appropriate and vigorous bed exercises, encouragement of oral fluid intake, and the use of bulk stool softeners, laxatives, suppositories, and enemas as required.

Serum hepatitis may follow any blood transfusion. Its risk (approximately 1%–1.5% at present) may be lessened by the use of volunteer (nonpaid) donors and by substituting packed red cells for whole blood whenever feasible. Gamma globulin administered in the early postoperative period may offer some prophylaxis. Symptoms, which may not appear for several weeks following transfusion, include anorexia, vague abdominal pain, nausea, and jaundice. There is no specific treatment. Corticosteroids may be necessary in life-threatening situations, and fatalities (5%–10% of cases) have occurred.[67] Acquired immune deficiency syndrome (AIDS) has occurred following blood transfusion. Careful screening of blood donors is the only known method of prevention.

Genitourinary. *Postoperative retention of urine* is quite common in patients after extensive surgery, especially if sitting or standing is not permitted. Administration of bethanechol chloride (Urecholine), applying warm packs to the abdomen, or running water from a faucet may be helpful, but catheterization (preferably intermittent and at 8- to 12-hour intervals) may be necessary. Having the patient practice using the urinal or bedpan in the supine position preoperatively may be of some prophylactic value.

Urinary tract infection, especially lower tract infection, may occur following catheterization or may appear later in the postoperative period without predisposing cause. Symptoms are urinary frequency, dysuria, and fever. Proper management includes a urine culture and sensitivity determination, phenazopyridine HCl (Pyridum) administration if necessary, and appropriate chemotherapy over a 10- to 14-day interval. Avoidance of continuous (Foley) catheterization, when possible, reduces the incidence.

Renal lithiasis (formation of renal or ureteral stones) may follow prolonged immobilization. Analgesics and hydration are useful. Avoidance of prolonged immobilization in patients with a history of stones, proper hydration, and appropriate bed exercises may prevent this complication. Although most stones pass spontaneously, urologic consultation is advisable.

Renal failure occasionally follows prolonged shock or hemolytic transfusion reactions. Oliguria is its trademark. Meticulous attention to fluid and electrolyte balance is mandatory. Urgent consultation with a nephrologist is advisable, and renal dialysis may be necessary.

Postoperative Psychosis. One of the most common postoperative psychoses is delirium tremens, which usually follows a 3- to 5-day abstinence from alcohol. Agitation, tremor, and hallucinations announce the problem, which requires careful attention to fluid and electrolyte balance, sedation, and appropriate consultation. We recommend providing alcohol on a prophylactic basis to any patient suspected of being a candidate. Other postoperative psychoses occur rarely.[73]

Death. The mortality rate for arthrodesis of the hip in patients less than 50 years old is less than 1%.[6,12,17,18,56,94,102] Most of the reported deaths have been due to either myocardial infarction or pulmonary embolization.

Regional

Wound disruption is a rare complication in young, healthy patients. It has occurred more commonly in patients taking steroid drugs over prolonged periods. Once it occurs, there are two options: one is to permit secondary healing, and the other is to excise the wound and close it secondarily over drains.

Wound hematoma is a relatively common complication. If it is extensive, evacuation under aseptic conditions may be required; otherwise, it is best left undisturbed. Antibiotics may be of some value. At the time of operation, careful attention to hemostasis, appropriate wound closure obliterating dead space, and the use of suction drainage reduces its incidence.

Stitch abscess (localized inflammation and infection) around skin and subcutaneous sutures occurs frequently. Removal of the offending suture cures. Use of less reactive materials for skin closure, such as monofilament nylon and stainless steel, reduces the incidence.

Wound infection may involve the surgical wound superficially (between the investing fascia and the skin) or deep to the investing fascia. Usually in the young, healthy patients undergoing hip fusion, a virulent organism such as hemolytic, coagulase-positive *Staphylococcus aureus* is required to initiate an invasive infection.

Host factors, such as diabetes mellitus, previous surgery with extensive scarring, or infection elsewhere in the body, may be important contributing factors. Most operative infections are believed to be initiated in the operating theater. Such factors as prolonged operating time, breaks in scrub (aseptic) technique, or personnel with infective lesions such as furuncles may be offenders. However, in most postoperative infections no obvious cause can be demonstrated. The use of implants for internal fixation increases the risk. We believe that shaving and washing the skin immediately before the operation begins, appropriate application of antiseptics, careful surgical technique, and operating as rapidly as feasible are most advantageous.

Appropriate wound irrigation, careful wound closure obliterating dead space, and use of perioperative antibiotics (bacteriocidal, starting 1 to 4 hours preoperatively and continuing 24 to 48 hours postoperatively) lower the incidence of infection. Superficial infections can usually be cured by opening the wound, administering appropriate antibiotics, and administering local wound care. The wound may be left to heal secondarily or closed later over drains, or a skin graft may be added, as deemed necessary.

Deep infections usually require more vigorous treatment in the operating theater. The wound should be opened wide; all purulent material and infected granulation tissue should be removed, and the wound either left open to heal secondarily or closed over a suction-irrigation apparatus. Appropriate systemic chemotherapy after culture and sensitivity determination is required. Most large series of hip fusions report infection to occur in approximately 5%.[12,17,18,56,94,102]

Superficial thrombophlebitis following surgery about the hip is not uncommon. It may occur in the upper extremity following intravenous therapy, especially with plastic catheters. The diagnosis is readily apparent, with localized pain and swelling, erythema, muscle tenderness, and palpable hardness along the course of the superficial vein. Pulmonary embolization rarely, if ever, follows this event. Most physicians favor the use of anticoagulant therapy; however, the majority of these episodes respond to elevation of the part, with application of warm compresses and administration of an anti-inflammatory agent such as phenylbutazone (Butazolidin) or aspirin. The offending plastic catheter must be removed.

Deep vein thrombosis (phlebothrombosis) occasionally complicates arthrodesis of the hip. Severe pain, massive swelling, and discoloration of the limb may follow. Treatment requires anticoagulants, and consultation is advisable.

Pressure sores are not uncommon, and any part of the body that rests on a surface such that the local pressure exceeds that of the perfusing capillaries (approximately 35 torr) for 6 to 8 hours may develop tissue necrosis manifested by an ulcer. Tissue ischemia is very painful, and patients will complain bitterly of local pain. Positioning the part or windowing the cast so that the pain is relieved is mandatory. The posterior aspect of the heel, presacral area, elbow, fibular head, and greater trochanter are most often involved. Most pressure sores heal satisfactorily by secondary intention, but a few require skin grafts.

Nerve palsy caused by complications of surgical exposure and operative techniques has been discussed previously. The most common postoperative palsies involve either the ulnar or peroneal nerves and are due to prolonged pressure over the subcutaneous portion of the nerves at the elbows and knees, respectively. Treatment involves early recognition and protection of the elbow and knee areas.

LATE POSTOPERATIVE COMPLICATIONS

Functional Limitations

Most young patients with hips fused in good position (30° of flexion, 0° of abduction, 10°–30° of external rotation) are able to lead full, vigorous lives with few significant restrictions.[102] However, the operation does lead to certain limitations. Most patients experience difficulty sitting in a low chair, and this may lead to inconvenience on a commode. Unless full knee flexion is regained, there may be difficulty in donning stockings and shoes and in maintaining foot hygiene. If there is only a little shortening, there may be difficulty in alternate-foot stair climbing. A few female patients describe awkwardness with sexual intercourse; however, many successful pregnancies and normal deliveries have been accomplished following hip fusion. Successful rehabilitation of the patient following ar-

throdesis of the hip involves frank discussion of these limitations before the operation and assistance by the surgeon and physical therapist afterward in explaining and minimizing these problems.

Failure of the Internal Fixation Device

The implants used in the internal fixation of hip arthrodeses bend and break with some frequency. Forces about the hip are strong: straight leg raising produces forces of twice the body weight on the hip, and unsupported slow walking produces stress of almost three times body weight. No implant is strong enough to withstand such forces over extended periods. The lesson seems clear: the arthrodesis must be suitably protected until union is secure.

Pseudarthrosis

Failure of the arthrodesis or of a concomitant proximal femoral osteotomy to unite with bone occurs in 10% to 15% of patients (Fig. 42-1).[17,18,56,94,102] Most pseudarthroses at either site are painful; however, we have followed several patients with fibrous ankylosis of the hip who have done well over prolonged periods. Thus, treatment must be individualized. We believe that many pseudarthroses are the result of technical error. Failure to use adequate systemic chemotherapy in tuberculous arthritis of the hip has led to increased pseudarthrosis, as has extensive postoperative pyogenic wound infection.

Malposition

There is some controversy as to the optimal position for hip fusion.[4,55,102] We believe this position to be 30° of flexion, 0° of abduction, and 10° to 30° of external rotation. It is often difficult at the time of surgery to be absolutely certain of the position of the hip. Some surgeons prefer low intertrochanteric osteotomy, wire loop fixation of the osteotomy, and postoperative spica cast support that can be wedged or changed if necessary. If the position is to be fixed by internal fixation at surgery, one must take great care to ensure that the position accepted is that deemed optimal for that patient. It is well known that arthrodesis of the hip in optimal position in a growing child may result in undesirable

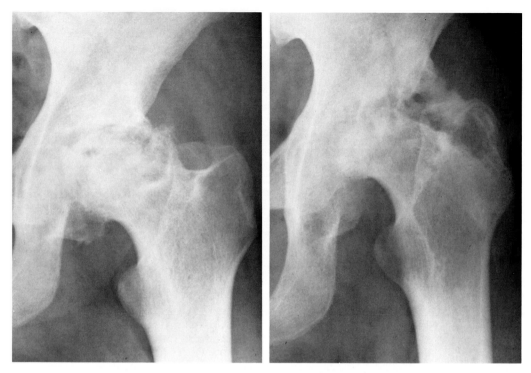

FIG. 42-1. Pseudarthrosis followed hip fusion in a patient with avascular necrosis of the femoral head. It is necessary to excise all of the necrotic bone and obtain good, healthy bone surfaces for fusion.

flexion and adduction with growth.[35] Fusion in the child does not prevent deformity from occurring owing to the constant pull of strong deforming muscle forces. We have followed patients with fused hips who had excessive flexion and adduction, and some have fared well over several years, but others were improved by a correcting osteotomy.

Fracture

Femoral neck fractures following hip fusion, especially at the base of the neck, are not rare. The internal fixation device must cross into the pelvis for adequate fixation. Femoral shaft fractures have been reported in as many as 10% of patients followed for long periods.[6,7,12,17,18,56,94,102] Reduction by closed means may be difficult. If treatment by open reduction is chosen, strong internal fixation is needed, since stresses at the fracture are increased by the fused hip (Fig. 42-2). Fractures of the graft in Brittain

extra-articular fusion have been reported, but most have apparently been secondary to technical error in positioning the graft.[18] Prolonged cast protection has resulted in union of most of these fractures, but occasionally reoperation has been necessary. We have little personal experience with this method.

Iliac Hernia

Following the use of a full-thickness iliac bone graft, iliac hernia may occur at the donor site.[33] We believe that it is less likely to occur if the graft is taken from the extreme anterior or posterior end of the ilium and if accurate repair of the detached muscle, periosteum, and fascia is performed. A hernia, if symptomatic, should be surgically corrected.[10] If the graft was originally taken from the middle of the ilium, the repair may require removal of a portion of the anterior or posterior ilium in case of a ring defect.

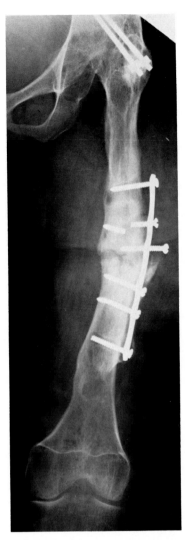

FIG. 42-2. Closed fracture of the femoral shaft on the side of a successful hip fusion resulted in nonunion after internal fixation. This illustrates the necessity for very strong internal fixation if an open reduction is to be done, since the forces on the fracture are increased considerably by the stiff hip.

Obstetric Problems

There have been many uneventful pregnancies and normal vaginal deliveries following unilateral hip fusion. However, several of our patients have required caesarean section, apparently because of pelvic deformities associated with the condition that necessitated arthrodesis of the hip.

Pediatric Problems

Malposition. Arthrodesis of a hip placed initially in good position in a child may become progressively flexed and adducted with growth,[35,76] and corrective osteotomy may be required. Some authors have suggested placing the hip in more abduction and extension at the time of arthrodesis to compensate for this inevitable change.

Slipped Capital Femoral Epiphysis. Slipping of the upper femoral epiphysis has been observed after hip fusion, although we have seen no such case at the Campbell Clinic. It would seem appropriate in surgical correction to use multiple pins, anchoring them in the pelvis and producing a closure of the proximal femoral epiphysis.

Deformity of the Knee. If the hip is fused in malposition and the epiphyses about the knee are open, deformity at the knee may occur. This complication must be unusual, for we are aware of no such occurrence at the Campbell Clinic.

Knee Ligament Laxity. With the hip fused in malposition, growth may lead to abnormal laxity of the protecting ligaments of the knee. Inadequate rehabilitation of the musculature about the knee and leg may contribute to this problem.

Increased Stress on Contiguous Joints

Pain in the Lumbar Spine. Hip fusion causes increased stresses on the lumbar spine,[28,37,54,79] and too little emphasis has been placed on rehabilitation of the abdominal musculature to support this stress. It has been estimated, however, that approximately half of the population of a developed Western country has significant backache, so it is not surprising that varying numbers of patients have reported having backache following hip fusions. There is even more stress on the lumbar spine if the hip is fused in malposition.[4,55] Of 20 patients followed at the Campbell Clinic for 10 years or longer after hip fusion, seven had significant backache, and four of these hips had been fused in malposition. Stewart and Coker, reviewing 109 patients with arthrodesis of the hip, found a substantial number whose back pain was improved after hip fusion.[94] Treatment involves intermittent rest, heat, abdominal strengthening exercises, and the occasional use of a suitable support, such as a lumbosacral corset. However, if the back pain is unrelenting and no other specific cause, such as ruptured disc, can be found, it may be justifiable to convert the hip fusion to a total hip arthroplasty.

Osteoarthritis of the Ipsilateral Knee. Hip fusion also puts increased stress on the knee,[8,79] and adequate rehabilitation of its protective musculature (quadriceps, hamstring, and "gastroc-soleus" groups) is necessary. We have observed significant problems with the ipsilateral knee in three of 20 patients with fused hips followed 10 years or longer. One of these was due to tuberculous involvement of the knee. Malposition of the fused hip increases the added stress on the ipsilateral knee.

Osteoarthritis of the Contralateral Hip. Hip fusion increases the stress on the opposite hip.[28,29,37,79] Malposition, especially excessive abduction, accentuates the stress. Two of 20 patients with fused hips followed 10 years or longer developed significant degenerative changes in the opposite hip. One of these had preexisting congenital dysplasia of the degenerating hip; the other had malposition of the fused hip. If conservative measures fail, the patient may require surgical intervention with appropriate arthroplasty. Conversion of the fused hip to total arthroplasty may also be considered.

Limited Motion in the Ipsilateral Knee. Limited knee motion following hip fusion has been mentioned by many authors.[17,18,56,94,102] Of our 20 patients followed 10 years, four had significant knee stiffness, one secondary to tuberculosis of the knee. In years past, when hip fusion required prolonged plaster immobilization, knee stiffness was much more a problem than it is today, since modern methods of arthrodesis rarely require prolonged plaster protection. Isometric exercises in the cast hasten recovery of knee motion.

Chronic Venous Insufficiency

The postphlebitis syndrome, with swelling, superficial varicosities, stasis dermatitis, and/or intermittent skin ulceration, may complicate arthrodesis. Treatment consists of intermittent elevation of the extremity, use of supportive stockings, and active foot and ankle exercises.

COMPLICATIONS OF ARTHRODESIS OF THE KNEE

INTRAOPERATIVE COMPLICATIONS

Injury to the popliteal vessels or to the peroneal or tibial nerves may occur. Prompt recognition and repair of the injured structure is required.

Tourniquet palsy rarely occurs if attention is paid to calibration of the pneumatic tourniquet and pressures in excess of 450 torr to 600 torr are avoided.[63] The tourniquet should not be inflated continuously for longer than 2 hours. If release becomes necessary, at least 20 minutes should elapse before the tourniquet is reinflated. Patients younger than 40 years can usually expect spontaneous resolution of a tourniquet palsy; older patients are more likely to have permanent impairment.

EARLY POSTOPERATIVE COMPLICATIONS

Systemic

Cardiopulmonary. Atelectasis, pneumonitis, pulmonary embolization, and myocardial infarction, which have all been discussed under Complications of Arthrodesis of the Hip, can also occur in knee arthrodesis. Pneumothorax has also been reported following arthrodesis of the knee.[38] Miliary tuberculosis and tuberculous meningitis have occurred following arthrodesis for tuberculous knee infections when adequate preliminary chemotherapy was not used.

Gastrointestinal. Other than constipation, gastrointestinal complications following arthrodesis of the knee are rare.

Genitourinary. Urinary retention following knee surgery is common. Catheterization may be required, and urinary tract infection may follow. Permitting the male patient to stand by his bed with help, if feasible in the early postoperative period, often enables him to void.

Postoperative Psychosis. Psychosis following arthrodesis of the knee has occurred. The patient's drug and alcohol habits must be known, and careful discussion of the implications of knee fusion and its aftercare should be accomplished before surgery.

Regional

Wound Disruption. Dehiscence following knee fusion is uncommon.

Wound Slough. Skin necrosis occurs frequently in the thin, atrophic skin of patients with rheumatoid arthritis, especially those on corticosteroids. Vasculitis may play a role. The use of gently curved or straight incisions and careful handling of the wound margins reduce its likelihood.

Wound Hematoma. Release of the tourniquet prior to wound closure, meticulous hemostasis, careful wound closure with the elimination of dead space, and appropriate (suction) drainage can lessen the incidence of wound hematoma.

Wound Infection. The manifestations of wound infection may involve stitch abscess or cellulitis, which, as a rule, clear with removal of the sutures. Superficial infection that does not extend beneath the investing fascia is cured by adequate drainage, with or without systemic antibiotics. Deep infection may require surgical debridement and drainage. The incidence of infection, superficial and deep, following arthrodesis of the knee is approximately 5%,[11,38,84] and though it may delay fusion, it seldom prevents the arthrodesis.

Peroneal Palsy. In the early postoperative period, peroneal palsy (as distinguished from tourniquet palsies) is presumably due to prolonged pressure over the peroneal nerve at the neck of the fibula. Its incidence can be reduced by attention to the application of the postoperative splints or plaster dressing and to the positioning of the limb in bed. The patient should not be permitted to lie supine for prolonged periods with the lower extremity externally rotated.

Compartment Syndromes. Following extensive surgery about the knee, one may see compartment syndromes in the lower extremity. Early recognition and fasciotomy are necessary.

Pin Tract Infection. Arthrodesis in which Charnley clamps are used is complicated by pin tract infection in 1% to 10% of patients; it may be the result of "burning" the bone by inserting the pins too rapidly.[28,38] Most infections resolve quite promptly following removal of the pins. Occasionally, a ring sequestrum occurs, which requires curettage and excision of the tract.

Pressure Sores. Pressure sores may occur under the cast, especially over the fibular head, patella, lateral malleolus, posterior aspect of the heel, and bunionette (the fifth metatarsal head). Careful attention to the initial padding and to the patient's complaints of local pain, followed by appropriate windowing of the cast, should reduce their occurrence.

LATE POSTOPERATIVE COMPLICATIONS

Functional Limitations

Inability to sit in a confined space presents the most serious inconvenience to the patient with a knee fusion.[27] Unless there is considerable shortening of the fused limb, difficulty in clearing the foot over obstacles, such as a curb, may be experienced. Climbing stairs foot over foot requires circumduction and trick movement of the extremity. Significant shortening may be compensated for by an appropriate lift on the shoe. The great majority of patients with knee fusions are entirely satisfied with their fused knee.[11,21,38,84] Most experience only slight alteration of their life style, and many participate in recreational athletics such as golf, tennis, bowling, dancing, and horseback riding.

Failure of the Internal Fixation Device

Problems such as pin breakage or cutting out in an osteopenic bone, bending, breaking or backing out of intramedullary nails, and absorption of bone with subsequent holding apart of arthrodesis surfaces by a plate or rods have been encountered. Careful attention to the technique of the arthrodesis chosen plus appropriate support of the limb should reduce the occurrence.

Pseudarthrosis

With currently available methods, successful knee fusion can be expected in at least 90% of patients. However, the neuropathic or Charcot knee presents a special problem. The literature suggests a 50% failure rate with standard methods. Drennan and colleagues achieved nine fusions in nine arthrodeses of Charcot knees by including in the technique meticulous excision of scarred capsule and synovium.[31] They believe that this excision prevents shunting of blood past the fusion surfaces and subsequent pseudarthrosis. Lucas and Murray achieved four of four knee arthrodeses in Charcot joints using their double-plating technique, suggesting that rigid immobilization also is necessary in this problem.[58]

Pseudarthrosis is also a significant problem in treating failed total knee arthroplasties, particularly those due to infection and those in which a large-stemmed implant (*i.e.,* hinged knee) has been used.[14,19,41,57,95,99] Use of external fixation combined with compression and judicious use of autologous bone grafts may reduce the incidence.

Fusion in Malposition

Optimal position for knee fusion is believed to be from 0° to 20° of flexion and slight valgus, with approximately 10° of external rotation.[20,92] Careful carpentry of fusion surfaces and suitable application of internal fixation achieve this position, provided that no strong deforming muscle force exists about the knee. If such a force exists, it should be released by tenotomy, myotomy, neurectomy, or bone resection. The combination of internal fixation device plus external support must be strong enough to support the fusion surfaces, and the support must be continued long enough for solid union to occur. The apparatus must not be a distracting or potentially distracting force, as in crossed pins (Fig. 42-3).

Increased Stress on Hip, Ankle, and Foot

There has been discussion of the consequences of increased stress on the ipsilateral hip, ankle, and foot following knee fusion, which may cause symptoms and degenerative arthritis. However, we have found little documentation,[27,42,88] and our experience tends to minimize this problem.

Fracture of the Femur or Tibia

Fractures of the ipsilateral femur or tibia following knee fusion have been reported in as many as 5% to 10% of patients followed for prolonged periods.[34,38] Most of these injuries have occurred at times remote from the arthrodesis. Treatment should be on an individual basis; it may be difficult to align femoral fractures above a stiff knee using standard traction methods.

COMPLICATIONS OF ARTHRODESIS OF THE ANKLE

INTRAOPERATIVE COMPLICATIONS

Consideration has been given in previous sections to complications of anesthesia and acute adrenal insufficiency. Injury to the anterior or posterior tibial vessels or to the tibial, sural, or peroneal nerves may occur during the surgical procedure. One or the other of the anterior or posterior tibial vessels may be ligated if injured, but the tibial nerve should be accurately repaired if divided.

EARLY POSTOPERATIVE COMPLICATIONS

Systemic

Systemic complications such as atelectasis, pneumonitis, pulmonary embolization, myocardial infarction, acute urinary retention, urinary tract infection, constipation, and postoperative psychoses have been discussed. Rare instances of tetanus following operations about the foot and ankle in patients with previous injury have occurred. Early recognition and vigorous use of systemic relaxants, as well as antibiotic, immunologic, local surgical, and supportive measures are indicated. Hyperbaric oxygen, if available, and K_3MnO_4 irrigation should be considered.

Regional

Excessive swelling of the foot and toes is common. Splitting or bivalving the cast and continously elevating the extremity higher than the head should relieve the situation. Preclosure release of the tourniquet with ligation of vessels and postoperative suction-drainage may help prevent swelling.

Wound disruption is uncommon. Skin slough, unfortunately, is not a rare occurrence. The use of straight or gently curved incisions with thick flaps and careful handling of wound margins should be routine.

FIG. 42-3. Malunion followed knee fusion in this patient with a marked flexion contracture of the knee. Strong deforming muscle forces must be eliminated prior to or at the time of arthrodesis to avoid this complication.

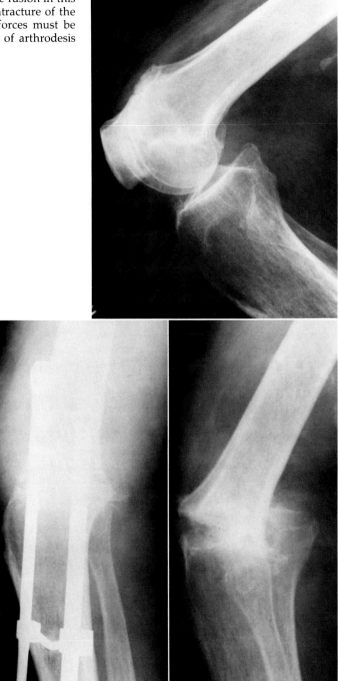

Wound hematoma, wound infection, peroneal palsy, pin tract infection, and pressure sores, which have been discussed under Complications of Arthrodesis of the Knee, also occur in the ankle. Wound infection in arthrodesis of the ankle has been reported in 3% to 23% of patients.[5,26,51,68,69,83,87,101] Although it is a delaying feature, infection has not, as a rule, prevented ankle arthrodesis.[93]

LATE POSTOPERATIVE COMPLICATIONS

Cosmetic and Functional Considerations

Many patients, and women particularly, have objected to the thickening and enlargement about the ankle following ankle fusions.[69] Stewart and colleagues have emphasized reduction in size by osteotomy and resection of the inner two thirds of the medial and lateral malleoli to minimize this objection.[93] Some difficulty in walking on irregular ground is common.[5,62,68]

Foot Problems

Forefoot strain, fatigue fracture, and hallux rigidus have been reported following ankle fusion; however, they are often associated with previous injury to the tarsal or metatarsal bones. Customary methods of treatment, such as rest, strapping, use of a metatarsal bar, and arch support, should help. Careful attention to the correct position of fusion should minimize these problems. It is important to maintain the foot at an angle of 90° to the tibia in most patients.

Although a few patients develop tarsal hypermobility following ankle fusion, most are stiffer about the midfoot and hindfoot.[9,47] This leads to added stresses on the foot and distal leg. For those patients in whom pain about the foot and lower leg is present following ankle fusion, the use of a rocker shoe and SACH ankle to simulate ankle motion has been helpful.[87]

Pseudarthrosis

With the methods currently available, successful fusion should occur in 90% to 95% of patients,[20,22,23,44,49,68,93,101] although Boobbyer reported fusion in only 78.4% of patients.[9] Patients with neuropathic (Charcot) ankles present a more difficult problem, and failure-of-fusion rates of 50% and higher have been reported.[15] It may well be that aggressive resection of the scarred capsule and synovium, as suggested by Drennan and colleagues for the knee,[31] along with rigid immobilization and prolonged postoperative support, will lead to more success.

Fusion in Malposition

We believe the optimal position for ankle fusion to be at 90° to the leg, with neutral varus-valgus angulation of the heel and rotation comparable to the normal foot. This position can best be achieved by consideration of the entire extremity from above the knee to the toes, careful carpentry of the fusion surfaces, and appropriate application of the fixation devices. Postoperative support should be carried out long enough to permit solid union—an average of 3 to 4 months.

Involvement of the Distal Tibial Epiphysis

Separation of the distal tibial epiphysis following ankle fusion in childhood occurs occasionally, but fractures about the ankle after fusion in adults are apparently uncommon. Arthrodesis of the ankle in children is best accomplished by the method of Chuinard[23] or Hatt's central bone graft.

COMPLICATIONS OF ARTHRODESIS OF THE SHOULDER

INTRAOPERATIVE COMPLICATIONS

Shoulder fusions are performed only occasionally today, and technical errors are best avoided by careful study of the anatomy and the technique of arthrodesis chosen. Anesthetic complications, which have been discussed previously, also occur in shoulder arthrodesis. Sufficient arrangements for blood replacement should be made prior to surgery.

EARLY POSTOPERATIVE COMPLICATIONS

Systemic

The problems of pulmonary atelectasis, pneumonitis, pulmonary embolization, and myocardial infarction, which have already been discussed, also occur in shoulder arthrodesis. The cast syndrome has occurred following immobilization in a shoulder spica cast.[45] Constipation is a common problem, as is urinary retention. Gastrointestinal and genitourinary complications, as well as postoperative psychosis, also occur and have been discussed previously.

Regional

Wound disruption, skin slough, wound hematoma, and infection (stitch abscess, cellulitis, superficial and deep infection) are similar to those in other major joints discussed previously. Infection (exclusive of pin tract infection) occurs in 3% to 5% of patients with arthrodesis of the shoulder. Pressure sores under a shoulder spica cast are not uncommon, and complaints of local pain must be investigated promptly. Traction palsies involving the ulnar and radial nerves have occurred following shoulder fusion.[75]

LATE POSTOPERATIVE COMPLICATIONS

Pseudarthrosis

Failure of fusion occurs in 5% to 20% of patients.[46,78,81,82,98] There is a small area of contact in the glenohumeral joint, and leverage of the upper extremity produces large forces. Indications for arthrodesis of the shoulder are few,[48,60,81,82] and no one surgeon has had much experience. Consequently, a multitude of techniques have been described. Thorough intra- and extra-articular arthrodesis with strong internal fixation, supplemental bone grafts, and suitable postoperative support should lead to more success.

Failure or Migration of the Internal Fixation Device

Breakage of implants used for internal fixation of the shoulder arthrodesis may occur if the extremity is not supported appropriately. Migration of such devices is not uncommon, and implants such as unthreaded Steinmann pins and Kirschner wires have been removed from the lung.[59,97] If pins are to be used about the shoulder, we suggest that they be threaded, as are screws, or if unthreaded, bent with a 90° hook on the lateral end to prevent medial migration.

Fusion in Malposition

There has been considerable discussion as to the optimal position for arthrodesis of the shoulder.[25,48,60,81,82] We believe that for paralytic conditions about the shoulder, the position recommended by the Research Committee of the American Orthopaedic Association is optimal.[78] This position is 50° of abduction, 15° to 25° of flexion, and 25° of internal rotation. Ingram and Miller have shown that this position is most accurately ascertained by preoperative and operative roentgenograms with the spine of the scapula used as the landmark.[46] This position causes some scapular winging, a mild cosmetic handicap, but it enhances function of the arm and hand.

Rowe has suggested that this position of abduction is excessive, especially in adults in whom arthrodesis has been done for nonparalytic conditions.[80] Using the clinical posture of the arm relative to the side of the body, Rowe proposes the following optimal position: 20° of abduction, 30° of flexion, and 40° of internal rotation. With excessive abduction, the arm does not reach the side of the body, and the scapula protrudes posteriorly, causing chronic strain of the posterior musculature, which may result in the development of pain.

Milgram, and later Pipkin, suggested resection of the distal end of the clavicle as a secondary operation following arthrodesis of the shoulder to allow more pectoral girdle movement and to compensate for the excessive abduction and its attendant problems.[75]

Fracture

Fracture of the humerus has been reported in 10% to 15% of patients.[25] Fracture of the tibial graft used in a Brittain fusion is not uncommon. Occasionally fracture has occurred at the site of fusion. Open reduction and internal fixation may be required.

Traction Neuritis and Posterior Shoulder Girdle Strain

Suprascapular traction neuritis may occur, especially in a position of excessive abduction. Humeral osteotomy, as suggested by Rowe,[80] or claviculectomy, as suggested by Pipkin,[75] may relieve these symptoms.

Acromioclavicular Luxation

Acromioclavicular luxation may occur following shoulder fusion.[75] Its occurrence has been used to support clavicular resection as an adjunct to shoulder arthrodesis.

Epiphyseal Problems

Premature fusion of the proximal humeral epiphysis or epiphysiolysis has occurred rarely following shoulder fusion in children. An internal fixation device used in an arthrodesis of a growing child should be removed after the fusion has healed. A central bone graft through the head of the humerus into the glenoid will not, as a rule, disturb epiphyseal growth.

COMPLICATIONS OF ARTHRODESIS OF THE ELBOW

Arthrodesis of the elbow is rarely required, and probably the only indication would be the presence of infection. The available English-language literature on arthrodesis of the elbow is meager, and the operation is apparently seldom performed.

INTRAOPERATIVE COMPLICATIONS

Anesthetic problems, tourniquet palsy, neural or vascular injury, and technical problems may occur, as in other arthrodeses.

EARLY POSTOPERATIVE COMPLICATIONS

Systemic

Systemic complications have been reported infrequently following arthrodesis of the elbow. However, the surgeon should be aware of such potential problems as miliary dissemination of tuberculosis, pulmonary atelectasis, pneumonitis, and urinary retention.

Regional

Volkmann's contracture may occur following any extensive surgery about the elbow, forearm, or wrist. We advise release of the tourniquet before closure and recommend fasciotomy if indicated. The problems of wound disruption, skin slough, hematoma, and infection, which have been discussed, also occur in elbow arthrodesis. An accurate incidence of wound infection for arthrodesis of the elbow has not been found. Ulnar palsy is avoided by not permitting excessive pressure over the ulnar nerve at the elbow. Stiffness of the shoulder and hand is prevented by early active motion of the joints.

LATE POSTOPERATIVE COMPLICATIONS

Pseudarthrosis

Failure of fusion has been reported in approximately half of attempted elbow arthrodeses.[50,91,92] The most successful operations have been those employing the principles of Brittain or Steindler.

Fusion in Malposition

We recommend 90° of flexion as the optimal position for elbow fusion if it is unilateral. In bilateral elbow fusions, standard texts suggest approximately 50° of extension in one elbow and 110° of flexion in the other,[92] although we found no reported case of bilateral elbow arthrodesis.

Fracture

Fractures through a successful arthrodesis of the elbow or in the distal humerus above the fusion have occurred in approximately 25% of patients.[50] Most fractures have been treated successfully by closed means.

Failure of Internal Fixation Devices

Breakage and migration of implants used for internal fixation in arthrodesis of the elbow have occurred when the arthrodesis failed to unite or if the extremity was not supported adequately postoperatively.

Limitation of Forearm Rotation

Restricted pronation and supination of the forearm have been common in patients with arthrodesis of the elbow. Quite probably, the injury or disease that prompted the operation played a significant role in most patients. Radial head resection may be helpful if there is painful forearm rotation following elbow fusion.

COMPLICATIONS OF ARTHRODESIS OF THE WRIST

INTRAOPERATIVE COMPLICATIONS

Problems of anesthesia and acute adrenocorticosteroid insufficiency have been discussed and apply to wrist arthrodesis as well. Wrist arthrodesis is commonly performed in patients with rheumatoid arthritis,[89,100] and a relatively common problem in these patients is stiffness and/or instability of the cervical spine. Endotracheal intubation may pose considerable difficulty in such a patient, and knowledge of these problems before surgery is mandatory. Block anesthesia may provide an effective alternative in these patients. Vessel or nerve injury and technical complications can be minimized by careful attention to the surgical exposure and to the method of arthrodesis selected. Tourniquet palsy, which has been discussed, also occurs in wrist arthrodesis.

EARLY POSTOPERATIVE COMPLICATIONS

Systemic

Systemic complications such as pulmonary atelectasis, gastric dilatation, acute urinary retention, and postoperative psychosis are rare following arthrodesis of the wrist. Rechnagel reports a case of miliary spread of tuberculosis following wrist arthrodesis.[77] We believe that such a complication can be eliminated by adequate preoperative chemotherapy.

Regional

Swelling. Marked swelling of the hand and fingers is common in the early postoperative period following arthrodesis of the wrist. The problem can be reduced by release of the tourniquet prior to wound closure, with ligation of points of bleeding, loose skin closure, and appropriate drainage if indicated. Constant elevation of the extremity and encouragement of finger motion for the first 48 to 72 hours following surgery is advisable. Once excessive swelling has occurred, the treatment is bivalving the cast down to the skin. If forearm compartment syndromes occur, fasciotomy may be required.

Wound Complications. Wound disruption and skin slough may occur, especially in the atrophic skin of patients with rheumatoid arthritis, as already discussed. Wound hematoma can be minimized by the measures already discussed. Wound

infections are uncommon following arthrodesis of the wrist.

Nerve Palsy. Carpal tunnel syndromes have occurred in the postoperative period following wrist arthrodesis, on occasion requiring section of the volar carpal ligament for relief. Ulnar palsies usually follow prolonged pressure on this nerve at the elbow. The patient should be advised of this possibility and taught correct positioning of the extremity.

Pin Tract Infection and Pin Migration. The use of pins for internal fixation in arthrodesis of the wrist has occasionally led to pin tract infection or pin migration. Usually neither leads to serious consequences.

Pressure Sores. Local skin necrosis may occur under the cast postoperatively. In our experience this has usually involved the humeral epicondyles or olecranon, the ulnar head, or the second metacarpal head. Prompt windowing of the cast over areas of local pain reduce the occurrence.

LATE POSTOPERATIVE COMPLICATIONS

Functional Limitations

Wrist fusion in good position usually produces a happy patient with good hand function, and pain is relieved in the majority of patients. There is controversy as to how far distal the fusion should extend. Riordan believes that the fusion should extend to the metacarpal bases,[78a] whereas Abbott and co-workers have fused successfully only to the proximal row of the carpus when the arthritic change was believed to be limited to the radiocarpal articulation.[2] Loss of wrist motion produces loss of manual dexterity, especially in the dominant hand, and many patients complain of clumsiness. Certain activities, such as using a hammer, are difficult except by trick maneuvers.

Pseudarthrosis. Arthrodesis is successful in 80% to 90% of patients.[2,24,40,64,65,100] Fibrous ankylosis may produce an acceptable result and be relatively painless.

Fusion in Malposition. For a unilateral wrist fusion we believe the optimal position is 10° to 15° of dorsiflexion, with the axis of the third metacarpal coinciding with the axis of the radius. For bilateral fusion we prefer one wrist in neutral dorsiflexion and the other in slight palmar flexion, maintaining the axis of the third metacarpal with the radial axis. Many authors believe that slight ulnar deviation of the wrist, so that the axis of the second metacarpal coincides with the axis of the radius, is the position of choice. Increased ulnar or radial drift of the fingers has been reported in patients with rheumatoid arthritis after wrist fusion.[64,74,89,100] Loss of power in finger flexion or extension may occur if the fusion is in the extremes of palmar flexion or dorsiflexion. There should be little difficulty in maintaining the chosen position if careful carpentry of the fusion surfaces and bone grafting with adequate internal fixation and suitable postoperative splinting are carried out.

Loss of Forearm Rotation. A properly performed arthrodesis of the wrist should not result in loss of forearm rotation unless distal radioulnar joint arthritis is present at the time of surgery. If distal radioulnar joint arthritis exists, resection of the distal ulna should be performed.

Sympathetic Dystrophy. Autonomic dysfunction has been reported following wrist fusion[77] and may require stellate ganglion block and possibly cervical sympathectomy.

Fracture. Although a theoretical possibility, fracture of a fused wrist or adjacent bones has seldom been reported.

Disturbance of Growth of the Distal Radial Epiphysis. Disturbance of growth of the distal radial epiphysis must be considered in children and has been reported following certain techniques of arthrodesis. Makin has reported bending of the arthrodesis and late dislocation of the distal radioulnar joint in children.[61]

REFERENCES

1. Abbott, L.C., and Lucas, D.B.: Arthrodesis of the hip in wide abduction. J. Bone Joint Surg., 36A:1129, 1954.
2. Abbott, L.C., Saunders, J.B., and Bost, F.C.: Arthrodesis of the wrist with the use of grafts of cancellous bone. J. Bone Joint Surg., 24:883, 1942.
3. Adams, J.C.: Vulnerability of the sciatic nerve in closed ischio-femoral arthrodesis by nail and graft. J. Bone Joint Surg., 46B:748, 1964.
4. Ahlback, S.E., and Lindahl, O.: Hip arthrodesis—
the connection between function and position. Acta Orthop. Scand., 37:77, 1966.
5. Ahlberg, A., and Henricson, A.S.: Late results of ankle fusion. Acta. Orthop. Scand., 52:103, 1982.
6. Barmada, R., Abraham, E., and Ray, R.D.: Hip fusion utilizing the cobra head plate. J. Bone Joint Surg., 58A:541, 1976.
7. Bazant, VonB., Popelka, S., Chodera, J.S., and Hadraba, I.: Femoral fractures in hips following arthrodesis. Z. Orthop., 99:322, 1964.
8. Boillett, R., and Delchef, J.: Arthrosis of the knee: A late consequence of hip ankylosis—a study of 40 cases. Acta Orthop. Belg., 34:947, 1968.
9. Boobbyer, G.N.: The long-term results of ankle arthrodesis. Acta Orthop. Scand., 52:107, 1981.
10. Bosworth, D.M.: Repair of hernias through iliac-crest defects. J. Bone Joint Surg., 37A:1069, 1955.
11. Brattstrom, H., and Brattstrom, M.: Long-term results in knee arthrodesis in rheumatoid arthritis. Reconstr. Surg. Traumatol., 12:125, 1971.
12. Breitenfelder, J., and Juke, B.: Fatigue fractures of the homolateral femur after hip arthrodesis. Arch. Orthop. Trauma Surg., 78:248, 1974.
13. Brittain, H.A.: Architectural Principles in Arthrodesis. Baltimore, Williams & Wilkins, 1942.
14. Brodersen, M.P., Fitzgerald, R.H., Peterson, L.F.A. et al.: Arthrodesis of the knee following failed total knee arthroplasty. J. Bone Joint Surg., 61A:181, 1979.
15. Brooks, A.L., and Saunders, E.A.: Fusion of the ankle in denervated extremities. South. Med. J., 60:30, 1967.
16. Burckhardt, A., and Taillard, W.: Study of weight bearing and electromyography after arthrodesis of the hip. Clin. Orthop. Rel. Res., 111:710, 1973.
17. Carter, P.J., and Wickstrom, J.: Arthrodesis of the hip: An assessment of results in 100 patients. South. Med. J., 64:451, 1971.
18. Chan, K.P., and Shin, J.S.: Brittain ischiofemoral arthrodesis for tuberculosis of the hip. J. Bone Joint Surg., 50A:1341, 1968.
19. Chand, K.: The knee joint in rheumatoid arthritis. V. The role of arthrodesis. Int. Surg., 60:154, 1975.
20. Charnley, J.: Compression Arthrodesis. Edinburgh, E. & S. Livingstone, 1953.
21. Charnley, J., and Howe, H.G.: A study of the end results of compression arthrodesis of the knee. J. Bone Joint Surg., 40B:633, 1958.
22. Christensen, S., Jensen, J.H., and Sørensen, S.S.: Ankle arthrodesis: A long-term follow-up study. Ugeskr. Laeger, 143:1652, 1981.
23. Chuinard, E.G., and Peterson, R.E.: Distraction-compression bone graft arthrodesis of the ankle: A method especially applicable in children. J. Bone Joint Surg., 45A:481, 1963.
24. Clendenin, M.B., and Green, D.P.: Arthrodesis of the wrist—complications and their management. J. Hand Surg., 6:253, 1982.
25. Cofield, R.H., and Briggs, B.T.: Glenohumeral arthrodesis: Operative and long-term functional results. J. Bone Joint Surg., 61A:668, 1979.
26. Davis, R.J., and Millis, M.B.: Ankle arthrodesis in the management of traumatic ankle arthrosis: A long-term retrospective study. J. Trauma, 20:674, 1980.

27. Dee, R.: The case for arthrodesis of the knee. Orthop. Clin. North Am., 10:249, 1979.
28. Dei Poli, N., and Fiandaca, A.: Physiopathology of compensating joints in hip arthrodesis. Minerva Orthop., 21:81, 1970.
29. DeMigneux, F., Rainaut, J.J., and Cedart, C.I.: Study of the effect of arthrodesis on the opposite hip. Rev. Chir. Orthop., 54:649, 1968.
30. Diehl, K., and Hort, W.: Static and dynamic investigations in compression arthrodesis of the knee. Z. Orthop., 3:919, 1973.
31. Drennan, D.B., Fahey, J.J., and Maylahn, D.J.: Important factors in achieving arthrodesis of the Charcot knee. J. Bone Joint Surg., 53A:1180, 1971.
32. Fjermeros, H., and Hagen, R.: Post-traumatic arthritis in the foot and ankle treated with arthrodesis. Acta Chir. Scand., 133:527, 1967.
33. Froimson, A.I., and Cummings, A.G., Jr.: Iliac hernia following hip arthrodesis. Clin. Orthop., 80:89, 1971.
34. Frymoyer, J.W., and Hoaglund, F.T.: The role of arthrodesis in reconstruction of the knee. Clin. Orthop., 101:82, 1974.
35. Fulkerson, J.P.: Arthrodesis for disabling hip pain in children and adolescents. Clin. Orthop., 128:296, 1977.
36. García Gonzales, G., Solares Ahedo, R., Villegas Ayala, F. et al.: Arthrodesis of the hip using a cobra plate: Comments on preliminary reports. Prensa Med. Mex., 41:235, 1976.
37. Gore, D.R., Murray, P.M., Sepic, S.B., and Gardner, C.M.: Walking patterns of men with unilateral surgical hip fusion. J. Bone Joint Surg., 57A:759, 1975.
38. Green, D.P., Parkes, J.C., and Stinchfield, F.E.: Arthrodesis of the knee—a follow-up study. J. Bone Joint Surg., 49A:1065, 1967.
39. Gschwend, N.: A little known complication of hip arthrodesis. Arch. Orthop. Trauma Surg., 62:263, 1967.
40. Haddad, R.J., and Riordan, D.C.: Arthrodesis of the wrist. J. Bone Joint Surg., 49A:950, 1967.
41. Hagemann, W.F., Wood, W., and Tullos, H.S.: Arthrodesis in failed total knee replacement. J. Bone Joint Surg., 60A:790, 1978.
42. Hamacher, R., and Koch, F.G.: Late onset sequelae of arthrodesis of knee. Z. Orthop., 3:441, 1973.
43. Hamilton, W.K., and Sokoll, M.: Tourniquet paralysis. J.A.M.A., 199:37, 1967.
44. Huckell, J.R., and Fuller, J.: Arthrodesis of the ankle. In Bateman, J.E. (Ed.): Foot Science. Philadelphia, W.B. Saunders, 1976.
45. Hughes, J.P., McEntire, J.E., and Setze, T.K.: Cast syndrome. Arch. Surg., 108:230, 1974.
46. Ingram, A.J., and Miller, T.R.: Arthrodesis of the shoulder. Unpublished, 1950.
47. Jackson, A., and Glasgow, M.: Tarsal hypermobility after ankle fusion—fact or fiction? J. Bone Joint Surg., 61B:470, 1979.
48. Kalamchi, A.: Arthrodesis for paralytic shoulder: Review of 10 patients. Orthopedics, 1:204, 1978.
49. King, H.W., Watkins, T.B., Jr., and Samuelson, K.M.: Analysis of foot position in ankle arthrodesis and its influence on gait. Foot Ankle, 1:44, 1980.
50. Koch, M., and Lipscomb, P.R.: Arthrodesis of the elbow. Clin. Orthop., 50:151, 1967.
51. Lance, E.M., Paval, A., Fries, I. et al.: Arthrodesis of the ankle joint: Follow-up study. Clin. Orthop., 142:146, 1979.
52. Lange, M.: Arthrodesis of the hip—a review of a series of more than 500 cases. J. Int. Coll. Surg., 29:638, 1958.
53. Lindahl, O.: Determination of hip adduction especially in arthrodesis. Acta Orthop. Scand., 36:280, 1965.
54. ————: Functional capacity after hip arthrodesis. Acta Orthop. Scand., 36:453, 1965.
55. ————: Hip-joint arthrodesis: To find the best position. Acta Orthop. Scand., 37:317, 1966.
56. Lipscomb, P.R., and McCaslin, F.E.: Arthrodesis of the hip—review of 371 cases. J. Bone Joint Surg., 43A:423, 1961.
57. Lortat-Jacob, A., Lelong, P., Benoit, J., and Ramadier, J.O.: Arthrodese du genou apres ablation de prothese totale selon une technique inspiree de la methode de Papineau. Rev. Chir. Orthop., 65:461, 1979.
58. Lucas, D.B., and Murray, W.R.: Arthrodesis of the knee by double plating. J. Bone Joint Surg., 43A:423, 1961.
59. McCaughan, J.S., and Miller, P.R.: Migration of Steinmann pin from shoulder to lung. J.A.M.A., 207:1917, 1969.
60. Makin, M.: Early arthrodesis for a flail shoulder in young children. J. Bone Joint Surg., 59A:317, 1977.
61. ————: Wrist arthrodesis in paralyzed arms of children. J. Bone Joint Surg., 59A:312, 1977.
62. Mazur, J.M., Schwartz, E., and Simon, S.R.: Ankle arthrodesis: Long-term follow-up with gait analysis. J. Bone Joint Surg., 61A:964, 1979.
63. Middleton, R.W.D., and Varian, J.P.: Tourniquet paralysis. Aust. N.Z. J. Surg., 44:124, 1974.
64. Mikkelsen, O.A.: Arthrodesis of the wrist joint in rheumatoid arthritis. Hand, 12:149, 1980.
65. Millender, L.H., and Nalebuff, E.A.: Arthrodesis of the rheumatoid wrist. J. Bone Joint Surg., 55A:1026, 1973.
66. Moldaver, J.: Tourniquet paralysis syndrome. Arch. Surg., 68:136, 1954.
67. Morgenstern, J.M., Hassman, G.C., and Keim, H.A.: Modifying post-transfusion hepatitis by gamma globulin in spinal surgery. Orthop. Rev., 4:29, 1975.
68. Morrey, B.F., and Wiedeman, G.P., Jr.: Complications and long-term results of ankle arthrodeses following trauma. J. Bone Joint Surg., 62A:777, 1980.
69. Morris, H.D., and Herrick, R.T.: Ankle arthrodesis. In Bateman, J.E. (Ed.): Foot Science. Philadelphia, W.B. Saunders, 1976.
70. Nelson, J.P., Ferris, D.O., and Ivins, J.C.: The cast syndrome. Postgrad. Med., 42:457, 1967.
71. Noble, R.P., Gregersen, M.I., Porter, P.M., and Buckman, A.: Blood volume in clinical shock. I. Mixing time and disappearance rate of T-1824 in normal subjects and in patients in shock: Determination of plasma volume in man from 10-minute sample. J. Clin. Invest., 25:158, 1946.
72. ————: Blood volume in clinical shock. II. The

extent and cause of blood volume reduction in traumatic, hemorrhagic and burn shock. J. Clin. Invest., 25:172, 1946.

73. Noh, E.: Mental problems of patients with arthrodesis of hip. Z. Orthop., 3:418, 1973.

74. Pahle, J.A., and Raunio, P.: The influence of wrist position on finger position in the rheumatoid hand. J. Bone Joint Surg., 51B:664, 1969.

75. Pipkin, G.: Claviculectomy as an adjunct to shoulder arthrodesis. Clin. Orthop., 54:145, 1967.

76. Price, C.T., and Lovell, W.W.: Thompson arthrodesis of the hip in children. J. Bone Joint Surg., 62A:1118, 1980.

77. Rechnagel, K.: Arthrodesis of the wrist joint. Scand. J. Plast. Reconstr. Surg., 5:120, 1971.

78. Research Committee of the American Orthopaedic Association: A survey of end results on the stabilization of the paralytic shoulder. J. Bone Joint Surg., 24:699, 1942.

78a. Haddad, R.J. Jr., and Riordan, D.C.: Arthrodesis of the wrist: A surgical technique. J. Bone Joint Surg., 49A:950, 1967.

79. Ronpe, G.: Late onset damages of neighboring joints following hip fusion. Z. Orthop., 3:435, 1973.

80. Rowe, C.R.: Re-evaluation of the position of the arm in arthrodesis of the shoulder in the adult. J. Bone Joint Surg., 56A:913, 1974.

81. Rybka, V., Raunio, P., and Vainio, K.: Arthrodesis of the shoulder in rheumatoid arthritis. J. Bone Joint Surg., 61B:155, 1979.

82. ———: Arthrodesis of the shoulder joint in rheumatoid arthritis. Acta Chir. Orthop. Traumatol. Cech., 46:135, 1979.

83. Said, E., Hunka, L., and Siller, T.N.: Where ankle fusion stands today. J. Bone Joint Surg., 60B:211, 1978.

84. Salenius, P., and Kivilaakso, R.: Followup examination of a series of arthrodesis of the knee joint. Acta Orthop. Scand., 39:91, 1968.

85. Sanders, R.: The tourniquet, instrument or weapon. Hand, 5:119, 1973.

86. Schwartz, D.R., and Wirka, H.W.: The cast syndrome: A case report and discussion of the literature. J. Bone Joint Surg., 46A:1549, 1964.

87. Scranton, P.E., Jr., Fu, F.H., and Brown, T.D.: Ankle arthrodesis: A comparative clinical and biomechanical evaluation. Clin. Orthop., 151:234, 1980.

88. Siller, T.N., and Hadjipavlou, A.: Knee arthrodesis: Long-term results. Can. J. Surg., 19:217, 1976.

89. Skak, S.V.: Arthrodesis of the wrist by the method of Mannerfelt: A follow-up of 19 patients. Acta Orthop. Scand., 53:557, 1982.

90. Soren, A.: Function of the foot following arthrodesis. Ann. Phys. Med., 9:63, 1967.

91. Staples, O.S.: Arthrodesis of the elbow joint. J. Bone Joint Surg., 34A:207, 1952.

92. Stewart, M.J.: Arthrodesis. In Edmonson, A.S., and Crenshaw, A.H. (Eds.): Campbell's Operative Orthopaedics, 6th ed. St. Louis, C.V. Mosby, 1980.

93. Stewart, M.J., Beeler, C.T., and McConnell, J.C.: Compression arthrodesis of the ankle: Evaluation of a cosmetic modification. J. Bone Joint Surg., 65A:219, 1983.

94. Stewart, M.J., and Coker, T.P.: Arthrodesis of the hip. Clin. Orthop., 62:136, 1969.

95. Stulberg, S.D.: Arthrodesis in failed total knee replacements. Orthop. Clin. North Am., 13:213, 1982.

96. Thal, A.P., Brown, E.B., Hermreck, A.S., and Bell, H.H.: Shock: A Physiologic Basis for Treatment. Chicago, Year Book Medical Publishers, 1971.

97. Tristan, T.A., and Daughtridge, T.G.: Migration of a metallic pin from the humerus into the lung. N. Engl. J. Med., 270:987, 1964.

98. Tyazhelkova, P.I.: Remote results of arthrodesis of the shoulder joint in children. Khirurgiia (Mosk), 43:106, 1967.

99. Vahvanen, V.: Arthrodesis in failed knee replacement in eight rheumatoid patients. Ann. Chir. Gynaecol., 68:57, 1979.

100. Vahvanen, V., and Kettunen, P.: Arthrodesis of the wrist in rheumatoid arthritis: A follow-up study of 62 cases. Ann. Chir. Gynaecol., 66:195, 1977.

101. Vahvanen, V., and Rokkanen, P.: Arthrodesis of the ankle—a follow-up study on 28 patients. Ann. Chir. Gynaecol. Fenn., 61:37, 1972.

102. Watson-Jones, R., and Robinson, W.C.: Arthrodesis of the osteoarthritic hip joint. J. Bone Joint Surg., 38B:353, 1956.

103. Waugh, W.: The functional consequences of arthrodesis. Egypt. Orthop. J., 7:255, 1972.

43 Musculoskeletal Changes Complicating Burns

E. Burke Evans

Classification of Musculoskeletal Changes Secondary to Burns

Alterations Limited to Bone
  Osteoporosis
  Periosteal new bone formation[7]
  Irregular ossification[7]
  Diaphyseal exostosis[7]
  Acromutilation of fingers[8]
  Pathologic fracture
  Osteomyelitis
  Necrosis and tangential sequestration
Alterations Involving Pericapsular Structures
  Pericapsular calcification
  Heterotopic para-articular ossification
  Osteophyte formation[7]
Alterations Involving the Joint Proper
  Dislocation
  Septic arthritis
  Spontaneous dissolution
  Ankylosis
Alterations Involving Muscles and Tendons
  Desiccation of tendons
  Fibrosis of muscles[21]
Alterations Secondary to Soft Tissue Contractures
  Muscle contractures
  Malposition of joints
  Scoliosis
Abnormalities of Growth[1,19]
  Acceleration
  Destruction of the growth plate
Nonviability of Extremity Leading to Amputation

Thermal burns mainly affect the skin, and, although burns are occasionally so severe as to alter or expose muscles, tendons, joints, and bones, these structures are usually secondarily affected. Musculoskeletal changes are less often complications of specific treatment than they are the results of failures of treatment or of failures to institute preventive measures. It is in this context that a classification of musculoskeletal changes secondary to burns is given and that selected changes affecting functional prognosis are discussed.

CHANGES LIMITED TO BONE

Osteoporosis

Generalized bone atrophy or osteoporosis occurs in burned patients who are confined to bed for long periods. It is a complication of severe burns and is nowadays rarely observed, since even severely burned patients are mobilized quickly. In the past, when many patients were kept in bed until grafts were stable, bone atrophy was part of the burn illness, and it deterred mobilization of patients, being often of such severity as to leave bones precariously fragile.

Other factors may favor deossification. Owens emphasizes the role of hyperemia.[17] Artz and Reiss mention adrenocortical activity.[2] Colson and associates credit, in addition, reflex vasomotor phenomena.[4]

Hyperemia is responsible, in part at least, for the local atrophy observed in burns limited to one extremity. Likewise, among patients with generalized burns the atrophy observed in an extensively burned extremity is often more intense than that of other bones affected only by generalized mineral loss (Fig. 43-1). The badly burned extremity suffers the double insult of hyperemia and limitation of motion.

Fracture

Fractures occurring at the time of a burn are not complications of treatment, but they

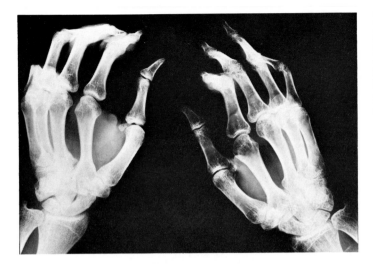

FIG. 43-1. Generalized osteoporosis in a 16-year-old boy following 40% third-degree burns and extended bed confinement. The more intense bone atrophy of the right hand reflects the greater severity of the burn on that side.

make overall care of the patient still more difficult. Such fractures can be managed by skeletal traction and often by external support (Fig. 43-2, *A* through *C*).[6] In a patient with severe burns, fractures that are nondeforming may not be recognized immediately (Fig. 43-2, *D*).

Pathological fractures due to the stress of exercise or weight bearing on atrophic bone are now rare (Fig. 43-3). They are usually of the compression type, and they heal rapidly if the patient has reached the anabolic phase of recovery.[5]

Osteomyelitis

Hematogenous osteomyelitis is not a common complication of burn care. Given the prevalence of bacteremia and the high incidence of septic states among the severely burned, this circumstance is difficult to explain. Likewise, when bones are exposed

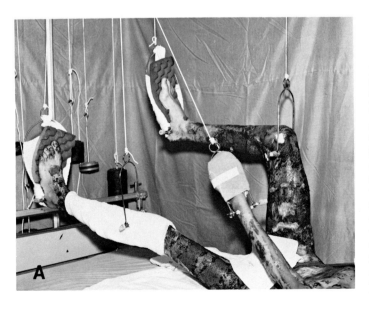

FIG. 43-2. (*A*) A 15-year-old boy with 45% third-degree burns and closed fractures of the right femur, left humerus, and left radius. The fractures, treated with skeletal traction initially and then with light cast, a thigh corset, and a sling, respectively, healed in 8 weeks. (*B*) Fracture of the humerus 3 weeks after injury. (*C*) Fracture of the femur 5 weeks after injury. (*D*) An occult torus fracture of the left radius was discovered during a roentgenographic check of pin position.

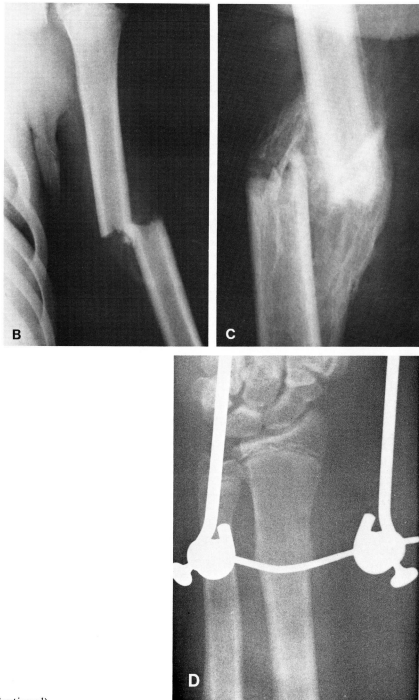

FIG. 43-2. (*Continued*)

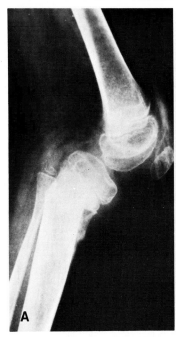
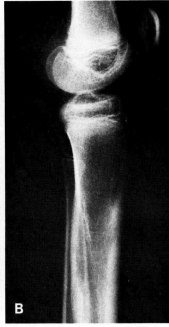

FIG. 43-3. (A) This pathologic fracture in the upper third of the tibia in a 5-year-old girl with 11% third-degree burns was the result of overzealous manipulation after long-term bed confinement. (B) Four years after fracture, limb lengths were equal, and the range of knee motion on the side of the fracture was normal.

by the burn or by the removal of eschar, osteomyelitis does not usually develop. If exposure is prolonged, the devitalized cortex forms a sequestrum tangentially. Drilling exposed bone to promote the development of surface granulation tissue involves little risk of bone infection.

Osteomyelitis is now observed as a complication of the skeletal suspension and traction used in the treatment of both acute and chronic burns. In acute burns, pins are inserted directly through burned skin eschar or granulation tissue, if necessary, and no amount of prior local cleaning is likely to sterilize the area of insertion. In our own experience, roentgenographically discernible osteomyelitis has occurred in approximately 5% of patients treated in traction (Fig. 43-4). The infections have remained localized and have resolved without specific antibiotic or surgical treatment.

Factors favoring pin tract infection are prolonged traction, excessive movement of the extremity leading to loosening of the pin, and sealing of pin sites. It is thus desirable to keep pin sites open and clean

while pins are in place, and for several days after they are removed. Skeletal traction should be discontinued if extremity motion is excessive and uncontrollable.

CHANGES INVOLVING PERICAPSULAR STRUCTURES: HETEROTOPIC OSSIFICATION

The cause of heterotopic para-articular calcification and ossification associated with burns is not known. The following factors are recognized as contributory: the severity and extent of the burn, the length of bed confinement, superimposed trauma, and familial predisposition.[5] The fact that heterotopic bone is seen in patients who have a third-degree burn involving 30% or more of the body surface is probably less important than the fact that patients with severe burns are often immobilized for a long time.

After extended bed confinement, heterotopic calcification or ossification may seem to occur quite rapidly and may appear at

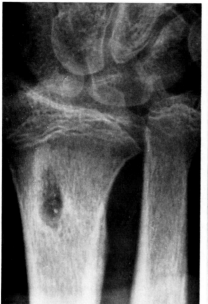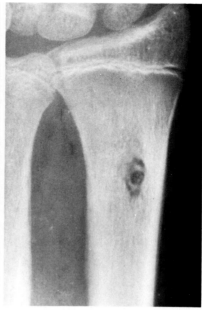

FIG. 43-4. Localized osteomyelitis in the radius of 7-year-old boy with 30% third-degree burns. There is a distinct cigarette sequestrum on the right. The upper extremities were in traction 15 days. The lesions healed uneventfully.

several joints simultaneously. It is as though some abrupt humoral phenomenon has triggered the mechanism. Although mobilization of mineral salts is often a roentgenographic certainty, serum calcium and phosphorus levels have not been found to be altered in relation to this phenomenon.[5] Koepke found alkaline phosphatase levels to be elevated in patients with extensive third-degree burns during the first few weeks after injury.* Four of the patients in his study of 100 consecutive admissions developed heterotopic bone as their phosphatase levels were declining. Calcium and phosphorus and other serum electrolytes were normal. Thus an elevated alkaline phosphatase level reflects the activity, but it does not disclose the reason for it.

The location of heterotopic bone is not determined by the distribution of burn.[12] The joints of slightly burned extremities may be affected as readily as those underlying a full-thickness burn. There is evidence that the joints of less severely burned extremities may be affected because of overuse of those extremities and superimposed trauma to the para-articular structures. Dislocation of a hip joint in one of our cases was thought to be responsible for the relatively more extensive involvement of that joint (Fig. 43-5).

Heterotopic calcification and ossification occur in only 2% to 3% of severely burned persons.[5] It is thus reasonable to suggest that individual idiosyncrasy or familial predisposition is a factor. Our experience with twin brothers supports this suggestion (Fig. 43-6). Neither brother was seriously burned. Both developed heterotopic bone in very much the same distribution.

Heterotopic ossification occurs at all major joints. In adults, the elbow is most frequently affected, bilateral involvement being the rule rather than the exception. Posteriorly the calcific or osseous bridge extends

(*Text continues on page 1314.*)

* Koepke, G.H.: Personal communication, 1976.

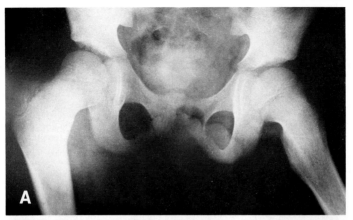

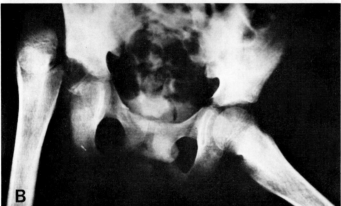

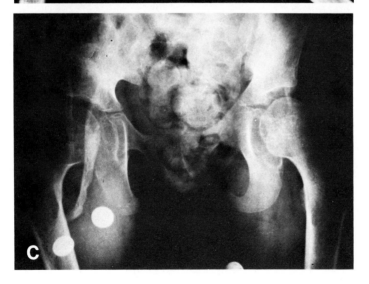

FIG. 43-5. (*A*) The adducted position of the right hip in this 5-year-old boy favored eventual displacement. There was 40% third-degree burn. (*B*) Two months after the burn the right hip dislocated during routine transfer to the dressing table. The dislocation was reduced with skeletal traction. (*C*) Two months after the dislocation there was extensive heterotopic bone formation on the right. (*D*) One year following the dislocation, most of the heterotopic bone had disappeared. The hips were functionally normal. (*D* from Evans, E.B.: Orthopaedic measures in the treatment of severe burns. J. Bone Joint Surg., 48A:662, 1966)

FIG. 43-5. (*Continued*)

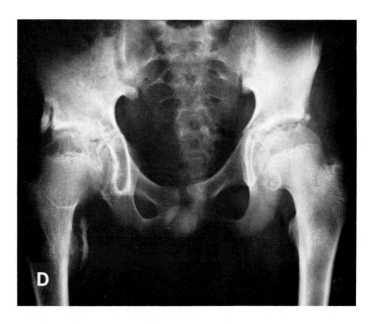

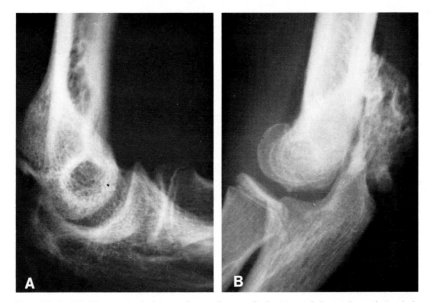

FIG. 43-6. (*A*) Heterotopic bone along the medial epicondylar ridge of the left humerus in a 12-year-old boy with a 14% third-degree burn that did not involve the affected extremity. (*B*) The twin brother of the patient in *A* with more extensive heterotopic bone in the same location on the left. He had 17% third-degree burns, the left arm being slightly involved near the elbow. The bone did not bridge the joint in either elbow, and it resorbed spontaneously.

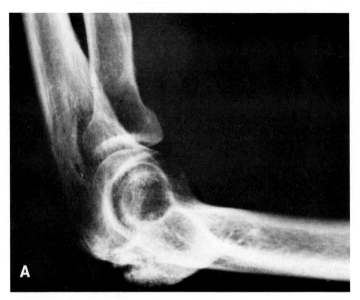

FIG. 43-7. (*A* and *C*) Hetero-topic bone extends from the olecranons to the medial epi-condylar ridges of the humeri in the elbows of a 37-year-old man. He had 20% third-de-gree burns, but the upper ex-tremities were only slightly burned. The joints were oth-erwise preserved, and pro-nation and supination were retained. (*B* and *D*) Roentgen-ograms made 3 weeks after excision of the heterotopic bone show the range of el-bow extension. Full range of motion was regained in 6 months. (Evans, E.B.: Ortho-paedic measures in the treat-ment of severe burns. J. Bone Joint Surg., 48A:666, 1966)

from the olecranon to the medial epicon-dylar ridge of the humerus (Fig. 43-7). Anterior bridging in the adult elbow is rare, but the radius occasionally becomes fixed to the ulna (see Fig. 43-10). The shoulder is the next most frequently involved joint in adults, whereas the hip is rarely affected. In children, hip and elbow are affected with about equal frequency (see Figs. 43-5 and 43-8). In the elbow, however, the bone is deposited anteriorly rather than posteriorly. We have not observed involvement of the shoulder in children.

Knowledge of five facts simplifies the handling of burn patients with heterotopic calcification and ossification: Para-articular calcification and ossification may increase in dimension as long as there are open granulating areas. When the burn has healed, if ectopic bone has not bridged the joint, it will in children gradually disappear; in adults it will become much smaller (see Figs. 43-5 and 43-9). Heterotopic bone that bridges a joint in one plane often spares the articulation. In this circumstance, if the offending bone is removed adequately after the burn has healed, it will not, as a rule,

re-form sufficiently to compromise motion, and it may not recur at all (see Fig. 43-7, *C* and *D*). If heterotopic bone bridges a joint in more than one plane, the prognosis for restoration of motion after resection of the bone diminishes as the extent of involve-ment increases, regardless of apparent spar-ing of the articulation. The articular surfaces of extensively involved joints will eventually be lost, and intra-articular ankylosis will occur (Fig. 43-10).

In recent years, paralleling the institution of early mobilization of burn patients, het-erotopic bone formation has become a rel-atively insignificant problem.

CHANGES INVOLVING THE JOINT PROPER

Dislocation

Luxations or subluxations may be due to destruction of support structures, faulty po-sitioning, or scar contracture. When a major joint such as the knee or elbow is exposed or its ligaments damaged by the burn, it

(*Text continues on page 1318.*)

FIG. 43-7. (*Continued*)

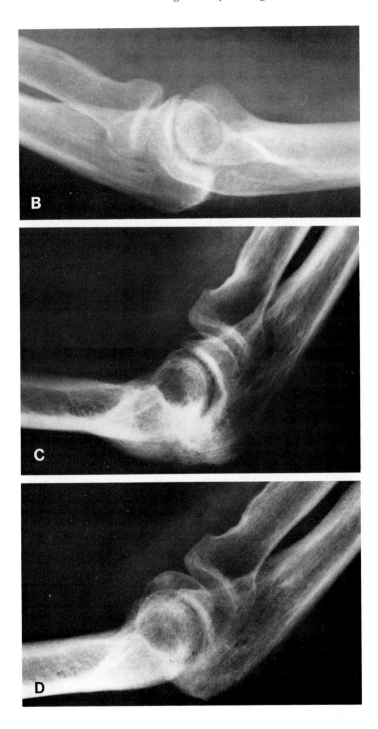

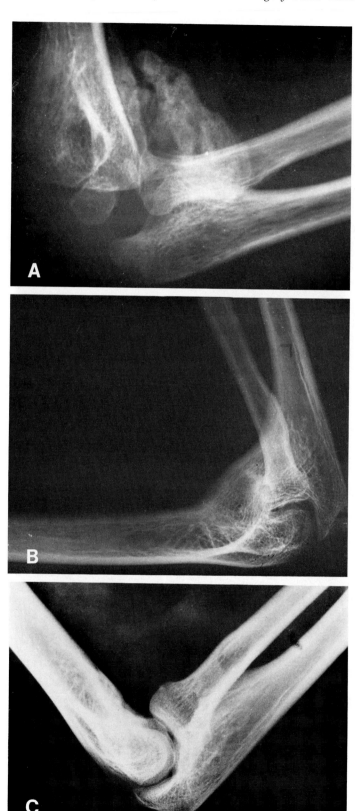

FIG. 43-8. (A) Immature heterotopic bone bridges the elbow of a 7-year-old girl with 50% third-degree burns, 2 months after injury. The bone lies in the plane of the brachialis tendon. Both upper extremities were burned. (B) Four months after the burn the heterotopic bone is mature. (C) One year after excision of the heterotopic bone, there has been no recurrence, and elbow motion is normal.

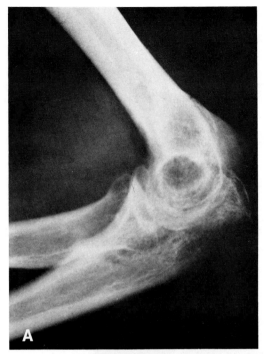

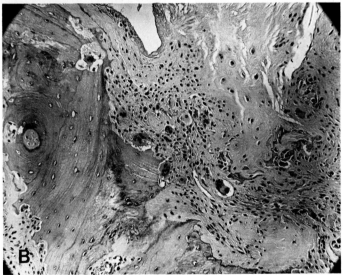

FIG. 43-9. (*A*) The small exostosis on the medial epicondylar ridge of the humerus of a 23-year-old man had begun to decrease in size after total skin coverage. It was excised to accelerate restoration of range of motion. (*B*) A section of removed exostosis shows osteoclastic activity at the margin. (Evans, E.B.: Orthopaedic measures in the treatment of severe burns. J. Bone Joint Surg., 48A:663, 1966)

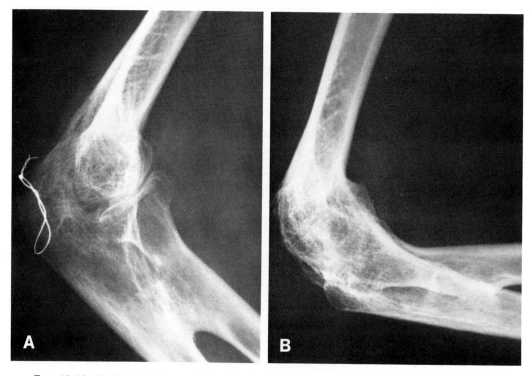

FIG. 43-10. (*A*) In this 33-year-old woman there were bridges of heterotopic bone from the humerus to the olecranon posteriorly and from the radius to the ulna at the level of the bicipital tuberosity. Cartilage space was markedly diminished in both joints. (*B*) Excision of the two osseous bridges did not restore joint motion, and intra-articular ankylosis occurred soon after surgery.

tends to slip into subluxation if it is not held in position by an external splint or by a brace transfixed to the bone above and below the joint. Subluxation or luxation likewise occurs in joints compromised by hematogenous septic arthritis if articular destruction is extensive. If the subluxation is fixed by scar contracture, alignment must be corrected by skeletal traction or surgery before the splinting device is applied (see Fig. 43-11, *B*). Optimal position must be held until the joint is covered with graft, and standard bracing can be used for protection. The elbow and the hip are susceptible to subluxation or luxation from poor positioning, particularly when a patient is in the catabolic phase and is relatively immobile.

Abduction and extension favor displacement of the head of the humerus. Thus the shoulder should be positioned in no more than 85° of abduction and in at least 20° to 25° of flexion. In tense or agitated patients the danger of dislocation is increased as they press their elbows into the bed and lever the head of the humerus forward. Treatment in the prone position may put the shoulders in jeopardy unless the trunk is elevated sufficiently to allow the arms to drop forward.

Since flexion and adduction favor posterior displacement of the head of the femur (see Fig. 43-5), hips should be positioned in extension and symmetric abduction of 15° to 20°.

Scar contracture alone may cause subluxation of metacarpophalangeal joints. The first and fifth digits are the ones most frequently affected. Displacement can be prevented by consistent accurate splinting. Correction entails scar release, capsulotomy, and postoperative splinting. Reduction can often be achieved by progressive, accurate splinting alone. Short-term constant pin traction may be helpful following capsulotomy, or it may be all that is needed to reduce the subluxation.

Septic Arthritis

Septic arthritis is inevitable if a joint is exposed at the time of the burn or when eschar is removed (Fig. 43-11). Such a joint must be stabilized by suitable splinting or traction and must be regularly and thoroughly irrigated and washed, preferably in a tub. In children, a high percentage of exposed joints can be saved. In adults, joints are less resilient.

Hematogenous joint infection is a rather common complication, usually occurring when a patient with extensive burns is acutely ill. The infection may remain occult or may be camouflaged by the surface wounds. There are no reliable diagnostic signs such as elevation of temperature or sedimentation rate, or localizing pain, heat, or swelling. Diagnosis may have to be made on suspicion alone. Roentgenograms may reveal only local cellulitis. Aspiration usually confirms the diagnosis but may not yield bacteria-containing material because these patients are often already receiving high doses of broad-spectrum antibiotics.

If an organism can be cultured from the aspirate, specific antibiotic therapy may be instituted instead of or in addition to what is already being given. Of far greater importance in the treatment is the exteriorization of the joint and the institution of vigorous lavage and tubbing, as for an exposed joint (Fig. 43-12). Unrecognized septic arthritis will progress to ankylosis of the joint (Fig. 43-13).

Preferred Positions for Major Joints

Neck: midline in neutral or slight extension
Shoulders: scapulothoracic retraction, 85° of glenohumeral abduction, 20° to 25° of glenohumeral flexion
Elbows: extension
Wrists: slight extension
Metacarpophalangeal joints, (2 through 5): 80° to 90° of flexion
Proximal and distal interphalangeal joints: full extension
Thumbs: carpometacarpal flexion and abduction, metacarpophalangeal flexion 5° to 10°, interphalangeal extension
Spine: extension without lateral bend
Hips: extension, 15° of symmetric abduction, slight external rotation
Knees: extension
Ankles: neutral
Feet: neutral

Contracture

The most common and troublesome complication of burns is scar contracture leading to malposition and limitation of joint motion. When a burn occurs, there are no contractures, and ideally there should be no contractures when the acute phase of treatment, including total grafting of the burn wound, is complete. Prevention of contracture involves proper positioning for each joint and maintenance of joint mobility.

Contractures of the skin are dermal and thus complicate the management of deep second- or third-degree burns. There is evidence that with early excision of the burn wound and split-thickness grafting, scarring is less severe, and contractures are less likely to occur.[1,3,11,16] Clearly, if grafting is delayed until separation of eschar, granulation tissue formation, and collagen proliferation, contracture is more likely to occur. Likewise, scarring and contracture are more likely to be problems if grafts are placed on fat or on unhealthy granulation tissue.

The most effective means of preventing scar contracture and hypertrophy is continuous consistent local pressure. Pressure is

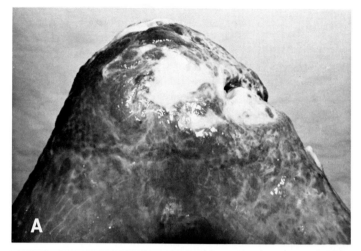

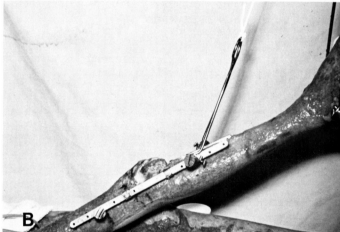

FIG. 43-11. (*A*) Right knee joint exposed by a full-thickness burn in a 12-year-old girl with 40% third-degree burns. (*B*) The knee-flexion contracture was corrected with skeletal traction through the calcaneus and tibia, and the corrected position was held by an adjustable external splint transfixed to bone above and below the joint. (*C*) The extremity was cleaned daily in a hypochlorite tub bath. The joint was lavaged regularly. Closure of the joint was achieved with split-thickness autogenous grafting after the defect was bridged by granulation tissue. (*D*) One year after removal of the splint, the knee could be flexed to 90° from neutral. (*E*) Roentgenogram made 1 year after closure of the joint shows a normal cartilage space and no osseous destruction.

likewise effective in reducing scar hypertrophy and contracture and thus in correcting deformity due to contracture. Pressure may be applied with elastic bandages for extremities, with sponges and elastic wraps for axillae, with special Jobst garments for hands, trunk, and extremities, with special masks for the face, and with isoprene splints for the neck (Figs. 43-14 and 43-15).[9,14,22] Larson and co-workers have shown that the minimum pressure required is 25 torr.[14]

Skeletal traction or periodic continuous stretching coupled with accurate splinting corrects most contractural deformities of the extremities (Fig. 43-16).[8,13,20,22]

CHANGES SECONDARY TO SOFT TISSUE CONTRACTURES

Scoliosis and Kyphosis

Scoliosis is transient in patients who have asymmetric trunk, axillary, or groin contracture if the contracture is surgically relieved before the spine develops structural changes (Fig. 43-17). Structural scoliosis is thus a rare complication, and we have had experience with only one case.[6]

Kyphosis occurs when there are third-degree or deep second-degree burns over the upper chest extending onto the shoul-

(*Text continues on page 1324.*)

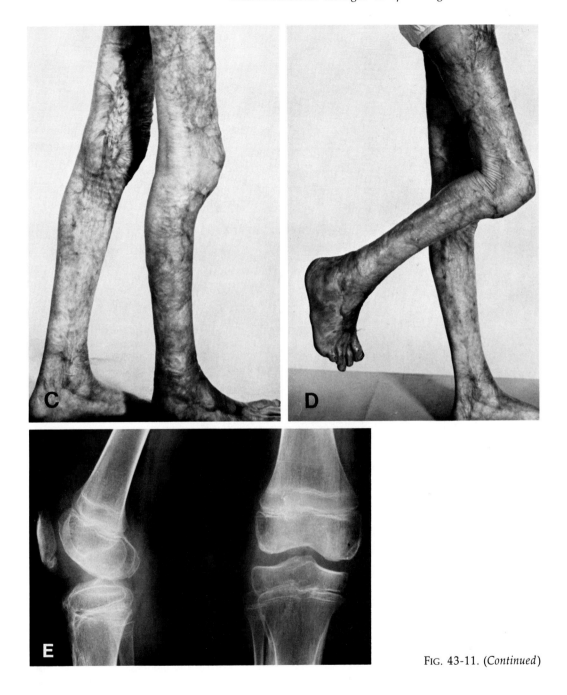

FIG. 43-11. (*Continued*)

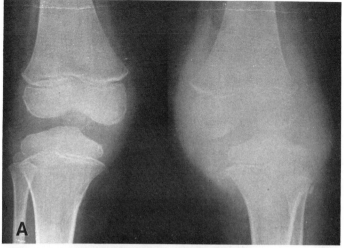

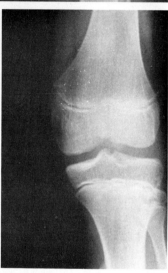

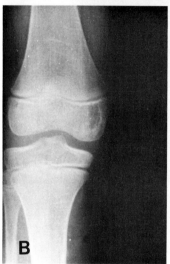

FIG. 43-12. (*A*) Hematogenous infection of the knee joint in a 10-year-old girl with 35% third-degree burns. The extremity of the affected knee was severely burned. The joint was exteriorized and lavaged regularly. (*B*) Three years after the infection the knee functioned normally. The roentgenogram shows minimal evidence of the previous disease.

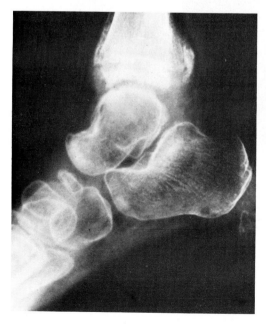

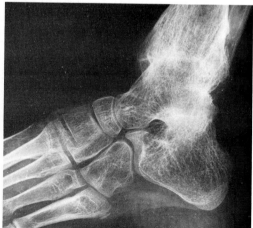

FIG. 43-13. Advanced septic arthritis in the ankle and subtalar joints of a 7-year-old girl with 50% third-degree burns, resulting in complete ankylosis of both joints.

FIG. 43-14. A 3-year-old girl with 59% third-degree burns, as she appeared after acute burn. Elastic bandages with sponge pads for the neck and axillae were used for pressure. The bandages were worn for 4 months more. The right side of the groin and both antecubital fossae required additional surgery.

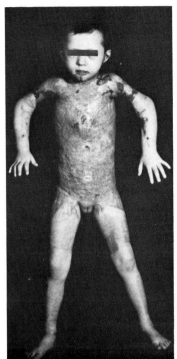 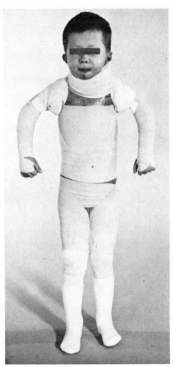

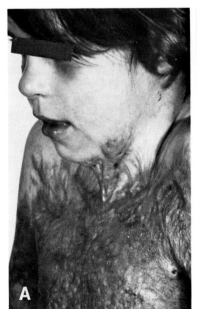 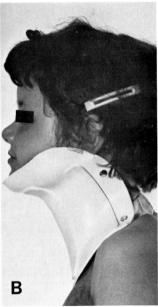 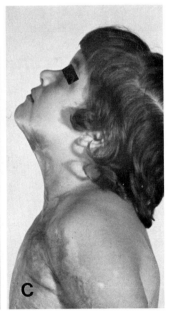

FIG. 43-15. (A) Severe contracture of the neck in a 10-year-old girl with 32% third-degree burns. (B) The deformity was corrected with isoprene splints that were replaced or remodeled as the scar flattened and the neck extended. (C) Appearance 1 year after treatment began. The splint was worn until the scarred area became soft and pliant. (Larson, D.L., Abston, S., Evans, E.B. et al.: Techniques for decreasing scar formation and contractures in the burned patient. J. Trauma, 11:818, 1971)

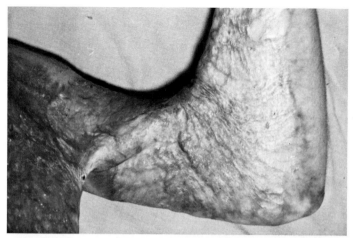

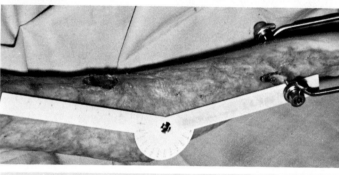

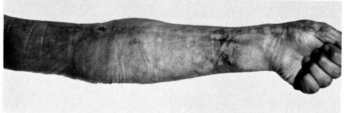

FIG. 43-16. A 100° flexion deformity of the left elbow due to scar hypertrophy and contracture was corrected by skeletal traction in 10 days. The position was maintained with a three-point aluminum splint, and the scar was controlled with an elastic bandage.

ders and neck. The recumbent position in bed favors protraction of the shoulders and flexion of the neck and thoracic spine. A roll or narrow pad placed between the shoulders helps to keep the shoulders retracted, the neck extended, and the thoracic spine flat. Once a deformity is established, the slump-shouldered, kyphotic posture tends to persist even after surgical correction of the contracture and softening or maturing of the scar. Bracing helps to prevent recurrence of the deformity (Fig. 43-18).

Hand Contractures

Deformities in burned hands are common. Typically in a burned hand allowed to heal unsupported, the metacarpal arch is reversed, the metacarpophalangeal joints are hyperextended, and the proximal interphalangeal joints are flexed.[5] The first metacarpal is extended and adducted (Fig. 43-19). The two most troublesome of these deformities are contracture of the first web space and loss of extension of the proximal interphalangeal joints of the medial four digits.

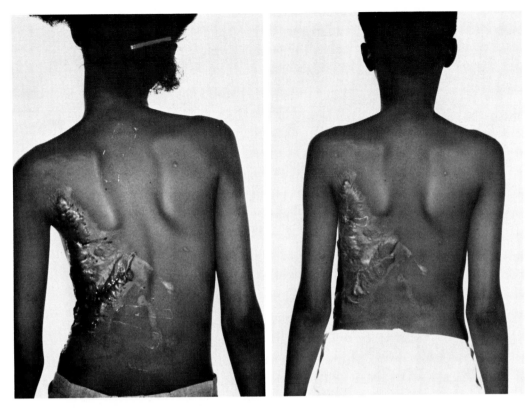

FIG. 42-17. Nonstructural scoliosis in this 11-year-old girl was corrected by release of the constricting hypertrophied scar.

Loss of the first intermetacarpal space can be prevented by splinting. The most common splinting error consists in applying pressure to the volar surface of the proximal phalanx rather than to the head of the metacarpal or to the medial surface of the first phalanx with the metacarpophalangeal joint in slight flexion. If the metacarpophalangeal joint is allowed to extend to neutral, it will quickly go into hyperextension, and the metacarpal will drift into adduction. Accurate, efficient splinting of the hands can easily be accomplished in adults and older children (Figs. 43-20 and 43-21). The hands of small children and infants are difficult to manage, and positioning—initially and for grafting—may best be accomplished by digital traction through pins

in the distal phalanges (Figs. 43-22 and 43-23).

An established adduction contracture can rarely be corrected by external splinting alone. Operative release is usually necessary. Splints or wrappings that create pressure in the first web space cause adduction of the first metacarpal and are likely to cause hyperextension of the metacarpophalangeal joint.

If the wrist is not supported in neutral position or in slight extension, the metacarpophalangeal joints of the medial four digits will extend, and the proximal interphalangeal joints will flex. If this posture is allowed to persist, proximal interphalangeal extension will be lost. In some digits the distal interphalangeal joint becomes fixed in ex-

(*Text continues on page 1329.*)

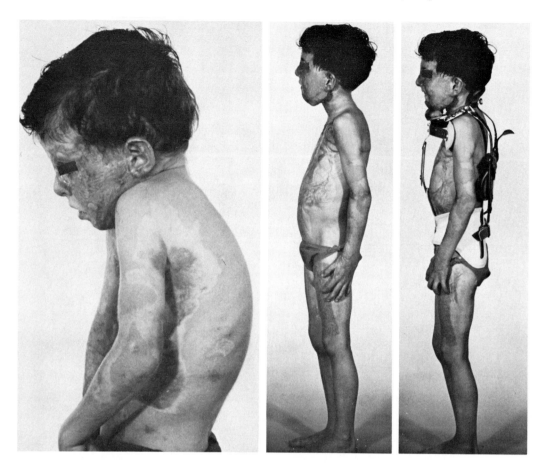

FIG. 43-18. Kyphosis was due to contracture of scars over the anterior chest and neck of this 4-year-old boy. After surgical correction, posture was controlled with a Milwaukee brace. (Evans, E.B., Larson, D.L., Abston, S., and Willis, B.: Prevention and correction of deformity after severe burns. Surg. Clin. North Am., 50:1366, 1970)

FIG. 43-19. A typical hand deformity developed in a 9-year-old girl 3 months after she sustained 60% third-degree burns. Note the extension of the metacarpophalangeal joints and the flexion of the proximal interphalangeal joints of the medial four digits and the extension and adduction of the first metacarpal.

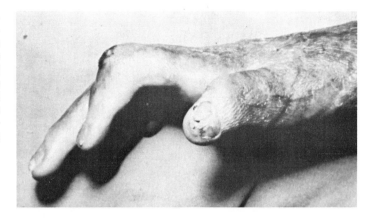

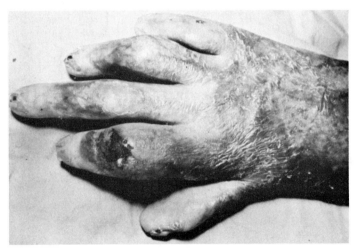

FIG. 43-20. A normal hand in an isoprene splint shows the wrist in slight extension, the metacarpophalangeal joints in flexion, the interphalangeal joints in extension, and the thumb in metacarpal abduction and flexion, and slight metacarpophalangeal flexion.

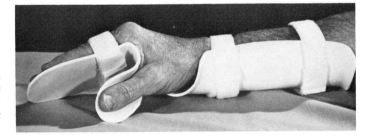

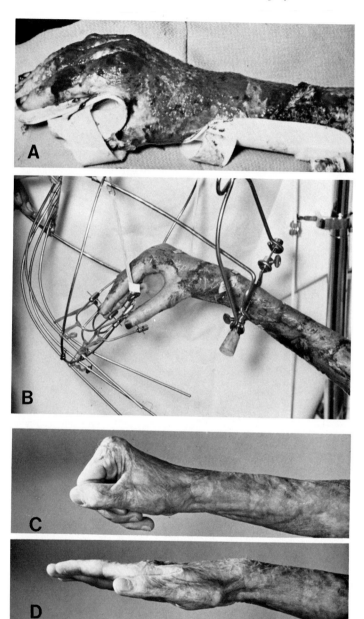

FIG. 43-21. (*A*) A hand with third-degree burns properly positioned in an isoprene splint. (*B*) The position was maintained in hay-rake splint for split-thickness skin grafting. Isoprene splints were used after grafting, with an elastic pressure wrap. (*C* and *D*) Final result, 2 years after the burn.

FIG. 43-22. An isoprene hand splint was fashioned for this 8-month-old boy with 3% deep second-degree burns restricted to the hands. The splint holds the hand in a position that only approximates the ideal but that, with careful wrapping, prevents deformity.

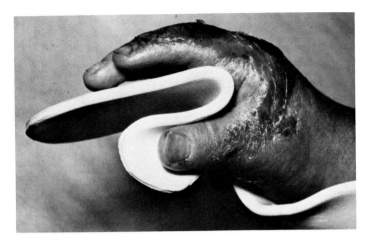

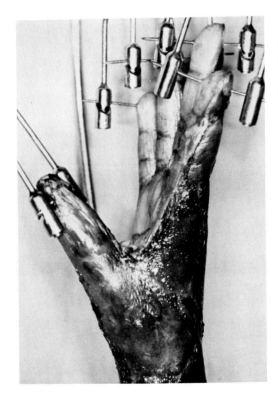

FIG. 43-23. The hand of this 4-year-old child is properly positioned in skeletal traction to facilitate grafting. The thumb is held in maximum intermetacarpal flexion and abduction.

tension, creating a boutonnière deformity. If the dorsal surface of the digits has been burned, the central slip over the proximal interphalangeal joint will be in jeopardy, and failure to keep the joint in full extension may result in severe stretching or complete loss of the slip. Occasionally the central slip is rendered nonviable by the burn and will be lost. In this circumstance the joint must be kept fully extended until it is covered by a skin graft (Fig. 43-24).

An established flexion deformity of the proximal interphalangeal joint may be corrected by progressive extension splinting or by pin traction followed by splinting. This treatment may be effective for long-standing deformities (Fig. 43-25). Even complete loss of the central slip need not require surgical reconstruction. Active extension is regained through improvement of lateral band efficiency, and apparently through reestablishment of continuity of the central slip.

Foot Deformity

When there is a deep burn of the dorsum of the foot extending to the toes, the resulting scar as it contracts can pull the toes into marked extension, creating a disabling deformity with the metatarsal heads deflected sharply plantarward. The contracture

(*Text continues on page 1333.*)

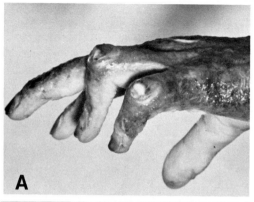

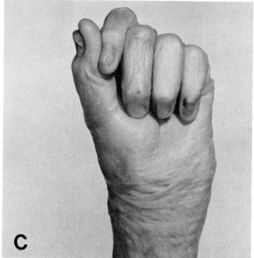

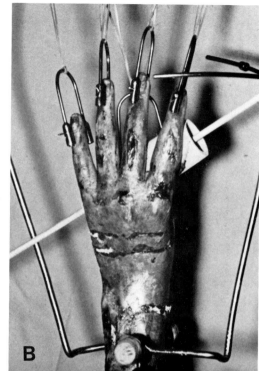

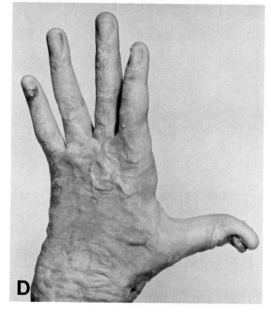

FIG. 43-24. (*A*) Exposure of the proximal interphalangeal joints of the fourth and fifth digits with complete loss of the central slip in both digits. (*B*) The deformity was corrected with skeletal traction, and the joints were closed with split-thickness skin grafts over a thin sheet of granulation tissue. (*C* and *D*) Proximal interphalangeal extension was restored without additional surgery.

FIG. 43-25. (*A*) Boutonnière-type deformity developed in all four fingers of this 34-year-old woman 6 months after a burn. (*B*) The deformity was corrected with skeletal traction in 10 days. (*C*) Proximal interphalangeal extension was regained without surgery. The hand was protected in an articulated isoprene splint for 3 months after traction.

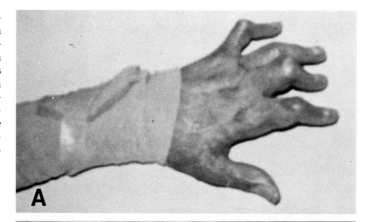

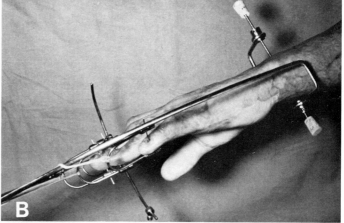

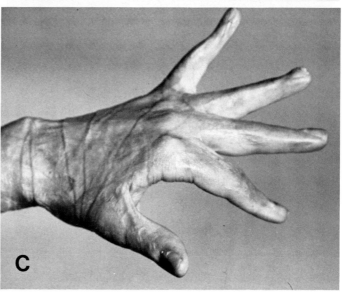

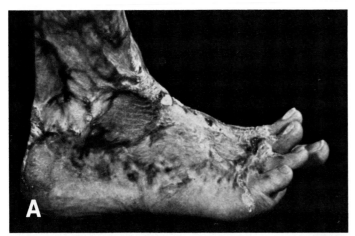

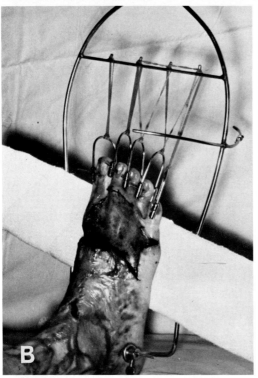

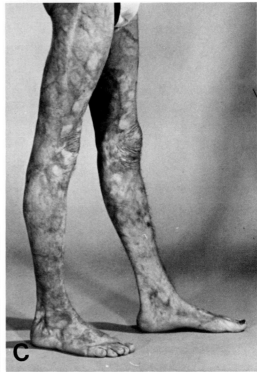

FIG. 43-26. (*A*) Extension deformity of the digits developed in a foot with dorsal contracture following third-degree burns. Both feet were affected. (*B*) After scar division and split-thickness grafting, the toes were held in a flexed position by skeletal traction until the graft was stable. (*C* and *D*) The postoperative correction was maintained with elastic wrapping and with well-fitted shoes with metatarsal bars.

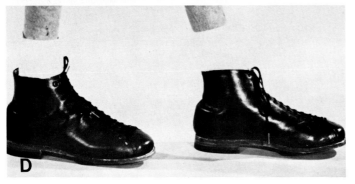

FIG. 43-27. In this acutely burned foot the flexed toe position was held with a modified hay rake throughout the period of primary split-thickness grafting.

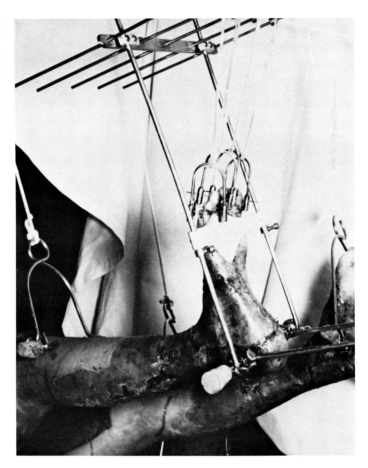

is easily corrected surgically, and the same measures necessary to prevent recurrence of the deformity after surgery will prevent its occuring in the first place (Figs. 43-26 and 43-27).

The ankle must be firmly supported in neutral position. Following surgical scar release or primary grafting if there has been any prior tendency for the digits to extend, the toes should be in a flexed position. Skeletal traction holds this position securely.[10] When the grafts are stable, the foot can be exercised and can be wrapped protectively for walking. A supportive shoe with a metatarsal bar will help maintain the correction (see Fig. 43-26, C and D). Scar contracture can cause the foot to deviate medially, laterally, and plantarward, but the deformity described is the one most frequently seen.

REFERENCES

1. Artz, C.P., and Moncrief, J.A.: The Treatment of Burns, 2nd ed. Philadelphia, W.B. Saunders, 1969.
2. Artz, C.P., and Reiss, E.: The Treatment of Burns, 1st ed. Philadelphia, W.B. Saunders, 1957.
3. Burke, J.F., Bondoc, C.C., and Quinby, W.C.: Primary burn excision and immediate grafting: a method of shortening illness. J. Trauma, 14:389, 1974.
4. Colson, P., Stagnara, P., and Houot, H.: L'ostéoporose chez les brûlés des membres. Lyon Chir., 48:950, 1953.
5. Evans, E.B.: Orthopaedic measures in the treatment of severe burns. J. Bone Joint Surg., 48A:643, 1966.
6. Evans, E.B., Larson, D.L., Abston, S., and Willis, B.: Prevention and correction of deformity after severe burns. Surg. Clin. North Am., 50:1361, 1970.
7. Evans, E.B., and Smith, J.R.: Bone and joint changes following burns. J. Bone Joint Surg., 41A:785, 1959.
8. Frantz, C.H., and Delgado, S.: Limb-length dis-

crepancy after third-degree burns about the foot and ankle. J. Bone Joint Surg., 48A:443, 1966.

9. Fujimore, R., Hiramoto, M., and Ofuji, S.: Sponge fixation method for treatment of early scars. Plast. Reconstr. Surg., 42:322, 1968.

10. Heimberger, R.A., Marten, E., Larson, D.L. et al.: Burned feet in children—acute and reconstructive care. Am. J. Surg., 125:575, 1973.

11. Janzekovic, Z.: A new concept in the early excision and immediate grafting of burns. J. Trauma, 10: 1103, 1970.

12. Johnson, J.T.H.: Atypical myositis ossificans. J. Bone Joint Surg., 39A:189, 1957.

13. Koepke, G.H., Feallock, B., and Feller, I.: Splinting the severely burned hand. Am. J. Occup. Ther., 17:147, 1963.

14. Larson, D.L., Abston, S., Evans, E.B. et al.: Techniques for decreasing scar formation and contractures in the burned patient. J. Trauma, 11:807, 1971.

15. Larson, D.L. et al.: Contracture and scar formation in the burn patient. Clin. Plast. Surg., 1:653, 1974.

16. Mahler, D., and Watson, J.: The early excision of burns. Burns, 1:65, 1974–1975.

17. Owens, N.: Osteoporosis following burns. Br. J. Plast. Surg., 1:245, 1949.

18. Rabinov, D.: Acromutilation of the fingers following severe burns. Radiology, 77:968, 1961.

19. Ritsilä, V., Sundell, B., and Alhopuro, S.: Severe growth retardation of the upper extremity resulting from burn contracture and its full recovery after release of the contracture. Br. J. Plast. Surg., 29: 53, 1976.

20. Robitaille, A., Halpern, D., Kottke, F.J. et al.: Correction of keloids and finger contractures in burn patients. Arch. Phys. Med. Rehabil., 54:515, 1973.

21. Salisbury, R.E., McKeel, D.W., and Mason, A.D.: Ischemic necrosis of the intrinsic muscles of the hand after thermal injuries. J. Bone Joint Surg., 56A:1701, 1974.

22. Willis, B.A., Larson, D.L., and Abston, S.: Positioning and splinting the burned patient. Heart Lung, 2:696, 1973.

44 Complications of Amputation Surgery

NEWTON C. MCCOLLOUGH III

Amputation, the most ancient of all surgical procedures, continues to be one of the most common operative procedures performed in modern times. It is estimated that there are 400,000 amputees in the United States and that this number is increasing by approximately 20,000 per year, of which about 85% are amputations of the lower limb.[100]

Common causes of operative amputation are vascular disease, trauma, infection, and tumor. Of these, the most common cause of amputation in the Western world today is peripheral vascular disease. In a well-documented Swedish study by Hansson, it is reported that while in 1926 only 2% of all lower-extremity amputations were due to vascular disease, by 1955 this category accounted for 57% of the total.[33] Furthermore, the incidence of lower-extremity amputation in males over 60 years of age was 34 per 100,000 in 1947 and rose to 129 per 100,000 by 1962 in this study. In a more recent survey of 6000 amputees seen for prosthetic fitting in the U.S. 70% of all patients had their amputations for vascular disease,[41] and 22.4% had amputations secondary to trauma. Other comprehensive clinical studies reveal that between 70% and 90% of all lower-limb amputations are performed for vascular disease.[67,82,86,103] Since the majority of all amputations, and especially the majority of lower-limb amputations, are due to vascular disease, it can be anticipated that complications secondary to amputation surgery are very frequently related to the effects of ischemia.

When an amputation is performed for a pathologic state, whatever the cause, it is done to eliminate the pathology and restore function that otherwise would not be possible. Amputation of a limb, however, introduces a new pathology, and it is of the utmost importance that this be minimized as much as is technically possible. Although ablative, the amputation must be thought of as a reconstructive procedure in that it eliminates a diseased or otherwise useless limb as a means of restoring functional use through prosthetic replacement. It should be recognized that the lower the level of amputation, the more successful will be the degree of functional prosthetic rehabilitation.

Recent energy-cost studies have confirmed the fact that the lower the level of amputation, the less the cost of energy consumption increases, particularly with regard to a comparison of below-knee amputees with above knee amputees.[30,104] In the case of upper-extremity amputees, the superiority of function in low-level amputations is self-evident. Conversely, the higher the level of amputation, the greater will be the functional loss and the complication rate. A guiding principle of amputation surgery is that an amputation should be performed at the lowest possible level consistent with tissue viability and good surgical judgment. This principle, when followed by the surgeon, helps to optimize functional recovery and minimize disability and complications.

Many amputations for peripheral vascular disease can be avoided by appropriate reconstructive arterial surgery. In one review of 244 consecutive patients presenting with limb ischemia, the overall 5-year cumulative limb salvage rate was 76%.[59] When amputation becomes necessary, many complications can be avoided by the proper selection of level to ensure optimal healing. Although the use of modern technology such as Doppler ultrasound, radioisotope assessment, segmental transcutaneous PO_2 measurements, and skin perfusion pressure are useful adjuncts to the determination of the optimal amputation level, this decision should be made primarily on the basis of bleeding of the skin edges at surgery. If skin bleeding is not observed within 3 minutes after the initial incision, the amputation should be done more proximally, at a level of adequate skin bleeding.

To avoid complications in amputations for vascular disease, the surgeon must recognize the desirability of gentle tissue handling, minimal dissection between tissue planes to preserve skin circulation, and avoidance of long flaps. In certain specific amputations a long flap may be desirable owing to the superior blood supply it provides (*e.g.*, the below-knee amputation technique advocated by Burgess). Meticulous hemostasis is also of prime importance in the prevention of hematoma formation, infection, and delayed healing.

In the case of amputation for trauma, the most important consideration is prevention of infection. Injuries that are severe enough to require amputation are nearly always heavily contaminated and associated with extensive tissue devitalization. The amputation, with rare exception, should be left open and appropriate revision done at a later date to minimize the risk of infection.

Complications of the amputation that occur later and that relate primarily to the amputee's residual limb are best managed by a team approach. The amputee clinic team is a combination of medical and paramedical professionals, each of whom has a particular area of expertise in amputee management and whose combined evaluation and judgment are used in solving the problems and complications of the amputee. Commonly, the team consists of an orthopaedic surgeon, a physical therapist, an occupational therapist, and a prosthetist, but others may also be involved, such as the social worker, the rehabilitation nurse, and the vocational counselor. Complications that arise may be solved or treated by medical or surgical approaches, by therapy, or by prosthesis revision or design, and frequently a combination of these treatment modalities is necessary to provide optimal treatment.

The prevention, as well as the treatment, of complications ensuing after amputation

has been enhanced tremendously by recent advances in the field of prosthetics. Not only have new materials, designs, and technology had an impact on the successful rehabilitation of the amputee, but the increasing competence of the prosthetist has also provided much improved problem-solving ability to the amputee clinic team. Surgical revision of problem amputation stumps is now needed much less frequently, since the art of prosthetics now has the wherewithal to fit the prosthesis to the stump rather than requiring the surgeon to tailor the stump to the prosthesis.

In this chapter, complications of amputation surgery are divided into early complications, which usually occur during the preprosthetic period, and late complications, or those that arise commonly in the period after the prosthesis has been fitted. In both the early and the later periods, complications are further categorized into general problems and local problems. Certain complications can be anticipated or expected with certain types and levels of amputation and are not true surgical complications but complications related to a specific level. For instance, certain complications arise with a very short below-knee stump. These are not only anticipated, but accepted as a worthwhile tradeoff for the additional pathology and loss of function that would result if an amputation site above the knee had been selected. Methods of dealing adequately with these expected complications frequently allow a lower and more functional level of amputation to be performed.

EARLY COMPLICATIONS

General

Mortality following amputation surgery varies according to the cause and circumstances of the amputation. Studies with well-documented mortality figures have been confined primarily to the lower-extremity amputee with peripheral vascular disease. The reported mortality following amputation in this group of patients ranges from 10% to 39%.[3,34,71,77,82,86,99]

Mortality rates for amputation below the knee are considerably less than for amputation carried out above the knee, and in one series, a reversal in the 2-to-1 ratio of above-knee amputees to below-knee amputees led to a drop in mortality from 24% to 10%.[82] In a recent review of 100 consecutive patients requiring above-knee amputation for arterial disease, the operative mortality rate was 15%, and an additional 26% mortality occurred during a 2-year follow-up period. Principal causes of death were sepsis (54%), heart disease (16%), and stroke (11%). The poor prognosis of patients requiring above-knee amputation appears to be related to progression of systemic disease and to generalized debility among these patients.[39] Ligation of the femoral vein has not proven successful in preventing pulmonary embolism.[99] The use of routine prophylaxis against thromboembolic disease, such as heparin or aspirin administration, could conceivably reduce the mortality rate from these vascular catastrophes.[77] Otteman and Stahlgren[71] report a significant difference in mortality rate when spinal anesthesia is used (25%), as compared with general anesthesia (43%).

Morbidity secondary to general complications has also been studied in a large series of patients undergoing amputation for peripheral vascular disease.[71] In order of frequency, serious complications include pneumonia (11.8%), myocardial infarction (7.2%), pulmonary embolism (6.3%), and cerebrovascular accident (5.4%). The median age of patients in this series was 67.4 years, and serious preoperative problems were identified in 71% of the 323 patients studied. In a study of 90 patients undergoing a total of 110 lower-limb amputations over a 4-year period, Potts and associates reported an overall complication rate of 40% and identified the patients at greatest risk as being above-knee amputees over 60 years of age with peripheral vascular disease.[74] In addition to the possibility of using prophylactic anticoagulation to decrease morbidity in this age group, early mobilization of the patient is of prime importance in reducing these complications. Because earlier restoration of functional activity can be achieved in patients with below-knee amputations than in those with above-knee amputations, making every effort to save the knee joint in this class of patient will lower the early postoperative morbidity.[82] Techniques of immediate postoperative fitting and early temporary fitting can also be expected to reduce postoperative complications of this nature, since they allow rapid mobilization of the patient.[67,79]

Postoperative Depression. A complication seen frequently in the postoperative phase is psychological depression due to loss of the body part.[20,27,38,85] The extent of grief and depression varies according to the patient, his age, the location and level of the amputation, his premorbid personality, his preoperative preparation, and his postoperative management and counseling. Psychological disturbances tend to be more profound in the adult, in the female, in upper-extremity amputees, and in those who have not had adequate preoperative preparation and postoperative counseling. Depression revolves about the loss of body image (loss of wholeness), disfigurement, loss of acquired skills, loss (or threat of loss) of economic security, and uncertainty of social acceptance. To a degree, these factors are beyond the control of the physician, but the complication of postamputation depression can be greatly minimized by preparing the patient for loss of the limb before the operation, and by enforcing a vigorous program of postoperative care. Preoperatively, the patient may frequently be relieved of some remorseful decision making about the amputation by giving him assurance that loss of the limb is an inevitable if not already accomplished fact, and that operation will serve to relieve his discomfort, lessen his overall risk, and provide him with function that he may not have had for some time. He should be made aware of the approximate level of function he will be able to achieve, the type of prosthesis he may expect, the length of time before receiving the final prosthesis, and the events that will transpire in the interim. The physician must be careful to express optimism without promising too much, and his predictions must be based on the level of anticipated amputation and the pre-illness level of function as well as any concomitant disabilities. Following these guidelines, the physician takes much of the uncertainty and the fear of amputation away from the patient. Postoperatively, the physician must impart his enthusiasm as to the rehabilitative aspects of amputation to the patient and emphasize positive aspects of the patient's abilities as he regains function with his prosthesis. In this regard, the technique of early postoperative fitting (or immediate postoperative fitting, when applicable) is invaluable. Interruption of function, whether that of grasp in the upper-limb amputee or locomotion in the lower-limb amputee, should be as brief as possible postoperatively. Association with successfully rehabilitated amputees should also be encouraged as a means of reducing depression and anxiety following loss of limb. When depression becomes severe, psychiatric or psychological counseling should be requested, but every surgeon should be aware of the possibility of preventing or ameliorating depression by his own relationship with the patient, beginning in the preoperative phase.

Local

Hematoma. The formation of a hematoma in an amputation stump may be a source of infection or pain, may embarrass circulation to the skin and result in gangrene of the skin edges, and may result in delayed healing or wound dehiscence. Meticulous hemostasis after the tourniquet has been released and before the wound is closed is essential to the prevention of this complication. Drains may also be effective in preventing hematoma formation. If a hematoma of significance is noted early, aspiration under aseptic conditions followed by use of a compressive wrap may be successful. Large hematomas that do not respond to aspiration should be surgically drained in the operating room, with prophylactic intravenous antibiotic coverage. Careful hemostasis should then be obtained prior to closure over a drain, and prophylactic intravenous antibiotics should be continued for 48 hours.

Wound Dehiscence. Wound dehiscence is most common in the amputee with vascular disease who has had premature removal of skin sutures and in whom early prosthetic weight-bearing ambulation has occurred. It may, of course, occur in any amputation as a consequence of infection. Uncomplicated wound dehiscence (Fig. 44-1) can be avoided in the amputee with vascular disease by the use of a good subcutaneous closure to minimize skin tension, and delay for at least 3 weeks— preferably 4 weeks—in removing skin sutures. This is particularly important when

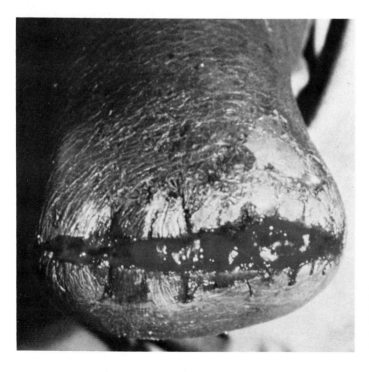

Fig. 44-1. Wound dehiscence 3 weeks after amputation, following premature removal of sutures in an amputee with vascular disease.

early weight bearing in the prosthesis is a part of the postoperative program, since shear forces on the sides of the stump are converted to tension forces at the suture line. Once major dehiscence has occurred, it should be surgically closed under sterile operating conditions after cleansing. If the dehiscence is more than 6 hours old, it should be left open and treated with saline compresses until the tissues are clean and healthy; then wound excision in the operating room should precede closure. Intravenous antibiotics before, during, and after surgery are recommended as a prophylactic measure.

Delayed Wound Healing. Delayed wound healing of the amputation stump is both a predisposing factor for infection and a result of infection when it occurs. It may occur especially in peripheral vascular amputations, due to borderline circulation to the skin edges. Meticulous coaptation of the skin edges with fine suture after tension has been minimized with subcutaneous closure, is the best method of avoiding this complication. Adverse factors in wound healing following amputation have been found to include poor quality of the femoral pulse, hypertension, a failed bypass procedure, and angiographic evidence of stenosis or occlusion of the common femoral or deep femoral artery.[93] Therefore, proximal reconstructive surgery may be indicated prior to amputation in patients with a diminished femoral pulse. In a recent Danish study the incidence of ipsilateral reamputation secondary to wound problems was reported as being 10.4% after 1 month, 16.5% after 3 months, and 18.8% after 6 months.[21] When delayed healing is noted, sutures should be allowed to remain for several weeks, and reinforcement with sterile adhesive coaptation strips may be helpful. Weight bearing should be postponed and sterility observed in care of the stump.

Gangrene of the Amputation Stump. Frank gangrene of an amputation stump occurs as a result of inadequate circulation to the skin flaps, either because the level selected was too low or because there has been additional thrombosis of proximal vessels that has raised the level of ischemia (Fig. 44-2). Careful evaluation of bleeding at the cut skin edges at the time of ampu-

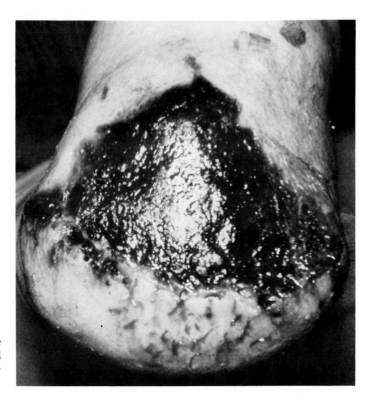

FIG. 44-2. Gangrene of the amputation stump occurred owing to inadequate circulation to the anterior flap.

tation and gentle handling of the tissues without forceps can serve to lessen the incidence of this complication. In amputation for acute arterial occlusion, one should wait several days in most cases, until the level of ischemia has become clearly demarcated, before proceeding with the surgical procedure. Once gangrene of the stump is recognized, reamputation at a higher level is the only alternative. In such cases, consultation with a vascular surgeon is desirable, since, if an obstructive lesion has recently formed and is amenable to surgery, the success of the second amputation may be greatly enhanced by restoration of circulation.

Necrosis of the skin margins at the site of incision is a relatively common complication of amputation surgery in vascular disease. The incidence of this complication may be reduced considerably by avoiding closure of the skin under excessive tension. All significant tension on the skin sutures should be reduced to a minimum by the use of a good subcutaneous closure, so that strangulation of the skin by sutures that are too tight will not occur (Fig. 44-3). If the necrosis of skin margins does not exceed ¼ inch, delayed healing by secondary in-

tention is feasible, and rehabilitation efforts can usually progress concomitant with wound healing. Daily or twice-daily cleansing of the stump with antiseptic soap helps prevent infection while wound healing occurs. If necrosis exceeds ¼ to ½ inch, however, revision of the stump frequently speeds the healing process and decreases the time to definitive fitting.[98]

Pressure Necrosis. Early in the postoperative period, excessive pressure of the rigid or soft compressive dressing over the bony prominences of the stump, particularly the tibia, may result in skin necrosis (Fig. 44-4). If the patient complains of pain in one particular area of the stump in the immediate postoperative period, the rigid dressing should be removed or the elastic wrap released for inspection of the stump. If an area of redness is present, appropriate soft padding should be placed over the area before the dressing is reapplied. If frank necrosis of skin is present, debridement and healing by secondary intention is recommended in small wounds, and stump revision should be undertaken in larger wounds that extend down to bone.

Wound Infection. Infection of the amputation stump occurs in up to 16% of

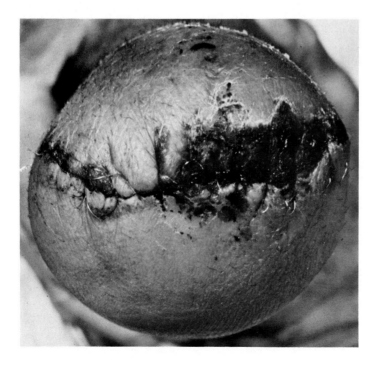

FIG. 44-3. Necrosis of the skin edges was probably secondary to excessive skin tension caused by widely spaced, strangulating sutures.

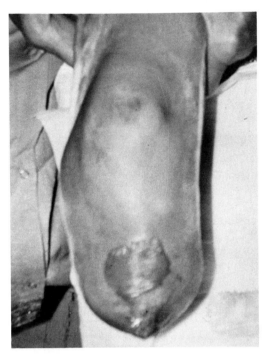

FIG. 44-4. Pressure necrosis of the skin was secondary to a poorly applied rigid dressing.

amputations performed for peripheral vascular disease,[71,99] and to a lesser extent in amputations from other causes. In amputation necessitated by acute infection, the incidence of wound infection can be reduced by leaving the amputation open and performing a secondary closure or reamputation at a later date. In amputations for chronic infection associated with peripheral vascular disease or diabetes, it is preferable to close the amputation at the level of healthy tissues, using intraoperatively and postoperatively the intravenous antibiotics of choice for the infection.[55]

Infections of the amputation stump may be superficial, in which case cellulitis is frequently associated with skin margin necrosis, or they may be deep, involving all tissue layers down to bone. In the former case, treatment with warm saline compresses and intravenous antibiotics may suffice. In the case of deep infection, all sutures should be removed and the tissues opened for adequate drainage. Soaks or irrigation with antibiotic or antiseptic solution should then be instituted, along with

the appropriate intravenous antibiotics as determined by the culture and sensitivity studies. This treatment should continue for several days up to 2 weeks, until the wound is clean and local reaction has subsided. At this time, the wound must be assessed and a decision made to continue the same treatment in hope of obtaining healing by secondary intention, or to amputate at a higher level through healthy tissues. If osteomyelitis is present, a second amputation is indicated. When a second amputation is necessary, the surgeon should strive to preserve the next proximal joint (*e.g.*, the knee joint in the infected below-knee stump). If this is not possible, disarticulation rather than amputation above the joint may be preferable.

If continued treatment and healing by secondary intention is the method of choice, the amputee should be up and as active as possible. I have used temporary prostheses with considerable success in this situation, since ambulation improves drainage, enhances circulation to the stump, and improves the physical condition of the amputee.

Anaerobic infection of the amputation stump can be a devastating complication, since proximal extension of the infectious process can result in progressively higher levels of amputation, with consequent reduction of functional capacity. Such infections are best managed by wide open drainage, intravenous antibiotics, and hyperbaric oxygen. Gas gangrene, although extremely rare as a complication of amputation surgery, has been reported in amputations for peripheral vascular disease.[83] A recent report associated *Clostridium perfringens* wound infections with the use of nonsterile elastic outer bandages in diabetic patients who have undergone lower-limb amputation for vascular insufficiency.[73] A similar regimen of intravenous antibiotics and hyperbaric oxygen after a second amputation through healthy tissues is the treatment of choice for this dreaded complication.

Edema. The presence of edema in the amputation stump in the postoperative period is detrimental to wound healing, and efforts to control the swelling should be made when it is recognized. The use of a rigid plastic dressing immediately postoperatively or the use of immediate postsurgical fitting is thought by many to prevent or minimize edema formation.[12,58,80,108,112] If this technique is not used, some type of compressive dressing such as soft gauze and elastic bandage is indicated. Stump wrapping with an elastic bandage, however, is critical, and one must be careful not to produce a tourniquet effect proximally, which will cause—not prevent—stump edema. Anchoring the bandage in place with adhesive tape prevents rolling of the bandage and a tourniquet effect in the immediate postoperative period. Later, as stump wrapping is performed for progressive shrinkage, it is important that the amputee have proper instruction in wrapping from distal to proximal with oblique turns to prevent constriction and choking of the stump. Wrapping should be repeated several times a day to eliminate the possibility of prolonged circumferential pressure in one area.

The introduction of early weight-bearing ambulation in a temporary prosthesis will also minimize edema formation and speed its resolution, if present, through intermittent compression of the stump and through muscle activity. It is important to add stump socks as necessary, since shrinkage of the stump occurs and edema subsides. When the patient is not using the prosthesis, the stump should be wrapped with an elastic bandage.

Systemic causes of edema, such as cardiac failure and electrolyte imbalance, should not be overlooked. The presence of pitting edema on the opposite side is suggestive of a systemic cause, and appropriate medical measures, such as the use of diuretics, should be instituted.

Pain that occurs in the amputation stump in the early postoperative period must be carefully evaluated. Nearly all amputees have moderate to severe pain as an early consequence of the amputation, but this normal response to injury is characterized by two factors. (1) The pain is diffuse over the amputation site, and the patient cannot localize it with a single finger. (2) The pain gradually diminishes over a period of several days. Any deviation from this pain pattern is cause for concern. Pain that can be localized by a single finger usually means

excessive pressure and impending skin necrosis, and the stump must be inspected. Pain that does not gradually lessen or becomes worse and continues to be diffuse is a sign of infection, particularly in association with fever. In this instance the wound should be inspected and appropriate measures carried out, as indicated previously for infection.

Immediate postsurgical fitting of the prosthesis and application of rigid plaster dressings in both upper- and lower-limb amputations are techniques that have contributed significantly to the reduction of postoperative pain.[10,12,80,108,112] Removal of the plaster for stump inspection is mandatory in the case of well-localized pain, increasing pain, or temperature elevation.

The presence of pain in the portion of the limb that has been amputated (phantom pain) is not unusual in the immediate postoperative period and may occur in as many as 35% of amputees.[62] It is particularly common in patients who have had an amputation for a chronic painful condition of the extremity. In most patients, it gradually subsides with the introduction of activity, and the use of early ambulation is valuable in this regard. There appears to be a low incidence of phantom pain phenomena in patients who undergo immediate postsurgical fitting.[102] In approximately 2% to 10% of patients, phantom pain persists as a difficult problem in management; this phenomenon is considered in detail later in this chapter.

Contracture. As is true for most complications, contractures are by far easier to prevent than to treat. The importance of guarding against joint contractures following amputation cannot be overemphasized. Established contracture can make successful prosthesis fitting difficult, if not impossible. Frequently, treatment of contractures by conservative measures is unsuccessful, and surgical release may constitute a major procedure that is poorly tolerated by the amputee who has vascular impairment owing to his borderline circulation and healing abilities. The shorter the amputation stump, the greater will be the tendency to contracture, and vigorous attempts to prevent contractures should be instituted in these patients early in the postoperative period.

Above-Knee Amputations. With amputation above the knee, the stump tends to go into flexion and abduction owing to the relative loss of hip extensors (hamstrings) and adductors. Also, the hip tends to go into flexion as a pain reflex. The more proximal the amputation, the greater will be the tendency to flexion and abduction. A permanent abduction or flexion contracture of more than a few degrees greatly increases the energy demands of walking with an above-knee prosthesis. Flexion contractures greater than 20° and abduction contractures greater than 10° may render the patient completely unsuitable for prosthesis fitting. To prevent contracture, postoperative pain should be well controlled, active extension and adduction exercises should be initiated in the first few postoperative days, and the patient should be encouraged to lie prone as frequently as possible. As pain diminishes, the patient should be started on active resistive exercises, as well as full passive range-of-motion exercises by the therapist or nurse. Time spent sitting in the wheelchair should be minimized, since this encourages flexion contracture. The patient should be up and about on parallel bars and then a walker or crutches in the first postoperative week, or ambulatory with the prosthesis in cases in which immediate postoperative fitting has been used. If immediate postoperative fitting has not been used, early fitting (10–14 days) with a temporary above-knee prosthesis is highly desirable.[57] As the activity level of the above-knee amputee increases, the propensity to develop contractures diminishes.

Treatment of the established contracture in an above-knee amputation stump is difficult, at best. Physical therapy should be used both for stretching the tight muscles and for strengthening the antagonist muscles. If the contracture is not so severe as to prohibit prosthesis fitting, the prosthesis should be fitted and maintained in the temporary adjustable state. This permits the amputee to exercise his stump while walking, and as the contracture diminishes, the alignment of the prosthesis can be changed. Frequently, the prosthesis can be aligned so as to encourage correction of the contracture while the patient is walking (*i.e.,*

reducing the amount of initial flexion in the socket so as to stretch the hip flexors when the patient steps forward with the opposite limb). If conservative management of the contracture is unsuccessful, surgical release may be indicated. In the case of hip flexion contractures, tenotomy of the psoas tendon at the pelvic brim should be performed, allowing the tendon to slide within the substance of the iliacus muscle. If the hip flexion contracture is not reduced following this, a sliding lengthening of the rectus femoris muscle and an anterior capsulotomy of the hip joint should be performed, depending on the tightness of these structures. In the case of abduction contracture, division of the iliotibial tract just below the level of the greater trochanter will be corrective. Postoperatively, a spica cast should be applied and worn for 3 weeks to hold the stump in the corrected position.

Below-Knee Amputations. In the case of below-knee amputations the short stump almost invariably has a tendency to go into flexion and develop a flexion contracture. When this occurs, the end of the stump and the incision become pressed against the mattress or underlying surface, and skin necrosis may follow. The use of a rigid plaster dressing postoperatively, immobilizing the knee in extension and providing a quiet protective bed for wound healing, obviates this problem.[66] Usually by the time the rigid dressing has been removed, some 10 to 14 days postoperatively, pain is no longer a significant factor in causing the stump to assume a flexion attitude. Quadriceps setting exercises should be done in conjunction with the use of the rigid dressing to strengthen extensor power. When the rigid dressing is removed, the therapist can then begin progressive resistive stump exercises, and the patient should begin walking in a temporary below-knee prosthesis. As in the case of the above-knee amputee, as the patient's activity level increases, the tendency for contracture diminishes.

When one is confronted with an established knee flexion contracture of short duration, conservative treatment may be successful, but if the contracture has been present for more than a few weeks, surgical release is usually indicated. Nonoperative treatment consists of passive stretching of the contracture by the therapist, as well as active resistive exercises of the quadriceps. Long-term electrical stimulation of the quadriceps has been helpful in a limited number of cases in reducing knee flexion contracture.* For electrical stimulation to be successful, however, a portable stimulator capable of cyclic transmission must be available for continuous use at home or in the hospital. In the case of below-knee flexion contractures not exceeding 30°, ambulation on a temporary prosthesis is a helpful adjunct to promoting reduction of the flexion contracture. The prosthesis may be aligned so as to extend the knee forcibly with each step by using a long toe lever arm or a soft heel cushion. As the contracture lessens, the prosthesis is adjusted accordingly.

Other means of straightening established knee flexion contractures, such as skeletal traction and cast wedging, have not proven successful. When an amputee with a short below-knee stump presents with a contracture that is resistant to nonoperative methods of correction, there are four alternatives to treatment.

With very short stumps and flexion contractures up to 40°, fitting can be accomplished with a standard total-contact, below-knee prosthesis with the socket aligned in the required amount of flexion. Gait is halting and not optimal, but this may be the treatment of choice in the "vascular disease" amputee whose walking is limited.

A "bent-knee prosthesis" may be used, enclosing the short stump in an above-knee socket with anterior opening and the knee flexed at 90°.[58] This requires the use of outside knee joints, and the patient is essentially treated as a knee disarticulation amputee with end bearing on the condyles, patella, and pretibial areas. Cosmesis is poor, and energy consumption is greatly increased owing to lack of normal knee motion. However, in the patient with vascular disease who may present a significant surgical risk for re-

vision, this may be the procedure of choice for short stumps with greater than 40° of flexion contracture.

Surgical release of the knee flexion contracture may be undertaken if the contracture is less than 60°. The skin incision should be vertical and midline across the posterior aspect of the knee joint without curving and without any transverse component. This incision ensures that the skin edges will be drawn together rather than separated when the knee is extended. Such a release requires a posterior capsulotomy of the knee joint, extending from the posteromedial to the posterolateral corner of the joint (Fig. 44-5), as well as hamstring lengthening. A rigid dressing with the knee in maximum extension is applied postoperatively, or in stumps that are difficult to control, transverse pins through the tibia and femur may be incorporated in plaster to maintain extension. This procedure requires

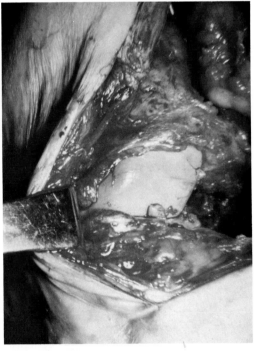

Fig. 44-5. Posterior capsular release of the knee joint was performed for a flexion contracture of a below-knee amputation stump. The capsular incision must extend around the posterolateral and posteromedial corners of the joint.

---

* Waters, R.L.: Personal communication, 1976.

considerable deep dissection and is not recommended for the amputee with vascular disease.

Surgical conversion to knee disarticulation or above-knee amputation may be done. I prefer knee disarticulation to the above-knee level, owing to the end-bearing qualities of this amputation and the superior strength of the stump. In the case of the very short stump, there may not be sufficient skin for coverage of the stump if a conventional incision is used. In this instance the technique of circular incision at the level of the tibial tuberosity with posterior closure is recommended (Fig. 44-6).[58] Conversion to knee disarticulation level has advantages over fitting with the bent-knee prosthesis in that better cosmesis is achieved and a four-bar-linkage hydraulic knee unit may be used, which provides excellent control over the swing and stance phases of gait. This operation is the procedure of choice for fixed contractures of the short stump greater than 60°.

Foot Amputations. Following certain amputations in the forefoot, such as the Lisfranc and Chopart levels, which are performed proximal to the insertion of the anterior tibial tendon, equinus deformity of the hindfoot frequently occurs. The presence of equinus deformity is an expected complication of this level of amputation, but it can be partially counteracted if the toe extensors and anterior tibial tendons are inserted into the dorsum of the remaining part of the foot at the time of definitive amputation.[98] These tendons should be inserted as far distally as possible on the remainder of the foot to obtain maximal mechanical advantage. Even with this technique, gradual equinus deformity may occur. In this situation, lengthening of the heel cord may result in a balanced foot. If not, the heel cord can be tenotomized or excised. Rarely, an ankle arthrodesis may be indicated to control this deformity. Finally, conversion to a Syme amputation may be considered if all else fails.

Upper-Limb Amputations. Development of contractures in the upper limb following amputation is relatively uncommon but is most likely in short below-elbow stumps. Adduction contracture may also occur in above-elbow amputations. The use of im-

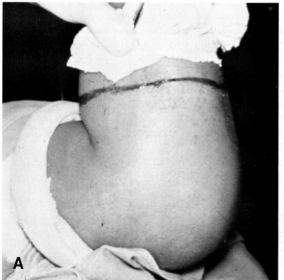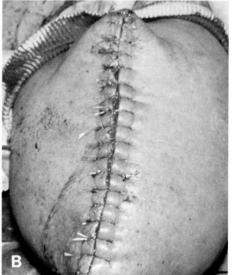

FIG. 44-6. (*A*) A circular incision is made at the level of the tibial tuberosity of knee disarticulation in an infected below-knee amputation stump. (*B*) Vertical posterior closure of the incision is particularly advantageous for the amputee with vascular disease because no flaps are created.

mediate postoperative fitting in the upper extremity tends to eliminate the tendency for contracture, because pain is reduced, and early functional activity may be instituted without delay.[10,81] Occasionally, in the case of the very short below-elbow amputation, a rigid dressing applied to maintain the elbow in extension may be preferred to immediate prosthesis fitting with a free elbow.

Principles of treatment of contractures of the upper-extremity amputation stump are identical to those given for contractures in the lower extremity. Flexion contracture of the below-elbow stump is generally not of functional significance unless it exceeds 30°. If surgical release of an elbow flexion contracture is desirable in more severe cases, anterior capsulotomy of the joint, combined with lengthening of the biceps brachii and the brachialis, is usually necessary.

LATE COMPLICATIONS

General

Our best insight into the long-term problems and complications of the amputee comes from the work of Solonen and coworkers, who studied 311 Finnish war amputees some 20 years after their amputations.[91] It was found that more than 60% were engaged in heavy or moderately heavy work at the time of follow-up. A control population was used, against which the amputee population was evaluated. The general physiological condition of the controls and the amputees was similar. Lower-limb amputees were found to have a significantly higher incidence of back pain and fatigue, scoliosis, and spondylosis of the lumbar spine than the control group. Arthrosis of the sound hip and the sound ankle was found to be more common among the amputees than among the controls. Also, the presence of flat foot on the sound side was extremely common in the amputee group as compared with the control population. In the case of upper-limb amputees, neck pain, cervical spondylosis, thoracic scoliosis, and periarthrosis of the sound shoulder were all significantly increased in the amputee group. Approximately 75% had satisfactory stumps, and phantom pain was most common in above-elbow and above-knee amputations. In general, the higher the level of the amputation, the more long-term complications were encountered. It is obvious from this study that amputation of a limb does produce long-range disability in other portions of the musculoskeletal system. Whether the current level of sophistication of prosthetic substitution will lessen these complications in the future is speculative. Suffice it to say that as surgeons, our only means of reducing this long-term complication rate is to endeavor to keep our amputation levels as low as possible, consistent with the principles of good surgical judgment. The occurrence of hypertension has been described as a long-term complication of lower-limb amputation. Labouret and associates, in comparing 106 men who had undergone amputation of one limb on account of war injury with 184 male controls of the same ages, found a significantly higher systolic pressure in the amputees.[51] Hypertension in amputees has been linked to increased levels of circulating norepinephrine secondary to mechanical irritation of the amputation stump by the prosthesis socket.[32]

With respect to the amputee with vascular disease, late mortality and morbidity are related primarily to the sequelae of vascular disease. The amputee who has lost his limb owing to peripheral vascular disease is also likely to have cerebrovascular disease, coronary artery disease, hypertension, and diabetes, not to mention peripheral vascular disease in the opposite limb. Kolind-Sorenson, in a follow-up of 121 amputees with vascular disease, found that only 50% were alive 2 years later.[46] Harris,[34] in a study of the fate of elderly amputees found that fewer than 50% survived 6 months. Others have found an extremely high late morbidity and mortality rate, secondary to myocardial infarction and cerebrovascular accidents.[18,71,99,111]

The diabetic who loses one limb to disease has a 20% to 50% chance of losing the second leg if he survives for 5 years.[13,84,89,111] In a study of more than 2000 amputations for arteriosclerotic and diabetic gangrene, Ebskov and Josephsen found the risk for contralateral amputation to be 11.9% within 1 year, 17.8% after 2 years, 27.2% after 3 years, and 44.3% after 4 years.[21] Since successful prosthetic rehabilitation of patients with bilateral below-knee amputations is the rule, even if they are elderly, every effort should be made to save the knee joint in the diabetic patient.[54,56]

Some have questioned the wisdom of prosthetic rehabilitation in the patient with vascular disease, since complications from vascular disease are prevalent, and the increased energy costs might be detrimental to his health. Others hold that restoration of functional activity in these patients enhances circulation and tends to improve the vascular status and the patient's wellbeing.[105] In general, prosthetic rehabilitation is favored for the dysvascular amputee to improve both his physiological and his psychological well-being. Judgment must be used, particularly with above-knee amputations secondary to vascular disease in patients who have serious coronary problems or severe hypertension. In these cases it may be wiser to encourage the amputee to use the wheelchair rather than burden a severely compromised cardiovascular system with the energy requirements of walking.[31]

Local

Local complications of the amputation stump that may occur in the early postoperative period have been described previously. Complications of the stump that occur later or in the postprosthetic fitting phase are not uncommon, and the surgeon must be keenly aware of the necessity of regular follow-up of all amputees to prevent or minimize these complications. The successful rehabilitation of an amputee depends on the satisfactory union of an adequately fashioned amputation stump to a prosthesis of sound design. Complications may thus result from defects of the amputation stump, from defects of prosthesis fitting and alignment, or from a combination of these two. In general, since the transmission of weight occurs through the stump–socket interface in lower-limb amputations, complications are more common in this group than in upper-limb amputations.

Skin Problems. Disorders affecting the skin of the amputation stump are the most common of all complications of lower-limb amputation and are relatively rare in the

patient who has lost his upper limb. The forces of weight bearing sustained by lower-limb amputation stumps, combined with the high incidence of amputation for ischemia in this group of patients, predispose amputees to numerous skin problems.

Abrasions and Blisters. The source of skin irritation or trauma may be a result either of underlying bony prominence or of poor prosthesis fit and alignment. Although abrasions and blisters may occur at any time during the life of the amputee, they appear most commonly in the first 6 months after permanent fitting of the prosthesis. During this time, the amputation stump continues to atrophy and shrink, though much less rapidly than in the preprosthetic period, and the fit of the prosthesis may not be adequate unless proper steps are taken. The modern use of total-contact sockets makes an accurate and intimate fit essential to the prevention of excessive pressures. In the amputee with vascular disease, particularly the diabetic, sensation may be sufficiently impaired that the amputee is unaware of a sore developing on the stump. For this reason, the lower-limb amputee must be taught to inspect his stump daily, using a mirror if necessary.

As the stump shrinks, owing either to natural atrophy or to amputee weight loss, the proximal weight-bearing areas lose their purchase on the prosthesis, and the stump migrates deeper into the socket, with resultant increased end-bearing. Additionally, the relative motion between the stump and socket increases, and friction becomes an etiologic factor. In the below-knee amputation the common sites of skin breakdown are over the subcutaneous crest of the tibia (especially distally), over the end of the stump, and over the fibular head. The solution to the problem is generally the addition of stump socks to regain better fit. Decreasing the anterior-posterior diameter by the addition of leather padding in the popliteal area may also be indicated. When the number of stump socks is 10-ply or more, the fit of the prosthesis becomes "sloppy," and a new prosthesis is indicated.

Skin trauma can also result from stump enlargement due to weight gain or other causes. In the below-knee amputee, this results in failure to insert the stump completely into the socket, and commonly, blistering or abrasion occurs over the tibial tuberosity, where the patellar tendon bridge impinges on it rather than on the patellar tendon. The fibular head no longer corresponds to its relief in the socket, and abrasion over this area may also result. An excellent method of evaluating socket fit in this situation is the use of weight-bearing roentgenograms of the stump of the prosthesis (Fig. 44-7). This frequently permits localization of the areas where the prosthesis impinges on the stump. Other methods used to detect areas of excessive pressure include the use of lipstick on the stump sock, which transfers to the socket on weight bearing, the use of a small ball of

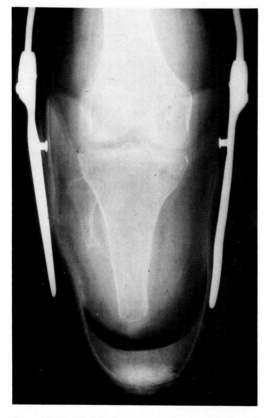

FIG. 44-7. Weight-bearing roentgenograms of the below-knee stump in the socket of the prosthesis are useful to determine the accuracy of fit of the prosthesis. Notice the lack of distal contact of the stump with the socket; the fibular head is superior to the area of socket relief for this bony prominence.

clay in the bottom of the socket to determine the extent of end-bearing, and the use of pressure-sensitive stump socks.[8]

If the stump enlargement is due to weight gain, a new prosthesis is required. If it is due to other, more transient causes, such as mild right-sided heart failure, wrapping the stump for a few days and using appropriate medical measures is indicated.

Skin trauma can also occur from an improperly formed socket. Failure to provide adequate relief for the bony prominences or a rough spot on the socket wall can be managed by grinding out the areas in question.

Improper prosthesis alignment can cause excessive skin pressures, resulting in skin breakdown. The most common errors in alignment in the below-knee amputee are insufficient flexion in the socket causing anterior distal tibial pressure, excessive valgus of the socket causing fibular head pressure, and excessive varus of the socket causing pressure over the distal fibula. Appropriate alignment corrections are the obvious solutions to skin sores from this source.

Surgically related causes of skin sores include failure to bevel the distal end of the tibia adequately, leaving the fibula longer than the tibia, and failure to provide sufficient soft tissue coverage over the end of the stump at the time of amputation. In some cases it may be possible to provide prosthetic solutions to these surgical errors. Foaming the end of the socket with silicone rubber or soft inserts may sufficiently relieve the pressure over these bony prominences. If these measures fail, stump revision becomes necessary. Whenever blisters or abrasions occur on the amputation stump from any of the above causes, prosthesis wear should be suspended and the stump washed daily with antiseptic soap solution, such as hexachlorophene or povidone-iodine. Only when the skin has healed and the appropriate corrective measures have been carried out should the amputee resume walking in his prosthesis. In the occasional below-knee amputation, the skin is excessively fragile, and skin breakdown may be a recurrent problem despite the corrective measures mentioned above. In such a case, the addition of a thigh corset for auxiliary weight bearing and reduction of the stump–socket interface pressures are indicated.

Ulceration. Full-thickness skin loss or ulceration is the result of unrecognized or untreated manifestations of excessive pressure, such as blistering or abrasion (Fig. 44-8). It occurs most commonly in amputees who have insensitive skin because of a primary disease process such as diabetes. These patients also frequently have other disabilities, such as poor vision and memory impairment. Prevention of this complication in this class of patient depends on adequate education of the patient and his family with regard to close stump inspection on a daily basis.

Ulceration occurs most commonly over the patellar tendon, over the tibial tuberosity, over the fibular head, and over the anterior distal aspect of the tibia. The causes are identical to those described above for more superficial skin lesions, but the trauma is of greater magnitude or has persisted over a longer period. Treatment consists of suspending the use of the prosthesis, debridement of any necrotic material at the base, implementing wet-to-dry saline or antibiotic soaks, and controlling any surrounding cellulitis with systemic antibiotics. When a clean granulating base has been achieved, one must decide whether the lesion would be best handled by allowing it to heal by secondary intention, or whether surgical measures are required. Larger, deeper ulcers are frequently better managed by excision of the margins and base of the ulcer, resection of underlying bone, and primary closure. This may involve excision of the fibular head or the entire fibula,[92] rebeveling of the tibia, or actually shortening the amputation stump. Resection of underlying bone removes the source of pressure and permits primary closure of the excised wound when the skin has been sufficiently mobilized. Prosthesis modification is usually required when there has been excision of bone, and fabrication of a new prosthesis is indicated if the stump shape has been significantly altered. In the case of full-thickness skin loss over the patellar tendon, the wound should always be excised and closed with good skin, since this is an area normally subjected to pressure during prosthesis wear, and good-quality skin is nec-

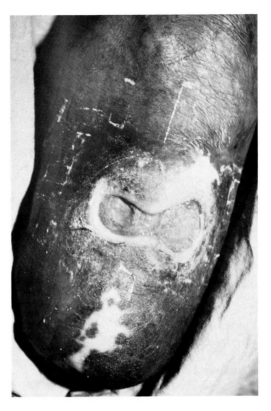

FIG. 44-8. Full-thickness skin ulceration over the tibial tuberosity was caused by poor fit of the prosthesis. In this instance the patellar tendon bridge of the prosthesis impinged on the insertion of the tendon rather than at its midpoint.

essary to tolerate the forces of weight bearing over this tendon.

Scarring. The presence of extensive scarring over the amputation stump is seen most frequently after amputation for trauma or burn. It is usually the result of attempting to save as much length of the injured limb as possible in the absence of adequate full-thickness skin for coverage. Such amputation stumps are not true complications of the surgical procedure but frequently represent successful salvage of a more functional level of amputation. Nevertheless, stumps with excessive scarring due to irregular closure of flaps, healing by secondary intention, or coverage by split-thickness grafts can pose significant problems to the prosthetic rehabilitation of the amputee.

While prevention of excessive stump scarring is a consideration from the time of initial management through the time of stump closure in amputations due to trauma, it is generally preferable to obtain wound healing at the lowest reasonable level and perform a secondary revision procedure at a later date if it becomes necessary. This is particularly true when higher amputation, to obtain good skin coverage, might result in loss of a knee or elbow joint or result in a very short amputation stump. Fortunately, the present level of prosthetic technology enables the amputee clinic team to manage many of these problem stump cases successfully without surgical revision.

Scarring of the stump tends to present more of a problem in lower-limb amputees than in upper-limb amputees owing to the shear forces imposed on the stump by weight bearing. In the case of the below-knee amputation, any scar present over the end of the stump or the subcutaneous portions of the tibia may break down owing to these forces. The same is true of scarring or poor skin over the patellar tendon. In the above-knee amputee, the areas of concern are over Scarpa's triangle anteriorly, where pressure must be exerted to keep the ischium over the posterior wall of the quadrilateral socket, and over the ischial area itself, which is the primary weight-bearing surface for the above-knee amputee. In the upper-limb amputee, scarring over the wrist disarticulation level of amputation may produce problems owing to compression forces at the end of the stump or shear forces imposed over the forearm with pronation and supination. In any amputee at any level, scarring can be a problem if nerve tissue is embedded in the scar and produces pain with use of the extremity.

As a general rule, once the scarred stump has healed and matured, prosthetic techniques should be used to prevent skin breakdown. Once stump breakdown has occurred, the stump should be allowed to heal and prosthetic techniques should be exhausted before surgical revision is contemplated, unless such revision would not significantly compromise the amputee's function.

In the below-knee amputee, the scarred stump requires the use of a soft liner, which may be of closed-cell polyethylene or silicone gel laminated between two layers of this material. Spenco,* a material made from closed-cell neoprene, may also be used in liner construction and has proven highly successful in reducing shear and friction forces on the stump. Another alternative to the use of a soft liner is the air-cushion socket.[11] This socket design is especially useful in preventing breakdown over the distal end of the stump. Developed by the University of California, it consists of a rigid outer socket and an elastic inner sleeve. Stump support is provided by the tension of the sleeve and by compression of the air between the sleeve and socket. In particularly resistant cases, in which breakdown occurs despite the above measures, the addition of a thigh corset for partial acceptance of weight bearing may be used. In extreme cases, the below-knee prosthesis may be made ischial weight bearing by the inclusion of a quadrilateral proximal brim. In addition to the above prosthetic measures, the inclusion of a "rotator" unit or torque-absorbing unit within the shank of the prosthesis may lessen torque shear forces between the skin and the socket wall or liner.

When these prosthetic solutions fail, or if their implementation significantly reduces the functional capacity of the amputee (*i.e.,* conversion to ischial weight bearing), surgical revision of the below-knee stump may be indicated. Excision of the scar with local advancement of full-thickness skin over the area is the preferred method of revision, if possible. Full-thickness skin can be advanced over prominent bony areas from soft tissue regions, which can then be grafted with split-thickness skin grafts. Scarring over the end of the stump may be managed by a second amputation at a slightly higher level if significant stump length remains. One should avoid, if at all possible, the use of cross-leg flaps for skin coverage of the below-knee stump. This procedure, while providing good-quality skin over the amputation stump, may compromise the opposite limb in appearance as well as function. Since the grafted skin is

---

* Spenco Medical Corporation, Waco, TX.

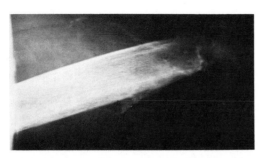

FIG. 44-11. Early bone spur formation in an above-knee amputation stump was probably of periosteal origin.

The presenting symptom of a bone spur is localized pain at the distal end of the stump with point tenderness on palpation. Spurs are not easily detected by clinical examination, so any amputee who presents with the symptom of localized distal stump pain should be x-rayed for appropriate diagnosis. The pain of a bone spur may frequently be related to an overlying bursa that is inflamed and may feel warm to the touch.

The complication may be minimized, but not entirely eliminated, by careful handling of the periosteum at the time of surgery.[98] Periosteum should not be stripped extensively proximally, and should be completely excised at the level of bone section or slightly above. This eliminates the possibility of retained periosteal tags giving rise to bone spurs. Some cases of bone spur formation are undoubtedly due to osseous metaplasia from muscle and fascial tissues adjacent to the bone, so a certain incidence of spur formation will occur even with the best amputation technique.

Treatment of the established symptomatic bone spur should consist of an initial attempt at nonoperative management followed by surgical removal in resistant cases. It is far better to solve the problem nonsurgically if possible, since the surgical trauma of removal may invite recurrent bone formation at the same site in certain patients who possess the so-called ossifying diathesis. Conservative treatment involves injection of the overlying bursa with anesthetic and corticosteroids, followed by a period of rest of the stump, and relieving, insofar as possible, direct pressure on the spur from the socket of the prosthesis. The occurrence of excessive distal end-bearing owing to poor socket fit may have activated a previously asymptomatic bone spur. This may occur following weight loss or stump atrophy. Closing in the proximal socket in the above-knee or below-knee amputation may serve to eliminate the problem by relieving weight bearing at the distal end. The addition of stump socks in the below-knee amputee may serve the same purpose. In other cases, relief of the socket by grinding out the polyester material directly over the spur may sufficiently reduce the pressure to result in elimination of symptoms.

When the above measures fail, surgical excision of the spur should be undertaken. In performing the surgery, gentle handling of the tissues tends to minimize the chance of recurrence. The spur should be removed extraperiosteally to the cortex of the parent bone. I prefer to use a small amount of bone wax on the exposed cortical surface at the site of removal to prevent reformation of the spur.

PAIN IN THE AMPUTEE

The painful amputation stump is the single most common complication following amputation surgery. Canty and Bleck, in a study of 7000 amputees treated over a 12-year period, found that all amputees suffer pain in the amputation stump at one time or another.[14] In a study of 1000 Finnish war amputees, Solonen found that only 15% were free of significant pain or tenderness in the stump.[90]

In the foregoing sections a number of specific complications that give rise to transient pain in the amputation stump have been discussed. For the most part, these conditions—infection, abrasions, scarring, edema, skin disorders, and bone spurs— are self evident and should be excluded first when one investigates the cause of pain in the amputated limb. This section deals with the chronic, more obscure causes of amputee pain and their treatment. This type of pain frequently cannot be measured or accurately located, and it appears to affect different patients with different intensities, so that surgeons may frequently be skeptical of its validity. The pain, however, is the very center of the patients' thoughts at home and at work. They long for pain-free sleep and the ability to do their work free of pain. The key to successful management of chronic stump pain is first of all to determine the origin of the pain stimulus, and second to eliminate the causative factor, if possible.

General Considerations

There are two types of pain in the amputated limb: pain in the stump and pain experienced in the phantom limb. The two types are not necessarily mutually exclusive. They may coexist, and either type may occur at any time in the life of the amputee; both have been noted to occur as long as 40 years later in a previously pain-free stump. The sensitivity of the amputated limb, as compared with the normal limb, has been shown by Aftana and Zubek[1] and by Korin and associates[47,48] to be heightened for both upper- and lower-limb amputees. Korin and co-workers found greater sensitivity in above-knee stumps than in below-knee ones.

In the approach to diagnosis of chronic, obscure amputee pain, one must first determine whether the pain is confined primarily to the tissues of the stump or whether it occurs in relation to the amputated part. Local factors to be explored in addition to the more obvious ones are bursitis, proximal nerve compression, ischemia, and neuromas. These factors should also be explored in cases of phantom limb pain, for the unrecognized presence of local stimuli may serve either to incite or to aggravate the painful phantom limb. Evaluation of phantom pain also includes a search for remote sources of pain (*e.g.,* angina, which may serve as a triggering mechanism), as well as psychological studies.

Diffuse Stump Pain

Generalized pain and tenderness of a mild to moderate degree in the amputation stump is common in the period immediately after the prosthesis is fitted. Unless there are specific localizing signs and symptoms, one can assume that this represents tenderness due to the unaccustomed pressure borne by the stump. The stump must go

through a period of conditioning and adjustment to socket pressures, and this is particularly true of the lower-limb amputee. Both tension and compression forces are at work on the soft tissues at the interface between the skin and the socket. Graduated increase in weight bearing and in the time spent on the limb usually resolves this problem within a few weeks. One should avoid removing the prosthesis in this situation, since tolerance to forces generated on the stump comes only with persistence in wearing the artificial limb.

Generalized stump pain in the amputee who has been doing well but suddenly becomes a problem case owing to pain must be investigated thoroughly. The following causes must be considered.

Bursitis. Formation of bursa over bony prominences, particularly over the end of the amputated bone, is common. Although this is a physiologic response on the part of the body in areas subjected to friction and pressure, inflammation of the bursa can result from excessive or prolonged forces. The pain perceived may be quite intense and frequently is poorly localized by the patient, causing tenderness throughout the distal portion of the stump. In myoplastic amputations, the bursae are located between the bone and the sutured muscle. Although amputation stump bursitis is distinctly more common in lower-limb amputees, it also occurs with amputations of the upper extremity, particularly when myoplasty rather than myodesis has been used. Bursitis in areas adjacent to the stump may also occur and cause radiating pain into the residual limb. Thus, the subdeltoid bursa may produce diffuse pain in the upper-arm amputation stump, and ischial or trochanteric bursitis may produce generalized or poorly localized pain in the above-knee stump.

Treatment of bursitis in amputees differs little from the methods used in the non-amputee. Injection of an anesthetic agent and corticosteroids, once or repeatedly, usually relieves pain. In more resistant cases the prosthesis should be discarded until pain has resolved. Systemic anti-inflammatory agents may also be used in conjunction with local injection. Ultrasound as a therapeutic agent has not been particularly successful in my experience. In rare cases, surgical excision of the bursa may be indicated together with myodesis if the inflamed bursa is located between the bone and muscle in a myoplastic amputation. In all instances, prosthesis fit must be evaluated and corrections made in cases in which poor fit is an etiologic factor.

Proximal Nerve Compression. Compression of a major nerve by the socket of the prosthesis may produce diffuse pain and paresthesias in the amputation stump.[16] Burning-type paresthesias are most common. The most common site of compression involves the sciatic nerve at the posterior brim of the socket, causing pain in the above-knee amputation stump. This occurs more often in elderly amputees who have insufficient subcutaneous tissue in the buttock and who sit more than they walk. In this situation the posterior wall of the socket should be gently rounded or even reduced in thickness to minimize pressure on the nerve.[57]

Compression of the peroneal nerve at the neck of the fibula by the socket of the below-knee prosthesis is another common source of stump pain. This is particularly true in the short below-knee stump because the weight-bearing surfaces of the stump are of necessity concentrated proximally. If adequate relief from pain cannot be achieved by adjustment of the prosthesis, resection of the peroneal nerve to a level above the popliteal fossa is indicated. Spira and Steinbach have recommended fibulectomy as well as peroneal nerve resection for this condition.[92] When fibulectomy is performed, however, a new socket must be fabricated to accommodate the change in stump shape.

Other common sites of proximal nerve compression include the posterior tibial nerve in the popliteal fossa, producing below-knee stump pain, and the ulnar nerve in the below-elbow amputee who wears a supracondylar suspension-type prosthesis, producing below-elbow stump pain. Appropriate alterations in the prosthesis to relieve excessive pressures caused by the brim of the socket usually resolve the problem in these instances.

Proximal nerve compression may also occur as a result of a herniated cervical or lumbar disc. When a ruptured disc produces compression of a nerve root in an amputee, the pattern of referred pain may differ from the normal dermatome distribution in the stump as well as in the phantom limb. It has been shown that irritation of segmental ligamentous innervation of the spine in amputees by the injection of hypertonic saline solution produces intense stump pain, as well as phantom pain, which may not correlate well with the dermatome involved.[26]

Amputation stump pain as a result of chronic proximal nerve root compression is usually treatable simply by removal of the source of compression. Most of the difficulty encountered in managing amputees with pain of this type lies in the failure to make an accurate diagnosis. A high index of clinical suspicion must be maintained to identify and treat these cases properly.

Ischemia. Impairment of circulation to the stump by a vascular event in the proximal circulation may be a source of generalized pain and tenderness in the amputation stump. Obviously, the occurrence of ischemia as an etiologic factor in the production of stump pain is more common in patients whose original amputation was for vascular disease of the lower limb. Increased coldness, skin color changes, and increased tenderness of the below-knee stump should suggest proximal arterial occlusion. If of sudden onset, rapid progression to frank gangrene of the stump may occur. In cases of stump pain thought to be due to a change in the circulatory status of the limb, consultation with a vascular surgeon and arteriography are indicated. Although severe ischemia occurring in the previously healed below-knee stump is a relatively rare event, it is of the utmost importance that it be recognized and diagnosed. Salvage of the below-knee stump, so important to successful ambulation in the elderly, may thus be achieved in some instances with appropriate vascular surgery.

Ischemia of another type has been recognized by some, notably Weiss and Wirski,[109] Burgess and colleagues,[11] and Dederich,[19] as a cause of pain in the amputation stump. These authors believe that myoplasty and myodesis are valuable procedures for the promotion of circulation throughout the stump. It is postulated that the continued activity of muscles so sutured promotes arterial circulation to the tissues of the stump and minimizes scar formation distally over the end of the bone. In a similar manner, continued muscle activity in the stabilized muscles during functional activities enhances venous return from the stump. Amputation stumps that have been formed without muscle stabilization and have the presenting symptoms of pain and tenderness, particularly with activity, may be suffering from the effects of local tissue ischemia. Dederich feels strongly that this type of ischemia may not only cause local stump pain, but causalgia and phantom pain as well.[19] In his study of 560 amputations and stump revisions, all cases of stump pain were relieved by revision of the amputation to a slightly higher level with a myoplastic closure technique.

I strongly believe that a properly performed myoplastic operation at the time of amputation, in the upper as well as the lower limb, significantly reduces the incidence of chronic stump pain in the amputee. Whether this occurs as a direct result of better circulation to the stump, as a result of better proprioceptive feedback, or as a result of providing adequate soft tissue padding over the distal stump is open to conjecture. Most likely, it is a combination of the three factors that enhances the general well-being of such an amputation stump. Myoplastic revision may be beneficial in certain amputees whose painful stumps defy identification of the cause and for whom no other successful treatment has been found.

Causalgia. Sympathetic reflex dystrophy occurs occasionally following amputation and is most common in distal amputations below the wrist and ankle. Causalgia-like states can also occur in below-knee and below-elbow stumps following trauma to the healed stump, but this condition is rarely if ever observed proximal to the knee and elbow. These patients frequently have a history of being cold-handed or cold-footed, with skin that sweats excessively and a labile emotional makeup. Sympathetic blocks should be used in such cases as a diagnostic tool. If good response is obtained from the block, sympathectomy is indicated

and has produced favorable and long-lasting results in the experience of some.[61,110] White and Sweet caution, however, that sympathectomy is rarely successful for stump pain above the wrist and ankle.[110]

Tumor. Recurrent tumor in the stumps of patients undergoing amputation surgery for malignancy may cause pain, and this should not be overlooked. Intense local stump pain may result, or the pain may be linked to the phantom limb. If the original tumor originated in bone, the bone scan can be useful in early detection of local recurrence. Detection of early recurrence of soft tissue tumors is more difficult, but radioisotope scanning and arteriography may be helpful.

Treatment may involve further amputation, radiation therapy, or chemotherapy, depending on the nature of the tumor and whether there has been distant metastasis.

Neuroma

One of the most common complications following amputation is the formation of sensitive neuromas, which usually produce well-localized and exquisite stump pain, in contrast to the diffuse type of pain just discussed. Neuromas form at the ends of all severed nerves and consist of bulbous enlargements containing a tangled mass of nerve fibers. They are a source of pain only when irritated, and thus, the more superficial the neuroma, the more likely it is to produce pain. Irritation of a neuroma may occur from direct pressure on the nerve end that is compressed against the wall of the socket, from friction between the socket of the prosthesis and the stump, or from tension on the nerve ending when it is embedded in scar at the amputation site.

The amputation surgeon should be cognizant of the potential problems of painful neuroma formation and should make every effort to ensure that the nerve endings are buried deep in the soft tissue at the time of amputation. The major nerves should be carefully identified, drawn distally, and severed as high as possible with a sharp scalpel, allowing them to retract deep into the soft tissues of the stump. No other special treatment of the nerve ends is necessary at the time of amputation, although ligature and injection of the nerve endings with phenol, alcohol, or formalin has been recommended by some.[37]

I prefer to ligate the larger nerves above the knee and above the elbow prior to allowing them to retract into the deep tissues, simply to avoid the bleeding from these nerves, which may be substantial. The use of myoplastic closure following deep retraction of the nerve ends also ensures that the neuromas that form will be well protected from pressure, as well as from entrapment in superficial scar.

The differential diagnosis of pain due to irritation of a neuroma includes bursitis and bone spur formation. Indeed, formation of a bone spur may be a causative factor in the production of a painful neuroma through chronic irritation of the nerve ending. The diagnosis of pain secondary to a neuroma may be made by performing a proximal nerve block of the nerve in question with local anesthetic. This relieves pain from a neuroma, but not from a local inflammatory process such as a bursitis.

Treatment of the painful neuroma may be quite simple but can be exceedingly difficult. The neuroma may have become symptomatic owing either to atrophy or to enlargement of the stump with consequent poor prosthesis fit. Fabrication of a new socket or modification of the socket to relieve pressure over the area in question may solve the problem. It is worthwhile to inject the neuroma directly with a local anesthetic and a corticosteroid preparation, since this alone may give long-lasting, or even permanent, relief of pain. The local application of dimethyl sulfoxide (DMSO) has also been reported to be somewhat effective in relieving painful neuromas.[94] Percussion of the sensitive neuroma has been recommended as a simple but effective measure in relieving stump pain. As described by Russell and Spalding,[78] the percussion technique consists of having the patient repeatedly pound a wooden applicator placed directly over the neuroma with a mallet, also made of wood, for up to 20 minutes several times a day.

Operative intervention is indicated for those painful neuromas that do not respond to conservative methods of management. Simple excision of the neuroma in question, allowing the freshly cut nerve end to retract deep into the soft tissues, is the method of choice. Unfortunately, in a certain number of cases, there may be recurrent pain after excision, which may be just as severe and of the same character as the original pain. For these cases, various means of preventing neuroma formation at reoperation have been advocated, including burying the nerve end in bone[111] and capping the nerve with metal,[17] acrylic,[22] or silicone.[28] None of these methods has met with consistent success. Perhaps more likely to succeed in cases of recurrent painful neuromas is proximal neurotomy. White and Sweet report a case in which proximal neurotomy of the sciatic nerve 45 cm above a peroneal neuroma gave dramatic relief when a previous proximal neurotomy 10 cm above the lesion had failed.[110] Farley has described a technique in which a segment of the proximal nerve is excised and then resutured as a free autograft, forming a natural point of terminal ingrowth for the nerve ends.[25] His experience with this method has been most encouraging. When the technique of proximal neurotomy is contemplated, however, one must be certain that the level of section will not result in denervation of valuable functioning muscle.

Perhaps the best method of surgical management of a painful neuroma is excision of the neuroma followed by nerve ligation. Battista and colleagues have shown that there is no histologic evidence of significant neuroma formation following ligation as long as 16 months after this operative procedure.[4]

Rarely, following failure of the above peripheral surgical methods to control pain of neuromatous origin that is limited to the tissues of the stump itself, anterolateral cordotomy is indicated. This procedure is generally successful for stump neuralgia but should be used as a last resort for extremely resistant cases.

PHANTOM PAIN IN THE LIMB

Severe, unremitting phantom pain, or persistent pain felt in the amputated part, is the most formidable and dreaded complication of amputation surgery. Fortunately, this complication occurs to a severe and incapacitating degree in only 2% to

15% of all amputees.[23,30,61,62,90,105] Phantom pain is to be distinguished from phantom limb, which is a natural sensation following amputation in 85% to 95% of all amputees.[9,30,90]

The phenomenon of the phantom limb was first recorded (insofar as is known) by Ambrose Paré in 1551.[43] Some three centuries later, the phenomenon of phantom limb and phantom pain was studied in American Civil War amputees by S. Weir Mitchell[65] in 1871, who commented

A person in this condition is haunted, as it were, by a constant or inconstant fractional phantom of so much of himself as has been lopped away—an unseen ghost of the lost part, and sometimes a presence made sorely inconvenient by the fact that while but faintly felt at times, it is at others acutely called to his attention by the pains or irritations which it appears to suffer from a blow on the stump or a change in the weather.

Ever since Mitchell's observations were recorded, there has appeared during the last century a voluminous literature on the subject—its characteristics, its etiology, and its treatment. A great deal is now known about phantom pain, but it continues to evade consistently succesful methods of treatment. Essential to the selection of proper treatment for these difficult cases is a knowledge of the characteristics of the phantom limb, the characteristics of the painful phantom, and the etiologic factors thought to be involved in the production of phantom pain.

CHARACTERISTICS OF THE PHANTOM LIMB

Immediately following amputation of a limb, the vast majority of patients (85%–95%) experience the feeling that the limb is still present. This may be associated with a tingling feeling of a rather pleasant nature. The presence of the limb is felt so strongly by some that they later may attempt to get out of bed on awakening, completely oblivious to the fact that they have but one leg to stand on. The phantom sensation is rarely reported in children under the age of 4 years or in persons with congenital absence of a limb.[87,106] In children this is presumably due to a lack of organization of body schemata in the brain.

The phantom limb is aligned with the remainder of the limb and seems to move with it. The most richly innervated parts of the limb (*i.e.*, the hand and foot) form the strongest and most enduring part of the phantom. Upper-limb phantoms tend to be stronger and last longer than lower-limb phantoms,[107] and the incidence of phantom sensation is higher after proximal than after distal amputations.[90] The phantom limb may be felt to move and assume different postures at different times, in contrast to the painful phantom, in which a fixed and unchanging position is common.[44] Similar phantom limb movements occur in patients with spinal cord injury,[7] and Melzack and Bromage[63] have demonstrated this same phenomenon in patients undergoing brachial block anesthesia.

Gradually, the phantom sensation weakens and the tingling feeling disappears. In most cases, disappearance of the phantom limb is associated with gradual telescoping of the limb, so that the parts of the limb between the end of the stump and the hand or foot are not felt, and the distalmost part of the limb feels as though it were an appendage of the stump. This telescoping phenomenon is reported in 80% of the amputees studied by Varna and colleagues.[101] Solonen,[90] however, in his study of 1000 Finnish war amputees, reported the telescoped phantom in only 21% of patients and the isolated phantom of the hand or foot felt at normal distance from the stump in 46% of the cases. It has been noted by Bors that telescoping does not occur in the paraplegic phantom, and furthermore, if amputation occurs at the same time as spinal cord injury or afterward, the phantom limb does not shrink or telescope, but behaves as a paraplegic phantom.[7]

A recent case is reported in which a paraplegic patient with full sensory ablation below the 11th thoracic level experienced phantom limb pain only after actual amputation of one of his legs. This suggests that the cause in this case could only be central.[15]

Phantom sensation eventually disappears in many patients, but a tremendous variation in both the rate of disappearance and the percentage of patients who become phantom-free has been reported. Weiss states that the phantom usually disappears in 2 to 3 years.[107] Varna and co-workers report an average duration of 3 months and 17 days, with a range from 10 days to 10 years.[101] Henderson and Smythe state that upper-limb phantoms usually persist from 24 to 30 months and lower-limb phantoms only 12 to 18 months.[36] In Solonen's study, only 15% of patients examined at 12 to 38 years after amputation were free of the sensation of phantom limb.[90]

The mechanism of production of the phantom limb is as yet unresolved. Some investigators feel that peripheral nerve stimuli form the basis for the phantom limb and for phantom pain.[24] The adherents of the "central theory," who are in the majority, invoke the body-image concept of Head and Holmes[35] and of Riddock[75] to explain the phantom phenomenon. As a result of various sensations experienced over the years, the patient builds up in his own mind an image of himself in relation to the external world. The more distal parts of the body, the fingers and toes, which are more richly supplied with sensory nerves, and which are in greater contact with the external environment, have a proportionally greater cortical body image representation. Riddock states that the image is actually formed from three components, based on sensory, kinesthetic, and visual perceptions, the last of which is the least important. In support of the central theory is the fact that persons born with an absent limb and traumatic amputees under 4 years of age rarely possess phantom extremities. Also, Appenzeller and Bicknell[3] have reported disappearance of the phantom sensation following central nervous system lesions in the distribution of the middle cerebral artery. Others have subscribed to the psychogenic theory, considering the phantom limb as a form of narcissism, in which the patient is incapable of accepting permanent loss of a body part. This is thought to be consistent with the high incidence of emotional disturbances found in patients with phantom pain.[44] The advocates of the organic peripheral and central etiologies, however, feel that the emotional aspects seen with phantom pain are secondary to the pain itself.

CHARACTERISTICS OF PHANTOM PAIN

According to Melzack,[62] pain in the phantom limb occurs at some time in 35% of amputees, but the persistent and debilitating type of phantom pain occurs in only 5% to 10%. Solonen describes this latter type of pain in only 3% of his 1000 war amputees.[90] In the majority of patients who develop incapacitating phantom pain, it develops immediately or very soon after amputation.[62,72,101] It is not uncommon, however, for a painful phantom to develop for the first time many years after the amputation, and Kolb[45] describes one patient with a 25-year delay of onset after ablation of the limb. Late onset of pain is usually accompanied by an observed physical defect such as angina, herniated intervertebral disc, arthritis, or significant trauma to the stump.[45,62]

Phantom pain tends to be more common in patients who have had chronic pain in the limb prior to amputation or in those with intense pain from an injury to the limb with a significant time lapse between injury and amputation. It is more common in upper-limb amputees than in lower-limb amputees and more common in proximal than in distal amputations.[9,91] It has been reported as being more severe at night than in the daytime.[72]

There are three broad types of phantom pain that stand out: a postural type of a cramping or squeezing character, a burning pain, and a pain of sharp, shooting, or lancinating character.[30,43] The cramping type is usually associated with a strong spatial impression of the phantom member, and the patient is usually able to describe in detail the contorted posture that the phantom has assumed. The burning type of pain is less common than the positional type but is apt to be more severe and unremitting. It tends to be more serious, since it is frequently progressive in its intensity, and the patient seems to make a less tolerable adjustment to its presence. The third, or lancinating, type is usually intermittent and transient but equally as severe and may be superimposed on the other types. This type may become cyclic, occurring at intervals of weeks or months and frequently associated with chronic muscular contractions of the stump.

In Solonen's study, amputees were interviewed with respect to the precipitating causes of attacks of phantom pain and the factors that tended to ameliorate the symptoms. The most common factors provoking phantom pain were strain on the stump and on the whole person, touching the trigger point on the stump, weather changes, poor prosthesis fit, and cold. Factors that tended to eliminate phantom pain were many and variable, including positioning of the stump, rest of the stump, movement of the stump, walking rapidly, walking slowly, swimming, shaking the stump, massaging the stump, beating the stump, use of heat, cold, alcohol, or drugs, wearing the prosthesis, and removing the prosthesis.

The premorbid personality of the patient who develops phantom pain has been studied by two separate investigators, who came to remarkably similar conclusions. According to Parkes[72] and Varna and co-workers,[101] such patients tend to be rigidly compulsive, self-reliant to an extreme, hard working, disciplined, dominant, and assertive. Kolb,[45] on the other hand, found no consistent personality pattern in the group of patients he studied. Correlation of premorbid personality with phantom pain phenomena, however, is probably a more valid approach than defining personality structure once it has become enmeshed with a chronic pain syndrome.

ETIOLOGY OF PHANTOM PAIN

Unfortunately, the etiology of phantom pain is not sufficiently clarified to permit a systematic and effective treatment plan. As noted in relation to the etiology of the phantom limb phenomenon, there are both peripheral and central theories to explain the organic cause of the pain, and a third school of thought holds that functional or psychogenic factors play the major role in its production. It is likely that these theories

are not necessarily mutually exclusive and that there may be, to varying degrees, peripheral, central, and psychogenic contributions to development of the phantom pain syndrome.

Mitchell,[65] Livingston,[53] and Falconer[24] subscribe to the theory of peripheral origin. They postulate that painful sensations from an infected stump or from a neuroma may start a chain of events that leads to a severe, persistent pain. Livingston states that as a result of incoming painful impulses, a reverberating circuit is set up in the internuncial pool of neurons, which travels cephalad until it reaches the thalamus. A vicious cycle is then set up between the thalamus and the cerebral cortex, which is self-perpetuating. Although initially in the pain sequence, removal of the peripheral source of pain may result in cure of the phantom pain, at this stage, ablation of the peripheral stimulus may no longer be effective. It is further postulated that these painful peripheral events may also set off autonomic disturbances, with vasospasm and a cold, clammy stump. The painful spasm of the blood vessels further increases the pain, establishing another vicious cycle. In some of these cases, early sympathetic block may be quite effective, the stump becoming warm and the painful phantom relieved. Also in favor of the peripheral theory is the fact that Bors observed that amputees with painful phantoms had disappearance of their phantom pain after spinal cord injury, although the phantom limb phenomenon persisted unchanged.[7] The peripheral theory, however, fails to account for the fact that the pain does not follow a peripheral nerve distribution and is not an anatomic representation of the part.

Support for the central theory of origin of the phantom pain is given by the observation of Head and Holmes[35] in which disappearance of a postamputation painful foot followed a vascular lesion of the opposite parietal lobe. Bornstein reported three cases of a similar nature, in which painful phantoms were relieved by (1) a self-inflicted wound in the opposite parietal cortex, (2) destruction of this area from metastasis of a hypernephroma, and (3) postictal cortical paralysis that periodically followed recurrent epileptic seizures.[6] Also in support of the central theory of origin is the well-known high percentage of failure with surgical attempts to interrupt peripheral sensory pathways to the brain.

That psychogenic factors play a part in the production and severity of any painful process is difficult to deny. Kolb, however, attributes a central role to the influence of psychogenic factors in the development of the painful phantom.[44] He cites nine patients of 22 studied whose painful phantom was induced by some cause of anxiety in their interpersonal life.

The exact cause of phantom pain remains an enigma. Peripheral, central, and psychogenic factors undoubtedly interrelate to some degree in both the production and the perpetuation of the phantom pain phenomenon. Pathologic conditions in the stump, in the conducting system between the stump and the brain, in the brain, and in the consciousness should be considered as different aspects of one continuum.[43]

TREATMENT OF PHANTOM PAIN

The treatment of phantom pain is difficult, at best, and has been directed at every level of the continuum from the stump to the brain. It is particularly frustrating to note that success has been reported with nearly every form of treatment reported for this condition, but no treatment has yielded a high percentage of success. The success is frequently dimmed by recurrence of phantom pain when follow-up of the patients treated is sufficiently long.

In developing a treatment program for phantom pain, one must first of all assess the patient very carefully for the presence of peripheral stimuli that may be contributing to the pain cycle. These peripheral events may be related to the stump itself or to a site of irritation remote from the stump such as angina pectoris, herniated nucleus pulposus, or prostatitis.[45,60,62] If the phantom pain is associated with stump pain, all possible effort should be devoted to elucidating the cause of the painful stump and treating it accordingly. Successful abolition of stump pain, whether from a neuroma, bursitis, ischemia, or a bone spur, may result in elimination or at least diminution of phantom limb pain. Successful

treatment of angina pectoris has been known to eliminate phantom pain.[70]

If no stump pain coexists with the phantom pain and no remote treatable sources of pain stimulus are identified, initial treatment alternatives consist of a number of medical or nonsurgical agents, none of which gives consistent results, but any of which may provide dramatic relief in an individual case. Psychotherapy is also an alternative in those cases in which psychological evaluation suggests a causal relationship. As a last resort, destructive neurosurgical procedures at locations in the nervous system from the peripheral nerves to the cerebral cortex may be indicated.

Nonsurgical Treatment

Drug Therapy. The standard non-narcotic analgesic drugs are usually of no value in the treatment of phantom pain. Although narcotics may offer some temporary relief, they are to be avoided in any chronic pain situation. Chlorpromazine,[64] LSD,[50] and DMSO[76,95] have been reported to have a favorable influence on phantom pain. I have had occasional success in decreasing, but not eliminating, phantom pain with the use of diphenylhydantoin (Dilantin) and occasional similar results with the use of carbamazepine (Tegretol).

Ultrasound. Anderson[2] has reported four cases of phantom pain occurring in young traumatic amputees that were successfully treated by the administration of ultrasound. Long-term follow-up results are not known.

Electrical Stimulation. Melzack has suggested the possibility of control of phantom pain by modulating the sensory input to the spinal cord and brain by either decreasing or increasing afferent impulses.[62] The latter may be done by implantation of electrodes directly on the spinal cord for electrical stimulation or by the use of long-term transcutaneous electrical stimulation. Good early results in the management of pain have been reported with the technique of deep brain stimulation in the mesencephalic lemniscus medialis by means of chronically implanted electrodes.[68] Although no long-term studies have been recorded, some early results of electrical stimulation have been encouraging.[42,49,69]

Psychotherapy. The role of psychotherapy in the treatment of phantom pain has yet to be defined, but the same can be said for any other modality of treatment for this condition. There is little question that in cases of intractable phantom pain, psychological studies are indicated as an integral part of the patient's evaluation. Psychotherapy is indicated when psychogenic factors are considered to be significant in the etiology of pain. Kolb[45] strongly believes that psychotherapy is a useful technique in the treatment of phantom pain, and Blood[5] also reports favorable results in two patients.

Surgical Treatment

Surgical procedures on the amputation stump are indicated to remove a source of local pain that may be a contributing factor to the perpetuation of phantom pain. Such procedures may involve excision of bone spurs, bursae, scars, or neuromas, which are local sources of discomfort. Proximal neurotomy may also be indicated in cases of persistent neuroma-like pain following neuroma excision.

Further amputation to a higher level is not successful in cases of pure phantom pain and serves only to decrease functional ability. A second amputation may have a place, however, in the treatment of phantom pain associated with a diffusely painful stump secondary to the effects of ischemia. Dederich[19] and Gillis[30] both advocate myoplastic revision in such cases to improve stump circulation and physiology. When myoplastic revision is contemplated, however, the second amputation should be done at the lowest possible level compatible with myoplastic closure to preserve functional length of the stump.

Neurosurgical Procedures. Proximal *Neurotomy and Posterior Rhizotomy.* Interruption of afferent impulses to the spinal cord by sectioning the peripheral nerve or dorsal roots has not been successful in relieving cases of pure phantom pain. These procedures may have some merit if stump pain is determined to be the causative factor in the phantom pain phenomenon. Such determination should be made on the basis of successful anesthetic blocks that eliminate not only stump pain, but the phantom pain as well.

Anterolateral cordotomy has been shown to be effective in relieving phantom pain in a proportion of patients. Falconer[24] reported successful treatment of nine out of 12 patients, who experienced relief of phantom pain up to 7 years. His results were equally good for upper- and lower-limb phantom pain. White and Sweet report successful relief, for up to 14 years, of lower-limb phantom pain in 11 of 18 patients treated by cordotomy.[110] Their results were poor, however, in four cases of upper-limb phantom pain. These authors believe, however, that anterolateral cordotomy is the neurosurgical treatment of choice for intractable phantom pain.

Sympathectomy. Results from sympathectomy for phantom pain have generally been unrewarding.[40,110] The procedure may be indicated in causalgia associated with phantom pain in which sympathetic blocks provide relief of both states, but the relief obtained from sympathectomy may be short-lived.

Postcentral Gyrectomy. Excision of the postcentral gyrus of the brain has been reported by Stone to be successful in the treatment of phantom pain.[96] The rationale for this procedure is based on the previously noted disappearance of phantom pain with certain lesions of the parietal lobe.[6,35] White and Sweet, however, have noted recurrence of phantom pain following this procedure, and they feel that it is an unreliable procedure, carrying a high risk of postoperative epileptic seizures.[110]

Frontal lobotomy has been recommended as a procedure of last resort but can rarely be accomplished without serious psychological damage.[44] This may be an instance in which the cure is worse than the disease.

Thalamotomy. Stereotactic thalamotomy has been reported by Talairach and co-workers[97] to have been successful in two patients and is viewed with optimism by White and Sweet.[110] No long-term results have been acquired, and the procedure does not have a large number of proponents.

CHOICE OF TREATMENT

It is apparent from the number of surgical and nonsurgical methods of treatment that have been described that no method is consistently successful, and none can be termed the treatment of choice for the disabling complication of phantom pain. Each case must be individually analyzed with regard to the relative magnitude of psychogenic, peripheral, and central etiologic factors. Nonoperative methods of management should be employed first, using drugs, transcutaneous nerve stimulation, or psychotherapy, if indicated. Contributing or initiating peripheral stimuli should be sought and the source eliminated. Stump revision should be entertained if the phantom pain is associated with localized stump pain or if the stump is of poor quality and could be improved in its end-bearing, proprioceptive, and circulatory characteristics by myoplastic amputation. Operations on the peripheral nerves, such as the implantation of electrical stimulators, should be considered prior to definitive central nervous system surgery in the more resistant cases. If all of these measures fail, anterolateral cordotomy may be the procedure of choice for phantom pain associated with a significant peripheral component. This procedure, though not uniformly successful, is sufficiently well standardized and offers relief in a sufficiently large percentage of cases to make it an acceptable surgical alternative for patients in whom all else has failed. Beyond the procedure of cordotomy, there is presently no neurosurgical procedure in which the risk factors involved justify the chance of success, at least on a statistical basis.

REFERENCES

1. Aftana, M., and Zubek, J.P.: Cutaneous sensitivity of unilateral arm amputees. Can. J. Psychol., 18: 101, 1974.
2. Anderson, M.: Four cases of phantom limb treated with ultrasound: Case report. Phys. Ther. Rev., 38:419, 1958.
3. Appenzeller, O., and Bicknell, J.M.: Effects of nervous system lesions on phantom experience in amputees. Neurology (Minneap.), 18:306, 1968.
4. Battista, A.F., Cravioto, H.M., and Budzilovich, G.N.: Painful neuroma: Changes produced in peripheral nerves after fasicoligation. Neurosurgery, 9:589, 1981.
5. Blood, A.M.: Psychotherapy of phantom limb pain in two patients. Psychiatr. Q., 30:114, 1956.
6. Bornstein, B.: Sur le phenomene de membre fantome. Encephale, 38:32, 1949.
7. Bors, E.: Phantom limbs of patients with spinal cord injury. Arch. Neurol. Psychiatr., 66:610, 1951.
8. Brand, P.W., and Ebner, J.D.: Pressure-sensitive devices for denervated hands and feet. J. Bone Joint Surg., 51A:109, 1969.
9. Brown, W.A.: Postamputation phantom pain. Dis. Nerv. Syst., 29:301, 1968.
10. Burgess, E.M., and Romano, R.L.: The management of lower extremity amputees using immediate postsurgical prostheses. Clin. Orthop., 57: 137, 1968.
11. Burgess, E.M., Romano, R.L., and Zettle, J.H.: The management of lower extremity amputations. Washington, Veteran's Administration, TR 10-6, 1969.
12. Burkhalter, W.E., Mayfield, G., and Carmona, L.D.: The upper extremity amputee: Early and immediate postsurgical fitting. J. Bone Joint Surg., 58A:46, 1976.
13. Cameron, H.C., Lennard-Jones, J.E., and Robinson, M.P.: Amputation in the diabetic: Outcome and survival. Lancet, 2:605, 1964.
14. Canty, T.J., and Bleck, E.E.: Amputation stump pain. U.S. Armed Forces Med. J., 9:635, 1958.
15. Catchlove, R.F.: Phantom pain following limb amputation in a paraplegic: A case report. Psychother. Psychosom., 39:89, 1983.
16. Christopher, P., and Koepke, G.H.: Peripheral nerve entrapment as a cause of phantom sensation and stump pain in lower extremity amputees. Arch. Phys. Med., 44:631, 1963.
17. Coburn, D.F.: Painful stumps and their treatment. Navy Med. Bull., 44:1194, 1945.
18. Cranley, J.J., Krause, R.J., Strasser, E.S., and Hafner, C.D.: Below the knee amputation for arteriosclerosis obliterans. Arch. Surg., 98:77, 1969.
19. Dederich, R.: Plastic treatment of the muscles and bone in amputation surgery. J. Bone Joint Surg., 45B:60, 1963.
20. Dembo, T., Leviton, G.T., and Wright, B.A.: Adjustment to misfortune: A problem of social psychological rehabilitation. Artif. Limbs, 3:4, 1956.
21. Ebskov, B., and Josephsen, P.: Incidence of reamputation and death after gangrene of the lower extremity. Prosthet. Orthot. Int., 4:77, 1980.
22. Edds, M.V., Jr.: Prevention of nerve regeneration and neuroma formation by caps of synthetic resin. J. Neurosurg., 2:507, 1945.
23. Ewalt, J.R., Randall, G.C., and Morris, H.: The phantom limb. Psychosomat. Med., 9:118, 1947.
24. Falconer, M.A.: Surgical treatment of intractable phantom limb pain. Br. Med. J., 1:299, 1953.
25. Farley, H.H.: Treatment of painful stump neuroma. Minnesota Med., 48:347, 1965.
26. Fernstein, B., Luce, J.C., and Langton, J.N.K.: The influence of phantom pain. In Klopsteg, P.A., and Wilson, P.D.: Human Limbs and their Substitutes. New York, McGraw-Hill, 1954.
27. Fishman, S.: Amputee needs, frustrations and behavior. Rehab. Lit., 20:322, 1959.
28. Fracketon, W.H., Teasley, J.L., and Tauras, A.: Neuromas in the hand treated by nerve transposition and silicone capping. J. Bone Joint Surg., 53A:813, 1971.
29. Gillis, L.: Infected traumatic epidermoid cysts— the result of rubbing by an artificial limb. Proc. Roy. Soc. Med., 47:9, 1954.

30. ———: The management of the painful amputation stump and a new theory for the phantom phenomenon. Br. J. Surg., 51:87, 1964.

31. Gonzalez, E.B., Corcoran, P.J., and Reyes, R.L.: Energy expenditure in below the knee amputees: Correlation with stump strength. Arch. Phys. Med. Rehabil., 55:111, 1974.

32. Groubeck-Loebenstein, B., Korn, A., and Waldausl, W.: The role of adrenergic mechanisms in the blood pressure regulation of leg amputees. Basic Res. Cardiol., 76:267, 1981.

33. Hansson, J.: The leg amputee: A clinical follow-up study. Acta Orthop. Scand., 69[Suppl.]:1, 1964.

34. Harris, E.E.: Prosthetic management of lower limb amputation. In Modern Trends in Vascular Surgery. London, Butterworths, 1970.

35. Head, H., and Holmes, G.: Sensory disturbances from cerebral lesions. Brain, 34:102, 1911.

36. Henderson, W.R., and Smythe, G.E.: The phantom limb. J. Neurol. Neurosurg. Psychiatr., 11:88, 1948.

37. Hermann, L.G., and Bollack, C.G.: Treatment of large nerves at the time of amputation of the extremity: A probable cause for persistent pain. Am. Surg., 22:696, 1956.

38. Hoover, R.M.: Problems and complications of amputees. Clin. Orthop., 37:47, 1964.

39. Houston, C.C., Bibbins, B.A., Ernst, C.B., and Griffen, W.O., Jr.: Morbid implications of above knee amputations: Report of a series and review of the literature. Arch. Surg., 115:165, 1980.

40. Kallio, K.E.: Permanency of the results obtained by sympathetic surgery in the treatment of phantom pain. Acta Orthop. Scand., 19:391, 1950.

41. Kay, H., and Newman, J.D.: Relative incidences of new amputations: Statistical comparisons of 6,000 new amputees. Orthot. Prosthet., 29:3, 1975.

42. Kirsch, W.M.: A new method of managing chronic pain. Med. Times, 102:115, 1974.

43. Klopsteg, P.A., and Wilson, P.D.: Human Limbs and Their Substitutes. New York, McGraw-Hill, 1954.

44. Kolb, L.C.: Psychiatric aspects of treatment for intractable pain in the phantom limb. Med. Clin. North Am., 34:1029, 1950.

45. ———: The Painful Phantom. Springfield, IL, Charles C Thomas, 1954.

46. Kolind-Sorenson, V.: Follow-up of lower limb amputees. Acta Orthop. Scand., 45:97, 1974.

47. Korin, H.: Altered tactile sensitivity in lower extremity stumps. Am. J. Phys. Med., 46:134, 1967.

48. Korin, H., Weiss, S.A., and Fishman, S.: Pain sensitivity of amputation extremities. J. Psychol., 55:345, 1963.

49. Krainick, J.N., Thoden, N., and Riechert, T.: Spinal cord stimulation in post amputation pain. Surg. Neurol., 4:167, 1975.

50. Kuromaru, S. et al.: The effect of LSD on the phantom limb phenomenon. Lancet, 87:22, 1967.

51. Labouret, G., Achimastos, A., Benetos, A. et al.: Hystolic arterial hypertension in patients amputated for injury. Presse Med., 12:1349, 1983.

52. Levy, S.W.: The skin problems of the lower extremity amputee. Artif. Limbs, 3:20, 1956.

53. Livingston, W.K.: Pain Mechanism: A Psychological Interpretation of Causalgia and Its Related States. New York, Macmillan, 1944.

54. McCollough, N.C. III: The bilateral lower extremity amputee. Orthop. Clin. North Am., 3:373, 1972.

55. ———: The dysvascular amputee. Orthop. Clin. North Am., 3:303, 1972.

56. McCollough, N.C. III, Jennings, J.J., and Sarmiento, A.: Bilateral below the knee amputation in patients over fifty years of age: Results in thirty-one patients. J. Bone Joint Surg., 54A:1217, 1972.

57. McCollough, N.C. III, Sarmiento, A., Williams, E.M., and Sinclair, W.F.: Some considerations in management of the above knee geriatric amputee. Artif. Limbs, 12:28, 1968.

58. McCollough, N.C. III, Shea, J.D., Warren, W.D., and Sarmiento, A.: The dysvascular amputee: Surgery and rehabilitation. Curr. Probl. Surg., October 1971, pp. 1–67.

59. Maini, B.S., and Mannick, J.A.: Effective arterial reconstruction on limb salvage: A ten year appraisal. Arch. Surg., 113:1297, 1978.

60. Maloney, P.K., Jr., and Darling, R.C.: Phantom-limb sensations evoked by palpation of inflamed prostate: Report of a case. Arch. Phys. Med., 47:360, 1966.

61. Maroon, J.C., and Janetta, P.J.: Pain following peripheral nerve injuries. Curr. Probl. Surg., 8:20, 1973.

62. Melzack, R.: Phantom limb pain: Amputations for treatment of pathologic pain. Anesthesiology, 35:409, 1971.

63. Melzack, R., and Bromage, P.R.: Experimental phantom limbs. Exper. Neurol., 39:261, 1973.

64. Miles, J.E.: Psychosis with phantom limb treated by chlorpromazine (phenothiazine derivitive). Am. J. Psychiatr., 112:1027, 1956.

65. Mitchell, S.W.: Phantom limbs. Lippincott's Magazine of Popular Literature and Science, 8:563, 1871.

66. Mooney, V., Harvey, J.P., Jr., McBride, E., and Snelson, R.: Comparison of postoperative stump management: Plaster versus soft dressings. J. Bone Joint Surg., 53A:241, 1971.

67. Moore, W.S. et al.: Below the knee amputation for ischemic gangrene. Am. J. Surg., 124:127, 1972.

68. Mundinger, F., and Salomao, J.F.: Deep brain stimulation in mesencephalic lemniscus medialis for chronic pain. Acta Neurochir. (Wien) (Suppl.), 30:245, 1980.

69. Nielson, K.D., Adams, J.E., and Hosobuchi, Y.: Phantom limb pain: Treatment with dorsal column stimulation. J. Neurosurg., 42:301, 1975.

70. Oille, W.A.: Beta-adrenergic blockade and the phantom limb. Ann. Intern. Med., 73:1044, 1970.

71. Otteman, M.G., and Stahlgren, L.H.: Evaluation of factors which influence mortality and morbidity following major lower extremity amputation for arteriosclerosis. Surg. Gynecol. Obstet., 120:1217, 1965.

72. Parkes, C.M.: Factors determining the persistence of phantom pain in the amputee. J. Psychosom. Res., 17:97, 1973.

73. Pearson, R.D., Valenti, W.M., and Steigbigel, R.T.: Clostridium perfringens wound infections associated with elastic bandages. J.A.M.A., 244: 1128, 1980.
74. Potts, J.R. III, Wendelken, J.R., Elkins, R.C., and Peyton, M.D.: Lower extremity amputation: Review of 110 cases. Am. J. Surg., 138:924, 1979.
75. Riddock, G.: Phantom limbs and body shape. Brain, 64:197, 1941.
76. Rosenbaum, W.M., Rosenbaum, E.E., and Jacob, S.W.: The use of dimethylsulfoxide (DMSO) for the treatment of intractable pain in the surgical patient. Surgery, 58:258, 1965.
77. Rosenberg, R., Adiarte, E., Bujdoso, L.J., and Backwinkel, K.D.: Mortality factors in major limb amputations for vascular disease: A study of 176 procedures. Surgery, 67:437, 1970.
78. Russell, W.R., and Spalding, J.M.K.: Treatment of painful amputation stumps. Br. Med. J., 2:68, 1950.
79. Sarmiento, A.: A functional below-the-knee brace for tibial fractures. J. Bone Joint Surg., 52A:295, 1970.
80. Sarmiento, A. et al.: Lower extremity amputation: The impact of immediate postsurgical prosthetic fitting. Clin. Orthop., 68:22, 1970.
81. Sarmiento, A., McCollough, N.C. III, Williams, E.M., and Sinclair, W.F.: Immediate postsurgical prosthetic fitting in the management of upper extremity amputees. Artif. Limbs, 12:14, 1968.
82. Sarmiento, A., and Warren, W.D.: A re-evaluation of lower extremity amputations. Surg. Gynecol. Obstet., 129:799, 1969.
83. Schraibman, I.G.: Gas gangrene after amputation for peripheral vascular disease. Postgrad. Med. J., 44:551, 1968.
84. Silbert, S.: Amputation of the lower extremity in diabetes mellitus: Follow-up of 294 cases. Diabetes, 1:297, 1952.
85. Siller, J., and Silverman, S.: Studies of the upper extremity amputee. VII. Psychological factors. Artif. Limbs, 5:88, 1958.
86. Silverstein, M.J. et al.: A study of amputations of the lower extremity. Surg. Gynecol. Obstet., 137:579, 1973.
87. Simmel, M.L.: Phantom experiences following amputation in childhood. J. Neurol. Neurosurg. Psychiatr., 25:69, 1962.
88. Slocum, D.B.: An Atlas of Amputations, pp. 254–288. St. Louis, C.V. Mosby, 1949.
89. Smith, B.C.: A twenty-year follow-up in fifty below knee amputations for gangrene in diabetes. Surg. Gynecol. Obstet., 103:625, 1966.
90. Solonen, K.A.: The phantom phenomenon in amputated Finnish war veterans. Acta Orthop. Scand., 54[Suppl.]:1, 1962.
91. Solonen, K.A. et al.: Late sequelae of amputation. Orthop. Pros. Appl. J., 19:316, 1965.
92. Spira, E., and Steinbach, T.: Fibulectomy and peroneal nerve resection in short tibial stumps. Acta Orthop. Scand., 44:589, 1973.
93. Squires, J.W., Johnson, W.C., Widrich, W.C., and Nabseth, D.C.: Cause of wound complications in elderly patients with above knee amputation. Am. J. Surg., 143:523, 1982.
94. Stewart, G., and Jacob, S.W.: Use of dimethylsulfoxide (DMSO) in the treatment of postamputation pain. Am. Surg., 31:460, 1965.
95. Stewart, J.D.M.: Traction and Orthopaedic Appliances. New York, Churchill Livingstone, 1975.
96. Stone, T.T.: Phantom limb pain and central pain: Relief by ablation of a portion of the posterior central cerebral convolution. Arch. Neurol. Psychiatr., 63:739, 1950.
97. Talairach, J., Tournoux, P., and Bancard, J.: Chirurgie parietale de la douleur. Acta Neurochir. (Wien), 8:153, 1960.
98. Thompson, R.G.: Complications of lower extremity amputations. Orthop. Clin. North Am., 3:323, 1972.
99. Thompson, R.G., Jr., Delblanco, T.L., and McAllister, F.F.: Complications following lower extremity amputations. Surg. Gynecol. Obstet., 120: 301, 1965.
100. Tooms, R.E.: Amputations. In Crenshaw, A. (ed): Campbell's Operative Orthopaedics. St. Louis, C.V. Mosby, 1971.
101. Varna, S.K., Lal, S.K., and Mukherjee, A.: A study of phantom experience in amputees. Indian J. Med., 26:185, 1972.
102. Vitale, M., and Redhead, R.G.: The modern concept of the general management of amputee rehabilitation including immediate postoperative fitting. Ann. R. Coll. Surg. Eng., 40:251, 1967.
103. Warren, R., and Kahn, R.: A survey of lower extremity amputations for ischemia. Surgery, 93: 107, 1968.
104. Waters, R.L., Perry, J., Antonelli, D., and Hislop, H.: Energy cost for walking of amputees: The influence of level of amputation. J. Bone Joint Surg., 58A:42, 1976.
105. Weaver, P.C., and Marshall, S.A.: A functional and social review of lower limb amputees. Br. J. Surg., 60:732, 1973.
106. Weinstein, S., and Sersen, E.A.: Phantoms in cases of congenital absence of limbs. Neurology, 11:905, 1961.
107. Weiss, A.A.: Phantom limb. Ann. Intern. Med., 44:668, 1956.
108. Weiss, M.: The prosthesis on the operating table from the neurophysiological point of view. (Report of workshop panel on lower extremity prosthetic fitting.) Committee on Prosthetics Research and Development, National Academy of Sciences, 1966.
109. Weiss, M., and Wirski, J.: Neurophysiology of the amputee. Prosthet. Internat., 2(6):9, 1966.
110. White, J.C., and Sweet, W.H.: Pain and the Neurosurgeon: A Forty-Year Experience. Springfield, IL, Charles C Thomas, 1969.
111. Whitehouse, I.W., Jurgensen, C., and Block, M.A.: The later life of the diabetic amputee: Another look at the second leg. Diabetes, 17:520, 1968.
112. Wilson, A.B., Jr.: New concepts in the management of lower extremity amputees. Artif. Limbs, 11:47, 1957.
113. Wilson, A.B.: Limb prosthetics—1970. Artif. Limbs, 14:1, 1970.
114. Young, F.: Posttraumatic epidermoid cysts. Lancet, 1:716, 1951.

45 Complications of Surgery for Neoplasms

JOHN A. MURRAY

Many of the complications that arise in patients who have undergone surgery directed at a neoplastic process are no different from those encountered after surgery of the musculoskeletal system for any other class of disease. The reader is referred to the other chapters of this work for other opinions and approaches to the management of these complications. This chapter will cover and perhaps reiterate completely some of the complications set down in previous chapters that have to do specifically with disease falling into the classification of neoplasms. As in all types and aspects of orthopaedic surgery, each case and each complication must be individualized. There is no substitution for good clinical judgment and experience.

CLASSIFICATION OF NEOPLASMS OF BONE

A classification of neoplasms of bone is outlined in Fig. 45-1. It is similar to many other classifications found in other standard texts and has proven useful for the clinician.

All neoplasms of bone are readily divisible into two broad groups: primary and secondary. By far the most common neoplasms encountered in the general practice of orthopaedic surgery are secondary lesions of bone. This category includes lesions metastatic by both distant spread and direct invasion. Those seen most frequently by distant spread are carcinoma of the breast in women and carcinoma of the prostate in men, and also carcinoma of the lung, kidney, and thyroid in both sexes. Direct secondary invasion by relapse of soft tissue sarcoma and the distant metastasis from osteosarcoma, Ewing's sarcoma, and some fibrosarcomas make up the sarcomatous types of spreads seen.

Clinically, primary neoplasms of bone may be broken down into three categories: benign, locally aggressive, and malignant. Under the malignant classification is a second division of frankly malignant tumors. These are very different in their histopathology and treatment and are classified as "small round cell lesions." In both the benign and malignant categories, the complications arising from each of the three major components making up bone (*i.e.*, bone, cartilage, and fibrous tissue) and two very minor types (neural and vascular) will be considered. The group classified as locally aggressive but late metastasizing will be considered separately. It is this latter group that so frequently presents the greatest challenge to the orthopaedic surgeon.

Each category will be considered in its systemic, regional, and local significance, as well as its early and late complications. An attempt will be made to indicate how the complication may be avoided and how it should be managed when it does occur.

BASIC APPROACH TO THE TREATMENT OF BONE NEOPLASMS

One can summarize a satisfactory philosophy in the approach to the management of neoplasms of bone as follows:

1. Eradicate the tumor without exception.
2. Avoid amputation whenever possible.
3. Preserve maximum function of the individual and the extremity.

There can be no compromise with the first goal. If the neoplasm cannot be eradicated, all other efforts are futile. Any procedure that is not directed at eradicating the tumor locally should be abandoned. It is most desirable to avoid, when possible, the mutilation of amputation. Regardless of the

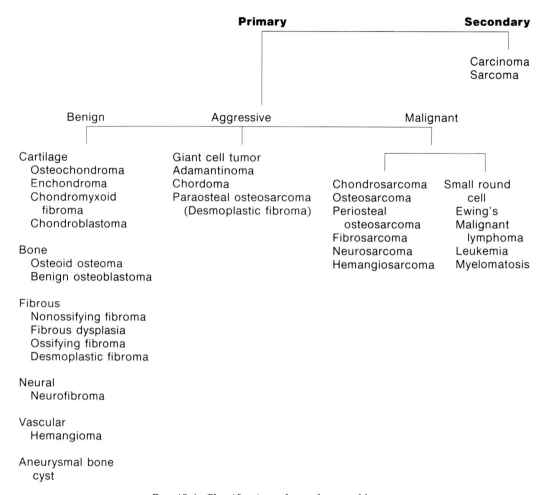

FIG. 45-1. Classification of neoplasms of bone.

quality and technical improvement in prosthetics today, the exoprosthesis is a poor substitute for the original extremity when sensation and motor activity can be preserved. Similarly, a useless extremity (*i.e.,* one without sensation or motor power) can be a hazard and a detriment to the patient. What constitutes preservation of maximum function is the area in which each case and individual patient must be evaluated. The exact types and techniques of reconstruction of an extremity after eradication of a large neoplasm of bone is a matter of judgment. The reader is referred to the abundant literature covering reconstruction of major bone and joint problems for aid in this area.[6–8] The capability of the orthopaedic or oncologic surgeon to satisfy the criteria

of the management of neoplasms of bone is clearly determined by the histopathology of the lesion in question, its exact anatomical site—not only of what bone but what part of bone (*i.e.,* diaphysis or epiphysis)—and the size that the lesion has obtained by the time it is detected and comes to treatment.

COMMON ERRORS TO BE AVOIDED AT THE INITIAL PROCEDURE

Many of the complications to be discussed in the subsequent pages, and some that have been mentioned in the preceding chapters, are extremely fundamental and could be obviated at the outset by careful initial evaluation.

The quality of the initial radiographic examination is crucial to the subsequent care and management of any lesion of bone and of neoplasms in particular. The technical quality of the initial images and the number of projections are extremely important in establishing the basic characteristics of the lesion. These characteristics direct the planning of any subsequent diagnostic procedure. There is no substitute for a quality roentgenogram.[2] One frequently encounters cases in which problems would have been easily avoidable if the clinician, radiologist, and pathologist had the ability, willingness, and interest to communicate with one another prior to the institution of any invasive procedure. The roentgenogram is the best study we have available for demonstrating the basic growth pattern and gross pathology of the lesion. The radiologist, in conjunction with the pathologist, can direct the inexperienced clinician to the areas where the yield from tissue obtained may be critical. If you are unable to find interested and enthusiastic consultants, the patient should be referred before any invasive procedure is instituted.

The pathologist is capable only of interpreting material forwarded to him. It is incumbent on the clinician to provide adequate and representative tissue for interpretation. It is incumbent on the pathologist to see that the material supplied is appropriately managed as to fixation and staining. In most centers the transmission electron microscope is available to the histopathologist, and he should be willing and able to provide for the electron microscopist tissue that may aid in the ultimate definition of the lesion. Electron microscopy is a clinical tool that should be available for your patients.

The biopsy procedure presents several unique problems and complications. Under certain circumstances, many definitive procedures are done on the basis of a frozen or quick section. It is certainly unwise to proceed with any definitive procedure when a frozen-section diagnosis is equivocal or when the pathologist is hesitant or uncomfortable about returning a firm opinion.

Advance, unhurried planning on the part of the operator is essential in avoiding the complications of biopsy. An inappropriately placed biopsy incision can jeopardize the definitive procedure because of implantation within the wound or embarrassment to the vasculature of an amputation flap. Even in the most aggressive lesions with the shortest tumor doubling times, there is plenty of time for careful planning before proceeding.

Once open biopsy has been elected, it is imperative that an adequate amount of tissue be obtained. It is equally important to avoid removing so much bone tissue that the structural stability of the bony unit is in jeopardy. With experience, needle biopsy can prove an easy and safe technique of obtaining tissue for histopathologic study. This is particularly true when the diagnosis of secondary neoplasm (metastatic carcinoma) is suspected. However, if the pathologist is not experienced, if you do not have fluoroscopic control, or if you suspect a primary lesion, open biopsy is the recommended choice.

Special care must be exercised in the technique of preparing the patient for the biopsy procedure. An infected biopsy site is the most restrictive complication in the further management of neoplasms of bone. Should an infection occur in a biopsy site, no definitive reconstructive procedure can be carried out until all infection has been eliminated. This could convert a potentially salvageable extremity to one for which only amputation could be offered. The time-proven regimen of adequate drainage, elimination of nonviable tissue, and administration of systemic antibiotics is the management of choice, should infection develop. Consultation with an infectious-disease specialist often proves beneficial. Only rarely is open biopsy under local anesthesia recommended in lesions suspected of being neoplastic. Local anesthesia is very limiting for a surgeon if any problem (*i.e.*, hemorrhage, large areas of necrotic tumor) arises during biopsy.

SECONDARY NEOPLASMS OF BONE

Surgical intervention in the management of secondary neoplasms of bone is of relatively recent origin. As late as 1950, amputation was recommended for the management of secondary neoplastic fracture of bones of the extremities. The surgical intervention and management of carcinoma secondarily involving bone are now well established. The basis for the selection of patients, from a systemic and regional point of view, remains basically unchanged: (1) that an open procedure will be more beneficial to the patient than any accepted closed technique, (2) that the patient's overall general condition and longevity justify the proposed and needed surgical procedure, (3) that adequate stability of the extremity can be obtained surgically by the use of internal appliances, and (4) that the proposed procedure will facilitate the patient's ability to cope with daily living and the management of the overall medical problem.[5,9]

The orthopaedist should be in close communication with the oncologist primarily responsible for the patient's overall care. Prior knowledge of the systemic effects of the primary neoplasm or the treatment already introduced (*e.g.*, thrombocytopenia and/or neutrophilopenia 2 to 4 weeks following a pulse of chemotherapy) may avoid complications.

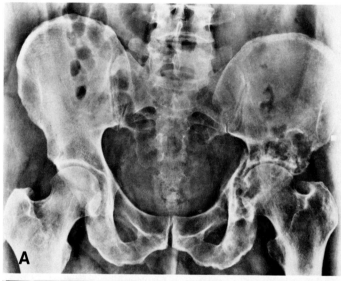

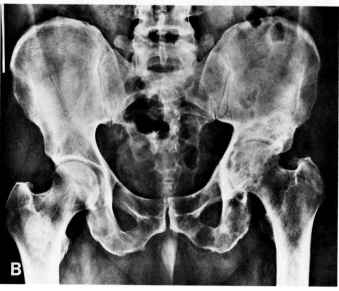

Fig. 45-2. This 42-year-old man had progressive hip pain over a 3-month period, 18 months after nephrectomy for hypernephroma. (*A*) A large metastatic lesion in the left acetabulum was treated with 4000 rad in 20 fractions through opposing ports over a 4-week period. (*B*) Fracture healing and reossification secondary to the radiotherapy 2 years after therapy. (*C*) The patient fell on the golf course, sustaining a second fracture of the pelvis 3 years after radiotherapy. (*D*) This was followed by rapid deterioration of the hip. In the film made 6 months after the fracture, note the large metastasis at the level of the sciatic notch.

Management of lesions involving the axial skeleton secondary to neoplasia does not normally involve orthopaedic surgery. However, the question of the suitability of stabilizing the spine following a decompressive or analgesic procedure may arise. Little experience is available to influence the decision, and each case must be judged individually. However, it is important to keep in mind that in many myeloproliferative diseases (*e.g.*, myeloma), almost all bone is involved; in diffuse carcinomatosis, many bones are involved, though there are no marked roentgenographic changes. In such cases it may be impossible to obtain satis-

factory quality of bone proximal and distal to the lesion to provide the stability necessary to benefit the patient.[4]

Secondary wound infection after fixation of a neoplastic fracture is a serious complication. Patients whose disease is advanced far enough to produce bony metastasis are frequently in no condition to withstand a serious local infection or the systemic effects of infection. Local wound management with drainage and systemic antibiotics may not be adequate to salvage the patient with this complication, and early amputation may be life-saving, palliative, and practical.

Fungation of cancer through a biopsy

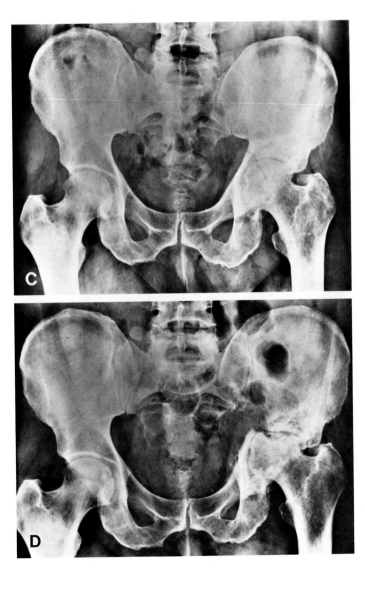

Fig. 45-2. (*Continued*)

incision or after fixation is a complication that may necessitate ablation of the extremity above the area of fungation to avoid secondary infection and septicemia. Meticulous care in wound closure and closure in layers with absorbable suture material will avoid the problem of tumor fungation in most instances. Postoperative radiotherapy and/or chemotherapy generally controls the growth of tumor, at least locally (Fig. 45-2).[1,5,9]

After the fixation of a secondary neoplastic fracture, every effort should be made to control the disease locally as well as systemically. If the disease is not controlled locally, you can reasonably expect loss of the stability of the fixation by continued bone destruction. In most instances in which this occurs, the life expectancy of the patient is such that reoperation is not justified.

Symptomatic management will suffice (Fig. 45-3).

With the addition of polymethylmethacrylate to the armamentarium of the orthopaedist, obtaining stable fixation is less of a problem than it once was.[3,5] Should stability or fixation be lost and the disease controlled systemically or locally, the patient's overall condition should be reevaluated. Refixation and restabilization can be accomplished as with any other neoplastic fracture, so long as the criteria for the selection of patients are followed (Fig. 45-4). A satisfactory result that will be beneficial to the patient can be expected. If further stability and altered fixation cannot be anticipated on the basis of local bony conditions, and if the patient has persistent disabling pain in the face of a good chance

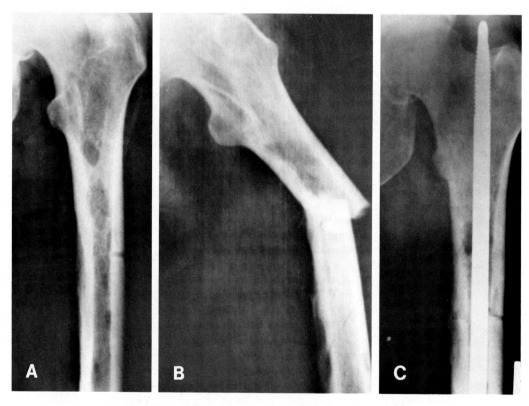

FIG. 45-3. This 56-year-old man had been diagnosed as having hypernephroma of the left kidney 3 years earlier. (*A*) Metastasis from the hypernephroma to the femur was proven by needle biopsy (note biopsy site). (*B*) The patient sustained a neoplastic fracture of the femur getting out of an automobile. (*C*) Open reduction and internal fixation was the treatment for the neoplastic fracture. (Note the fracture through the needle biopsy site—a "stress raiser.")

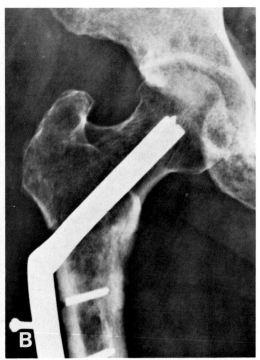

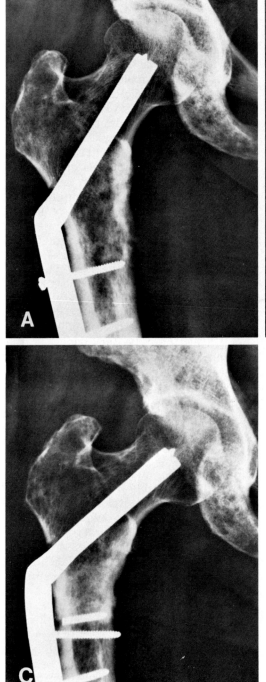

FIG. 45-4. This 62-year-old woman had carcinoma of the breast. (A) Six months after prophylactic nailing and postoperative radiotherapy
for a large metastasis at the level of the lesser
trochanter, note the loss of purchase in the
diseased bone by the proximal screw. (B) Later,
all screws fractured, and there was lateral angulation of the femur at the level of the lesser
trochanter. (C) The Jewett appliance was reattached, and more radiation and chemotherapy
were added. The patient was ambulatory with
a walker until death.

of survival, then a neurosurgical pain-con-
trol procedure is recommended. This is
often very palliative.

Many sarcomas metastasize to bone in
their natural course. These are often terminal events, and the overall condition and

life expectancy of the patient preclude an aggressive approach. The direct-extension type of metastasis of soft tissue sarcomas to bone presents a unique problem. Good results are obtained by high-dose radiotherapy following "debulking" (removal of all gross tumor) from soft tissue lesions. However, if, following this, local relapse occurs, ablative surgery is the only recourse—again, provided that the patient's overall outlook justifies this aggressive approach. Distant metastasis of sarcomas to bone, whether arising in soft tissue or from other bones, would be managed essentially the same as distant metastasis to bone from carcinomas. On the basis of our experience, however, it is extremely unusual that surgery is necessary.

The use of methylmethacrylate makes correct placement of medullary fixation critical. After polymerization of the cement, any attempt to manipulate the rod threatens the stability. Radiographic control is very important in the operating room (Fig. 45-5).

PRIMARY BENIGN NEOPLASMS

It is the area of primary benign tumors of bone that the orthopaedic surgeon has the most to offer in the overall management of the patient. It is necessary to reiterate the approach to management. Again, there can be no exception or compromise to the first point in management.

Approach to Management of Bone Neoplasms

1. Eradicate the tumor without exception.
2. Avoid amputation whenever possible.
3. Preserve maximum function of the individual and the extremity.

Eradication of the tumor is most consistently accomplished by wide or radical excision and reconstruction as dictated by the defect created. The reconstruction is frequently a matter of philosophy and the availability of material. The techniques for these procedures are readily available in the orthopaedic literature.[6–8] Once the initial procedure has been accomplished and complications develop, a new situation exists. If the tumor has been completely eradicated, the secondary complications of infection, fracture, contracture, and postoperative pain

are managed in the same manner as similar complications occurring with other diseases.

One must be certain, however, that there has not been a relapse of the original lesion to explain or add to the complication. Relapse of the original lesion is, of course, the most significant complication to be considered here. This indicates that the tumor was not completely eradicated, and complete reassessment of the situation is necessary. The surgeon is advised to proceed with appropriate dispatch, but not in haste. Each relapse dictates that the original procedure and tissue be totally reassessed. Consultation with pathologists is often necessary and is recommended. If the diagnosis is indeed reconfirmed, the basic management of the tumor needs reassessment.

If the size of the relapse and its anatomical location, as well as the tissue diagnosis, make amputation necessary, this must be offered. If it is decided after careful consideration that the lesion can be eradicated, if amputation can be avoided, and if significant function can be maintained in the extremity, a second local attack on the lesion is recommended. All relapses must be excised widely (Fig. 45-6). It is important to keep in mind that some lesions may dedifferentiate and change their actual biology to be more aggressive, either secondary to the surgical manipulation or with the passage of time.

Repeat biopsy and frozen-section interpretation, if possible, are necessary with every relapse. When a definitive diagnosis cannot be made, the definitive surgery should be delayed pending permanent-section diagnosis. Should no basic change be noted between frozen section and the previous permanent section, definitive surgery can proceed.

Large grafts, whether autograft or allograft, frequently fracture. Regrafting or supplementing the original graft with further autograft and/or allograft should be considered after evaluation of the local condition of the graft and the demonstration of no local or distant relapse.

As a general rule, very few lesions should be managed by curettage. Most are best handled by excision with a margin of normal tissue. Any tumor in relapse, regardless of its apparent benignity, should be considered for wide local excision (Fig. 45-7).

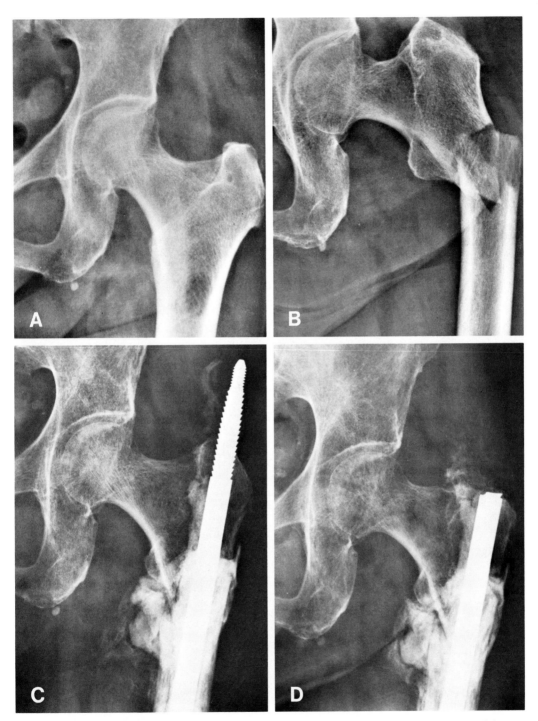

FIG. 45-5. This 58-year-old woman with carcinoma of the breast had been treated by radical mastectomy 18 months before fracture. (*A*) A metastasis in the left proximal femur was discovered during a skeletal survey. (*B*) The patient incurred a fracture through the metastasis during the course of chemotherapy. (*C*) It was treated by open reduction, internal fixation, and application of methylmethacrylate. At the time of surgery, it was not appreciated that the position of the rod at the greater trochanter would prevent the patient from sitting without pain. The rod was shortened *in situ* with a carborundum wheel on a high-speed drill. (*D*) The shortened rod is stable in the femur.

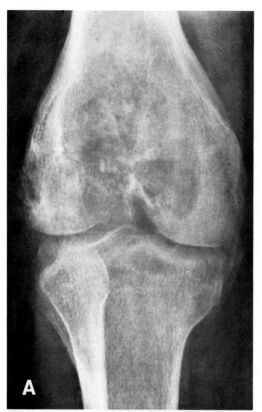

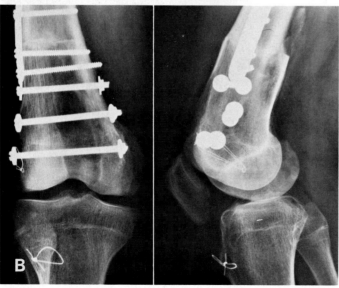

FIG. 45-6. This 15-year-old boy with a diagnosis of chondroblastoma of the right distal femur was treated by curettage and autograft packing. (*A*) Six months later he presented with profound synovitis and restriction of knee motion. The previous graft had resorbed, and there was increased destruction. Treatment was by resection of the distal femur, with the exception of a thin medial cortical strip with the medial collateral ligament attached, and allograft transplantation. Three years postoperatively (*B*), the graft had united; the knee was stable with motion from neutral to 90° of flexion.

PRIMARY MALIGNANT NEOPLASMS

In considering the surgical management of any primary malignant tumor of bone, one must keep in mind the necessity of eradicating it. Today, many highly malignant tumors of bone can be eradicated and amputation avoided. This involves preoperative control of the tumor with chemotherapy. Then, effective wide local excision

FIG. 45-7. This 35-year-old woman developed pain in her left knee. A diagnosis of giant cell bone tumor (A) was made at surgery. It was treated by curettage and packing with autograft chips. There was prompt recrudescence of the giant cell tumor anteriorly and medially (B), which was again treated by curettage and autograft packing. (C) Again there was prompt recrudescence of the tumor medially and anteriorly, but this time with skin invasion that precluded further limb salvage. An above-knee amputation was recommended.

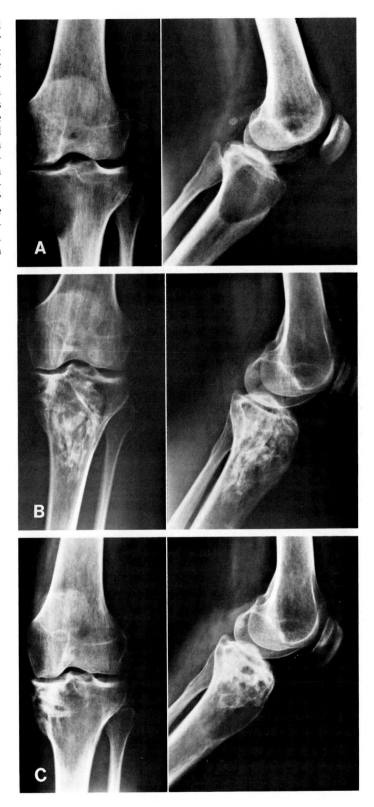

is adequate for tumor control. An inappropriate or misplaced biopsy incision is unacceptable and would dictate amputation rather than attempted limb salvage.

The question of transmedullary amputation versus disarticulation (clearing the whole bone) as the ideal level of ablation has been evaluated in the past. The majority of authorities in the field agreed that with good staging and judgment, transmedullary amputation is a safe and adequate procedure. From a purely philosophical point of view, the better oncologic procedure is clearly the disarticulation, or "clearing-the-whole-bone" technique, as opposed to transmedullary amputation. There is no proof that a relapse in a stump increases the mortality rate. With the development of a stump relapse, prompt amputation at a higher level to avoid fungation or possible pulmonary seeding is generally adequate.

The justification of amputation in the face of pulmonary metastasis must be based purely on the clinical judgment of the physicians involved in the patient's care. It must be kept in mind that extremity tumors of bone and soft tissue origin become quite large, extremely painful, and disabling. They frequently fungate and fracture prior to the death of the patient. It is accepted that mutilating surgery (*i.e.,* amputation) is clearly justified in the face of pulmonary metastasis, should the patient's life expectancy and overall condition justify the procedure. A palliative amputation is an important part of the armamentarium of the oncologic surgeon.

In evaluating the initial presentation of a patient it is also important to keep in mind that tumors that have been tampered with, (*i.e.,* surgically attacked but not eradicated) can differentiate to a more aggressive character. Some chondrosarcomas are reportedly notorious for this behavior. Should local relapse develop, either in the surgical incision or in the stump of a previous amputation, reamputation at a higher level is necessary if surgically feasible.

For lesions that are malignant but of low grade (*i.e.,* well-differentiated chondrosarcomas and fibrosarcomas), amputation can be avoided by the use of wide local excision of the tumor-bearing bone, resecting in continuity the previous surgical incision and

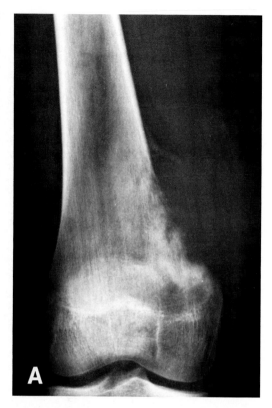

FIG. 45-8. This 17-year-old boy with osteosarcoma of the distal right femur (*A*), a metaphyseal lesion, a large soft tissue mass, Codman's triangle, cortical destruction, and new bone formation was treated by disarticulation. (*B*) He was referred to M. D. Anderson Hospital 9 months after the amputation with pulmonary metastases. (*C*) Nine months after the start of chemotherapy (Cytoxan, vincristine, Adriamycin-dimethyl triazeno imidazole carboxamide), there was complete remission of the metastatic disease. The disease relapsed, however, and the patient died of metastatic osteosarcoma.

the surgical tract. Reconstruction of the resulting defect varies from surgeon to surgeon and from institution to institution. The technique used should be individualized by the operator, who should choose the one available to him with which he feels most comfortable and that he feels will be the most functional for his patient.

At present there are no chemotherapy programs for chondrosarcoma or fibrosarcoma. In metastatic lesions, however, some effort at palliation with chemotherapy has been recommended. Similarly, radiotherapy

FIG. 45-8. (*Continued*)

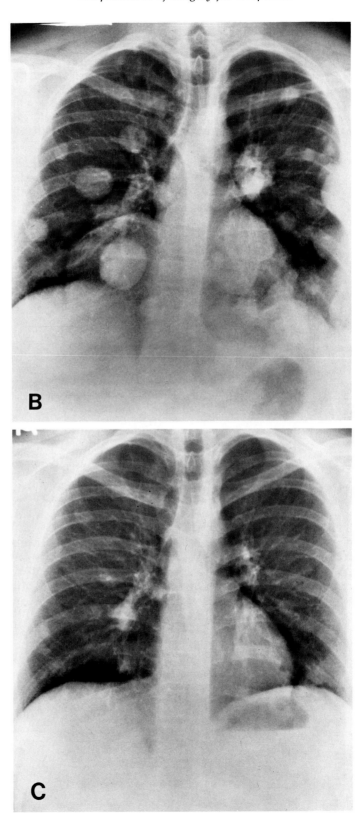

has no place in the primary management of malignant bone lesions but can prove beneficial as palliation for secondary deposits of these tumors and tumor inaccessible to the surgeon.

Pulmonary metastasis following control of the local disease is not necessarily a preterminal event (Fig. 45-8). If, after careful evaluation, the patient is felt to be capable of withstanding the necessary pulmonary surgery to resect the demonstrable lesions, and if the tumor doubling time justifies so aggressive an approach, the patient should be recommended for resection of the pulmonary metastases. This is not a decision to be made by the orthopaedic surgeon but by a pulmonary surgeon experienced in this aspect of oncology.

SMALL ROUND CELL LESIONS

Small round cell lesions include Ewing's sarcoma, malignant lymphoma, both Hodgkin's and non-Hodgkin's lymphomas, leukemia, and multiple myeloma. Because of the difficulty in differentiating these entities from neuroblastoma and rhabdomyosarcoma on the basis of the histopathology, the latter two are frequently included in this classification.

As a rule the surgeon has little to offer in the management of these lesions other than the acquisition of material for the establishment of the diagnosis. The current management of these lesions is multidrug chemotherapy and radiotherapy in various combinations and sequences. Only primary small cell lesions of the foot, distal fibula, and perhaps distal tibia require surgical ablation. In patients under the age of 9 years in whom the irradiation fields must cross the epiphyseal plate, amputation is preferable to irradiation. The injury to and resultant deformity of the epiphyseal plate make amputation more functional.

The complications secondary to the disease and the treatment may necessitate intervention by the orthopaedist. Secondary fracture as a complication of the radiotherapy, either through a previous biopsy site or in an area of radionecrosis, presents a challenging problem to the surgeon. The local condition in the extremity and the overall condition and predictable longevity of the patient are first considerations. Local or systemic problems may necessitate the use of amputation to eradicate the problem and allow the continued mobility of the patient.

When malignant lymphoma or Hodgkin's disease involves bone, it is important to realize that this usually constitutes a Stage IV level of the disease. In planning any type of reconstructive procedure, one must look carefully at the overall life expectancy of the patient. It should appear obvious that no curative local procedure is available at that point. Similarly, when neuroblastoma involves bone, it is Stage IV disease, and life expectancy and overall medical management should dictate treatment. If the clinical judgment is to make an attempt at reconstruction, fixation with the local addition of methylmethacrylate should be considered (Fig. 45-9). In Ewing's sarcoma, if the patient is considered disease free, the addition of autograft at the fracture site in heavily irradiated bone is important to establish union.

Multiple myeloma is the most common malignant disease arising in bone, though it is generally not classified as a primary tumor of bone. The techniques used in overall management of the problem arising secondary to multiple myeloma are essentially those used in the management of carcinoma metastatic to bone. Of special importance is the recognition that myelomatosis is a very destructive disease involving bone diffusely. This may make stabilization of bone difficult. A basic characteristic of this disease is the depression of normal immunoglobin, and one must be careful to avoid any infection, since the host's ability to prevent and control infection is severely impaired. If high-quality remission has been induced by chemotherapy, the patient most likely has normal immunoglobins and coagulation mechanisms.

SPECIAL CONSIDERATIONS

All of the complications and problems secondary to any type of reconstructive procedure can and do occur after the basic techniques are used in the management of neoplastic disease. The major concern of the orthopaedist should be to be assured that the tumor is eradicated. With the new techniques available in the diagnostic eval-

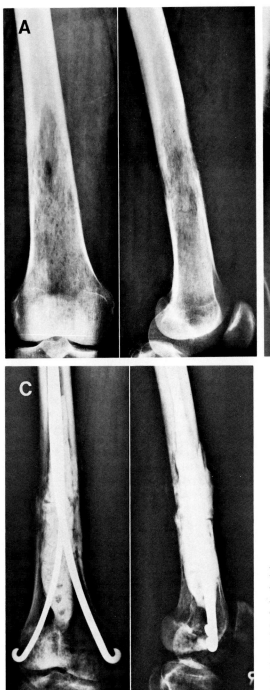

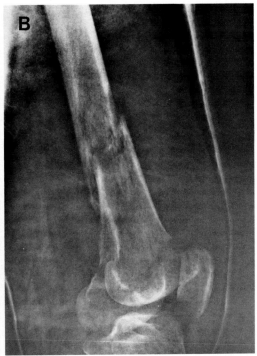

FIG. 45-9. This 55-year-old man was diagnosed as having Stage IIB_e malignant lymphoma. (*A*) After biopsy he was started on Cytoxan, hydroxyurea, Oncovin, and prednisone-bleomycin. (*B*) He suffered a fracture of the distal femur at home and was told that the bone was "too soft for surgery." He was placed in a spica and returned to M. D. Anderson Hospital. Staging was changed to Stage IV. (*C*) Crossed Rush rods and 80 g of cement supplied enough stability to enable the patient to walk with crutches.

uation of lesions (*i.e.*, polytomography, CT scanning, needle biopsy, and angiography), one can normally be quite certain that the tumor has been eradicated. In the absence of relapse, the management of a painful prosthesis, an infected or painful stump, or an infected or fractured bone graft is no different than for similar complications in conditions other than neoplasm. The reader is referred, therefore, to the preceding chapters for elucidation of the management of these complications.

The complications in bone secondary to high-dose radiotherapy are not truly considered complications of the neoplasm but are indeed complications of disease management. The changes in bone secondary to high-dose radiotherapy are directly related to the radiation dose given over a specific period, as well as to the source of radiation. The discernible changes are immediate or delayed death of all cells, arrest of cell division, abnormal repair, a new neoplasm, and loss of vasculature due to secondary soft tissue changes. All of these changes are also discernible in a child, with the addition of cessation of chondrogenesis in regions where growth is active (*i.e.,* epiphysis and epiphyseal plate). In addition, the changes are related to the age and growth potential of the child at the time he undergoes radiotherapy. Exactly how heavily-irradiated bone will respond to reconstructive orthopaedics is not known at present. The surgeon is cautioned to exercise care in the evaluation of complaints in the musculoskeletal system in regions of previously irradiated neoplasms. Reconstruction of bone and joint may be complicated by infection or nonunion, for instance, and thus may be difficult to manage. It may be best to accept disability from these problems rather than risk serious complications following a reconstructive procedure.

REFERENCES

1. Dahlin, D.C.: Bone Tumors, 2nd ed. Springfield, IL, Charles C Thomas, 1967.
2. Edeiken, J., and Hodes, P.J.: Roentgen Diagnosis of Diseases of Bone, 2nd ed. Baltimore, Williams & Wilkins, 1973.
3. Harrington, K.D., Johnson, J.O., Turner, R.H., and Green, D.L.: The use of methylmethacrylate as an adjunct in the internal fixation of malignant neoplaastic fracture. J. Bone Joint Surg., 54A:1665, 1972.
4. Murray, J.A.: Multiple myeloma. Curr. Pract. Orthop. Surg., 6:145, 1975.
5. Murray, J.A., and Parrish, F.F.: Surgical management of secondary neoplastic fractures about the hip. Orthop. Clin. North Am., 5:887, 1974.
6. Ottolengie, C.E.: Massive osteo- and osteoarticular bone grafts. Clin. Orthop., 87:156, 1972.
7. Parrish, F.F.: Treatment of bone tumors by total excision and replacement with massive autologous and homologous graft. J. Bone Joint Surg., 48A:968, 1966.
8. ———: Allograft replacement of all or part of the end of a long bone following excision of a tumor. J. Bone Joint Surg., 55A:1, 1973.
9. Parrish, F.F., and Murray, J.A.: Surgical treatment for secondary neoplastic fractures. J. Bone Joint Surg., 52A:665, 1970.

46 Complications of Allograft Surgery

AARON G. ROSENBERG AND HENRY J. MANKIN

With increasing desire and ability on the part of tumor surgeons to perform limb-sparing procedures in patients with malignant or aggressive bone tumors, systems for filling of the massive defects left in their wake must be devised, tested, and improved if the surgery is to achieve some measure of success and acceptance.[1-5,7,12,16,17,19,21,22,25,27,29] Current systems include the time-honored use of autograft implantation, either with or without microvascular anastamosis; but as is clearly evident both on theoretical grounds and on the basis of several recent studies, the supply of graft is limited, arthrodesis is required if a joint is resected, and the results are not as predictable as one would like, particularly as to rate of union and freedom from complications.[6,7,24,27] Metallic implants are of major benefit in elderly patients, especially around the hip, but the custom-made devices that have in recent years been implanted into the limbs of younger patients have a predictably high failure rate and are also inadequate in that they have no attachment sites for resected muscles and retaining ligaments for the joint.[2,3,21,27]

Segmental allografts, on the other hand, clearly have great advantages in this type of surgery: the supply is, in theory at least, unlimited (although numerous publications have attested to the need for improved publicity campaigns, harvest techniques, and storage facilities, suggesting that this aspect remains as a major problem;[8,9,10,11,16,17,22,23,26,28] the parts have the attachment sites for resected motors and joint stabilizers; through adequate banking facilities, a large stock of sizes may be available when needed; and perhaps most intriguing of all, if the procedure is successful and the host "accepts" the donor part, the graft behaves in some ways like an autograft and becomes a living part of the host tissues (theoretically, an ideal solution to the problem).

Since the first descriptions of the results of allograft implantation in the management of neoplastic and degenerative conditions of bone, the procedure has periodically been attempted with variable success.[13,14] The studies of Volkov in the Soviet Union[25] and Parrish in the United States[20] ushered in the modern era of allotransplantation of massive bone segments, mostly for the management of bone tumors or large defects resulting from trauma. Since these two major studies in the 1970s, numerous reports have appeared in the recent literature, suggesting not only that the procedure is feasible, but that a high degree of success could be achieved with it.

In the past decade, sufficient interest has been aroused in the orthopaedic community to warrant three sponsored invitational conferences, publication of a volume detailing the proceedings of one of them,[10] American Academy of Orthopaedic Surgeons instructional courses,[9] and a series of guidelines for banking of bone promulgated by the Musculoskeletal Council of the American Association of Tissue Banks.[8] Research presentations at various forums have suggested an enthusiastic interest of a small but growing group of investigators, who have, through the use of animal models, started to explore the immunology of implanted allograft segments, the pathologic sequence of events that the grafts undergo, and numerous approaches to improved banking of parts, with special emphasis on cryopreservation and infection control.

This chapter was supported in part by Grant #AM-21896 from the National Institutes of Health.

The problems encountered with massive allografting of osteoarticular segments, however, suggest that the "ideal" is as yet not attainable. Although success rates in our series have remained at approximately 70% to 80%, the incidence of significant complications of the procedure is sufficiently high to be of concern[15,16] and dictates continued exploration of ways to reduce or eliminate them.

The purpose of this chapter, then, is to review the incidence and possible causes of these complications. Based on the knowledge of the biology of alloimplantation of bone and the somewhat less well understood immunologic factors affecting the system, we also hope to provide some solutions, or at least avenues of further exploration, that may in the future make the procedure more predictable and universally accepted.

THE PATIENT SERIES

Between November 1971 and February 1984, the Orthopaedic Oncology Service of the Massachusetts General Hospital (MGH) performed 222 allograft transplantations in patients with a large variety of aggressive and malignant neoplasms of bone, as well as a smaller number of skeletal defects resulting from trauma, osteonecrosis, and other skeletal diseases.

Patients with bone tumors were selected for the skeletal resection and allograft replacement protocol from the population referred to the MGH Orthopaedic Oncology Unit and represent only a small fraction of the average of approximately 250 primary tumors seen per year, the bulk of which are treated by conventional means. As a prerequisite for inclusion in the program, all patients had full staging studies to assess the extent of the lesion and the presence or absence of distant metastases. An incisional biopsy was performed prior to the surgery and the diagnosis established on the basis of permanent paraffin sections. Because the procedure had a potentially high complication rate, we initially reserved it principally for patients in whom other methods of treatment were clearly less advantageous or less likely to succeed. Increasing familiarity with the technical aspects of the procedure and gratifying early results have led us to extend the indications for the procedure to include such problems as massive bone loss following trauma, osteonecrosis, and failed total hip replacement.

The diagnoses for the patients are shown in Table 46-1, and, as can be noted, the bulk of the neoplastic lesions are low grade (including 76 giant cell tumors, 20 low-grade chondrosarcomas, and 18 parosteal osteosarcomas). In recent years, however, we have chosen to perform the surgery in patients with more aggressive lesions such as central osteosarcomas, Ewing's sarcoma, and high-grade fibrosarcomas. In fact, at the present time, almost 20% of the lesions are high grade (Stage 2A and 2B, according

Table 46-1. Diagnosis in 222 Patients Selected for Allograft Transplantation

DIAGNOSIS	NO. OF CASES
TUMORS	
Giant cell tumor	76
Chondrosarcoma	39
Central osteosarcoma	20
Parosteal osteosarcoma	18
Fibrosarcoma	7
Metastatic carcinoma	7
Adamantinoma	7
Chondroblastoma (recurrent)	6
Aggressive osteoblastoma	4
Ewing's sarcoma	4
Desmoplastic fibroma	3
Lymphoma	2
Myeloma	2
Pigmented villonodular synovitis	2
Aneurysmal bone cyst, chondromyxoid fibroma, liposarcoma, and malignant fibrous histiocytoma (1 each)	4
Total	201
NONTUMOROUS CONDITIONS	
Trauma	8
Osteonecrosis	6
Failed total hip replacement	2
Gaucher's disease	2
Fibrous dysplasia	2
Paget's disease	1
Total	21

to the staging scheme proposed by Enneking[5]). We have also extended the indications for resection followed by allograft replacement in 11 of the patients (5.4%) presenting with an osseous metastatic focus of a primary solid tumor of the kidney, thyroid, prostate, or breast (Stage 3) (Table 46-2). The mean age of the patients included in the series was 31.2, with a range of 11 to 70. Ninety-three of the patients were male, 129 female.

The operative procedure for resection of the neoplasm does not differ from that used for other techniques. When indicated, we perform wide or, occasionally, marginal resection surgery, removing the tumor-containing bone, periosteum, adjacent muscular and ligamentous tissues, and, on occasion, neurovascular structures to provide a cuff of normal tissue on all sides of the lesion. The skin and soft tissue tract of the prior biopsy site is resected in continuity with the specimen. Following successful resection, the appropriate-sized allograft segment is obtained from our bone bank, thawed, and then inserted with rigid internal fixation (usually AO plates and screws or, on occasion, intramedullary rods). Soft tissue attachments to the bone are reconstituted with nonabsorbable sutures, with special attention paid to covering the graft with viable muscle and to reestablishing the continuity of important muscle groups: the rotator cuff, deltoid, and pectoralis major in the shoulder, the gluteus medius and iliopsoas around the hip, and so forth. We pay special attention to the joint stabilizers and make every effort to obtain a tight anastomosis of allograft and host collateral ligaments and posterior capsule in the knee joint, and dorsal and volar capsule in the wrist. A typical operative procedure is illustrated in Figure 46-1.

Postoperative management of patients in whom an allograft has been inserted differs little from that for other patients in whom a massive local resection has been performed. Suction drains are used for approximately 2 to 4 days to minimize dead space, and the patient is treated with intravenous antibiotics for at least a week. Anticoagulants are used as indicated.

Following initial healing of the wound, the limb is immobilized in a cast for approximately 2 to 3 months for lower extremities (a shorter period is usually sufficient for the arm) and is usually allowed partial weight bearing. After removal of the cast, a cast-type polypropylene orthosis is fitted, and the patient is treated with active and passive range-of-motion and gentle exercises until a satisfactory range of motion and good return of strength have been achieved. Unrestricted use of the extremity is not advocated until healing is satisfactory at the host–donor junction and the joint is stable, usually at about 7 to 9 months.

The patient is followed regularly by serial radiographic studies to assess the fate of the graft and the presence of local recurrence or distant metastases. Laboratory data are obtained as necessary, and a baseline bone scan is obtained at about 3 months and then every 4 to 6 months for the first 2 years to assess vascular ingrowth.

THE BONE BANK

As can be readily appreciated, the success of this procedure is in large measure dependent on the maintenance of a well-stocked bone bank that not only provides a wide assortment of parts in different sizes and ensures sterility and structural stability of the graft, but maintains adequate records of the transactions (both deposits and withdrawals). Our bank was established in 1973 and has grown proportionately with the demands of the oncology unit. The bank has an estimated 320 parts frozen at −80°C. It is operated through a computerized inventory system, and the hospital is currently experimenting with a computer-based sizing system. The interested reader is referred to

(*Text continues on page 1391.*)

Table 46-2. Stage of 201 Tumors in Patients Selected for Allograft Transplantation

STAGE	NO. OF TUMORS
0	9 (4.5%)
1A	40 (19.9%)
1B	99 (49.3%)
2A	3 (1.5%)
2B	39 (19.4%)
3	11 (5.4%)

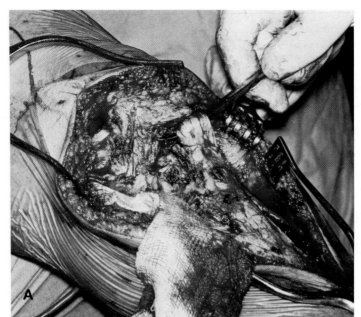

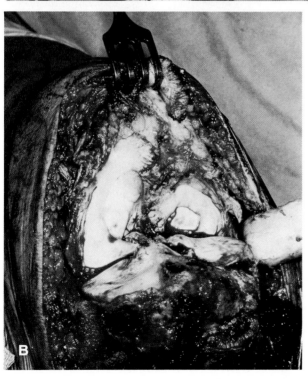

FIG. 46-1. Operative procedure. Resection and replacement of the proximal tibia for giant cell tumor. (*A*) Severing the patellar tendon insertion. (*B*) Appearance after sectioning the cruciate and collateral ligaments. (*C*) Sectioning the tibia distal to the lesion. (*D*) Diagram of the defect following removal of the proximal tibia. (*E*) Careful "vest-over-pants" anastomosis of the capsular and ligamentous soft tissues at the knee. (*F*) Bone anastomosis with the standard fixation technique. (*G*) Early postoperative result.

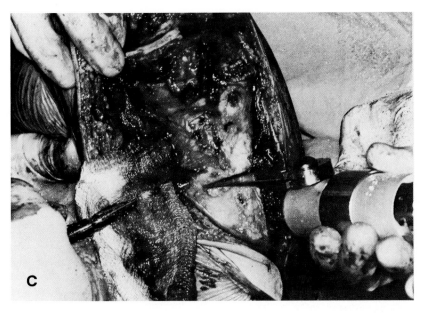

C

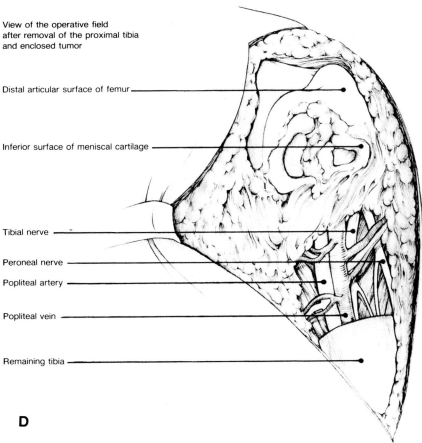

View of the operative field
after removal of the proximal tibia
and enclosed tumor

Distal articular surface of femur

Inferior surface of meniscal cartilage

Tibial nerve

Peroneal nerve
Popliteal artery

Popliteal vein

Remaining tibia

D

FIG. 46-1. (*Continued*)

FIG. 46-1. (*Continued*)

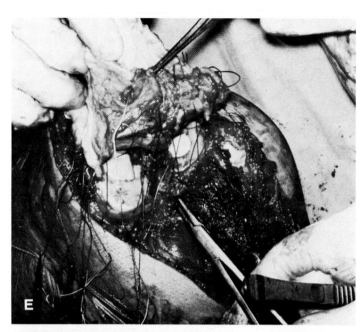

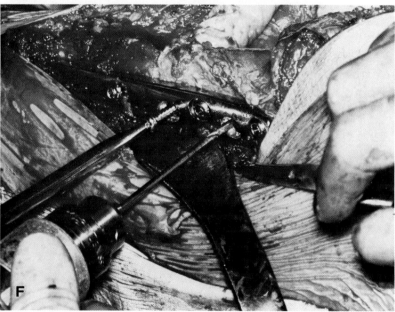

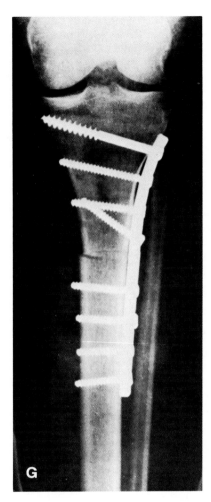

FIG. 46-1. (*Continued*)

plasms in the older. Antemortem treatment with corticosteroids or maintenance on a respirator for longer than 1 week usually disqualifies the donor on the basis of the high incidence of microabscesses and diffuse infection. Our bank takes special pains to secure permission from the next of kin, and special donor forms are available for that purpose. Whenever possible, we prefer to work with other transplant teams, since harvesting the bones adds only a short period to the procedure, and the information gained from the typing laboratory is helpful in our currently retrospective (but, we hope, soon prospective) matching.

The procurement takes place in the operating room, with all standard sterile procedures and precautions in effect. Through long extensile incisions the bones are removed and stripped of their muscular attachments, with care taken to leave all ligamentous attachments and capsular structures at least 2 cm long. The cadaver is reconstructed with wooden dowels and plaster of paris, and after we submit specimens for serologic tests for hepatitis and syphilis, we refer the cadaver to the pathology department for autopsy.

Cultures are obtained of the surface and medullary cavity of each of the bones, as well as the heart blood, pleural cavity, urine, and cryopreservative solution. The cartilaginous ends of the bones are soaked in 8% DMSO in Ringer's lactate, according to a technique previously described and supported by *in vitro* experimentation.[10] The segments are placed into gas-sterilized polyethylene bags, wrapped in sterile towels and drapes, placed in the refrigerator at 4°C overnight, and then frozen to −80°C. Radiographs in two planes are obtained with a radiopaque sizing marker as a control for magnification, and these are later used for either visual or computer sizing to determine the most appropriate segment for a specific patient. The bones are thawed just prior to use with warm Ringer's lactate solution to which antibiotics have been added after additional surface and medullary cavity cultures have been obtained.

It should be evident from the foregoing that the use of cadaveric allografts involves a complex system embracing graft procure-

several articles describing the banking procedure.[9,10,23]

Bones are obtained for deposit in the bank at a special "harvest" on carefully screened and selected donors, most of whom are recruited from the neurosurgical or the emergency wards of MGH. To be eligible for donation, a potential donor should have been declared dead no longer than 12 hours prior to harvest, and the history and laboratory data should reveal no evidence of infection, neoplasm, viral disease, or syphilis. We prefer donors between the ages of 15 and 45 to avoid the problems of open epiphyseal plates in the younger ages and osteopenia or occult neo-

ment and banking, patient staging and selection, resective surgery, selection and implantation of the graft, aftercare, rehabilitation, and follow-up. Since each case is different, particularly in terms of the anatomical structures that are sacrificed to remove the tumor, it is difficult to develop a standardized evaluation or even to obtain descriptive statistics. It is also difficult to compare anatomical sites (distal femur vs. midshaft of the humerus, for instance). To carry out such comparisons and also to provide information on the value of the operative procedures, we have arrived at a series of simple groupings and evaluative techniques.

The patients are grouped according to the *type* of graft, defined by the anatomy of the segment implanted. Grafts that involve a joint (usually one articular surface, such as the distal femur, proximal tibia, hemipelvis, etc.) are termed *osteoarticular* (*OA*) and include as a subcategory those grafts in which less than the full articular surface is implanted as *hemiosteoarticular* allografts. Grafts that do not involve a joint but are interposed between the resected ends of a single bone (midshaft of the humerus, proximal femur, etc.) are called *intercalary* (*IC*). Those in which a prosthetic implant such as a bipolar, Austin-Moore, or total joint arthroplasty is used along with the allograft are known as *allograft + prosthesis* (*AP*). In recent procedures we have added another category, in which allograft is introduced across a resected joint. These are called *allograft-arthrodeses* (*AAs*). Table 46-3 shows the distribution of patients according to type and anatomical site of the graft.

Although we are currently attempting to develop a rating scale analogous to those available for total joint replacements for the purpose of this study, we still adhere to the functional rating system outlined in our original description.[15] *Excellent* results are those in which the patient has no evident disease (NED), has no pain, enjoys full function of the part, and carries on most of life's activities without significant impairment. All of these patients returned to their presurgical occupational level, and although none are encouraged to participate

Table 46-3. Distribution of 222 Cases of Allograft Transplantation by Type and Anatomical Site

TYPE AND SITE	NO. OF PATIENTS
OSTEOARTICULAR	
Distal femur	59 (29 hemi-)
Proximal tibia	33 (17 hemi-)
Proximal humerus	19 (1 hemi-)
Proximal femur	14
Distal radius	13
Hemipelvis	6
Hemipelvis and proximal femur	4
Distal humerus	4 (1 hemi-)
Distal humerus-proximal ulna	2
Proximal ulna	3
Distal tibia	1
Total	158
INTERCALARY	
Tibial shaft	19
Femoral shaft	15
Humeral shaft	5
Ulna	1
Hemipelvis	1
Total	41
ALLOGRAFT + PROSTHESIS	
Proximal femur and Austin-Moore or bipolar prosthesis	6
Hemipelvis and Austin Moore or bipolar prosthesis	4
Proximal femur and total hip replacement	4
Hemipelvis and total hip replacement	2
Total	16
ALLOGRAFT-ARTHRODESIS	
Distal femur-proximal tibia	4
Proximal humerus-glenoid	3
Total	7

actively in sports, many do. A *good* result is one in which the patient remains NED and has no pain but shows a reduced range of motion. Although the patient is still able to perform many work-related tasks without difficulty and does not use a support or assistive device, he is unable to participate in sports and notices some limitations in lifestyle.

A *fair* result is one in which the patient remains NED, but either has significant pain or displays a major reduction in functional capacity. A brace, crutches, or a crane is required for function, and the ability to participate in the activities of daily living is reduced. Approximately half of the patients graded as *fair* returned to their preoperative work level. A patient is graded as a *failure* when tumor has recurred, metastasized, or caused death. Patients who have had to undergo amputation or resection of the graft for any reason are also classified as failures.

In consideration of the time to assessment of the "end-results," it should be apparent that when one is dealing with aggressive tumors of bone, some of which are very slow to recur locally or metastasize quite late in the course, that even for our longest follow-up (now approaching 14 years), the result must be considered, by some standards, preliminary. Furthermore, since the natural history of allograft implants is not really well known, it is obvious that several years should elapse before the evaluation is meaningful. We have chosen the figure of 2 years as the minimum follow-up period for this patient series, with the recognition that some of the patients may alter their status. Of the 222 patients now entered in the series, all have been followed closely throughout their course, and at this time 143 have been followed at least 2 years (or until death). These 143 patients constitute this study and are the subjects of the statistical evaluation and analysis of complications contributing to their current status.

RESULTS OF THE PATIENT SERIES

Table 46-4 defines the results of allograft transplantation in 143 patients followed for 2 or more years. The data are reported according to type of graft (osteoarticular, 103; intercalary, 29; allograft + prosthesis, 10; and allograft-arthrodesis, 1) and anatomical site in order of descending frequency. As can be readily noted, the excellent and good results (considered by most patients—and indeed by the evaluating physician—to be highly satisfactory) vary according to the type and size of the graft. Thus, for the osteoarticular implants, 80% of the patients with distal femoral and proximal tibial grafts were rated as excellent or good, those with proximal humeral and distal radius grafts did slighty less well (74% and 69%, respectively), and only three of nine hemipelvis, one of four proximal femoral, and one of three distal humeral grafts fell into the acceptable range. Part of the explanation for the poor rate of acceptable results for the hemipelvis patients was the high rate of tumor recurrence, metastases, and death (4/9 tumor failures, to be discussed further below). The summary data for the 103 patients with osteoarticular grafts show that 41% were graded as excellent and 28% good, with an overall "success" rate of 69% (despite a 13% tumor failure rate).

Examination of the results of the intercalary grafts shows that the overall rate of success is higher than for the osteoarticular grafts (in part owing to the low rate of tumor failures [2/29; 7%]) and that the three major anatomical sites (tibia, femur, and humerus) performed almost equally well, with excellent and good results achieved in greater than 80% of the patients. Patients in whom allografts and prostheses were inserted fared somewhat less well (the three hemipelvis patients all did poorly), but the single patient with an allograft arthrodesis followed longer than 2 years has done well (though still rated as good rather than excellent, since the absence of motion in the knee causes some disability).

The total values for the entire group of 143 patients are shown in the lower part of Table 46-4. Fifty percent of the patients were rated as excellent and another 22% as good, with a 72% total success rate for the procedure. Since the purpose of this study (indeed, of the entire system) is to define the efficacy of the allograft transplantation technique, it is appropriate to evaluate the remaining patients after the 16 tumor failures (11%) are deleted. These are shown on the bottom line of Table 46-4 and demonstrate that 69 of 127 patients (54%) achieved an excellent result from their procedure, and 31 of 127 (24%) were rated as good, for an overall success rate of 78%.

Further study of the table provides some insight into some of the problems encoun-tered in dealing with specific groups of patients. Hemipelvis transplants performed poorly in all three types of grafts, for a total of only three excellent or good results out of the entire group of 13 patients in whom the operation was performed. Had we not performed this particularly chal-lenging surgical procedure, the success rate

Table 46-4. Status of 143 Patients by Site and Type of Graft After Allograft Transplantation

PROCEDURE	NUM-BER	RESULTS				NO. OF TUMOR FAILURES
		EXCELLENT	GOOD	FAIR	FAILURE	
OSTEOARTICULAR						
Distal femur	35	20 (57%)	8 (23%)	3 (9%)	4 (11%)	3 (9%)
Proximal tibia	21	11 (52%)	6 (29%)	3 (14%)	1 (5%)	2 (10%)
Proximal humerus	15	1 (7%)	10 (67%)	1 (7%)	3 (20%)	3 (20%)
Distal radius	12	5 (42%)	2 (17%)	2 (17%)	3 (25%)	1 (8%)
Hemipelvis	9	2 (22%)	1 (11%)	1 (11%)	5 (56%)	4 (44%)
Proximal femur	4	0 (0%)	1 (25%)	2 (50%)	1 (25%)	0 (0%)
Distal humerus	3	0 (0%)	1 (33%)	1 (33%)	1 (33%)	0 (0%)
Proximal ulna	3	2 (67%)	0 (0%)	0 (0%)	1 (33%)	0 (0%)
Distal tibia	1	1 (100%)	0 (0%)	0 (0%)	0 (0%)	0 (0%)
Total	103	42 (41%)	29 (28%)	13 (13%)	19 (18%)	13 (13%)
INTERCALARY						
Tibia	12	9 (75%)	1 (8%)	1 (8%)	1 (8%)	0 (0%)
Femur	8	7 (88%)	0 (0%)	0 (0%)	1 (12%)	1 (12%)
Humerus	7	6 (86%)	0 (0%)	1 (14%)	0 (0%)	0 (0%)
Hemipelvis	1	0 (0%)	0 (0%)	0 (0%)	1 (0%)	1 (100%)
Ulna	1	1 (100%)	0 (0%)	0 (0%)	0 (0%)	0 (0%)
Total	29	23 (79%)	1 (3%)	2 (7%)	3 (10%)	2 (7%)
ALLOGRAFT + PROSTHESIS						
Proximal femur and Austin-Moore	5	4 (80%)	1 (20%)	0 (0%)	0 (0%)	0 (0%)
Proximal femur and total hip replacement	2	2 (100%)	0 (0%)	0 (0%)	0 (0%)	0 (0%)
Hemipelvis and total hip replacement	2	0 (0%)	0 (0%)	0 (0%)	2 (100%)	0 (0%)
Hemipelvis and Austin-Moore	1	0 (0%)	0 (0%)	1 (100%)	0 (0%)	1 (100%)
Total	10	6 (60%)	1 (10%)	1 (10%)	2 (20%)	1 (10%)
ALLOGRAFT-ARTHRODESIS						
Distal femur-proximal tibia	1	0 (0%)	1 (100%)	0 (0%)	0 (0%)	0 (0%)
Total for series	143	71 (50%)	32 (22%)	16 (11%)	24 (17%)	16 (11%)
If 16 tumor failures are deleted						
Total	127	69 (54%)	31 (24%)	13 (10%)	14 (11%)	

for the series would have been 77% (with a tumor failure rate of only 8%). For the group in which the tumor failures were deleted, the success rate would have risen to 82%. Of equal interest are the findings in Table 46-5, comparing the results for hemiosteoarticular grafts with those of the "totals," in which the entire joint surface covering the end of a long bone was included with the transplant. These data show that the hemigrafts had a significantly increased success rate and a markedly reduced complication rate as compared with the more extensive operation. Part of the explanation for this rests in the extent of the surgery and in the stage of the lesions treated (hemigrafts are obviously inappropriate in the treatment of Stage 2 lesions). It is also obvious that the graft is more likely to be vascularized rapidly when opposed to a broad corticocancellous metaphyseal surface than when the host–donor junction lies transverse in the narrow cortical diaphysis (Fig. 46-2).

As indicated above, it is also important to consider the diagnosis for which the patient was treated. The success rate (excellent and good results) for benign lesions (including nontumorous conditions) was 86% in 22 patients so categorized, the value for 102 patients with low-grade tumors was 75%, and that for the 19 patients with high-grade lesions (Stage 2A, 2B, or 3) fell to 37%. It is significant in considering these values that of 16 tumor failures, only five occurred in the 102 patients with low-grade lesions (6%), while the remaining 11 occurred in the 19 patients with high-grade lesions (58%).

COMPLICATIONS

As indicated above, wide or marginal resection of an aggressive or malignant tumor of bone is generally a formidable operative procedure, often resulting in extensive loss of bone, muscle, ligamentous and tendinous structures, and skin, and frequently requiring from 3 to 6 hours of surgery and considerable blood loss. The incisions are long and sometimes rather complicated, based on the requirement for most tumors that the tract of the prior biopsy be excised in continuity with the specimen. If part of a joint is resected with the specimen, the synovial tissues and joint stabilizers must also be sectioned, and to resect some tumors it may be necessary to transect major vascular channels and nerves, increasing both the extent of the surgery and the complexity of the repair. Once the tumor has been removed from the wound, the surgeon performing allograft replacement surgery (or for that matter, any other reconstructive procedure) must now face the equally demanding task of fitting, shaping, and internally fixing the graft to the host bone and restoring the continuity of divided musculotendinous and ligamentous structures.

It would be ideal in a study designed to define the complications encountered in allotransplantation of massive segments of bone to be able to distinguish clearly those complications attributable to the tumor resection from those associated with the allograft resection. Unfortunately, as will be seen below, this is not always possible. In fact, the technical demands of resection

Table 46-5. Comparison of Results of "Hemi" and "Total" Allografts About the Knee

Location	No. of Patients	Excellent	Good	Fair	Failure
Distal femur					
"Total"	16	4 (25%)	6 (38%)	2 (13%)	4 (25%)
"Hemi"	19	16 (84%)	2 (11%)	1 (5%)	
Proximal tibia					
"Total"	9	5 (56%)	1 (11%)	2 (22%)	1 (11%)
"Hemi"	12	6 (50%)	5 (42%)		1 (8%)

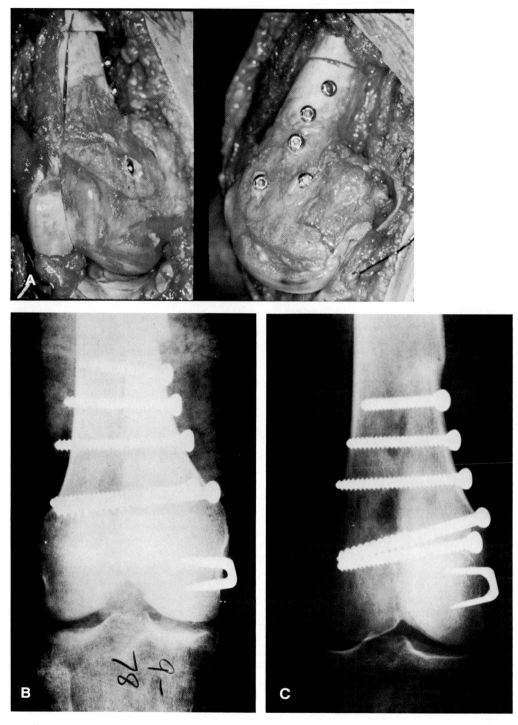

FIG. 46-2. Rapid healing of a broad metaphyseal allograft surface. (*A*) Intraoperative view of a distal femoral hemiallograft. (*B*) Immediate postoperative appearance. (*C*) Appearance at 1 year. (*D*) Appearance at 2 years. There is almost complete healing throughout the osteosynthesis site.

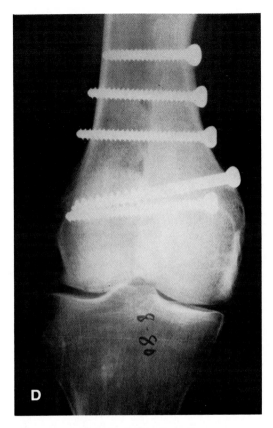

FIG. 46-2. (*Continued*)

history of the alloimplant and to demonstrate methods of improving the technique.

EARLY

The major early complications associated with the 143 surgical procedures described in this series are shown in Table 46-6. There were no operative deaths in the series, and there have been none to date. One patient suffered a cardiac arrest early in the course of a resection. Following resuscitation, the wound was rapidly closed and the procedure performed successfully 1 week later. This patient ultimately developed a deep wound infection and subsequently required an amputation. Five of the patients suffered massive hemorrhages, either at the time of surgery or in the immediate postoperative period. We do not use a tourniquet during our tumor resections (for the almost theoretical reason of limiting the likelihood of clumping of the tumor cells at the tourniquet margin and thus decreasing the size and presumed "viability" of micrometastases to the lungs as a result of intraoperative tumor manipulation), so that particularly with the larger resections, hemorrhage for 4 to 8 units is not uncommon. In the patients included in Table 46-6, the blood loss far exceeded these values

surgery, the sometimes poorly vascularized, muscle-deficient bed into which the graft is inserted, and the occasional need for preoperative or postoperative radiation or adjuvant chemotherapy all conspire to make the system a "worst case" for the allograft part, not only in terms of potential for healing and subsequent incorporation by the host system, but also with regard to the problems of rehabilitation and restoration of function. Ample testimony to this statement is offered by the data in Table 46-5 and in the analysis of the effect of malignancy of the tumor on end-result, described above. Both support the concept that the more complex the surgery, the more likely the graft system is to fail. Nevertheless, we have made an attempt to separate and explore the complications associated with the allograft implant, since in theory (and in practice), such an approach is likely to yield important information on the natural

Table 46-6. Early Complications of Allograft Transplantation in 143 Patients Followed for 2 or More Years*

COMPLICATION	NO. OF CASES
Death	0
Cardiac arrest	1
Wound hemorrhage	6
Arterial laceration	5
Nerve palsy (transient)	4
Nerve palsy (permanent)	3
Skin slough	9
Hepatitis	4
Cytomegalovirus infection	1
Deep venous thrombosis	5
Pulmonary embolism	1

* In interpreting these data, it is important to note that some of the patients had more than one complication, so the values are not additive.

and in one case required reoperation to ligate the profunda femoris vessel to control bleeding. In four patients (including one platelet-deficient patient with Gaucher's disease who required transfusions with HL-A matched platelets) the blood loss slowly diminished with correction of clotting factors, and in one, transarterial angiographic embolization was successful in clotting two small bleeding points. The largest blood loss encountered in the series (52 units) occurred in a 63-year-old obese woman undergoing a hemiplevic resection and implantation of an allograft + prosthesis (THR) for a Stage 2B chondrosarcoma. Two angiographic studies failed to demonstrate the bleeding site(s). Following cessation of the bleeding, the patient developed a massive deep hematoma, skin slough and wound infection, eventually requiring resection of the graft.

In five patients, inadvertent laceration of a major arterial trunk occurred in the course of tumor resection (in contradistinction to several patients in the series in whom the surgical plan included resection of the vessel in continuity with the tumor followed by saphenous vein reconstruction). In each case the vessel was identified, isolated, and repaired, usually with an interposed vein segment. Three of these five patients developed additional complications, one with a nerve palsy and deep wound infection, one with a skin slough and wound infection, and another with subsequent pulmonary metastases.

Four of the 143 patients developed transient nerve palsies, two peroneal, one radial, and one femoral. All recovered in a relatively short period and left no sequelae. In addition to patients in whom the nerves were sacrificed as part of the resection (one sciatic, one ulnar, and one radial), three patients with pelvic surgery had inadvertent injury to the roots or trunks that constitute the sciatic nerve and subsequently developed permanent palsies. None were complete or grossly disabling, though one patient required a posterior tibial transfer to compensate for a drop foot and has since done well.

Skin problems are very serious in patients in whom allografts have been implanted, chiefly because the nonviable graft has no defenses against infection and is useless as a bed for skin grafting. In early cases we were less concerned about skin coverage but soon learned that a skin slough is a disaster of major proportions. In this series of 143 cases there were nine skin sloughs, and in seven of these a deep wound infection occurred. The results for this group of patients are dismal, with six of the nine patients either losing their grafts or requiring amputations. Since this early experience we have gone to great lengths to achieve good muscle coverage of the graft (by transposing muscles on vascular pedicles if needed). Poor skin coverage is also treated by appropriate flap and grafting techniques when required.

Four of our patients developed hepatitis and one a cytomegalovirus infection. Given the age and activities of the patients and the number of blood transfusions they received, this hardly seems excessive for 143 operative procedures. None of the infections were severe, and all of the patients recovered without sequelae. There remains, however, a nagging concern that the viruses may have been transmitted not by the usual routes, but by the graft. There is certainly no way to prove or disprove this theory, but it is of such importance that our bank diligently seeks to obtain a history of such illnesses from the donor's past medical records and family. If it is suspected, or if the serologic studies are positive, we disqualify the bones from use.

All of our patients are anticoagulated with appropriate regimens in the postoperative period, and very few have developed clinical evidence of deep vein thrombosis. Our current policy is to use low-dose warfarin sodium (Coumadin) in the postoperative period (with the prothrombin time maintained at approximately 60%) for women and patients at high risk, and aspirin for men. Five of our patients developed unequivocal clinical evidence of deep vein thromboses and one a small pulmonary embolus. There were no sequelae of these problems in the series.

LATE

Table 46-7 lists the late complications encountered in the 143 patients included

Table 46-7. Late Complications of Allograft Transplantation in 143 Patients Followed for 2 or More Years*

COMPLICATION	NO. OF CASES
Tumor failure (recurrence or metastases)	16 (11%)
Deep infection	19 (13%)
Allograft fracture	16 (11%)
Delayed union or nonunion	10 (7%)
Joint instability	5 (3%)

* In interpreting these data, it is important to note that some of these patients had more than one complication, so the values shown are not additive.

in the series. The major complications encountered in the series were tumor failure (recurrence or metastasis), deep wound infection, allograft fracture, delayed union or nonunion at the host–donor graft junction, and joint instability. As noted in the footnote to the table, some of the patients had more than one complication, so the values displayed cannot be added to obtain a total figure for the series. In fact, 87 of the 143 patients (61%) had no late problems, and the 66 complications cited in the table occurred in 53 patients (37% of the total).

Tumor Failure

Data for the 16 patients with tumor failure are shown in Table 46-8. As can be seen, five of the patients developed a local recurrence of their tumor, four had both recurrence and metastases, and the remaining seven developed pulmonary metastases. Seven of the patients are dead, two are alive with disease, and the remaining seven are without current evidence of tumor (NED). As far as the success of the operative procedure is concerned, three are rated excellent or good, three are fair, and the remaining ten were considered to represent failures.

Although tumor failure occurred in 16 of the 143 patients (11%), as indicated above, this is not an accurate reflection of the "safety" and efficacy of the operative procedures for several reasons. First, it should be noted that 22 of the patients had either benign tumors or nontumorous lesions, so

only 121 of the patients were at risk for this complication (increasing the true tumor failure rate to 13%). The overall failure rate (5%) for the low-grade lesions (mostly giant cell tumors, 4%; low-grade chondrosarcomas, 5%; and parosteal osteosarcomas, 13%) is generally quite acceptable and compares favorably with other series. In fact, 11 of the 16 tumor failures occurred in the 19 patients in the series with high-grade sarcomas or metastatic carcinomas, with the failure rate for this group at 58%. It should be noted, however, that four of the tumor failures occurred in the group of five patients with metastatic carcinoma. If one discounts this group as being at very high risk (and, in fact, out of the control of the treatment protocol), the risk of failure for the 14 patients with Stage 2A and 2B lesions declines to the more respectable value of 50%, which is consistent with our results for high-grade sarcomas treated by other means. Since the number of patients with pelvic sarcomas is quite high in this group, the values are actually considerably lower than in our larger series treated by amputation. However, since the indications for surgery may have differed, the comparison is not valid.

One final note of caution is required in the interpretation. Although some of the patients have been followed for a long period, the cut-off for entry into the series is 2 years, and the mean length of follow-up is 42 months. For some of the lesions included (such as adamantinoma, parosteal osteosarcoma, chondrosarcoma, and even giant cell tumor), late recurrences and/or metastases are reported, and it would therefore be appropriate to consider the results defined in this series as preliminary. With that caveat, and on the basis of the discussion and statistics provided in the foregoing section, we have concluded that the procedure as described is far safer and more efficacious in the management of low-grade tumors than are intralesional procedures, and it is essentially equivalent to wide amputation or other appropriate resective procedures for high-grade tumors.

Deep Wound Infections

The most serious and prevalent of the nontumor-related complications is deep

Table 46-8. Status of 16 Tumor Failures in 143 Patients (11%) Followed for 2 or More Years After Allograft Transplantation

CASE NO.	AGE	SEX	DIAGNOSIS	STAGE	DATE OF SURGERY	PROCEDURE (TYPE)	TYPE OF FAILURE	TIME TO FAILURE (MO)	TREATMENT	PATIENT STATUS	CURRENT GRAFT STATUS
4	63	M	Metastatic CA (unknown)	3	10/73	Proximal humerus (OA)	Metastases	16	Chemotherapy	Dead	
15	38	F	Chondrosarcoma (Ollier's)	2B	5/75	Proximal humerus (OA)	Recurrence/ metastases	29	Chemotherapy/ radiation	Dead	
21	19	F	Osteosarcoma	2B	3/76	Distal femur (OA)	Metastases	8	Chemotherapy	Dead	
24	21	F	Giant cell tumor	1B	6/76	Proximal tibia (OA)	Recurrence	18	Resection/radiation	NED	Fair
43	28	M	Parosteal osteosarcoma	1B	8/77	Distal femur (OA)	Recurrence	72	Resection	NED	Fair
44	25	F	Fibrosarcoma	1B	8/77	Distal radius (OA)	Recurrence	12	Amputation	NED	Failure
53	18	M	Giant cell tumor	1A	6/78	"Hemi," proximal tibia (OA)	Recurrence/ metastases	36	Resection/allograft/ chest surgery	NED	Good
54	54	F	Metastatic CA (thyroid)	3	6/78	Proximal femur (AP)	Metastasis	2	Radiation/resection/ chemotherapy	Alive with disease	Excellent
72	69	F	Metastatic CA (kidney)	3	8/79	Hemipelvis (IC)	Metastasis	12	Resection/radiation	NED	Failure
75	18	M	Ewing's sarcoma	2B	10/79	Hemipelvis (OA)	Metastasis	6	Radiation/ chemotherapy	Dead	
77	17	M	Osteosarcoma	2B	10/79	Hemipelvis (OA)	Metastasis	7	Radiation/ chemotherapy	Dead	
84	40	F	Fibrosarcoma	2B	4/80	Hemipelvis (OA)	Metastasis	8	Radiation/ chemotherapy	Dead	
85	30	M	Chondrosarcoma	1B	5/80	Distal femur (IC)	Recurrence	36	Resection/allograft	NED	Excellent
96	58	F	Metastatic CA (thyroid)	3	12/80	Hemipelvis (OA)	Recurrence/ metastasis	12	Resection/radiation chemotherapy	Dead	
119	59	F	Chondrosarcoma	2B	9/81	Hemipelvis (AP)	Recurrence/ metastasis	12	Radiation/ chemotherapy	Alive with disease	Fair
138	31	M	Chondrosarcoma	2B	3/82	Proximal humerus (OA)	Recurrence	12	Amputation	NED	Failure

wound infection, which occurred in 19 of the 143 patients in the series (13%). Table 46-9 shows the data for this group of patients and clearly demonstrates some of the major problems encountered in this unfortunate group. In considering the high rate of this problem in our patients, it should first be pointed out that the value of the procedure stands out in striking contrast to the low overall infection rate at MGH for clean, non-tumor orthopaedic cases (<1%) and, in fact, for the surgery of tumors managed by more conservative measures (approximately 5%). A careful analysis of the cases shown demonstrates some important mitigating factors that are, at least in part, unrelated to the graft. Seven of the patients had skin sloughs, and in one a loop of large bowel was perforated by the rough margin of an intercalary hemipelvic allograft. Three of the patients received adjuvant chemotherapy and presumably at times had significant periods of profound leukopenia. In three patients the infection was manifested only at the time of or subsequent to reoperation for nonunion of the host–donor junction. In one patient treated very early in the series (before we had established adequate bacteriologic controls for the bank), the donor heart blood was found to contain a *Pseudomonas* species that subsequently appeared in the graft site 2 months following the surgical procedure. In fact, only seven of the 19 wound infections occurred without some apparent underlying cause, and if the one "uncomplicated" reoperation for nonunion (case #29) is added, the infection rate is 8/132 (6%). Even this value is too high, however, and the bacteriologic data suggest the possibility that some of these late-appearing infections with low-grade organisms may be consistent with immunologic "rejection."

All of the deep wound infections occurred within the first 2 years, and almost all were encountered by 6 months. The nature of the original lesion treated is of some consequence. The infection rate for Stage 2A, 2B, and 3 tumors is 26%, for Stage 1A and 1B tumors 13%, and for benign conditions 5%. A disproportionately high number occurred in high-grade lesions (five), but only one occurred in a patient with a benign

lesion. Furthermore, only one of the osteoarticular hemiallografts showed this complication. All of these data support the concept that the infection rate is highest in patients undergoing more radical surgery and lowest in those in whom the least amount of normal tissue is sacrificed.

Of perhaps greatest consequence is the effect that deep wound infection has on the patient's course and outcome. There is little doubt that an infected allograft represents an unmitigated disaster, and this impression is strongly borne out by the data, which demonstrate that 47% of this group of patients were classified as failures, and only 5 of 19 (26%) ultimately achieved excellent or good results.

The treatment of deep wound infection in patients with allografts is complicated. There appears to be little value in incision and drainage or standard wound debridement with appropriate antibiotic coverage, as are advocated for the usual postoperative wound infections occurring in viable tissue. Free or pedicle-based vascularized myocutaneous flaps are indicated for some wounds in which a skin defect overlies a "clean" graft. The most efficacious system, however, is the one used in six of our patients, in which the graft is resected, the limb maintained at length in an external fixator (or by a hanging cast, for a proximal humeral allograft infection) for 6 weeks to 6 months while the patient receives antibiotics, the soft tissue bed sterilized, and then a new allograft inserted (Fig. 46-3). Using this system, we have been able to "salvage" five of the six patients, and thus far, all but one of this group remain free of infection, with functional grafts.

Allograft Fracture

Sixteen of the 143 patients (11%) developed a fracture of the allograft segment. In addition, there were two patients in whom the host bone fractured (both healed uneventfully with immobilization in a plaster cast). The data for this group are shown in Table 46-10. As can be readily noted, the fractures occurred considerably later in the course than did tumor recurrence, metastasis, or deep wound infection. Two of these occurred as a result of significant trauma. Patient #13 fell from a window on

(*Text continues on page 1405.*)

Table 46-9. Status of 19 Patients (11%) With Deep Wound Infections From 143 Patients Followed for 2 or More Years After Allograft Transplantation

Case No.	Age	Sex	Diagnosis	Stage	Date of Surgery	Procedure (Type)	Time of Appearance of Infection (Mo)	Organisms Recovered	Surgical Treatment	Current Graft Status	Remarks
7	22	M	Giant cell tumor	1A	3/74	Distal femur (OA)	1	Staphylococcus aureus	Repeated debridements, amputation	Failure	Cardiac arrest during surgery
12	25	F	Chondrosarcoma	1B	9/74	Proximal humerus (OA)	2	Pseudomonas sp.	Repeated debridements, resection of graft, repeat allograft	Fair	Infected allograft
23	43	F	Malignant fibrous histiocytoma	2B	4/76	Proximal ulna (OA)	7	Escherichia coli, Pseudomonas	Repeated debridements, resection of graft	Failure	Skin slough, chemotherapy
27	18	F	Osteosarcoma	2B	7/76	Distal femur (OA)	1	E. coli, S. aureus	Repeated debridements, skin grafts, amputation	Failure	Arterial laceration, skin slough, chemotherapy
28	39	F	Giant cell tumor	1A	8/76	Distal femur (OA)	1	S. epidermidis	Debridement, resection of graft, reallograft, amputation	Failure	
29	28	F	Giant cell tumor	1B	1/77	Distal femur (OA)	10	S. epidermidis	Debridement	Good, periodic drainage	Reoperation for nonunion
38	25	M	Giant cell tumor	1B	6/77	Proximal tibia (OA)	6	S. epidermidis	Debridement	Good	Skin slough, reoperation for nonunion
45	17	M	Chondrosarcoma	1B	10/77	Hemipelvis and total hip replacement (AP)	11	Multiple-grain organisms	Repeated debridements, graft resected	Failure	Massive hemorrhage, skin slough
59	56	F	Adamantinoma	1B	11/78	Tibial shaft (IC)	42	Alpha Streptococcus	Incision and drainage	Fair	Infection developed 5 months after grafting for nonunion.

Case	Age	Sex	Diagnosis	Stage	Date	Location	No.	Organism	Treatment	Result	Complications
66	63	F	Chondrosarcoma	2B	6/79	Hemipelvis and total hip replacement (AP)	1	*Enterococcus, Proteus, Pseudomonas*	Drainage, resection of graft	Failure	Skin slough
67	19	M	Malignant osteoblastoma	1B	6/79	Hemipelvis (OA)	3	*Bacteroides*	Drainage, skin grafting, resection of graft	Failure	Skin slough, chemotherapy
70	15	M	Adamantinoma	1B	7/79	Tibial shaft (IC)	3	*Staphylococcus*	Repeated incision and debridement, removal of hardware	Good	
72	69	F	Metastatic carcinoma	3	8/78	Hemipelvis (IC)	3	*Enterobacter*	Resection of graft	Failure	Segment of graft perforated colon
81	36	F	Parosteal osteosarcoma	1B	2/80	Tibial shaft (IC)	2	*Proteus*	Repeated incision and debridement, amputation	Failure	Skin slough
101	30	F	Giant cell tumor	1B	7/81	Proximal humerus (OA)	1	Beta *Streptococcus, Proteus, Bacteroides*	Repeated incision and debridement, resection of graft, reallografting	Good	
110	26	F	Parosteal osteosarcoma	1B	4/81	Distal humerus (OA)	2	*Staphylococcus epidermidis*	Repeated incision and debridement, resection of graft, reallografting	Good	
112	15	F	Chondroblastoma	0	5/81	Proximal tibia (OA)	5	*Staphylococcus epidermidis*	Repeated incision and debridement, antibiotics, resection, reallografting	Too soon to judge	
120	52	F	Myeloma	3	9/81	Proximal femur (OA)	20	*Staphylococcus epidermidis*	Debridement	Too soon to judge	Infection developed 2 months after reoperation for nonunion.
140	21	F	Giant cell tumor	1A	4/82	Proximal tibia ("hemi") (OA)	3	*Enterobacter, enterococcus*	Debridements, resection of graft, reallografting	Too soon to judge	

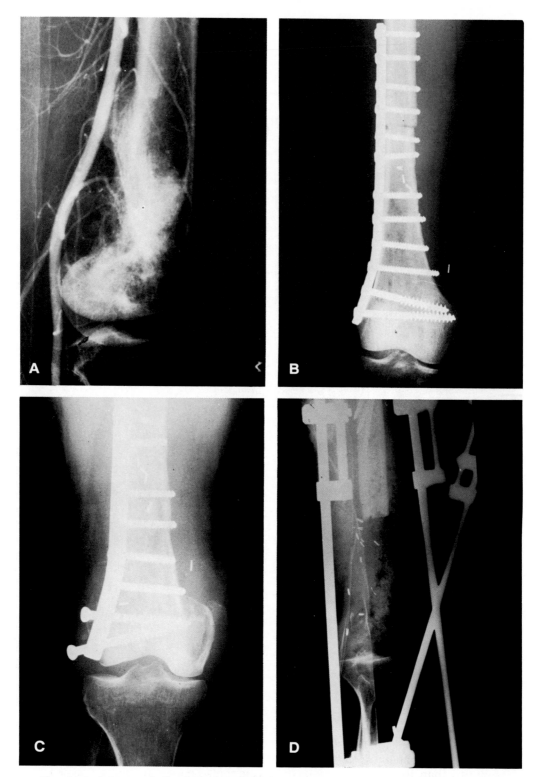

FIG. 46-3. Salvage of allograft infection. (A) Distal femur resected for fibrosarcoma. (B) Appearance immediately following allograft replacement of the distal femur. (C) By 9 months the graft has collapsed, and aspiration of the knee is positive for *Staphylococcus aureus*. (D) Appearance following removal of the graft and hardware with the limb in an external fixator. (E) Three months later, a new graft segment was inserted. It has functioned well over a 2-year follow-up, when this film was taken.

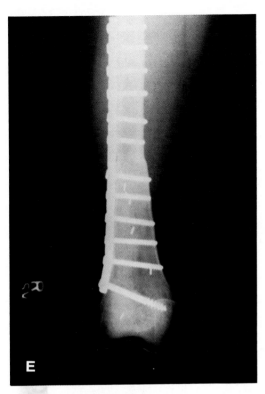

FIG. 46-3. (*Continued*)

his outstretched right hand at 111 months following successful allograft transplantation of the distal radius for a giant cell tumor. Patient #50 struck her right wrist violently against a dashboard during an automobile accident that occurred 36 months after implantation of a distal radial allograft. If these two cases are excluded, the incidence of fractures is reduced to 10%, and the mean time of occurrence is 23 months, with a range of 7 to 42 months. More than 50% of the fractures occurred in the first 2 years after surgery and all but two by 3 years. In rather sharp contrast to the data for tumor failures and infection, none of the patients in this group were treated for high-grade lesions.

The fractures were generally one of two types. The first form, joint fragmentation, occurred in five patients somewhat later (31 months) than the mean for the series. The cases were equally distributed among the sites, with two occurring in the distal femur and one each in the proximal tibia, distal radius, and distal humerus (Fig. 46-4). One of these occurred in a 31-year-old

man with uncontrolled diabetes and severe peripheral neuropathy and probably, in part at least, represents a Charcot's arthropathy. The second type of fracture was in the shaft and was either transverse or through the screw holes of the fixation device. The eleven patients who showed this complication included the two who were injured late in their course, and if these are discounted, the mean time to fracture (21 months) is considerably shorter than that for joint fragmentation group. In contrast with fragmentation, this type of fracture seems to be most prevalent in the proximal humerus (three of nine); given that proximal humeral grafts accounted for only 10% of the total series, this would seem to be inordinately high for this graft segment. The remainder of the nine fractures were distributed more proportionally, with two in the tibial shaft and one each in the distal femur, distal radius, hemipelvis, and proximal femur. One of the patients with a distal radial transplant for a giant cell tumor showed an extraordinarily rapid disintegration of the graft, presumably immunologically directed, at 8 months following the surgery (Fig. 46-5). Only one other patient, classified as a nonunion (see below) showed a similar pattern of rapid dissolution.

The fate of the patients who sustained fractures of their allografts is shown in Table 46-11. Excluding one case, that is too soon after treatment to evaluate, but including the two patients who sustained major trauma to their wrists, six of 15 (40%) were graded as excellent or good, six (40%) as fair, and three (20%) as failures. It is apparent from these data that allograft fracture significantly affects the outcome of the procedure but does not carry as grim a prognosis as either tumor failure or deep wound infection.

The treatment of allograft fracture varies considerably, depending on the type of injury sustained. For joint fragmentation we have successfully introduced conventional total joint replacement components in three of the five patients, and to date, these are holding up well. Of some interest is the absence of a radiolucent line at the cement–bone interface (in both these and other patients in whom the devices were implanted as a primary procedure), suggesting that in the absence of the cellular

Table 46-10. Status of 16 Patients (11%) With Allograft Fractures From 143 Patients Followed for 2 or More Years After Allograft Transplantation

CASE NO.	AGE	SEX	DIAGNOSIS	STAGE	DATE OF SURGERY	PROCEDURE (TYPE)	TIME OF APPEARANCE OF FRACTURE (MO)	TYPE OF FRACTURE	COURSE AND TREATMENT	REMARKS	CURRENT STATUS OF ORIGINAL IMPLANT
8	22	M	Giant cell tumor	1A	3/74	Distal radius (OA)	24	Joint fragmentation	Wrist replacement arthroplasty		Good
11	19	M	Multicentric giant cell tumor	1B	3/74	Distal femur (OA)	36	Joint fragmentation	Total knee replacement		Fair
13	23	M	Giant cell tumor	1B	9/74	Distal radius (OA)	111	Transverse fracture	Resection of graft and arthrodesis of the wrist	Fall from height	Failure
16	17	F	Giant cell tumor	1B	10/75	Distal humerus (OA)	15	Joint fragmentation (freeze-dried graft)	Resection and replacement with frozen graft	Healed	Fair
31	31	M	Pigmented villonodular synovitis	0A	1/77	Proximal tibia (OA)	36	Joint fragmentation	Brace	Diabetic neuropathy	Fair
33	29	M	Parosteal osteosarcoma	1B	3/77	Proximal humerus (OA)	17	Coronal-plane screw-hole	ORIF with autograft	Healed	Good
39	24	M	Giant cell tumor	1B	6/77	Proximal humerus (OA)	18	Anatomical neck	ORIF with autograft	Healed	Good
43	28	M	Parosteal osteosarcoma	1B	8/77	Distal femur (OA)	7	Coronal-plane screw-hole	ORIF with autograft, vascularized fibular autograft	Healed	Fair
42	28	F	Giant cell tumor	1A	7/77	Distal femur (OA)	42	Joint fragmentation	Total knee replacement		Good
50	34	F	Giant cell tumor	1B	2/78	Distal radius (OA)	38	Transverse fracture of graft	ORIF with autograft and arthrodesis of wrist	Auto accident	Fair

59	56	F	Adamantinoma	11/78	Mid-tibia (IC)	1B	34	Transverse fracture of graft	ORIF with autograft	Healed	Fair
76	18	F	Giant cell tumor	10/79	Hemipelvis (OA)	1B	21	Acetabular and femoral head fractures	Total hip replacement—poor result		Failure
78	20	M	Adamantinoma	11/79	Mid-tibia (IC)	1B	13	Transverse fracture of graft	ORIF with autograft	Healed	Excellent
83	48	F	Chondrosarcoma	4/80	Proximal humerus (OA)	1B	20	Surgical neck	Neer prosthesis		Good
91	22	M	Giant cell tumor	9/80	Proximal femur (OA)	1B	35	Femoral neck	ORIF with autograft		Too soon to judge
115	32	M	Giant cell tumor	6/81	Distal radius (OA)	1B	8	Disintegration of graft	Resection and arthrodesis with iliac graft	Solid arthrodesis	Failure

ORIF, open reduction and internal fixation.

mechanisms presumed, at least in part, responsible for loosening, these joints may hold up even better than those in living bone. In one of these patients, the fragmented freeze-dried distal humeral segment (obtained because none of the right size were available in our bank) was replaced at 15 months by a fresh frozen segment that has functioned well for an additional 7.5 years. The remaining patient, with diabetic arthropathy, has been treated with a long leg brace and remains disabled, but the fractured part has showed no increased disintegration in 3 years.

For nine of the 11 patients with shaft fractures the treatment has been open reduction, replacement of the hardware, and addition of copious quantities of iliac crest autograft. Outcome for one of these patients is too soon to evaluate, but in the remaining eight, this technique has resulted in healing of the fracture in six (75%). In one, a patient with a distal radial fracture, the procedure failed, and the graft was resected and replaced by a full-thickness iliac crest autograft that was fused to the wrist. In another, the nonunion of the fracture through the distal femoral allograft persisted, and a vascularized fibular autograft was implanted, resulting in prompt healing (Fig. 46-6). The two remaining patients in this group were one with a proximal humeral fracture treated with insertion of a Neer endoprosthesis and the patient with the distal radial segment that had disintegrated, in whom the graft was resected and replaced with an autogenous iliac crest segment fused to the carpus. Both of these procedures have been successful in restoring continuity to the extremity.

Nonunion or Delayed Union at the Host–Donor Junction

Only 10 (7%) of the 143 patients in the series exhibited nonunion or delayed union, and in general, it was the easiest to deal with and yielded the best long-term results. Two of the patients had their surgery too recently to evaluate, but of the remaining eight, six are classified as good, one excellent, and one a failure (see Table 46-11). In the final evaluation of this group, the overall success rate is 88%, even higher than the mean value for the entire series. All of

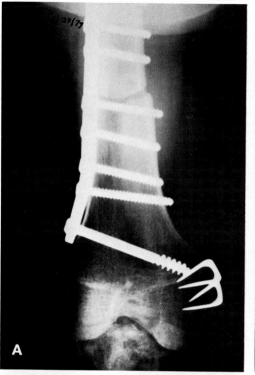

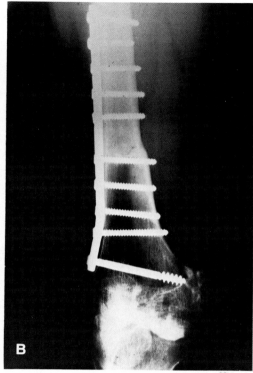

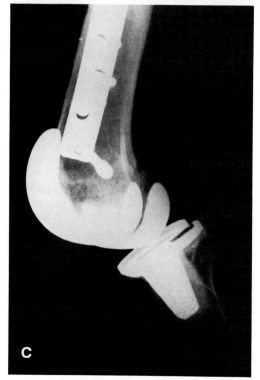

FIG. 46-4. Salvage of a fragmented allograft with total joint resurfacing. (*A*) Appearance 3 months following resection of the distal femur and replacement with an allograft segment. The bone has not healed at the anastomotic site. The joint space is preserved, and function is good. (*B*) Four years later, the anastomosis is well healed but fragmentation of the articular end of the graft has resulted in poor function. (*C*) Excellent function resulted from joint resurfacing.

these patients were treated at approximately 1 year after surgery with reapplication of plates and screws and insertion of autograft bone obtained from the iliac crest (Fig. 46-7). The failed case was a 31-year-old woman in whom the distal humerus and proximal ulna were replaced for a giant cell tumor that arose in the humerus and invaded the olecranon. The articulated allograft segment healed well at the humeral side but failed to unite on the ulnar side despite two separate procedures in which autograft was inserted. The segment was so badly disintegrated as a result of multiple placements of the hardware that it was finally resected, leaving the patient with a flail elbow that is satisfactorily controlled with a brace.

In considering the possible implications of the immune reaction to the alloimplant, it would seem logical to consider those patients in whom the graft was either slow or failed to unite to the host bone at high risk for failure of the system on the basis of "rejection" of the graft. The data do not support this contention, but the numbers are small and require further correlative study of the healing rate (*i.e.*, when the host–donor junction was obliterated on serial radiographs) with other factors for final judgment. In addition, it should be pointed out that none of the hemigrafts showed delayed union or nonunion and that we have a strong impression that when we obtain good compression of two closely apposed congruent surfaces, the rate of healing is far faster than when a gap remains.

Joint Instability

Only five patients showed significant joint instability. Not all of the patients in the series are at risk for this complication, and, in fact, only the osteoarticular and allograft + prosthesis groups involve articular surfaces (and the risk for the latter group is sharply reduced owing to constraints imposed by the geometry of the prosthesis). Thus the actual rate for this complication is greater than that shown in Table 46-7, and depending on which of the values is chosen for the denominator, falls at either 4% or 5%. In most of the 56 grafts inserted around the knee joint, at least one collateral ligament and a portion of the capsular

structures were sacrificed (for the "hemis"), and for many, all of the ligamentous support, including both cruciates, was lost. Coupled with the loss of quadriceps function associated with resective surgery of large parts of that muscle group and the damage to the menisci, the patients should predictably demonstrate a much greater incidence of this complication than we have observed. Much of the success of this phase of the procedure, however, is predicated on the meticulous repair of the transected ligaments to the ligamentous and capsular structures of the allograft. We do not repair or replace cruciate ligaments about the knee, and although some of our patients show some anteroposterior laxity, their functional deficit is minimal. Repair is based on a very tight "vest-over-pants" repair of the posterior capsule (under direct vision), which for the most part substitutes nicely during standard walking or light exercise. It is doubtful that these repairs would hold up under vigorous exercise or excessive torsional moments, so patients are strongly cautioned against such activities as skiing.

The treatment of ligamentous laxity for the five patients who have manifested this to an excessive degree has been principally bracing or avoidance of stress. Despite the problem, three (60%) are classified as successful procedures.

Of considerable interest is the rather striking fact that few of the patients show changes consistent with osteoarthritis of the joints. None of them, even the group followed for 10 or more years, show radiographic evidence of severe degenerative joint disease, and although many of the patients complain of morning stiffness and decreased mobility, none have as yet required a resurfacing procedure for this problem. We nevertheless anticipate that such a disorder will eventually occur, since the cartilaginous surfaces are unlikely to resist both the immune and degenerative biologic processes, and in many cases the joint surfaces are not congruent.

DISCUSSION

On the basis of the data presented above, there should be little doubt that the allograft transplantation system described in this re-

(*Text continues on page 1412.*)

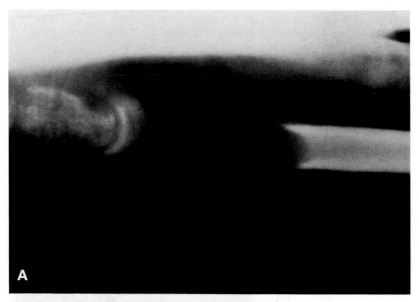

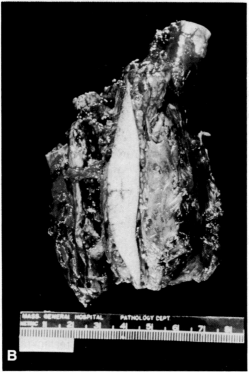

FIG. 46-5. Rapid allograft dissolution salvaged with arthrodesis. (A) Tomogram of the distal radius shows a giant cell tumor. (B) Resection specimen. (C) Appearance following a distal radial allograft. (D) Four months after replacement, the graft is fracturing. (E) By 6 months, total collapse is noted. (F) Salvage was accomplished by iliac crest autograft-arthrodesis.

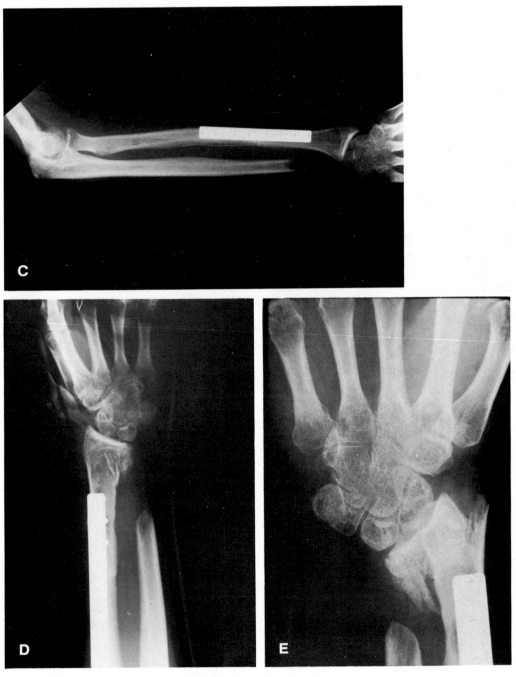

FIG. 46-5. (*Continued*)

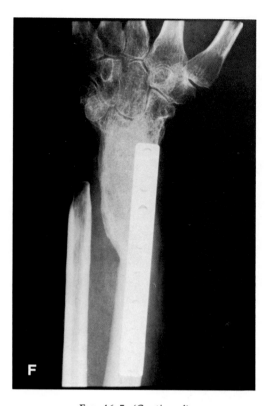

FIG. 46-5. *(Continued)*

view has merit, particularly in dealing with young patients with massive defects in the skeleton created as a result of resection for sarcoma or as a result of major trauma or severe skeletal disease. Despite the rigors of the operative treatment for the majority of the tumor patients in this series, almost three fourths of them (103 of 143) were restored to reasonable function, and in several studies to date,[10,15,16] we have established that their state remains essentially unchanged with time (at least up to the almost 14 years of follow-up of the patients in this series). Furthermore, when the 16-member tumor-failure group is viewed as resulting from a failure of the treatment system to deal with the neoplasm, rather than a fault with the alloimplantation technique, the procedure appears to be successful in almost 80% of the candidates.

Despite these rather glowing estimates of the value of the technique, it is quite apparent that some serious problems remain in the application, and these appear to lie

principally with the complications. Table 46-12 clearly illustrates this point. As can be noted in this table, which compares the results for the 143 patients in the total series with those for 87 patients who showed no complications and for the smaller groups of patients who sustained the five major complications reported in detail in this presentation, there are clear statistical differences in these subsets. What is even more striking is the fact that if the patients display no complications of the procedure, the likelihood of a successful outcome is almost 100%, while the presence of any of the complicating factors sharply reduces this value.

There are several areas of discussion that would seem appropriate in a final review of these data. First is the possibility that all of the "uncomplicated" patients—and, hence, successful results—are the recent ones and that the patient series will deteriorate with time. As is shown in our prior reports and, in fact, can be easily gleaned from study of the tabular description of the complications observed in this series, this is clearly not the case. The most serious complication of all, infection, appears prior to the first year, and fracture, the second most prevalent and serious threat that the patients face, occurs in years two and three (with the major share occurring in the second year). These data strongly suggest that if the patient passes the hurdles of infection in the first year and allograft fracture in the second and third year, the likelihood of a continued successful and functional graft is quite high. We anticipate osteoarthritic changes as a late sequela of the procedure, but to date we have been impressed by the absence of a significant degree of impairment as a result of this problem.

A second issue is whether any of these complications are related to the immune process. Clearly, the tumor failures are not, although it is striking that the local recurrences of the tumor have not been in the graft but in the adjacent bone and soft tissue, suggesting that the tumor tissue, no matter how aggressive, has considerable difficulty maintaining itself in the dead (or just barely viable) graft. Some of the infections, however, may in fact be manifesta-

(Text continues on page 1416.)

Table 46-11. Status of 16 Patients (11%) With Allograft Fractures From 143 Patients Followed for 2 or More Years After Allograft Transplantation

CASE NO.	AGE	SEX	DIAGNOSIS	STAGE	DATE OF SURGERY	PROCEDURE (TYPE)	TREATMENT OF NONUNION	REMARKS	CURRENT STATUS OF ORIGINAL IMPLANT
5	53	M	Chondrosarcoma	1A	2/74	Proximal humerus (OA)	ORIF with autograft		Good
6	32	F	Chondrosarcoma	1B	3/74	Mid-humerus (IC)	ORIF with autograft × 2		Excellent
18	25	F	Giant cell tumor	1B	10/75	Distal femur (OA)	ORIF with autograft	Mild varus deformity	Good
26	15	F	Giant cell tumor	1B	7/76	Distal radius (OA)	ORIF with autograft		Good
29	28	F	Giant cell tumor	1B	1/77	Distal femur (OA)	ORIF with autograft	Postop. wound infection	Good
38	25	M	Giant cell tumor	1B	6/77	Proximal tibia (OA)	ORIF with autograft	Postop. wound infection	Good
68	33	F	Ewing's sarcoma	2B	7/79	Proximal ulna (IC)	ORIF with autograft	Adjunctive chemotherapy	Good
74	31	F	Giant cell tumor	1B	10/79	Distal humerus and proximal ulna (OA)	ORIF with autograft ×2 ulnar resection	Short ulnar segment fragmented	Failure
116	43	F	Chondrosarcoma	1A	7/81	Proximal humerus (IC)	ORIF with autograft ×3	Still recovering from third procedure	?
120	52	F	Myeloma	3	9/81	Proximal femur (OA)	ORIF with autograft	Postop. wound infection	?

ORIF, open reduction and internal fixation

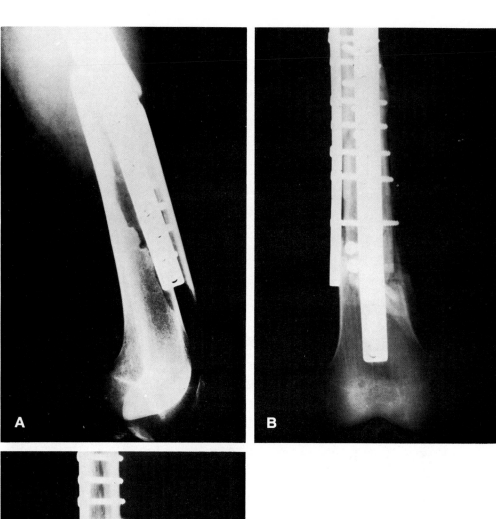

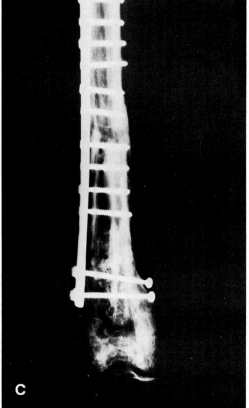

FIG. 46-6. Graft fracture and nonunion treated with a vascularized autograft. (*A*) Seven months after replacement of the distal femur for parosteal osteosarcoma, the allograft has fractured. (*B*) Salvage was attempted with replating of the fracture and addition of an iliac crest autograft. (*C*) Nonunion of the fracture and proximal anastomosis persisted, and 3 years after initial allograft placement, a vascularized fibular graft resulted in healing and good function.

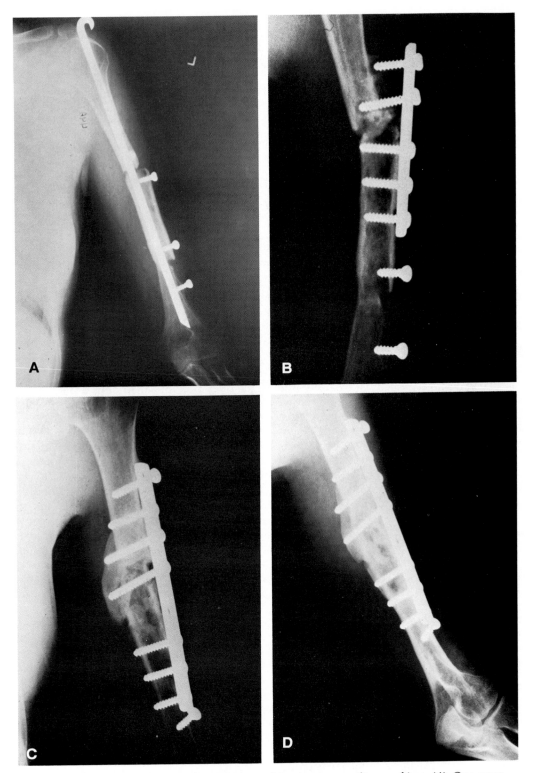

FIG. 46-7. Salvage of allograft nonunion with autogenous iliac grafting. (A) One year following intercalary allograft replacement at the humeral shaft, proximal nonunion is present. (B) One year following bone grafting and compression plating of the proximal anastomosis, the nonunion persists and the plate is loose. (C) A new plate was applied and fresh graft added. (D) One year later and 3 years after initial allograft replacement, excellent union was finally achieved.

**Table 46-12. Effect of Complications on End-Results in 143 Patients
Followed for 2 or More Years After Allograft Transplantation***

RESULT	TOTAL SERIES	PATIENTS WITH NO COMPLICATIONS	TUMOR FAILURE	INFECTION	FRACTURE	NONUNION	INSTABILITY
Excellent or good	103 (72%)	86 (99%)	3 (19%)	5 (26%)	6 (38%)	7 (70%)	3 (60%)
Fair	16 (11%)	0 (0%)	3 (19%)	5 (26%)†	7 (44%)†	2 (20%)†	2 (40%)
Failure	24 (17%)	1 (1%)‡	10 (63%)	9 (47%)	3 (19%)	1 (10%)	0 (0%)
Total	143	87	16	19	16	10	5

* Because some of the patients had two or more complications, the values are not additive.
† Includes three patients with infection, one patient with allograft fracture, and two with nonunions whose treatment has been too recent to judge the end-result
‡ In a patient with Gaucher's disease the proximal femoral allograft remained intact, but the acetabulum disintegrated as a result of pelvic osteonecrosis.

tions of the immune response, perhaps not directly, but as a result of a resistance to vascular invasion (which is basically the best protection against invasion by low-grade pathogens). The graft, like a total joint replacement, may serve as a "locus resistentia minoris" for showers of bacteria associated with infectious processes, and we suggest that patients observe the same safeguards against bacteremic states as should patients with metal and plastic parts.

Fracture is probably in large measure a result of the variable nature of the process of vascular invasion, which surely must be associated with the host's immune response. One can speculate that the earlier-appearing shaft fractures represent "too rapid" replacement with host tissue and that the weakening of the bone is a result of invasion of the bony donor tissue with blood vessels without concomitant new bone formation. This process is similar to the results for autograft implantation reported by Burchardt and associates,[6] although as can be anticipated, the time sequence is somewhat different. The later fractures, which are principally those of joint fragmentation, possibly represent the opposite problem, in which the bone resists vascular invasion by the host and undergoes stress fracture at the sites unprotected by the plates and screws used to retain the allograft.

Similarly, the rate of healing of the host–donor junction should be even a more

definitive function of the host's immune response to the foreign protein of the graft. This does not appear to be the case in our series, possibly because there are so many other variables, mostly related to the surgery and the reconstruction. When the probably inevitable osteoarthritic changes appear, it is likely that these will in part be immune directed, since cartilage is known to be adversely affected by cytotoxic antibodies. However, at this point the problems of congruity and ligamentous stability of the graft appear to be more important in dictating the quality and range of joint motion.

Based on the data reported in this study, it would seem crucial to direct our research and clinical innovation toward eliminating the complications cited above. If the procedure can be rendered free of infection, allograft fracture, nonunion, delayed union, and instability of the transplanted joint, there is good reason to expect that the applications for this technique will broaden, and it will be added to the armamentarium of the orthopaedist as a front-line technique in the management of a wide assortment of skeletal disorders.

REFERENCES

1. Andersson, G.B.J., Gaechter, A., Galante, J.O., and Rostoker, W.: Segmental replacement of long bones in baboons using a fiber titanium implant. J. Bone Joint Surg., 60A:31, 1978.
2. Burrows, H.J., Wilson, J.N., and Scales, J.T.: Exci-

sion of tumours of humerus and femur with restoration by internal prosthesis. J. Bone Joint Surg., 57B:148, 1975.

3. Chao, E.Y., and Ivins, J.C.: Tumour Prosthesis for Bone and Joint Reconstruction. New York, Thieme-Stratton, 1983.

4. Clark, K.: A case of replacement of upper end of the humerus by a fibular graft reviewed after 29 years. J. Bone Joint Surg., 41B:365, 1959.

5. Enneking, W.F.: Musculoskeletal Tumour Surgery. New York, Churchill Livingstone, 1983.

6. Enneking, W.F., Eady, J.L., and Burchardt, H.: Autogenous cortical bone grafts in the reconstruction of segmental skeletal defects. J. Bone Joint Surg., 62A:1039, 1980.

7. Enneking, W.F., and Shirley, P.D.: Resection-arthrodesis for malignant and potentially malignant lesions about the knee using an intermedullary rod and local bone grafts. J. Bone Joint Surg., 59A:223, 1977.

8. Friedlaender, G., and Mankin, H.J.: Guidelines for the banking of musculoskeletal tissues. Newsletter Am. Assoc. Tissue Banks 3:2, 1979.

9. ————: Bone banking: Current methods and suggested guidelines. Instr. Course Lect., 30:36, 1981.

10. Friedlaender, G., Mankin, H.J., and Sell, K.W.: Osteochondral Allografts. Boston, Little, Brown & Co., 1983.

11. Gross, E.E., McKee, N.H., Pritcher, M.P.W., and Langer, F.: Reconstruction of skeletal deficits of the knee. Clin. Orthop., 174:96, 1983.

12. Johnson, J.T.: Reconstruction of the pelvic ring following tumor resection. J. Bone Joint Surg., 60A:747, 1978.

13. Lexer, E.: Joint transplantation and arthroplasty. Surg. Gynecol. Obstet., 40:782, 1925.

14. ————: Die Verwendung Der Freien Knochenplastic Nebst Versuchen Über Gelenkversteifung und Gelenk-transplantation. Arch. Klin. Chir., 86:939, 1980.

15. Mankin, H.J., Doppelt, S.H., Sullivan, T.R., and Tomford, W.W.: Osteoarticular and intercalary allograft transplantation in the management of malignant tumours of bone. Cancer, 50:613, 1982.

16. Mankin, H.J., Doppelt, S., and Tomford, W.: Clin-

ical experience with allograft implantation. Clin. Orthop., 174:69, 1983.

17. Marcove, R.: En bloc resection for osteogenic sarcoma. Can. J. Surg., 20:521, 1977.

18. Meyer, M.H., Jones, R.E., Bucholz, R.W., and Wenger, D.R.: Fresh autogenous grafts and osteochondral allografts for treatment of segmental collapse in osteonecrosis of the hip. Clin. Orthop., 174:107, 1983.

19. Miller, R.C., and Phalen G.S.: The repair of defects of the radius with fibular bone grafts. J. Bone Joint Surg., 29:629, 1947.

20. Parrish, F.F.: Treatment of bone tumors by total excision and replacement with massive autologous and homologous grafts. J. Bone Joint Surg., 48A:968, 1966.

21. Scales, J.T.: Massive bone and joint replacement involving the upper femur, acetabulum and iliac bone. In The Hip: Proceedings of the Third Open Scientific Meeting of the Hip Society, pp. 245–275. St. Louis, C.V. Mosby, 1975.

22. Sijbranij, S.: Resection and reconstruction for bone tumors. Acta Orthop. Scand. 49:249, 1978.

23. Tomford, W.W., Doppelt, S.H., Mankin, H.J., and Friedlaender, G.E.: Bone banking procedures. Clin. Orthop., 174:15, 1983.

24. Tuli, S.M.: Bridging of bone defects by massive bone grafts in tumorous conditions and in osteomyelitis. Clin. Orthop., 87:60, 1972.

25. Volkov, M.: Allotransplantation of joints. J. Bone Joint Surg., 52B:49, 1970.

26. Watari, S., Ikuta, Y., Adachi, N., et al.: Vascular pedicle fibular transplantation as treatment for bone tumors. Clin. Orthop., 133:158, 1978.

27. Weiland, A.S., Moore, J., Russell, D., and Rollin, K.: Vascularized bone autografts. Clin. Orthop., 174:87, 1983.

28. Wilson, P.D., Jr.: A clinical study of the biomechanical behavior of massive bone transplants used to reconstruct large bone defects. Clin. Orthop., 87:81, 1972.

29. Wilson, P.D., Jr., and Lance, E.M.: Surgical reconstruction of the skeleton following segmental resection for bone tumors. J. Bone Joint Surg., 47A:1629, 1975.

Index

The letter *f* after a page number indicates a figure;
t following a page number indicates tabular material.

ankle *(continued)*
    reflex of, in spinal cord injury, 736
    replacement of. *See* ankle, arthroplasty in
    skin of
        anatomy of, 599–600, 600f
        effect of trauma on, 600–601
    stiffness of
        in femoral shaft fracture, 534
        in lower extremity fracture, 591
    strapping of, 963
    synovitis of, 962
    tendons of, injury to, 614–615
    tibial angulation and, 131–132, 133f
ankylosing spondylitis
    in cervical spinal injury, 689–690, 691f, 695
    diagnosis of, 1181, 1182f
ankylosis
    artificial. *See* arthrodesis
    of elbow, 319–321, 319f–321f, 994–996
    following hip arthroplasty, 1093–1094
anterior cruciate ligament
    instability of, 954–957, 957f–959f
    release of, 563
    repair of, 573
anterior interosseus artery, injury to, in fracture, 586
anterior spinal artery, injury to, 733–734, 740
    in gunshot wound, 731–732
anterior tibial compartment syndrome, 961–962
anterior tibial tendon
    injury to, 614
    rupture of, 658
    transfer of, in flatfoot, 1256, 1257f
antibiotics
    in amputation stump infection, 1341
    anesthesia and, 58
    in ankle fracture, 607–608
    in cement, 198–199
    in femoral shaft fracture, 527
        open, 531
    in forearm fracture, 328
    in gas gangrene, 31–32
    in hip arthrodesis, 1292
    in hip arthroplasty, 197–199, 1086–1088, 1087t
    in irrigation solutions, 189
    in knee arthroplasty, 1112, 1114, 1120
    misuse of, 189
    in open fractures, 186–187, 191
    in phlebitis prevention, 23
    prophylactic use of, in joint replacement, 187–189
    in spinal injury, 780–781
    in spinal surgery, 1211, 1228–1229
    in tetanus, 34
anticholinesterase drugs, anesthesia and, 58
anticoagulants
    in allograft surgery, 1398
    in ankle edema, 602

    in hip arthrodesis, 1291–1293
    in hip arthroplasty, 1081, 1083
    in knee arthroplasty, 1116–1117
    in knee surgery, 561
    in microvascular surgery, 849
    nonunion and, 216
    in pulmonary embolism, 29
    in spinal surgery, 1233–1234
    in thrombosis, deep vein, 26–28
        with spinal injury, 771–772
anticonvulsants in anesthesia reaction, 64
antihistamines in contrast media allergy, 69
anti-inflammatory agents. *See* corticosteroids
antiplatelet agents in thrombotic thrombocytopenic purpura, 22
antithrombic agents. *See* anticoagulants
antithrombin III, 18, 19f
    in disseminated intravascular coagulation, 21
antitoxin in gas gangrene, 32
anulus, penetration of, in disc surgery, 1197
aorta
    aneurysm of, spinal cord ischemia and, 740–741
    injury to, 836
        during disc removal, 1197
aortoenteric fistula following arterial repair, 841–842
apophysis, 931–932
    disorders of, in Little League elbow, 932–933
    of ischium, lesions of, 935, 938f–939f
    of tibial tuberosity, inflammation of, 935–936, 940f
appendix, injury to, in spinal surgery, 1198
arachnoiditis
    adhesive, in epidural block, 66
    following myelography, 77, 1185
arcade of Frohse, 318
Arfonad (trimethaphan camsylate) in autonomic dysreflexia, 776
arm. *See also* forearm
    amputation of, contracture in, 1345–1346
    anatomy of, 277–278
    ischemia of. *See* Volkmann's ischemia
    throwing, disorders of, 932–935, 932f–937f
arterectomy in knee dislocation, 568
arteria intumescentia lumbalis (vessel of Adamkiewicz), 741
arteriography, 78
    in brachial vessel damage, 288–289
    in knee dislocation, 566–568, 567f
    in pelvic fracture, 806
arteriosclerosis. *See also* atherosclerosis
    arterial repair and, 838
        thrombosis of, 824
arteriovenous fistula
    following arterial repair, 838–840, 839f
    formation of, during disc removal, 1197
    in hand, 461, 462f–463f
    following replantation, 855, 856f

bladder
distension of, in autonomic dysreflexia, 775–776
injury to, in pelvic fracture, 809–811, 812f
neurogenic, management of, 781–782
Blair procedure, 660, 660f
bleeding. *See* blood vessels, injury to; hemorrhage
bleeding disorders. *See also* coagulopathy
spinal surgery and, 1183
blindness, cortical, in cervical spine surgery, 702, 705
blisters
in amputation stump, 1347–1349, 1348f
fracture, in ankle injury, 601–603
blood
coagulation of. *See* coagulation; coagulopathy
loss of. *See* hemorrhage
replacement of. *See* blood transfusion
typing of, 5, 910
whole, in shock, 5, 7
blood-brain barrier, antibiotics and, 780–781
blood clotting, mechanism of, 18, 19f
blood flow
digital, measurement of, 888
maintenance of, in microvascular surgery, 848–849
nonunion and, 216–217
restoration of, following replantation, 852
in tissue transfer, 857–858
blood pressure. *See also* hypertension; hypotension; shock
in corticosteroid therapy, 40
effect of bone cement on, 1060–1061
monitoring in hemorrhagic shock, 8–9
blood supply
cerclage wires and, 156–157
effect of intramedullary nails on, 167
effect of plates on, 163–164
healing and, with implant use, 155–156
of scaphoid, 368
to skin of foot, 649
of spinal cord. *See* spinal cord, blood supply of
blood transfusion
autologous, 63
in hip arthroplasty, 1081
in spinal surgery, 1227
complications of, 1080–1081
in hemorrhage control, 911, 913
massive, 7
retroperitoneal, 807
in hip arthrodesis, 1289–1290
reactions to, 5, 7
risks of, 911, 913
in spinal surgery, 1227
universal donor, 5
blood vessels. *See also* artery(ies); vein(s)
compression of, in hip dislocation, 487

of foot, surgery on, 1251, 1252f–1253f
of hand, surgery on, 460–461, 462f–463f
injury to
in cervical spine surgery, 701–702, 705, 707f–709f
in clavicle injury, 253–254
in elbow arthroplasty, 993
in external fixation, 110–112, 111f
in hip arthrodesis, 1289–1290
in humeral shaft fracture, 287–289
in knee dislocation, 566–569, 567f
in lumbar disc removal, 1197–1198, 1197f
in microvascular surgery, 845–846
in shoulder dislocation, 258
in sternoclavicular joint dislocation, 237
in tibial condyle fracture, 549
unrecognized, 1170–1171
repair of. *See also* microvascular surgery
amputation following, 819t, 833–834, 834t–835t
with associated injury and disease, 840–842, 841t
complications of, 815–820, 816f–818f, 819t, 820f, 821t
delayed, 838–840, 839f
history of, 820–822, 822t
infection following, 827t, 828–832, 828t, 829f, 830t
long-term changes in, 837–838
mortality rate in, 835–837, 835t–836t
stenosis following, 832–833
thrombosis following, 822–828, 825f, 827t–828t
blood volume
in shock, 4
nonunion and, 212
body cast. *See* cast, body; cast syndrome
body movement, recognition of, in nerve injury assessment, 878
Böhler-Braun frame, 86–87
bolts, extrusion of, from knee prosthesis, 1134–1135
bone(s)
accessory, of foot, 679
biopsy of, 78
demineralization of, in reflex sympathetic dystrophy. *See* reflex sympathetic dystrophy
density of, in avascular necrosis, 225–226
disorders of, in amputation stump, 1345–1355, 1335f
ectopic, in elbow, 319–321, 319f–321f
effect of corticosteroids on, 40–41
injury to
with arterial injury, 840–841
thermal, in cement curing, 1078–1079
loss of, in humeral shaft nonunion, 1015, 1019, 1020f
neoplasms of. *See* neoplasms
rehabilitation of, in implant use, 153–155, 154f

hypercalcemia, 35–38
  calcitonin in, 37
  conditions predisposing to, 36
  corticosteroids in, 36–37
  diagnosis of, 36
  diphosphonate in, 37
  diuretics in, 36
  fluid replacement in, 36
  in hip spica cast, 94
  inorganic phosphate in, 36
  mithramycin in, 36
  parathyroid tumors and, 37
  pathogenesis of, 36
  saline diuresis in, 36
  signs and symptoms of, 36
  treatment of, 36–38
hyperemia, osteoporosis and, 1307, 1308f
hyperkalemia
  cardiac arrest and, 61–62
  in spinal cord injury, 743–744
hyperpathia, 886
  electrical stimulation in, 889
hypertension
  following amputation, 1346
  in autonomic dysreflexia, 775–776
  in knee flexion contracture, 563
  in spinal cord injury treatment, 741
hyperthermia, malignant, 61
hypnosis in pain relief, 891
hypotension. *See also* shock
  in cardiac tamponade, 10
  in conduction anesthesia, 65
  in knee arthroplasty, 1119
  in pelvic injury, 805–806
  in shock, 4–5, 7–8
  in spinal injury, 770
  in spinal surgery, 1226
hypothermia
  following blood transfusion, 913
  during emergence from anesthesia, 63
  in spinal injury, 770
hypoxemia in fat embolism syndrome, 13,
    15–17

ICLH ankle prosthesis, failure of, 1150, 1152f
ileus
  following hip arthrodesis, 1290–1291
  following spinal fracture, 718
  following spinal surgery, 1230
iliac crest
  as donor site, 1199–1200
  transfer of, with tissue, 861
ilium
  hernia of, in hip arthrodesis, 1294
  nonunion of, arthrodesis in, 803
immobilization. *See also* bedrest; traction
  in ankle injury, chondrolysis and, 605–606
  in cervical spine injury, 685–689, 689f

failure of
  in skin attachment traction, 82, 82f–83f
  in spinal orthosis, 97, 97f
  figure-eight, in sternoclavicular joint
      dislocation, 247, 249
  of hand joints, 456
  hypercalcemia in, 36
  inadequate, nonunion and, 215
  kidney stone formation and, 517
  of knee, 558, 572–573
  of scaphoid fracture, 371–372
  in spinal surgery, 1241–1242
immune response
  allograft and, 1412, 1416
  following blood transfusion, 911
immunization in tetanus, 33–35, 35f
impedance plethysmography in deep vein
    thrombosis, 24
implant, 149–178. *See also specific type*
  bone rehabilitation and, 153–155, 154f
  cerclage wires and, 156–158, 158f–160f,
      160–161
  external fixation. *See* external fixation
  failure of, 149–150, 150f
    brittle, 151f, 152
    fatigue, 152–153, 152f–154f
    plastic, 151–152, 151f
  fracture healing and, 155–156
  history of, 149
  intramedullary nails and, 166–170, 169f
  life of, 149
  load on, 152–153, 152f
  load-deflection curve for, 151, 151f
  long-term, 152
  peritrochanteric, 170–171, 172f, 173–175,
      174f–175f
  plates and, 163–166, 165f–167f
  screws and, 161–163, 163f
implant trinity, 149, 150f
impotence following lumbar disc surgery, 1199
incisions, 433–434, 433f
  in ankle injury, 602
  in cervical spine injury, 1200
  complications of, 1174
  in elbow arthroplasty, 993
  in foot sole, 650–651, 651f
  in foot surgery, 1251
  in spinal surgery, 1191–1192
  in tibial fracture, 588, 588f
infection. *See also* osteomyelitis
  in acromioclavicular joint injury, 256
  in allograft surgery, 1399, 1401, 1402f–1403f,
      1412
  in amputation stump, 1340–1341
    in hair follicles, 1353
  in ankle arthrodesis, 1299–1300
  in ankle fracture, 607–608, 609f
    in children, 638
  in ankle injury, 608, 610
    diabetes mellitus and, 641

in tibial condyle fracture, 554–555
trochanteric, 171, 172f
  in hip arthroplasty, 198–199, 1084–1086, 1085f
  infected, 198–199
os trigonum, fracture of, 664, 664f
overflow phenomenon in motor neuron disorder, 1268
oxacillin
  in meningitis, 781
  in spinal surgery, 1228
oxygen administration
  in chemonucleolysis, 1210
  during emergence from anesthesia, 63
  in fat embolism syndrome, 15
  hyperbaric, in gas gangrene, 32
  in intertrochanteric fracture, 499–500
  in knee arthroplasty, 1119
  in malignant hyperthermia, 61
oxygen tension
  arterial, in fat embolism syndrome, 14–15
  nonunion and, 211–212
  in pneumonitis, chemical, 60

pacemaker in cardiac arrest, 13
pads
  for cast in lower extremity fracture, 591
  mobile, on digit, 463
  with traction device, 81–82, 87
pain. *See also specfic disorder*
  in amputation stump, 1355–1359
    diffuse, 1356–1358
    evaluation of, 1342
    from neuroma, 1358–1359
  in arthrography, 69
  following arthroscopy, 72
  back, 1181–1183, 1182f
    in hip arthrodesis, 1295–1296
    in myelography, 73
    from scoliosis, 1217–1218
  in bone neoplasms, 1374–1376
  burning, 774
  in cancer, 890–891
  central, 890
  chronic, 884
  in compartment syndrome, 82
  discography in, 78
  functional activity restoration in, 891–892
  from Harrington instrumentation, 1235
  inflammatory or systemic, 890
  in knee arthroplasty, 1137
  medical impairment classification and, 891
  mentioned, 774
  in nonunion, 218–219
  following patellar fracture, 548
  patellofemoral, 1131–1132, 1132f
  in peripheral nerve injury, 883–892
    differential diagnosis of, 885

  reflex sympathetic overflow in, 886, 888–890, 887f
  personality dysfunction and, 891
  phantom. *See* phantom limb, pain in
  prevention of, 884–885
  Raynaud's symptoms associated with, 888
  in reflex sympathetic dystrophy of foot, 652–654
  following replantation, 855, 856f
  in spinal injury, 774–775
  threshold of, 883–884
  tolerance of, 884
pain dysfunction syndrome in Colles' fracture, 359–361, 360f
pallor in compartment syndrome, 1171
palm, ligament release in, 1178
palmar flexion instability, 394, 396f
palmar-shelf arthroplasty, 1012–1013, 1013f
pancreatitis in corticosteroid therapy, 40
Pantopaque. *See* iophendylate
Papineau technique in tibial fracture, 593, 594f
paralysis from tourniquet use, 605
paranoia in spinal surgery, 1232–1233
paraplegia. *See also* spinal cord, injury to
  ascending neurological loss in, 733–734, 734f
  caloric intake in, 780
  fracture and wound healing in, 772–773
  hip flexion deformity and, 778
  respiration in, 768
  scoliosis in, 774
  from spinal blood supply interruption, 740–741
  in spinal deformity, 1221
  in spinal surgery for scoliosis, 1224–1226
parathyroid tumor, hypercalcemia and, 38
paresthesia
  in epidural block, 66
  in spinal cord injury, 774–775
Parham bands, 158, 158f
pars interarticularis, fracture of, 969
parturition, pelvic joint subluxation and, 803
patella
  dislocation of, 564–566, 565f
    in knee arthroplasty, 1131
  fracture of, 544–548, 546f–547f, 1121–1123
  neuroma in, 571
  subluxation of, 1132–1133
  tilting of, following hemipatellectomy, 545–546
patellar reflex in spinal cord injury, 736
patellar tendon
  avulsion of, in knee arthroplasty, 1120–1121, 1121f–1122f
  necrosis of, 1121
  realignment of, 564
patellectomy, 545–546
  in nonunion, 547
  pain following, 1131–1132
patellofemoral joint, chondromalacia of, 565–566

in phantom pain relief, 1363
pHisohex in knee arthroplasty, 1112
phlebitis, 22. *See also* thrombophlebitis
 septic, 910
 in skeletal traction, 84
phlebography, ascending, 25
phleborrheography, 24–25
phlebothrombosis in hip arthrodesis, 1291–1293
phosphatase, alkaline. *See* alkaline phosphatase
phosphate in hypercalcemia, 37
phosphorus, deficiency of, nonunion and, 211
Phospho-Soda in hypercalcemia, 37
physical therapy
 in above-knee amputation, 1343
 in below-knee amputation, 1343–1344
 in deep vein thrombosis, 25–26
 following spinal surgery, 1246
pick-up test, Moberg's, 883
pin. *See also* external fixation
 contact with bone of, 112–113, 113f
 in femoral shaft fracture, 520
 fracture of, after removal, 119–120
 infection at, 1310
  in femoral shaft fracture, 514, 514f
  in knee arthrodesis, 1297
 insertion of
  for halo traction, 1223
  for halo-pelvic traction, 1223–1224
 loosening of, 112–116, 113f
  in femoral shaft fracture, 514, 514f
 migration of
  in acromioclavicular joint injury, 255
  in clavicle dislocation, 248
  in shoulder arthrodesis, 1301
 motion of, 113–114
 in skeletal traction, 83–84, 84f
 spacer, in hand fracture, 420
 Steinmann. *See* Steinmann pins
 threaded, 113
 tract of
  contamination of, 114–116, 115f
  problems with, 112–116, 113f, 115f
pinch
 abnormality of, following peripheral nerve injury, 892
 key, tendon transfer in, 898
 measurement of, 882–883
 restoration of, in median-ulnar palsy, 901, 902t
 weakened, in ulnar nerve injury, 454–455, 455f
piperacillin in meningitis, 781
pisiform, fracture of, 405–406, 407f
pitching, mechanics of, 935
pitching arm, disorders of, 932–935, 932f–937f
planovalgus foot, 1253–1256, 1254f–1255f, 1257f
plantar digital nerves, excision of, 1285–1286, 1285f–1286f

plantar fascia, release of, 1177–1178
plantar nerves, injury to, 656
plasma expanders in shock, 7–8
plaster, burns from, 603
plaster cast. *See* cast, plaster
plate
 advantages of, 163
 application of, 164–166
 blood supply and, 163–164
 bone graft and, 165
 compression, 164
 conversion of, from load-bearing to load-sharing, 164
 disadvantages of, 165–166, 165f–167f
 dual, in femoral shaft fracture, 529
 failure of, 164–166, 165f–167f
 in femoral shaft fracture, 527–529, 528f–530f
 in fibular shaft fracture, 621
 in humeral shaft nonunion, 292
 use with screws, 162, 174f–175f
 time of removal, 215
platysma, contracture of, 1200
plethysmography in knee arthroplasty, 1117
pleural cavity, injury to, in spinal surgery, 1229
pneumonia in aspiration, 60
pneumonitis
 in aspiration, 60
 in hip arthrodesis, 1290
 in spinal surgery, 1229–1230
pneumoscrotum following arthroscopy, 72
pneumothorax
 in spinal injury, 767
 in spinal surgery, 1229
 from tracheal intubation, 59
poliomyelitis
 foot deformity in, 1267–1268
 scoliosis and, 1221
polyethylene knee prosthesis, deformation of, 1134, 1135f
Polymyxin B in irrigation solution, 1086
porous coating knee arthroplasty, 1141
Pontocaine, hypersensitivity to, 64
popliteal artery
 injury to
  during arthroscopy, 72
  in knee arthroplasty, 1117–1118
  in knee dislocation, 566–569, 567f
  in meniscectomy, 575, 1171
 thrombosis of, in knee injury, 957–959, 960f
popliteal fossa, trauma to, 90
popliteal vessels, injury to, in tibial condyle fracture, 549
porphyria, barbiturates and, 62
positioning of patient for surgery, 62
 spinal, 1190–1191, 1191f–1192f
positive end-expiratory pressure in fat embolism syndrome, 16
posterior interosseus nerve, injury to
 in elbow arthroplasty, 994
 in elbow fracture, 318

injury to
    in athletics, 968–970, 970f–972f
    diagnosis of, 681–682, 682f–685f
    Minerva cast for, 91
    pillar view of, 1188–1189, 1190f
    spondylolisthesis of, 969–970
    spondylolysis of, 969
curvature of. *See* kyphosis; scoliosis
degenerative changes in, following surgery,
    1212–1213
dorsolumbar
    anatomy of, 734–735, 735f
    fracture of
        Harrington instrumentation in,
            748f–751f, 752, 753f–754f, 754, 756
        internal fixation failure in, 759–760,
            761f–762f
        internal fixation methods for, 751–752
        Maurig-Williams plates in, 759, 760f
        orthosis for, 760–762, 763f–766f,
            764–765
        stable, 717–718
        types of, 717
        unstable, 718, 719f–721f, 721–722
        Weiss springs in, 755f–756f, 756–757,
            758f, 759
    fracture-dislocation of, 722, 745, 746f,
        747
    in hip arthrodesis, 1295–1296
    injury to
        abdominal injury with, 768–770
        amyloidosis following, 776
        assessment of, 735–738, 735f, 736t
        atraumatic, 717
        autonomic dysreflexia and, 775–776
        chest trauma and, 767–768, 768t
        etiology of, 715–722, 716t, 719f–721f
        heterotopic ossification and, 776–779
        history of treatment in, 749–751
        hyperextension in, 714
        hyperflexion in, 719, 721–722
        infection in, 728, 729f
        long-bone fracture with, 772–773
        mortality in, 767–768, 768t, 789–790,
            790f
        open, 728, 729f
        pain in, 774–775
        pulmonary embolism in, 770–772
        scoliosis following, 773–774
        spinal stenosis and, 779–780
        surgical decompression and, 744–745,
            746f, 747
        systemic injury incidence and, 765–767,
            766t
        manipulation of, 742, 742f–744f
        myelography of, 722–723, 1186, 1187f
    gunshot wounds of, 728, 730–732, 730f,
        732f
    hematoma of, in myelography, 73–74
    injury to, nucleus pulposus and, 723

instrumentation for. *See also* Dwyer
        instrumentation; Harrington
        instrumentation
    segmental, 1237–1238, 1238f
internal fixation devices for, biomechanics
    of, 787–788, 787f–788f
lumbar. *See also* spine, dorsolumbar
    dislocation of, 724–725, 725f–726f
    fracture-dislocation of, 724–727, 725f–727f
lumbosacral, 725f–726f, 727–728
malalignment of, effect on spinal artery,
    731–732
manipulation of, 714
neoplasms of, 1373
orthosis for, 96–97, 97f
stability of, in accident victims, 910–911
stenosis of, 779–780
    diagnosis of, 1181, 1186, 1187f–1188f
    following injury, 779–780
    following surgery, 1212–1213
surgery on
    cast syndrome and. *See* cast syndrome
    contraindications to, 747–749, 747f
    in discogenic disease and spon-
        dylolisthesis. *See* discogenic disease
        and spondylolisthesis
    incisions for, 1191–1192
    repeated, 1213
    in scoliosis. *See* scoliosis
thoracolumbar, injury to, 715–716
splanchnic vessels, autonomic dysreflexia
    and, 775–776
splayfoot
    with bunion, 1269, 1269f
    surgery for 1278–1282, 1280f–1281f
splint
    abduction, 98
    in ankle injury, 611–613
    in boutonnière deformity, 448–449
    in burn treatment, 1320, 1323f–1324f
        of hand, 1325, 1327f–1329f, 1329
    in cervical spine injury during x-ray, 681
    in clavicle injury, 250
    in hand contracture, 456
    in mallet finger, 447
    in nerve injury, 892
    pillow, in paraplegics, 773
    sugar-tong, 92–93, 93f
    in tendon graft, 441
    Thomas, 85–86, 85f
    in volar plate-injury, 457
spondylolisthesis. *See also* discogenic disease
        and spondylolisthesis
    of cervical spine, 969–970
    congenital, surgery for, 1193, 1193f
    diagnosis of, 1188, 1189f
    following spinal surgery, 1245
spondylolysis
    of cervical spine, 969
    following spinal surgery, 1212

implant in
    fracture of, 1052
    refracture of, 154–155, 154f
  movement of, at wrist, 1007–1008
  styloid of, fracture of, 364, 365f, 366–367
  translation of, 394, 397f
  translocation of, in elbow dislocation, 313
ulnar artery, thrombosis of, 461
ulnar nerve
  injury to
    in amputation stump, 1357
    in auto accident, 1184, 1184f
    with Colles' fracture, 343f, 344
    in elbow arthroplasty, 993–994
    in elbow dislocation, 312–313
    in elbow injury, 318–319
    in hand, 452–455, 455f
    in hip arthrodesis, 1293
    in wrist arthrodesis, 1303
  palsy of
    in elbow fracture, 305, 306f–307f
    with median palsy, 901, 902t
    with radial palsy, 901, 902t, 903
    tendon transfer in, 892, 894f, 897–898
  protection of, in spinal surgery, 1191
  in U-loop graft, 876
ulnar sleeve, 143–144, 146f–147f
ultrasound
  in deep vein thrombosis, 25
  in phantom pain, 1363
ultraviolet light in operating room, 183
umbrella filter in pulmonary embolism, 29
union
  delayed, 207–221
    in allograft surgery, 1407, 1409, 1413t,
      1415f
    causes of, 210–218
    of clavicle, 252
    in Colles' fracture, 353, 355f
    definition of, 207
    effect of kidney function on, 285–286,
      286f
    of femoral condyle, 539, 540f–541f, 541
    of femoral shaft, 518–520
    with forearm brace, 147
    with humeral brace, 143
    of humeral shaft, 282–286, 283f–286f
    incidence of, 209–210
    in internal fixation, 116–119, 118f
    in intertrochanteric fracture, 500f–501f,
      500–501
    of patella, 546
    pathogenesis of, 209
    in pelvic injury, 799–801
    of scaphoid, 368, 370f, 371–372
    with tibial brace, 133, 135f
    of tibia, 589
    of tibial condyle, 553
  slow, 207
    causes of, 213

Unna's paste boot, edema and, 602
Urecholine in urinary retention, 1291
ureter, injury to, in spinal surgery, 1232
urethra, injury to, in pelvic fracture, 809–811,
      810f
urinary tract
  anatomy of, 797
  disorders of, in spinal surgery, 1232
  infection of
    amyloidosis and, 776
    in hip arthrodesis, 1291
    in hip replacement, 198
    in paraplegics, 781–782
    following pelvic surgery, 811
    in spinal surgery, 1232
  injury to
    in hip injury, 490
    in pelvic fracture, 809–811, 810f, 812f
urine, retention of
  anesthesia and, 63–64
  in epidural block, 66
  in hemorrhagic shock, 9
  in hip arthrodesis, 1291
  in knee arthrodesis, 1296

Valium in tetanus, 35
vasodilation, peripheral, in microvascular
      surgery, 848–849
vasodilators in shock, 8, 10
vasopressors in hemorrhagic shock, 8
vasospasm in knee dislocation, 568
vehicular accident, 3–4. *See also* emergency
      treatment
vein(s)
  graft of, in microvascular surgery, 847–848
  insufficiency of, chronic, 842f, 843
  intravasation of, in myelography, 73
  repair of, 842–843, 842f
  thrombectomy of, in pulmonary embolism,
      29
  thrombosis of. *See* thrombosis
Velpeau bandage, 93, 93f
vena cava, injury to, during disc removal,
      1197
venography, 78
  intradural, in spinal disease diagnosis,
      1185–1186
  in knee arthroplasty, 1117
ventilation
  mechanical, in fat embolism syndrome,
      15–16
  during spinal surgery, 1227, 1246
vertebra. *See also* spine
  compression fracture of, 717–718
vertebral artery, injury to, in cervical spine
      surgery, 702, 705, 1201, 1202f
vessel of Adamkiewicz, injury to, 741
Vietnam War, injuries during. *See* blood ves-
      sels, repair of